Image Reconstruction in Radiology

Author

J. Anthony Parker, M.D., Ph.D.
Radiologist
Division of Nuclear Medicine
Beth Israel Hospital
and
Associate Professor of Radiology
Harvard Medical School
Boston, Massachusetts

CRC Press
Boca Raton   Ann Arbor   Boston

Library of Congress Cataloging-in-Publication Data

Parker, J. Anthony.
    Image reconstruction in radiology/author, J. Anthony Parker.
      p. cm.
    Includes bibliographical references.
    ISBN 0-8493-0150-5
    1. Diagnostic imaging--Digital techniques--Mathematics.
  [1. Radiographic Image Enhancement.   2. Technology, Radiologic.]
  I. Title
    [DNLM: WN 160 P241i]
  RC78.7.D53P36   1990
  616.07'57--dc20
  DNLM/DLC
  for Library of Congress   89-22062
                                                       CIP

Direct all inquiries to CRC Press, Inc., 2000 Corporate Blvd., N.W., Boca Raton, Florida, 33431.

© 1990 by CRC Press, Inc.

International Standard Book Number 0-8493-0150-5
Library of Congress Card Number 89-22062

Printed in the United States of America   3 4 5 6 7 8 9 0

Printed on acid-free paper

PREFACE

Sophisticated mathematical methods are being used more and more frequently in radiology. The physics of radiology has always been quantitative, but it has been only recently that common medical imaging procedures rely on complex mathematical methods. The goal of this book is to provide the radiologist with a practical introduction to these mathematical methods so that he may better understand the potentials and the limitations of the images he uses to make diagnoses.

This book is intended to be used as a text for a course given to radiology residents on image processing and image reconstruction methods. The book may also be of value to the practicing radiologist since the material is self contained. This book is not primarily intended for a hospital physicist or for the engineer interested in medical image processing; however, these professionals may find the analogies and examples useful when they are called on to explain mathematical methods to clinicians.

This book assumes that the reader has taken a course in college calculus. To refresh the memory, Chapter 2 provides a review of the basic mathematical principles which will be needed later in the book. The level of the presentation is meant to be appropriate for a radiology resident. Emphasis is placed on understanding principles, but some mathematical logic is important to this understanding. Where possible, ease of understanding has been chosen over mathematical rigor. Many diagrams and analogies are used in place of mathematical proofs.

This book seeks to bring together in a readable fashion results from a number of areas in mathematics. Although inclusion of several different mathematical methods increases the length of the book, together they provide better insight into the basic principles. Different methods often highlight different aspects of the same principle. In some cases, a principle is more easily understood with one method while in another case a principle is best explained with another method. The analogies between methods often improve the understanding of each. For example, we shall find that our natural geometric intuition will be useful in understanding the Fourier transform operation.

All of the material in this book is available in more complete form in mathematical or engineering texts. However, these texts are usually not written at a level appropriate for the radiologist, and they contain a great deal of material which is not directly applicable to radiology. Texts from various fields of mathematics use different symbols for similar concepts. For the experienced mathematician, the choice of symbols is inconsequential. However, for the non-mathematician this lack of uniformity can be bewildering. In this book an attempt has been made to use similar symbols for similar concepts across the various fields. Appendix A provides the reader with a quick reference to symbol usage.

An important part of most mathematical texts is solution of problems. The goal of the problems is to allow the reader to become facile with use of the method which is being presented. The goal of this book is not to teach the reader how to use the methods presented. Rather, it is intended to provide him with a general understanding of the methods so that he can understand and identify clinically important effects of the mathematics. This book does not seek to train the reader as an engineer; rather, it seeks to make the reader a better radiologist. Therefore, problems have not been not included.

The book is divided into four parts. Part I (System Models) introduces the various mathematical models which will be used to describe image collection and processing systems. Part II (Transformations) explains transform methods, particularly the Fourier transform. Our natural experience with the frequencies in sound will be useful in understanding the frequency representation of images provided by the Fourier transform. Transform methods will simplify the understanding of reconstruction techniques. Part III (Filtering) describes filtering operations including image enhancement. Filtering operations allow *a priori* knowledge about noise to be incorporated with the image reconstruction techniques. And Part IV (Reconstruction) describes the various types of image reconstruction. The most important applications are in Part IV, but throughout the book, the mathematical methods are placed in a radiological context.

Although one of the objects of the book is to emphasize the correlations between methods, the reader may wish to read only a portion of the book. For example, the reader who was only interested in understanding nuclear magnetic resonance data collection and reconstruction could read Chapters 1 to 6, 14 to 16, and 29. The reader who already has some mathematical background may wish to just read the summary chapters at the end of the first three parts and then read Part IV in greater detail. Chapter 1 attempts to indicate how the material in the various chapters is organized and how the chapters depend upon each other.

I wish to thank several people who have helped me during the writing of this book. B. Leonard Holman and Henry D. Royal have helped by reviewing portions of the book. Gerald M. Kolodny and Sven Paulin have provided a productive environment in which to work. Much of my understanding of the mathematics of radiology and best ideas in this book come from David A. Chesler. Several radiology residents have provided useful suggestions. In particular, I wish to thank Zaim Badra, Ed Cronin, Jean Gregoire, and Martin Charron. Parts of this book have been used in a course taught with Robert E. Zimmerman and Marie F. Kijewski. I should like to take credit for any ingenious explanations, and blame these individuals for any mistakes.

J. Anthony Parker

THE AUTHOR

J. Anthony Parker, M.D., Ph.D. is a Radiologist in the Division of Nuclear Medicine at the Beth Israel Hospital, and an Associate Professor of Radiology at Harvard Medical School, Boston, MA.

Dr. Parker graduated in 1968 from Yale College, New Haven, CT with a B.A. in Physics; he obtained his M.D. degree in 1972 from Washington University, St. Louis, MO, and his Ph.D. in Biomedical Engineering in 1983 from the Massachusetts Institute of Technology, Cambridge, MA. From residency training until the present, he has been at Harvard Medical School in The Joint Program in Nuclear Medicine.

Dr. Parker is a member of The Society of Nuclear Medicine, The Institute of Electrical and Electronic Engineers, The Society of Magnetic Resonance Imaging, The Society of Magnetic Resonance in Medicine, and The North American Society for Cardiac Radiology. He was the recipient of a Picker Scholarship and a Research Career Development Award.

Dr. Parker is the author of 65 papers and the co-author of a book on computer applications in cardiovascular nuclear medicine. His current research interests relate to application of biomedical engineering in cardiovascular radiology.

To Scott, Meg, and Bridget

TABLE OF CONTENTS

I. SYSTEM MODELS
Chapter 1
Introduction 3
I.   Structure of the Book 3
      A.   Part I. System Models 3
      B.   Part II. Transformation 4
      C.   Part III. Filtering 5
      D.   Part IV. Reconstruction 5
II.   Relationship of the Chapters 5
III. Further Reading 6
References 7

Chapter 2
Review of Basic Concepts 9
I.   Function 9
      A.   Continuous, Discrete, and Digital 11
      B.   Two-Dimensional Functions 12
      C.   Multi-Dimensional Functions 13
II.   Vectors 14
III. Operations 15
      A.   Operations on the Independent Variable 15
      B.   Difference 17
      C.   Derivative 17
      D.   Partial Derivative 18
      E.   Sum 18
      F.   Integral 19
      G.   Powers and Roots 22
      H.   Exponentials and Logarithms 22
IV.   Special Functions 25
      A.   Step Function 25
      B.   Delta Function 25
V.   Power Series Expansion 26
VI.   Summary 27
VII. Further Reading 27
References 27

Chapter 3
Convolution 29
I.   Description of Convolution 29
II.   Mathematical Description of Convolution 31
      A.   Basis Functions 33
      B.   Convolution Integral 35
      C.   Equivalence of the Input Signal and the System Function 35
      D.   Two-Dimensional Convolution 36
III. Examples of Convolution 38
      A.   Lung Time Activity Curve 38
      B.   X-ray Cassette 39
      C.   Audio Amplifier 39
      D.   Radioactive Decay 40

IV.   Summary 42
V.   Further Reading... 42
References.. 42

Chapter 4
Systems 43
I.   Mathematical Description of a System.. 43
II.   Examples of Systems 43
III.   Properties of Systems 44
        A.   Linearity... 44
        B.   Linearizable Systems 46
        C.   Time Invariance 46
IV.   Linear, Time Invariant Systems... 47
V.   System Complexity 50
VI.   Summary 51
VII.   Further Reading.. 51

Chapter 5
Eigenfunctions... 53
I.   Definition of Eigenfunctions 53
II.   Examples of Eigenfunctions 53
        A.   Audio Amplifier... 53
        B.   Nuclear Magnetic Resonance Spectroscopy............................... 54
        C.   Eigenvectors.. 56
III.   Eigenfunctions as Basis Functions 56
IV.   The Eigenfunctions of Linear, Time Invariant Systems 58
V.   Summary 59
VI.   Further Reading.. 59

Chapter 6
Complex Numbers 61
I   Number Systems... 61
        A.   Other Number Systems.. 61
        B.   Complex Number System 61
        C.   Applications of Complex Numbers 62
II.   Complex Number Representations 63
III.   Operations on Complex Numbers 65
        A.   Complex Conjugate 66
        B.   Complex Exponential... 66
IV.   Uses of the Complex Exponential.. 70
        A.   Trigonometric Relationships... 70
        B.   Mathematical Operations 70
        C.   Sinusoidal Functions 71
        D.   Plane Waves 74
        E.   Tissue Impedence to Ultrasound.. 75
V.   Functions of a Complex Variable 76
        A.   Analytic Functions 77
        B.   Derivatives of Complex Functions of Complex Variables 77
VI.   Eigenfunctions of Linear, Time Invariant Systems............................... 78
VII.   Summary 79
VIII.   Further Reading.. 79
Reference.. 79

Chapter 7
Differential Equations 81
I. Definition of a Differential Equation 81
II. Examples of Systems Described by Differential Equations 82
    A. Radioactive Decay 82
    B. Mass on a Spring 85
III. Additional Constraints 89
IV. Properties of Linear Differential Equations with Constant Coefficients 90
    A. Linear, Time Invariant Systems 90
    B. Natural and Forced Solutions 91
    C. Eigenfunctions 92
    D. Resonance 92
    E. System Function 93
    F. State 93
V. Summary 94
VI. Further Reading 95
References 95

Chapter 8
Linear Algebra 97
I. Solution of Simultaneous Linear Equations 97
II. Vector and Matrix Notation 99
III. Operations with Matrices 101
    A. Matrix Addition 101
    B. Scalar Multiplication 101
    C. Matrix Multiplication 101
    D. Associative and Commutative Properties 102
    E. Multiplication of a Matrix Times a Vector 103
    F. Image Arithmetic 103
IV. Simultaneous Linear Equations in Matrix Notation 103
V. More Operations with Matrices 103
    A. Matrix Inverse 103
    B. Transpose of a Matrix 105
    C. Vector Multiplication 106
VI. Vector Space 109
    A. Examples of Vector Spaces 109
    B. Complexity of Vector Space Versus a Signal 109
    C. Vector Subspace 110
    D. Projection 111
    E. Orthogonality 113
VII. Summary 114
VIII. Further Reading 114
Reference 115

Chapter 9
Linear Algebra Description of Systems 117
I. Linear Algebra Model of a System 117
    A. Comparison between Linear, and Linear, Time Invariant
        Models 118
    B. Two-Dimensional Signals 119

II.   Basis Vectors 119
     A.   Definition of a Vector Space in Terms of a Set of Basis
           Vectors...122
     B.   Linear Independence 124
     C.   Examples of Vector Spaces 124
III.   Signals Which Pass Through a System 125
     A.   Vector Spaces Associated with a Matrix 125
     B.   Examples of the Vector Spaces Associated with Matrices 129
IV.   Eigenvectors of a Linear System..131
V.   Summary 134
VI.   Further Reading..134
References...134

Chapter 10
Random Variables 135
I.   Probability Density Function...135
II.   Random Variables 136
     A.   Sum of Two Random Variables 136
     B.   Mean 137
     C.   Some Concepts about the Expectation Operator 139
     D.   Variance..140
     E.   Second Moment 141
     F.   Standard Deviation 141
     G.   Power and Energy..142
III.   Two Random Variables..143
     A.   Correlation of Deviations...143
     B.   Correlation 144
     C.   Independent, Orthogonal, and Uncorrelated Variables..................144
     D.   Sum of Two Uncorrelated Random Variables 146
IV.   Random Vectors 147
     A.   Energy and Length 147
V.   Normally Distributed Random Variables.................................149
VI.   Summary 150
VII. Further Reading..150
References...150

Chapter 11
Stochastic Processes..151
I.   Probability Density Function...151
II.   Examples of Stochastic Processes...152
III.   Mean 155
IV.   Autocorrelation 155
V.   Crosscorrelation...156
VI.   Stationarity..156
VII. Ergodicity...157
VIII. Poisson Process 158
IX.   Summary 159
X.   Further Reading..160
References...160

Chapter 12

Linear, Least Mean Square Estimation 161

I.   Model.. 161

II.   Linear Estimation.. 162

III.   Least Mean Square Error 164

IV.   Projection of a Vector onto a Second Vector 165

V.   Linear, Mean Square Estimation from Multiple Measurements 168

VI.   Estimation of the Data... 170

       A.   Algebraic Derivation 170

       B.   Geometric Derivation.. 171

       C.   Examples of Estimation of the Data............................... 172

       D.   What Is Wrong with Estimation of the Data? 173

VII.   Estimation of the Unknown.. 174

       A.   Unknown, Measurement, and Estimation Subspaces 175

       B.   Geometric Derivation.. 176

       C.   Algebraic Derivation 179

       D.   Example of Estimation of the Unknown.......................... 180

VIII.   Summary 182

IX.   Further Reading.. 182

References.. 182

Chapter 13

Summary of System Models 183

I.   Classification of Systems 183

II.   Representation of Signals in Terms of Basis Functions 185

III.   Complexity of System Models.. 186

IV.   Eigenfunctions 187

V.   State 188

VI.   Energy, Correlation, Orthogonality, and Vector Product................. 188

VII.   Estimation 189

VIII.   Summary 189

II. TRANSFORMATIONS

Chapter 14

Introduction to the Fourier Transform 193

I.   Hearing and Sight.. 193

II.   Spectroscopy.. 195

       A.   Optical Spectroscopy 195

       B.   Nuclear Magnetic Resonance Spectroscopy...................... 195

III.   Frequency Domain Representation of a Signal............................ 196

IV.   The Fourier Transform.. 199

       A.   The Two Domains... 199

       B.   Calculation of the Fourier Transform............................. 200

V.   Fourier Transform as a Correlation 200

VI.   Response of a System to an Imaginary Exponential...................... 202

       A.   Modulation Transfer Function 202

VII.   Real and Imaginary Parts of the Fourier Transform..................... 203

VIII.   Magnitude and Phase of the Fourier Transform.......................... 205

IX.   Two-Dimensional Fourier Transform 208

X.   Summary 208

XI.   Further Reading.. 209

References.. 210

Chapter 15
Fourier Transform 211
I.   Linearity 211
II.   Duality...212
III.   Orthogonality of the Imaginary Exponentials 213
IV.   The Integral of an Imaginary Exponential..............................217
V.   "Proof" of the Fourier Transform Relationships 219
VI.   Completeness 220
VII.   Summary 221
VIII.   Further Reading...222
References...222

Chapter 16
Properties of the Fourier Transform 223
I.   Mapping of Convolution to Multiplication 223
      A.   Response of a System to a Delta Function Input 225
      B.   Audio Component System.......................................225
      C.   Sequence of Systems 226
      D.   Mapping of Deconvolution to Division 228
II.   Shift/Modulation 229
      A.   Modulation of a Carrier 231
III.   Change in Scale..233
IV.   Mapping of Differential Equations to Polynomial Equations 234
V.   Fourier Transform of Even and Odd Signals............................235
      A.   Quadrature Signals 238
VI.   The Sinc Function 240
VII.   Value at the Origin and the Integral in the Other Domain 241
VIII.   Conservation of Energy...242
IX.   Uncertainty Principle...243
X.   Heuristics 245
XI.   Summary 246
XII.   Further Reading...246
References...246

Chapter 17
Polynomial Transform 247
I.   Signals of Limited Complexity...247
II.   Polynomial Representation of a Signal...................................247
III.   Sample Representation of a Signal.......................................249
IV.   Evaluation 250
V.   Interpolation 251
VI.   Polynomial Multiplication..252
VII.   Mapping of a Convolution to Multiplication 253
VIII.   Summary 255
IX.   Further Reading..256
References...256

Chapter 18
Discrete Fourier Transform 257
I.   Continuous, Discrete, Digital 257

II.   Periodic Signals...258
       A.   Representation of a Limited Extent Signal by a Periodic Signal........258
       B.   Shifting...259
III.   Discrete Fourier Transform 260
       A.   Examples of Discrete Fourier Transform Pairs 260
       B.   Basis Functions..261
       C.   Periodicity of the Discrete Fourier Transform 262
       D.   Definition of the Discrete Fourier Transform on any N Point
             Interval...263
IV.   Sum of Basis Functions..264
V.   Proof of the Discrete Fourier Transform Relation...........................265
VI.   Analogy between Vectors and the Discrete Signals 266
VII.   Fast Fourier Transform 267
VIII. Summary 268
IX.   Further Reading...269
References..269

Chapter 19
Vector Space Rotation 271
I.   Example of a Rotation Operation 271
II.   Rotation of a Vector Space 275
III.   The Discrete Fourier Transform as a Rotation 277
IV.   Matrix Rotation...279
V.   Rotation to an Eigenvectors Basis 281
VI.   Example of the Rotation of a System to an Eigenvector Basis................283
VII.   Analogy between Matrix Rotations and Linear Systems 284
VIII. Summary 285
IX.   Further Reading...285
References..285

Chapter 20
Other Transforms...287
I.   Multi-Dimensional Fourier Transforms 287
       A.   Rotation of a Signal and Its Transform..............................288
II.   Correspondence between the Continuous and the Discrete Fourier
       Transforms...291
       A.   Discrete Fourier Transform: Discrete Time, Discrete Frequency 292
       B.   Fourier Series: Continuous Time, Discrete Frequency.................292
       C.   Dual of the Fourier Series: Discrete Time, Continuous
             Frequency 294
       D.   Fourier Transform: Continuous Time, Continuous Frequency 296
III.   Laplace Transform...297
IV.   Path of Integration in the Complex Plane 299
V.   Complexity of the Signals Represented by Various Transforms................301
VI.   Hankel Transforms...302
VII.   Radon Transform 302
VIII. Summary 302
IX.   Further Reading...303
References..303

Chapter 21
Summary of Transformations 305
I.   The Frequency Domain 305
II.   Properties of the Fourier Transform... 306
III.   Selected Fourier Transform Pairs 308
IV.   Basis Functions 309
V.   Transformation, Correlation, and Projection 310
VI.   Transformations and Rotations.. 310
VII.   Eigenfunctions 311
VIII.   Mapping of Convolution to Multiplication 311
IX.   Relation of Discrete and Continuous Signals................................ 312
X.   Sequence of Systems.. 312
XI.   Summary 313

III. FILTERING
Chapter 22
Introduction to Filtering 317
I.   Definition of Filtering... 317
II.   Implementation 318
III.   Spatial Filtering 320
IV.   Windowing 323
V.   Ideal Low Pass Filter 327
        A.   Modulation, Demodulation 327
VI.   Band Pass Filter 329
VII.   Approximate Low Pass Filters 329
        A.   Hanning Window.. 330
        B.   Hamming Window 331
        C.   Butterworth Filter 331
        D.   Gaussian Filter 332
VIII.   Summary 332
IX.   Further Reading... 332
References.. 333

Chapter 23
Sampling.. 335
I.   Aliasing.. 335
II.   Comb Signal 337
III.   Sampling Using the Comb Function 343
IV.   Interpolation 345
V.   Sampling Theorem.. 347
VI.   Prevention of Aliasing in Under-Sampled Signals 348
VII.   Implementation of Sampling 348
VIII.   Summary 350
IX.   Further Reading... 350
References.. 350

Chapter 24
Filtering Stochastic Processes... 351
I.   Stochastic Processes 351
II.   Power Spectral Density Function 352
III.   Definition of Filtering a Stochastic Process 353
IV.   Mean of an Output Process 354

V.   Autocorrelation of an Output Process 355
VI.   Power Spectral Density Function of an Output Process 356
VII. Power Spectral Localization 357
VIII. Noise 359
IX.   Signal to Noise Ratio 362
X.   Summary 362
XI.   Further Reading 364
References 364

Chapter 25
Normal Equations 365
I.   Projection of a Vector onto a Subspace 365
II.   Model 371
III. Estimation of the Data 373
IV.   Iterative Solution 377
V.   Summary 379
VI.   Further Reading 379
References 379

Chapter 26
Wiener Filtering 381
I.   Models 381
II.   Wiener Filtering 383
      A.   Heuristics 383
      B.   Orthogonality 384
      C.   Mathematical Derivation of the Orthogonality Principle 384
      D.   Solution 385
      E.   Summary of Wiener Filtering 388
III. Wiener Deconvolution, Simplified Model 389
IV.   Wiener Deconvolution 391
V.   Summary 393
VI.   Further Reading 394
References 395

Chapter 27
Image Enhancement 395
I.   Image Enhancement and Image Restoration 395
II.   Examples of Image Enhancement 395
      A.   Smoothing 395
      B.   Edge Enhancement 396
      C.   Unsharp Masking 396
      D.   Low-Frequency Attenuation 396
III. Some Comments about Visual Physiology 398
IV.   Homomorphic Signal Processing 398
V.   Image Information 399
VI.   Summary 401
VII. Further Reading 401
References 402

Chapter 28
Summary of Filtering 403
I.   Filtering and Convolution 403

II. Sampling...404
III. Power Spectral Density Function 405
IV. Estimation of a Signal 405
    A. Orthogonality Principle..405
    B. The Normal Equations of Linear Algegra 406
    C. The Wiener Filter 408
    D. Wiener Deconvolution...408
V. Image Enhancement 408
VI. Summary 408

IV. RECONSTRUCTION

Chapter 29

Deconvolution: First Pass Radionuclide Angiocardiography 411

I. First Pass Radionuclide Angiocardiography.....................................411
II. Model...412
III. Noiseless Deconvolution..414
IV. Deconvolution with High Pass Filtering 415
VI. Wiener Filtering 415
VI. *A Priori* Information 416
VII. Linear Algebra Model 417
    A. Iterative Solution 419
VIII. Summary 420
IX. Further Reading...421
References...421

Chapter 30

Reconstruction from Fourier Samples: Nuclear Magnetic Resonance Imaging.....423

I. Physics and Instrumentation 423
II. Vector Addition of Magnetic Moments 425
III. Free Induction Decay and Spectrum 425
IV. Image, Spectrum Domain..426
V. Time, Frequency, Space, and Spatial Frequency..............................429
VI. Free Induction Decay, Spatial Frequency Domain 429
VII. Two-Dimensional Encoding..431
VIII. Alternate Data Collection Protocols...434
IX. Reconstruction 435
X. Chemical Shift Imaging..435
XI. Velocity Imaging 436
XII. Summary 438
XIII. Further Reading..439
References...439

Chapter 31

Reconstruction from Noiseless Projections 441

I. Data Collection Model..441
II. Back Projection 443
III. Projection, Slice Theorem 446
IV. Projection, Back Projection as Spatial Frequency Samples...................448
V. Reconstruction Filter..449
VI. Fourier Transform Reconstruction 450
VII. Convolution, Back Projection Reconstruction..................................450
VIII. Summary 451

IX.   Further Reading...452

References...452

Chapter 32
Reconstruction from Noisy Projections: Computed Tomography...................453
I.   Model...453
        A.   Data Collection...453
        B.   Back Projection 454
        C.   Back Projected Noise..454
        D.   Back Projected Noise Power Spectral Density.......................455
        E.   Back Projected Signal Power Spectral Density 456
        F.   Reconstruction Model 457
II.   Image Reconstruction 457
III.   Implementation 459
IV.   Summary 461
V.   Further Reading...462

References...462

Chapter 33
Iterative Reconstruction: Single Photon Emission Computed Tomography 463
I.   Single Photon Emission Computed Tomography................................463
II.   Point Source Attenuation Correction 464
III.   Image Collection Model 465
        A.   Linear System Model...466
        B.   Linear Algebra Model 469
IV.   Heuristics 470
        A.   Attenuation Viewed as Smoothing of the Spatial Frequencies 470
        B.   Constant Attenuation 470
V.   Linear, Shift Invariant Reconstruction Methods...........................475
        A.   Modification of the Projected Values..............................475
        B.   Post-Reconstruction Correction 476
        C.   Exponential Back Projection.......................................476
VI.   Iterative Reconstruction 478
VII.   Summary 481
VIII.   Further Reading 481

References...481

Chapter 34
Reconstruction from Multiple Samples: Multi-Detector Scanner 483
I.   Multi-Detector Scanner 483
II.   Model...485
III.   Linear, Shift Invariant Model...486
IV.   Review of Estimation of an Unknown from Multiple Samples..................488
V.   Reconstruction of Multiple Linear, Shift Invariant Samples................492
VI.   Comparison to the Normal Equations of Linear Algebra......................493
VII.   X-ray Computed Tomography 494
VIII.   Time-of-Flight Positron Emission Computed Tomography......................495
IX.   Summary 495
X.   Further Reading...496

References...496

Chapter 35

Summary of Reconstruction

Summary of Reconstruction 497
I.   Models...497
II.   *A Priori* Information 498
III.   Correlation Between Models 498
IV.   Eigenfunctions 499
V.   Back Projection 499
VI.   Exact Reconstruction, Noise Reduction, and Image Enhancement 500
VII.   Summary of Data Collection and Image Reconstruction 500
VIII.   Summary 502

Appendix: symbols...503

INDEX 507

I. System Models

Chapter 1

INTRODUCTION

The primary goal of this book is to explain the mathematical methods used for image reconstruction. Image reconstruction has become increasingly important in Radiology as computer performance has made image processing practical for day-to-day operation. It is likely that these methods will become even more important in the future.

The presentation of mathematical methods in this book is most similar to that in an area called signal processing in electrical engineering. In electrical engineering many of the signals of interest are one dimensional. Although images are two-dimensional signals, almost all of the one-dimensional signal processing methods can be directly extended to two dimensions. Consequently, the first three parts of the book will deal mostly with one-dimensional signals. In the last part of the book these methods will be applied to the task of image reconstruction.

Signal processing methods find a wider application in Radiology than image reconstruction. For example, these methods are very useful for understanding tracer kinetics and for understanding nuclear magnetic resonance spectroscopy. Hence, many of the examples in the first three parts of the book will come from nonimaging applications.

I. STRUCTURE OF THE BOOK

This book is divided into four parts — System Models, Transformations, Filtering, and Reconstruction. The object of the first three parts of the book is to provide a background for Part IV which explains image reconstruction. However, the methods described in the first three parts are useful in themselves for understanding several aspects of radiology. Throughout the book, an attempt will be made to show how the mathematical methods apply to radiological problems.

We assume that the reader has taken a college calculus course. However, since some of the mathematics may be only dimly remembered, Chapter 2 provides a brief review of the calculus which will be used in the rest of the book. Other mathematical background material, necessary to understand reconstruction, is described in greater detail — complex numbers in Chapter 6, vectors and matrices in Chapters 8 and 9, and statistics in Chapters 10, 11, and 12.

A. PART I. SYSTEM MODELS

Part I, System Models, deals with the various models which can be used to describe a system. The concept of a system is central to this book. Anytime one signal depends upon another signal, the relationship can be modeled as a system. The system is said to transform one signal, the input signal, into the other signal, the output signal. For example, the set of attenuation coefficients in a cross section of the body could be an input signal. The system could be a computed tomographic scanner. The output signal would then be the computed tomographic image.

Part I will explain the concept of a system by developing several different models of systems. The major models are convolution, simultaneous linear equations, and stochastic processes (noisy signals). In addition, differential equations are briefly mentioned in order to explain the idea of resonant signals.

Convolution is a method of describing simple linear systems. Convolution and Fourier transforms come from the field called linear systems theory. Chapters 3 through 6 deal with linear systems theory. Simultaneous linear equations provide a second method of describing linear systems. Simultaneous linear equations come from the field called linear algebra. Chapters 8 and 9 deal with linear algebra. We shall learn that a major feature of both of these models is that they assume that a system is linear.

For both convolution and simultaneous linear equations, we shall learn that there are special signals, called eigenfunctions, which do not change form as they pass through a system. These signals are described in Chapter 5. The concept of eigenfunction is often described in more complicated mathematical texts. We shall try to show that the basic concept of an eigenfunction is quite simple and will help in understanding how systems effect signals. Furthermore, in Part II, we shall find that eigenfunctions provide insights into the operation of the Fourier transform.

Complex numbers greatly simplify the description of linear systems and of the Fourier transform. Most readers either will have never heard of complex numbers or will have only a superficial acquaintance with complex numbers. In Chapter 6 we shall try to familiarize the reader with complex numbers. Although learning about complex numbers requires some mental anguish, the reward will be that much of the rest of the book will be considerably simplified.

Both convolution and simultaneous linear equations need to be combined with the idea of measurement noise in order to be useful for radiological applications. Chapter 10 introduces some basic statistical methods. Chapter 11 introduces statistical signals (stochastic processes). In Part IV, stochastic processes will be used to model both noisy measurements and reconstructed images.

Chapter 12 introduces the idea of estimation from a set of noisy measurements. Part III will combine the concept of a signals with estimation. Estimation is very important for real image reconstruction problems where the data include measurement noise.

B. PART II. TRANSFORMATIONS

Part II, Transformations, deals with the various transformation methods. The best known and most useful of these methods is the Fourier transform. The Fourier transform provides a method of describing signals in terms of frequencies. Although we do not have a natural context for understanding frequencies in terms of images, we do naturally understand frequencies in terms of sound. We shall stress the analogy to sound in order to help give some intuition about the frequency description of images.

Chapters 14 through 16 describe the Fourier transform. We shall find that the Fourier transform is very useful for understanding the operation of systems. It will also be key to an understanding of image reconstruction methods in Part IV. Chapter 17, which describes the polynomial transform, provides insight into the most important property of the Fourier transform, changing the complicated convolution operation into a simple multiplication operation.

Chapter 18 describes the discrete Fourier transform. The discrete Fourier transform is important for two reasons. First, it describes how digital computers perform the Fourier transform operation. Second, the relationship between the Fourier transform and the discrete Fourier transform helps to explain sampling, an important part of measurement. Sampling and the artifacts which can be caused by improper sampling are described more fully in Chapter 23.

Chapter 19 describes vector space rotation. Vector space rotation will provide the reader with a geometrical analogy for transform operations. This chapter will tie the transformation operation from the linear systems model with the rotation operation from the linear algebra model.

Chapter 20 describes the two-dimensional Fourier transform, the Laplace transform, and the z transform. The two-dimensional Fourier transform is a simple extension of the Fourier transform for use with images. The other transformation operations provide insight into the basic ideas underlying the Fourier transformation.

Except for Chapter 19, the material in this part depends only on the linear systems model (Chapters 3 to 6). Chapter 19 relates the Fourier transform to linear algebra (Chapters 8 and

9). The reader who is interested in a brief introduction to Fourier transforms could read Chapters 3 to 6 and 14.

C. PART III. FILTERING

Part III, Filtering, deals with methods for modifying signals to enhance certain features and suppress other features. For example, it is often desirable to filter an image to reduce the noise in the image as much as possible with the least reduction in the image information. At other times it is desirable to enhance some aspect of an image, such as the edges in the image. The primary application of filtering in this book is as a part of reconstruction process, but Chapter 27 presents a brief introduction to image enhancement.

Filtering stochastic signals, which is important for understanding image reconstruction in the presence of noise, is described in Chapter 24. Chapter 25 develops the analogy between linear algebra methods and stochastic filtering. Wiener filtering, Chapter 26, is an optimal method for suppressing noise. Wiener filtering is not only an important method of image enhancement, but also it is useful for understanding image reconstruction in the presence of noise.

Filtering is dependent on an understanding of the Fourier transformation. Except for Chapter 25, the necessary background for Part III is Chapters 3 to 6 and 14 to 16. Chapter 25, which draws an analogy between linear algebra and filtering, also depends upon Chapters 8 and 9.

D. PART IV. RECONSTRUCTION

Part IV, Reconstruction, deals with image reconstruction. The other parts of the book are a prelude to this part. The real meat of the Radiologic applications is presented in this part of the book. Part IV starts with a one-dimensional, deconvolution in tracer kinetics. Then the major reconstruction methods are explained in reference to an application where the methods are most useful.

Reconstruction from Fourier samples, Chapter 30, is the primary method used in nuclear magnetic resonance. Reconstruction from noisy projections, Chapter 32, is used in computed tomography. Iterative reconstruction (Chapter 33) can be used in many reconstruction problems. It allows more difficult reconstruction tasks to be performed, at the expense of additional computational complexity. Single photon emission computed tomography is an area where the added complexity is particularly beneficial.

Most of the discussion of reconstruction is in terms of the linear systems model. Reconstruction from Fourier samples and reconstruction from noiseless projections (Chapters 30 and 31) depend only on Chapters 3 to 6 and 14 to 16. Deconvolution, reconstruction from noisy projections, and reconstruction from multiple samples (Chapters 29, 32, and 34) also depend upon Chapters 22, 24, and 26 in Part III. Iterative reconstruction, described in Chapter 33, also depends upon the linear algebra model (Chapters 8, 9, 19, and 25).

Although the book is organized in a logical fashion, not everyone will choose to read it from beginning to end. By indicating how the chapters depend upon each other, hopefully the reader can extract efficiently the material of most interest. After reading selected portions of the book, he may then be interested in going back to read other chapters in order to expand the understanding of these mathematical methods.

II. RELATIONSHIP OF THE CHAPTERS

Table 1.1 attempts to show the most important relationships between the various chapters. It is organized in terms of the four parts of the book and the three major topics — linear systems, linear algebra, and stochastic processes. The lines indicate which previous chapters are required in order to understand a new chapter. A theme of this book is that the different

TABLE 1.1

Relation of Chapters

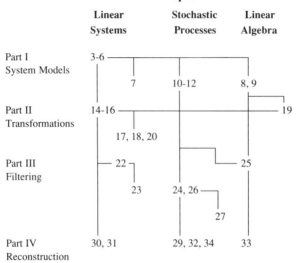

	Linear Systems	Stochastic Processes	Linear Algebra
Part I System Models	3-6		
	7	10-12	8, 9
Part II Transformations	14-16		19
	17, 18, 20		
Part III Filtering	22	25	
	23	24, 26	
		27	
Part IV Reconstruction	30, 31	29, 32, 34	33

topics each help to explain a part of a problem, so that all of the chapters are interrelated; however, Table 1.1 shows the major relations.

There are two ways this information may be used. First, the reader who is interested in a particular topic can read only those chapters upon which that topic depends. Second, the reader who is anxious to get to an application may decide to first take a quick path to Part IV, and subsequently to fill in more of the basic material.

Chapter 30, Reconstruction from Fourier Samples: Nuclear Magnetic Resonance Imaging, and Chapter 31, Reconstruction from Noiseless Projections, both depend only on Chapters 3 to 6 and 14 to 16. Reading just these eight chapters will provide an introduction to nuclear magnetic resonance imaging and to the basics of computed tomographic reconstruction.

The algorithm used in Chapter 33, Iterative Reconstruction: Single Photon Emission Computer Tomography, is most dependent on the chapters which explain linear algebra (Chapters 8 and 9) and the chapters which explain estimation (Chapters 12 and 25). However, the understanding of this material also depends on the chapters on linear systems.

Chapter 29, Deconvolution: First Pass Radionuclide Angiocardiography, Chapter 32, Reconstruction from Noisy Projection: Computed Tomography, and Chapter 34, Reconstruction from Multiple Samples: Multi-Detector Scanner, all involve reconstruction when noise is present. They require an understanding of stochastic processes (Chapters 10, 11, 12, 24, and 26).

Chapter 27, Image Enhancement, logically belongs in Part III, Filtering, but it is also an application. This chapter depends upon the linear system and stochastic process chapters.

Chapters 7, 17, 18, 19, 20, and 23 provide a deeper understanding of the mathematics, but are not necessary for understanding the radiological applications. The reader may wish to skip these chapters on first reading, and then return to them to gain additional understanding of the reconstruction process.

III. FURTHER READING

Except for the summary chapters, each of the chapters in this book will end with suggestions for further reading on the topics covered. Many of the chapters cover subjects which are typically covered in a whole book. The suggestions for further reading will be most useful for the reader who has a particular interest in one of the topics covered.

The treatment of signal processing in this book is similar to the treatment in the field of electrical engineering. There are several excellent books in that field. The book by Oppenheim and Willsky[1] is an excellent introduction. More advanced texts are referenced in subsequent chapters.

Several of the examples which are used in the first parts of the book deal with tracer kinetics. Although the methods in this book are useful for tracer kinetics, this book is not primarily intended as a text on tracer kinetics. The reader who is only interested in tracer kinetics is referred to the book by Lassen and Perl[2].

Image reconstruction in radiology is explained in many texts. A descriptive explanation of reconstruction is included in several computed tomography and nuclear magnetic resonance books. More mathematical explanations are found in the books by Robb[3], Barrett and Swindell[4], Herman[5,6], and Kak and Slaney[7].

REFERENCES

1. **Oppenheim, A. V. and Willsky, A. S.**, *Signals and Systems*, Prentice-Hall, Englewood Cliffs, NJ, 1983.
2. **Lassen, N. A. and Perl, W.**, *Tracer Kinetic Methods in Medical Physiology*, Raven Press, New York, 1979.
3. **Robb, R. A.**, Ed., *Three-Dimensional Biomedical Imaging*, CRC Press, Boca Raton, FL, 1985.
4. **Barrett, H. H., and Swindell, W.**, *Radiological Imaging: The Theory of Image Formation, Detection, and Processing*, Academic Press, New York, 1981.
5. **Herman, G. T.**, Ed., *Image Reconstruction from Projections: Implementation and Applications*, Springer-Verlag, Berlin, 1979.
6. **Herman, G. T.**, *Image Reconstruction from Projections: The Fundamentals of Computerized Tomography*, Academic Press, New York, 1980.
7. **Kak, A. C. and Slaney, M.**, *Principles of Computerized Tomographic Imaging*, IEEE Press, New York, 1987.

Chapter 2

REVIEW OF BASIC CONCEPTS

This chapter reviews several elementary mathematical concepts. We assume that this material has been studied in the past, but that it may not be fresh in your mind. We shall begin by defining a function, and show how a function can be used to represent one- and two-dimensional data. We shall distinguish between functions which are continuous, discrete, and digital. Vectors will be introduced briefly. The analogy between vectors and discrete functions will be used later in the book to provide geometrical insights into mathematical operations. There are several operations which can be performed on functions. Two operations, the derivative and the integral, will be of considerable importance throughout the book. Two useful functions, the step function and the delta functions, will be introduced.

I. FUNCTION

A function is often displayed in graphical form as shown in Figure 2.1. A function, f(t), assigns a value to the **dependent variable**, f, for each value of the **independent variable**, t. Frequently, the independent variable is time and the function represents the change in value of some parameter with time. For example, Figure 2.1 represents the signal from a nuclear magnetic resonance (NMR) experiment. The dependent variable, f, represents the current in the probe. The independent variable, t, represents time. Figure 2.2 represents the decay of a radioactive sample. The dependent variable represents the radioactivity in the sample at each point in time.

In this book we shall only consider **single-valued** functions. A single valued function has one and only one value of the dependent variable for each value of the independent variable. At each instant in time there is only one value of the NMR signal, and there is only one level of radioactivity emitting from the radioactive source. An example of a graph which does not represent a single-valued function is shown in Figure 2.3. At several points in time, there are two values of the dependent variable.

The reverse relation is different. Each value of the dependent variable may be related to none, one, or many values of the independent variable. In Figure 2.1, we can see that some NMR signal intensities occur at many times during the experiment, and some intensities never occur. In the case of radioactive decay, a particular decay rate occurs at only one point in time. However, some decay rates do not occur; for example, negative decay rates never occur.

The value of a function depends on only a single value of the independent variable, t. Given a time value, the value of the function can be calculated. This property may seem obvious, but it is very important. It is the basis of the major distinctions between functions and systems. The value of a function depends on a single input value while the value of a system may depend on many input values.

A graph is one way to represent the values of a function. A second method is to construct a mathematical relationship between the independent variable and the value of the function. For example,

$$f(t) = sin(t) \tag{2.1}$$

defines a function where the value of the dependent variable is equal to the sine of the independent variable. A graph representing the same function is shown in Figure 2.4. The value of a function is represented for only a small interval of time by a graph. The value of the function can be calculated for any time by applying its equation.

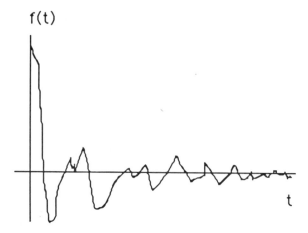

FIGURE 2.1.   Graphical representation of a function: the function,
f(t), assigns a value to the dependent variable, f, for each value of
the independent variable, t. This function represents the free induction
decay for a nuclear magnetic resonance experiment.

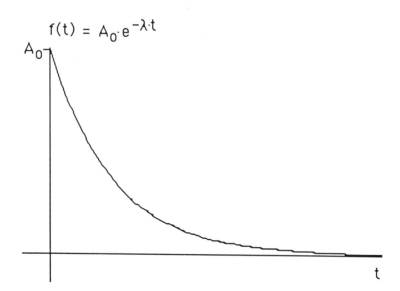

FIGURE 2.2.   Radioactive decay: this figure shows the decay of a radioactive substance. A_0 is the initial amount of activity. The radioactivity decays according to the
exponential, $e^{-\lambda t}$.

A third way to describe a function is to enumerate the value of the function for a sequence
of values of the independent variable. For example, the radioactivity of a sample could be
listed for each second from 0 to 50 sec. This method has the same problem as the graphical
method. The interval over which the function can be enumerated must be finite. With the
mathematical method, the description is not limited to any particular interval. A second
problem with enumeration is that a function can only be given at discrete points along the
time axis. It is not possible to divide the time axis up into infinitely small intervals.

It would seem that the mathematical description of a function is the most versatile of
the three methods. Let us not, however, so quickly discard the method of enumeration. In
most practical radiological situations, adequately fine sampling over the interval of interest
can be chosen. In fact all computer applications use the method of enumeration.

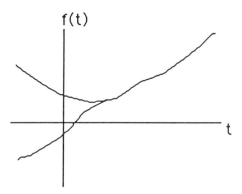

FIGURE 2.3. Multi-valued function: this figure shows a multi-valued function, f(t). For many of the values of t, this function has two separate values.

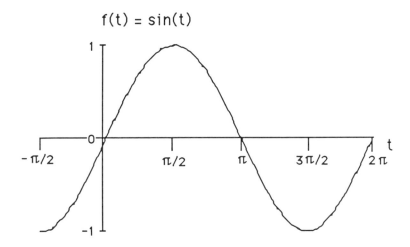

FIGURE 2.4. Sine function: the sine function has a period of 2π.

A. CONTINUOUS, DISCRETE, AND DIGITAL

These ideas can be put on a more sound mathematical footing by defining continuous and discrete functions. A **continuous function** is defined at every point along the independent variable; the time axis can be divided into infinitely small intervals. A **discrete function** is defined at only discrete points along the independent variable. In this book we shall use discrete functions which are defined at integer values of the independent variable, i.e., 0, 1, 2, etc. A discrete function can be shown in graphical form as a series of points. Figure 2.5 shows the discrete representation of the same sine function which is shown in Figure 2.4.

We shall use a different notation for continuous and discrete functions. Continuous functions will be indicated with parentheses around the independent variable, f(t). Discrete functions will be indicated with square brackets around the independent variable, f[n]. We shall also frequently use different symbols for continuous and discrete independent variables. We shall use t to indicate a continuous independent variable, and n to indicate a discrete independent variable. t can take on any value; n can only have integer values. We shall commonly refer to both t and n as time variables.

For both continuous and discrete functions, the dependent variable, f, can take on any

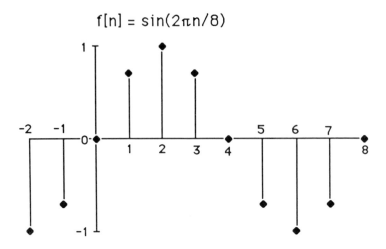

FIGURE 2.5.   Discrete sine function: this graph shows a discrete representation of the sine function shown in Figure 2.4. The discrete representation is defined for only a discrete set of values of the independent variable, n.

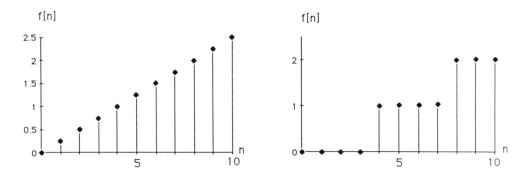

FIGURE 2.6.   Discrete and digital functions: the graph on the left shows a discrete ramp function. The value of the function is defined for only a discrete point along the independent variable. The value of the function can take on a continuous set of values. The graph on the right shows the same function represented as a digital function. The values of both the independent and dependent variable can have only discrete values.

value — the dependent variable is continuous. If both the dependent and independent variables are restricted to have only discrete values, the function is called a **digital function**. Figure 2.6 shows a discrete function on the left and a similar digital function on the right. Notice that the digital function can only have certain values.

All measurements have errors, so that the accuracy of the values is always limited. Therefore, it is reasonable to use digital functions to represent real data. Since digital computers can only represent numbers with a finite accuracy, the computer represents all functions as digital functions. Practical implementation of most radiological problems involves digital functions. However, the major goal of this book is to explain basic mathematical concepts. These concepts are best understood in terms of continuous functions. Therefore, most emphasis will be placed on continuous functions. Discrete functions will be required to explain certain concepts. Digital functions will not be used in this book.

B. TWO-DIMENSIONAL FUNCTIONS

Most of the applications in this book deal with pictures. A picture can be described as a function with two independent variables. One variable represents the horizontal axis and

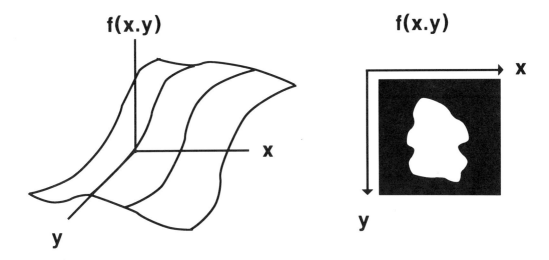

FIGURE 2.7. Two-dimensional function: on the left, a two-dimensional function, f(x,y), is shown as a three-dimensional graph. On the right, a similar function is shown as an image, where the intensity of the image is related to the value of the function.

one variable represents the vertical axis. The **two-dimensional function** assigns a value, the picture intensity, to each point within the picture. We shall use f(x,y) to represent a two-dimensional function, where x represents the horizontal position, y represents the vertical position, and f represents the picture intensity.

Figure 2.7 shows two ways that a two-dimensional function can be displayed. On the left, the function is shown in graphical form. A two-dimensional function requires a three-dimensional graph. For simple functions this type of graph can be very useful, but for more complicated functions this type of graph is difficult to understand and difficult to draw. One the right, the function is shown as a picture, where the value of the function at any point corresponds to the brightness of the image at that point. In radiology, this presentation is obviously much more common.

Two-dimensional functions are like one-dimensional functions except that the functions are defined for a pair of independent variables. For each pair of independent variables, there is one and only one value of the function. Two-dimensional functions can be continuous, discrete, or digital. Later in the book we shall encounter a few special features of two-dimensional functions; however, in general they are very similar to one dimensional function.

C. MULTI-DIMENSIONAL FUNCTIONS

A function can have any number of dimensions, including an infinite number of dimensions. For example, f(x,y,z) describes a function in three dimensions. An example of a three-dimensional function is the proton density in the head as measured by an NMR scanner. For each location in three dimensions, there is one value for the proton density.

For higher dimension functions our geometric intuition breaks down. It is difficult to conceptualize a function in four dimensions. However, such functions occur naturally in radiology. For example, the hydrogen spectrum as a function of position has four dimensions — three space dimensions, x,y,z, and one chemical shift dimension, ω. ω is an angular frequency variable. At each point in the three-dimensional space there is a spectrum, f(x,y,z,ω). The values of the independent variables give the position and the chemical shift. The dependent variable gives the value of the spectrum at that point and chemical shift. Figure 2.8 is highly diagrammatic representation of this function. It is very difficult to draw a picture of functions with more than three dimensions.

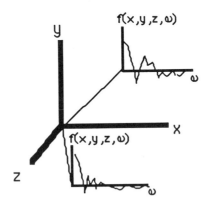

FIGURE 2.8.   Four-dimensional function: this figure shows a highly diagrammatic representation of a four dimensional function. The three space dimensions are given by x, y, and z. At each point in space the value of the function is also a function of ω. This diagram shows the function with respect to ω at two points in space.

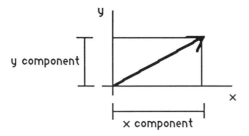

FIGURE 2.9.   Components of a vector: this figure shows a vector starting at the origin of a x,y coordinate system. The x and y components of the vector are the distances along the x and y axes to the end of the vector.

II. VECTORS

In this book, vectors will be used as another method to represent signals. The most common way of drawing a vector is an arrow from the origin to a point. Figure 2.9 shows a vector in a two-dimensional coordinate system. This vector has two components which represent its length along the x and y axes. Vectors with two components can be used to represent a point in a two-dimensional space. Similarly, a vector with three components could be used to define a point in a three-dimensional vector space.

In Chapter 8, we shall discuss vectors defined to have any number of dimensions including an infinite number of dimensions. It is not possible to draw vectors with more than three dimensions; however, we shall frequently appeal to our geometric intuition in three dimensions to understand vectors in multiple dimension.

Later, we shall make an analogy between a vector and a one-dimensional function which has been defined by enumeration. The sequence of values which define the function can be thought of as the components of a vector in a multi-dimensional space. The multiple points in a one-dimensional function are analogous to the components of a multi-dimensional vector. We shall find that a one-dimensional function is similar to a point in a multi-dimensional space.

Figure 2.10 shows a very simple example of this analogy. The function with two points shown on the left is analogous to the vector with two components shown on the right. The value of the function at zero, f[0], is equal to the x component of the vector, and the value at 1, f [1], is equal to the y component.

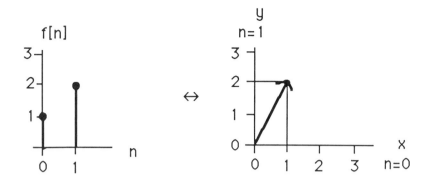

FIGURE 2.10. Vector representation of a discrete function: the figure on the left shows a discrete function which is defined for only two values, 0 and 1. The figure on the right shows a vector in the x,y coordinate system. A function defined for two point can be represented by a vector in two dimensions. The x component of the vector, 1, is equal to the value of the function for n = 0. The y component of the vector, 2, is equal to the value of the function for n = 1. The x axis can also be called the n = 0 axis; the y axis can also be called the n = 1 axis.

We shall find that many operations which can be performed on functions are analogous to operations which can be performed on vectors. It will be possible to apply our geometric intuition about vectors to understanding operations on functions. In Part II we shall make an analogy between the Fourier transform and vector rotation. The main reason for including the different models of systems in this book is the understanding that the different models provide about each other — but more of this later.

III. OPERATIONS

There are several operations which can be performed element by element on a function. For example, we can multiply a function by a constant to produce a new function:

$$g(t) = a \cdot f(t) \tag{2.2}$$

Each element of the new function is equal to the same element of the old function multiplied by the constant, a. Similarly, a new function could be defined as the sine of the sum of a function plus 5:

$$g(t) = \sin(f(t) + 5) \tag{2.3}$$

Two functions can be combined with simple mathematical operations. For example, two functions can be multiplied together:

$$g(t) = f_1(t) \cdot f_2(t) \tag{2.4}$$

Each element of g(t) is equal to the value of $f_1(t)$ times $f_2(t)$ at the same point. These simple operations are expressed by equations such as those given above.

A. OPERATIONS ON THE INDEPENDENT VARIABLE

Instead of operating on the dependent variables, it is also possible to define operations which involve the independent variables. An example of an operation on the independent variable is a shifting operation:

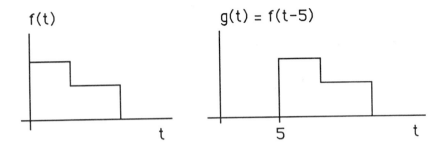

FIGURE 2.11.   Shifting: the graph on the left shows a function, f(t). The graph on the right shows a function, g(t), which is equal to f(t) shifted 5 units to the right.

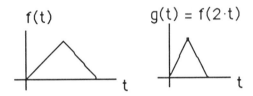

FIGURE 2.12.   Scaling the independent variable: the graph on the left shows a function, f(t). The graph on the right shows a function, g(t), which is equal to f(2 · t). When the independent variable is scaled, the function shrinks or expands along the independent variable.

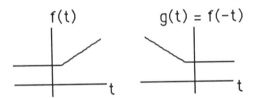

FIGURE 2.13.   Time reversal: changing the sign of the independent variable, flips the function about the ordinate. The graph on the left shows a function, f(t). The graph on the right shows a function, g(t), which is equal to f(−t).

$$g(t) = f(t - 5) \tag{2.5}$$

Figure 2.11 shows an example of two functions where one function is shifted to the right by 5 units. The value of g(·) at t equal to 1 is the same as the value of f(·) at t equal to 6. We shall use the notation, g(·), with the dot when we are referring specifically to a property of the function and are not concerned with the specific independent variable.

Another example of an operation on the independent variable is the scaling operation:

$$g(t) = f(2 \cdot t) \tag{2.6}$$

Figure 2.12 shows an example of this operation. By multiplying the independent variable by −1, the scaling operation can be used to flip a function about the f axis:

$$g(t) = f(-t) \tag{2.7}$$

Figure 2.13 shows an example of this operation.

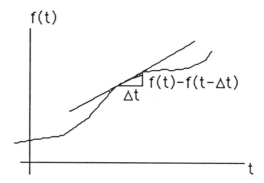

FIGURE 2.14.   Derivative: the derivative of a function, f(t), is equal to the slope of a line which is a tangent to the function. The slope of the line is the ratio of the change in the ordinate, f(t) − f(t − Δt), to the change in the abscissa, Δt. This ratio is used in the definition of the derivative (Equation 2.9).

B. DIFFERENCE

A new function can be produced from a discrete function, f[n], by subtracting the value of the preceding element from each element of the function. This **difference** operation can be written mathematically:

$$g[n] = f[n] - f[n - 1] \qquad (2.8)$$

The difference operation is of interest for determining the rate of change of a function over time. For example, if f[n] represents the volume of the left ventricle at 50-msec intervals, then g[n] gives the rate of left ventricular ejection during systole and the rate of filling during diastole.

C. DERIVATIVE

Sometimes it is useful to determine the rate of change of a continuous function. In that case, the difference operation is only an approximation. However, the difference operation can be extended to the continuous case using a limiting operation. The **derivative** is defined as:

$$df(t)/dt = \lim_{\Delta t \to 0} \{f(t) - f(t - \Delta t)\}/\Delta t \qquad (2.9)$$

The quotient inside the limit is the difference of the function over a small time interval, Δt, divided by that time interval. This quotient approaches the derivative, as the interval Δt gets smaller and smaller. Mathematicians are particularly concerned about when the limit in Equation 2.9 exists and when it does not exist. We shall largely ignore these mathematical concerns.

We can rewrite Equation 2.8, the equation for the difference operation, to emphasize the similarity between the difference and the derivative operations:

$$g[n] = \{f[n] - f[n - 1]\}/1 \qquad (2.10)$$

Δt in the derivative is analogous to 1 in the difference. The derivative operation for continuous function shares many properties with the difference operation for discrete functions.

Figure 2.14 shows the derivative operation graphically. The quotient in the limiting operation is the slope of a line between the two points, f(t-Δt) and f(t). As the interval becomes very short, the quotient is equal to the instantaneous slope of the line at a point.

TABLE 2.1
Derivatives

Function	Derivative
t	1
$a \cdot t$	a
t^n	$n \cdot t^{n-1}$
e^t	e^t
$e^{a \cdot t}$	$a \cdot e^{a \cdot t}$
$\ln(t)$	$1/t$
$f(t) + g(t)$	$df(t)/dt + dg(t)/dt$
$f(t) \cdot g(t)$	$f(t) \cdot dg(t)/dt + g(t) \cdot df(t)/dt$

Table 2.1 reviews some common functions and their derivatives. The following section can be skipped without loss of continuity.

D. PARTIAL DERIVATIVE

For a function, $f(x,y)$, with two independent variables, the **partial derivative** of $f(x,y)$ with respect to x is defined:

$$\partial f(x,y)/\partial x = \lim_{\Delta x \to 0} \{f(x,y) - f(x - \Delta x,y)\}/\Delta x \qquad (2.11)$$

The definition of the partial derivative (Equation 2.11) is very similar to the definition of the derivative (Equation 2.9). The key feature is that the other independent variable is held constant.

The **total differential** is defined as the sum of the partial derivatives times the respective differentials:

$$df(x,y) = [\partial f(x,y)/\partial x] \cdot dx + [\partial f(x,y)/\partial y] \cdot dy \qquad (2.12)$$

If the distinction between the derivative, the partial derivatives, and total differential are too abstract, do not worry. We shall have only very minor need of the total differential.

In many situations, it is not necessary to be rigorous about the distinction between a derivative and a partial derivative. However, when the independent variables are themselves functions of some other variable, such as t, then the partial derivative formalism becomes important. In this case we can write the derivative of $f(x,y)$ with respect to t in terms of the partial derivatives:

$$df(x,y)/dt = [\partial f(x,y)/\partial x] \cdot dx/dt + [\partial f(x,y)/\partial y] \cdot dy/dt \qquad (2.13)$$

E. SUM

The special symbol, Σ, is used to indicate the sum of a sequence of value of a discrete function. The values over which the function is to be summed are written above and below the Σ symbol. For example,

$$\sum_{n=1}^{5} f[n] = f[1] + f[2] + f[3] + f[4] + f[5] \qquad (2.14)$$

One or the other of the limits may be infinity, ∞. When the limits of the summation are obvious, they are often omitted.

Using the summing operation, we can define a function which is the sum of all of the values of a function prior to some time, n:

$$f[n] = \sum_{m=-\infty}^{n} g[m] \qquad (2.15)$$

The summation for f[n] has one more element, g[n], than the summation for f[n−1]. Therefore,

$$f[n] - f[n - 1] = g[n] \qquad (2.16)$$

This equation is the same as the definition of the difference, Equation 2.8. Thus, the summation operation with the proper limits is the opposite of the difference operation.

The summation operation is used frequently in radiology. If g[m] represents the X-ray attenuation coefficients along an X-ray beam, then the sum, f[n], gives the signal which would be measured during computed tomographic data collection. Measurement operation in radiology often involves a sum of components.

F. INTEGRAL

The integral operation applied to continuous functions is analogous to the summation operation on discrete functions. The integral is written:

$$\int_{a}^{b} f(t) \, dt \qquad (2.17)$$

a and b are the limits of the integration. The function f(t), is integrated from t equal a to t equal to b. dt indicates that the integration is performed with respect to the variable, t.

Like the derivative, the integral is defined using a limiting operation:

$$\int_{a}^{b} f(t) \, dt = \lim_{\Delta t \to 0} \sum_{n=0}^{(b-a)/\Delta t} f(a + n \cdot \Delta t) \cdot \Delta t \qquad (2.18)$$

This limit is somewhat complicated. Inside the limit is the sum of the value of f(·) at the values of t between a and b times the value, Δt. As Δt becomes smaller, the number of points in the summation becomes larger. In the limit of an infinite number of terms in the sum, the value of the sum approaches the integral. Mathematicians are very concerned about when this limit exists, and when it does not exist. Again we shall largely ignore these types of questions.

Figure 2.15 shows the integration operation graphically. On the interval between a and b, the function f(·) is approximated by a series of rectangles. The height of the rectangles is equal to the value of the function, and the width is equal to Δt. The area of each little rectangle is $f(a + n \cdot \Delta t) \cdot \Delta t$. The sum in Equation 2.18 is the sum of each of all of the areas of the rectangles. Thus the integral gives the area under the curve, f(t), between the points a and b. Table 2.2 gives the integrals of some common functions.

On occasion we shall find it necessary to switch the limits of the integration. Instead of integrating from a to b, we shall want to integrate from b to a. Switching the direction of integration, switches the intervals from Δt to $-\Delta t$. Therefore the sign of the integral changes:

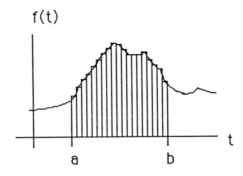

FIGURE 2.15.   Integral: the integral of the function, f(t), from a to b is the area under the curve. The rectangles shown in this figure approximate the area under the curve. As the rectangles get smaller, the area is approximated more accurately. This process is equivalent to the definition of the integral in Equation 2.18.

TABLE 2.2
Integrals

Function	Integral
1	$t + c$
t^n	$[1/(n+1)] \cdot t^{n+1} + c$
e^{at}	$(1/a) \cdot e^{at} + c$
$f(t) + g(t)$	$\int_{-\infty}^{+\infty} f(t)\, dt + \int_{-\infty}^{+\infty} g(t)\, dt$

Note: c = Constant.

$$\int_a^b f(t)\, dt = -\int_b^a f(t)\, dt \tag{2.19}$$

We can use the integral operation to define a function, g(t), which is equal to the area of a function, f(t), up to time, t. This function can be defined by the equation:

$$f(t) = \int_{-\infty}^t g(\tau)\, d\tau \tag{2.20}$$

t, the independent variable associated with f is one of the limits of integration. It would be too confusing to also use t for the function, $g(\cdot)$. Therefore, we have used τ as the independent variable in the integration. It is frequently necessary to change the variable in the integration. When we change the variable inside the integral, the new variable, τ, is called a **dummy variable of the integration.**

The integral in Equation 2.20 is analogous to the summation in Equation 2.15. That summation operation was the opposite of the difference operation, Equation 2.8. Similarly, the integral in Equation 2.20 is the opposite of the derivative operation given by:

$$df(t)/dt = g(t) \tag{2.21}$$

The substation of a dummy variable of integration in Equation 2.20 was quite simple. However, the operation is more complicated if the new variable is not equal to the original variable. For example, let us suppose that we wish to substitute:

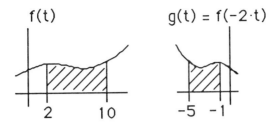

FIGURE 2.16. Change of variables: the area under the curve on the left is equal to the integral on the left side of Equation 2.26. The area under the curve on the right is equal to the integral on the right side of Equation 2.26.

$$c \cdot \tau = t \tag{2.22}$$

Then,

$$\int_a^b f(t)\,dt = \int_{a/c}^{b/c} f(c \cdot \tau)\,dc \cdot \tau = c \cdot \int_{a/c}^{b/c} f(c \cdot \tau)\,d\tau \tag{2.23}$$

It is necessary both to substitute for t and to change the limits of integration.

One additional complication arises when the scaling factor is negative. For example consider:

$$-c \cdot \tau = t \tag{2.24}$$

Then,

$$\int_a^b f(t)\,dt = -c \cdot \int_{-a/c}^{-b/c} f(-c \cdot \tau)\,d\tau = c \cdot \int_{-b/c}^{-a/c} f(-c \cdot \tau)\,d\tau \tag{2.25}$$

Since $-c \cdot a$ is larger than $-c \cdot b$, we have switched the order of integration in the last inequality (see Equation 2.19). Figure 2.16 shows an example given by:

$$\int_2^{10} f(t)\,dt = 2 \cdot \int_{-5}^{-1} f(-2 \cdot \tau)\,d\tau \tag{2.26}$$

where $-c$ is equal to -2.

A function with more than one variable can be integrated with respect to one or more of its variables. Integration with respect to one variable results in an output function with one less variable:

$$g(x) = \int_{-\infty}^{+\infty} f(x,y)\,dy \tag{2.27}$$

The meaning of this equation is that for each position, x, g(x) is equal to the area under the two-dimensional function, f(x,y), in the y direction.

Integration with respect to both variables gives the total area under the function:

$$h = \int_{-\infty}^{+\infty} \int_{-\infty}^{+\infty} f(x,y)\,dy dx \tag{2.28}$$

TABLE 2.3
Power and Roots

$$t^n \cdot t^m = t^{n+m}$$

$$t^n/t^m = t^{n-m}$$

$$(t^n)^m = t^{n \cdot m}$$

$$t^0 = 1$$

The output is a single number, h. The two operations are performed sequentially. First, the inner integral is evaluated with respect to y, then the outer integral is evaluated with respect to x. Equation 2.28 is obtained from Equation 2.27 by integration with respect to x.

G. POWERS AND ROOTS

Repetitive multiplication of a number can be written using the power notation:

$$2 \cdot 2 \cdot 2 \cdot 2 \cdot = 2^4 \qquad (2.29)$$

The superscript indicates the number of times that the number is multiplied by itself. The equation of a power function is:

$$f(t) = t^n \qquad (2.30)$$

With n equal to 1, this equation defines a line; with n equal to 2, it defines a parabola, etc.

A negative number in the exponent is used to indicate the reciprocal:

$$f(t) = t^{-n} = 1/t^n \qquad (2.31)$$

A root is given by a reciprocal in the exponent.

$$f(t) = t^{1/n} \qquad (2.32)$$

With n equal to 2, this equation defines the square root; with n equal to 3 this equation defines the cube root, etc. Table 2.3 shows some common operations using powers and roots. Using these operations we can show that the root is the opposite of the power function:

$$(t^n)^{1/n} = t^{n \cdot 1/n} = t^1 = t \qquad (2.33)$$

H. EXPONENTIALS AND LOGARITHMS

The definition of a power function can be extended to include any number in the exponent:

$$f(t) = a^t \qquad (2.34)$$

The symbol, a, represents a constant. It is called the **base of the exponential.** As t increases, the function, f(t), gives the different powers of a.

Any number can be used for the base of the exponential, but a common choice is the number, e.

$$f(t) = e^t \qquad (2.35)$$

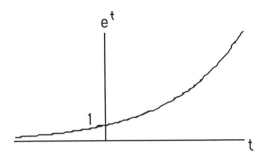

FIGURE 2.17. Exponential function: this figure shows the graph of an exponential function, e^t. The value of the exponential at t equal to 0 is 1.

e is approximately equal to 2.7183. Using e as the base of the exponential results in several very convenient properties. One of these properties is that e^t is its own derivative (see Table 2.1).

Figure 2.17 shows an example of an exponential function. This function increases very rapidly for large values of the independent variable. Radioactive decay is represented by an exponential function with a negative exponent:

$$f(t) = A_0 \cdot e^{-\lambda t} \tag{2.36}$$

This exponential function decreases with time (see Figure 2.2). It approaches zero rapidly for large values of t.

In computer applications a common base is the number two. The basic unit of computer storage is the bit, which can store two different values. There are four possible values which can be stored in two bits, and eight values which can be stored in three bits. In general, the number of different values which can be stored in n bits is given by the discrete function:

$$f[n] = 2^n \tag{2.37}$$

The opposite of the exponential is the logarithm. If

$$e^a = b \tag{2.38}$$

then

$$\log_e(b) = a \tag{2.39}$$

The most common bases for the logarithm are 10, e, and 2. Base 10 logarithms are commonly written without a subscript, log(b). The special symbol, ln, is commonly used for base e logarithms, ln(b). Base 2 logarithms are commonly written using the subscript notation, $\log_2(b)$.

The logarithm can be used to define a function:

$$f(t) = \ln(t) \tag{2.40}$$

An example of a logarithmic function is shown in Figure 2.18. The value of the function goes to negative infinity as t goes to zero. The value of the function increases very slowly when the independent variable is greater than 1.

Some common operations with logarithms are shown in Table 2.4. These operations

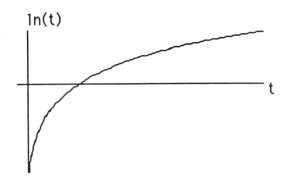

FIGURE 2.18. Logarithmic function: this figure shows the logarithmic function ln(t). The logarithm crosses the x axis at t equal to 1.

TABLE 2.4
Logarithms

$$\log(a \cdot b) = \log(a) + \log(b)$$
$$\log(a/b) = \log(a) - \log(b)$$
$$\log(a^n) = n \cdot \log(a)$$
$$e^{\ln(a)} = a$$
$$\ln(e^a) = a$$
$$\log(1) = 0$$

Note: $\ln = \log_e$.

can be used to shed light on the radioactive decay equation. Radioactive decay can be written in terms of half lives using a base $1/2$ exponential:

$$f(t) = A_0 \cdot \left(\frac{1}{2}\right)^{t/T_{1/2}} \tag{2.41}$$

After one half-life t equals $T_{1/2}$; therefore,

$$f(T_{1/2}) = A_0 \cdot \left(\frac{1}{2}\right)^1 = \frac{1}{2} \cdot A_0 \tag{2.42}$$

After two half-lives:

$$f(2 \cdot T_{1/2}) = A_0 \cdot \left(\frac{1}{2}\right)^2 = \frac{1}{4} \cdot A_0 \tag{2.43}$$

And so on for successive half lives.

Equation 2.41 can be transformed into the form given by Equation 2.36 using the relations in Tables 2.3 and 2.4:

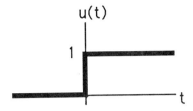

FIGURE 2.19. Step function: the step function, u(t), is equal to 0 for t less than zero and 1 for t greater than 1.

$$f(t) = A_0 \cdot (2^{-1})^{t/T_{1/2}}$$

$$= A_0 \cdot 2^{-t/T_{1/2}}$$

$$= A_0 \cdot (e^{\ln(2)})^{-t/T_{1/2}}$$

$$= A_0 \cdot e^{-\ln(2)t/T_{1/2}}$$

$$= A_0 \cdot e^{-\lambda t} \qquad (2.44)$$

where λ is equal to $\ln(2)/T_{1/2}$. The constant $\ln(2)$, which relates the decay constant to the half life, is approximately equal to .693.

Equation 2.41, which uses a base $1/2$ exponential, expresses the decay equation naturally in terms of the half life, $T_{1/2}$. Equation 2.36, which uses a base e exponential, expresses the decay equation naturally in terms of the decay constant, λ. This derivation shows that the somewhat mysterious constant, .693, is simply due to a change in the base of the exponential used to define the decay equation.

IV. SPECIAL FUNCTIONS

A. STEP FUNCTION
The step function, shown in Figure 2.19, has the value, 0, for times less than zero and the value, 1, for times greater than zero. We shall use the symbol, u(t), for the step function. The step function is often used in combination with another function to indicate the onset of the function.

For example, consider the equation for radioactive decay (Equation 2.44). For negative times, $A_0 \cdot e^{-\lambda t}$ is greater than A_0, the activity at time zero. As t become more negative, the f(t) becomes very large. However, these large values do not have any meaning. In a real situation, what usually happens is that a certain amount of radioactivity is produced at time zero, and then decays. With the step function we can give a more realistic description of this situation:

$$f(t) = u(t) \cdot A_0 \cdot e^{-\lambda t} \qquad (2.45)$$

This function is 0 for t less than zero and follows exponential decay for t greater than 0. In addition to providing a more accurate description of the experiment, use of the step function will be important in signal processing applications later in the book.

B. DELTA FUNCTION
The delta or impulse function is the mathematical equivalent of a bolus. It is nonzero for only an infinitesimal period of time. Mathematically, the delta function is zero for all times except for t equal to 0; at t equal to zero, it has an infinite value, and the integral of

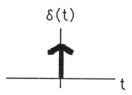

FIGURE 2.20.   Delta function: the delta function is equal to infinity for t equal to zero, and it is equal to 0 elsewhere. The integral of the delta function is equal to 1. We shall represent the delta function with an arrow.

the delta function is equal to 1. The delta function is a bit of a thorn in the side of mathematicians. We shall gloss over the mathematical problems with defining an infinitely large infinitely narrow function. In all radiological applications, we could use a function which approximates a delta function, for example, a Gaussian function with a very small standard deviation.

Sometimes, the delta function is described by a limiting process, where the delta function is equal to the limit of a series of functions which are progressively more narrow and tall. There is a firm mathematical footing on the delta function in the theory of generalized functions; however, for our purposes we shall simply consider the delta function to be a very narrow function. We shall ignore the fact that in some cases the mathematical methods used are not strictly correct.

We shall use the symbol, $\delta(t)$, to indicate the delta function. Figure 2.20 shows a delta function diagrammatically. We shall use an arrow pointing upward to indicate the delta function.

In the next chapter and in the rest of the book, the principle method of defining a system will be by its response to a delta function input. In radiology we frequently use a bolus to define biological systems. Contrast is injected as a bolus and then the response of some organ over time is observed. The delta function is an idealized version of this type of input.

V. POWER SERIES EXPANSION

Power series are important since many functions of interest in radiology can be expressed in terms of power series. Furthermore, power series representation of an exponential function will be used in Chapter 6 for deriving a generalization of the exponential in terms of complex numbers. The complex exponential will be used extensively in our description of the Fourier transform operation.

Many functions are writing directly in terms of a power series, e.g.:

$$f(t) = t + 4t^2 + 2t^3 + 5 \tag{2.46}$$

Other functions are not so clearly related to power series, but can be related to power series mathematically.

Reasonably well behaved functions can be expressed using the Taylor series expansion. (A mathematician would say functions that are infinitely differentiable can be expressed using a Taylor series expansion). The Taylor series expands a function about a point in terms of the derivatives of the function at that point and powers of the independent variable. Although the Taylor series may result in an infinite number of terms, often only the first few terms are necessary to obtain a good representation of the function over the interval of interest.

Some useful Taylor series expansions are given in Table 2.5. The power series expansion allows unfamiliar functions such as the exponential, the cosine, and the sine to be expressed

TABLE 2.5
Taylor Series Expansions

$$e^t = 1 + t + t^2/2! + t^3/3! + t^4/4! + \ldots$$
$$\cos(t) = 1 - t^2/2! + t^4/4! - t^6/6! + \ldots$$
$$\sin(t) = t - t^3/3! + t^5/5! - t^7/7! + \ldots$$

Note: $n! = n \cdot (n-1) \cdot (n-2) \cdot (n-3) \ldots$

in terms of more familiar functions. The **factorial** notation, n!, used in the table is defined by:

$$n! = n \cdot (n - 1) \cdot (n - 2) \cdot (n - 3) \ldots \tag{2.47}$$

0! is specially defined to be equal to 1.

Another advantage of the power series formulation is that it is sometimes possible to prove relationships which are difficult to prove otherwise. For example:

$$de^t/dt = 0 + 1 + 2 \cdot t^1/2! + 3 \cdot t^2/3! + 4 \cdot t^3/4! + \ldots$$
$$= 1 + t + t^2/2! + t^3/3! + t^4/4! + \ldots$$
$$= e^t \tag{2.48}$$

Thus, the derivative of e^t is e^t.

VI. SUMMARY

This chapter has briefly discussed several elementary concepts which will be used in the rest of the book. There is a relatively long description of the difference between continuous and discrete functions, since this distinction will be important in the rest of the book. Most of this material should be familiar to you. We shall use derivatives and integrals throughout the rest of the book.

VII. FURTHER READING

The material on derivatives and integrals is covered in any college calculus course. A discussion of the difference between continuous, discrete, and digital signals can be found in the book by Oppenheim and Willsky.[1]

REFERENCE

1. **Oppenheim, A. V. and Willsky, A. S.,** *Signals and Systems,* Prentice-Hall, Englewood Cliffs, NJ, 1983.

Chapter 3

CONVOLUTION

Convolution is a mathematical method for describing how a system transforms an input signal into an output signal. This technique was developed by electrical engineers. As a result, the terminology has a distinctly engineering flavor. Despite its engineering veneer, convolution is a general mathematical approach which is useful for a wide variety of applications. The average radiologist only knows of convolution as a mathematical technique that is somehow related to computed tomographic reconstruction. However, convolution can be used to describe many everyday radiologic processes. For example, the blurring of a film caused by a cassette can be easily described by convolution.

In this chapter, we shall describe a number of systems which can be described using the concept of convolution and show how this process can be written mathematically. Although convolution is a complex concept, the systems which can be described by convolution are quite familiar. One of the major objectives of the second part of the book will be to develop mathematical techniques which allow us to understand convolution in simpler terms. However, the immediate task at hand is to gain some familiarity with convolution and with the systems described by convolution.

I. DESCRIPTION OF CONVOLUTION

Most of the image processing applications in Part IV deal with two-dimensional convolution. However, one-dimensional convolution is very similar to two-dimensional convolution, and it is somewhat easier to understand. Many examples of one dimensional convolution come from tracer kinetics. We shall start with the excretion of a radiopharmaceutical by the kidney.

At any time after injection, the radioactivity in the kidney is due to two factors — the delivery of radiopharmaceutical to the kidney and the handling of the radiopharmaceutical by the kidney. The delivery of radiopharmaceutical to the kidney is described by blood time activity curve. To describe the handling of the radiopharmaceutical by the kidney, we can image a bolus input to the kidney. (A bolus can be modeled as a delta function described in Chapter 2; the blood time activity curve is nonzero for an infinitesimally brief time). In that case, the handling of radiopharmaceutical by the kidney could be measured from a time activity curve over the kidney.

The top curve in Figure 3.1, f(t), represents the blood time activity curve, the second curve represents the handling of the radiopharmaceutical by the kidney after a bolus input, h(t), the third curve represents actual kidney time activity curve, g(t). The process of combining the blood time activity curve with the handling of activity by the kidney to obtain the actual kidney time activity curve is an example of a system which can be described by convolution.

The blood time activity curve is called the **input** signal. It is the input of radiopharmaceutical to the kidney. The handling of the radiopharmaceutical by the kidney, is called the **system** function. The system function describes what the kidney time activity curve would be if the input were a bolus. The kidney time activity curve for any input is called the **output** function. It represents how the kidney responds to the given input.

Convolution of this complicated input signal with the system function is difficult to describe. A much simpler example is shown in Figure 3.2. The input signal, f(t), consists of two boluses of activity. The first bolus produces a portion of the output, $g_1(t)$, shown in the second panel. The second bolus produces a portion of the output, $g_2(t)$, shown in the third panel. Each of these portions of the output has the form of a system function. However,

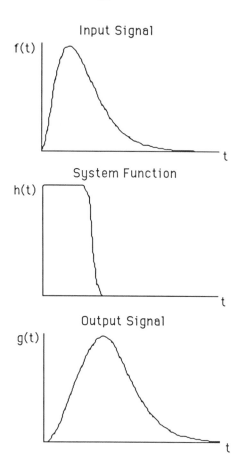

FIGURE 3.1. Renal excretion of an radiopharmaceutical: the input signal, f(t), is the time activity curve for the radiopharmaceutical in the arterial blood (top panel). The system function, h(t), is time activity curve from the kidney for an idealized bolus of activity injected into the renal artery (middle panel). The output signal, g(t), is the actual time activity curve from the kidney when the input is the arterial time activity curve shown in the top panel (bottom panel).

for each of these outputs the system function is shifted according to the position of the bolus and scaled according to the size of the bolus.

The output of the system in response to an input which is two boluses will be the sum of these two signals. The output, g(t), is shown in last panel of Figure 3.2. The output is the sum of the contributions from each part of the input. The process of convolution can be summarized as **shift, scale, and add.**

Let us now return to the more complicated example shown in Figure 3.1. We can imagine that the input signal is made up of a large number of individual boluses of activity as shown in the first panel of Figure 3.3. The responses of the system to the first three boluses are shown in the second, third, and fourth panels of Figure 3.3. Each component of the input gives rise to a shifted and scaled system function. The output is the sum of a large number of shifted and scaled system functions. We can appreciate that shifting scaling and adding this large number of system functions is a complicated and time consuming task. It is even reasonably time consuming for a computer.

In this example, we are most interested in the system function, the handling of the radiopharmaceutical by the kidney. What we are able to measure is the input and output signals, the blood and kidney time activity curves. The process of deconvolution described in Part IV is a method for recovering the system function from the input and output functions.

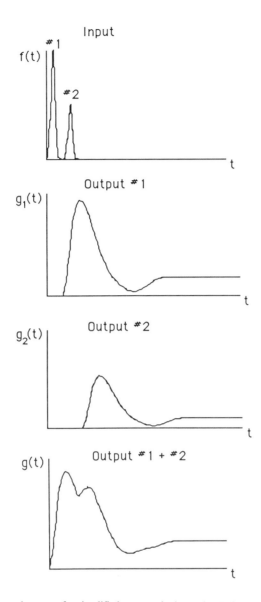

FIGURE 3.2.   Input and output of a simplified system: the input signal, f(t), consists of two boluses of activity, #1 and #2, where the second bolus is half the size of the first bolus. The outputs, $g_1(t)$ and $g_2(t)$, are due to boluses #1 and #2, respectively. The two outputs are the same except that the second output is shifted in time and is one-half the size of the first output. The total output, g(t), is the sum of the outputs due to each portion of the input (bottom panel).

II. MATHEMATICAL DESCRIPTION OF CONVOLUTION

Figure 3.4 shows the diagram which we shall use to represent a system. The input signal is represented by the function, f(t). The output signal is represented by the function, g(t). The system is represented by a box which has the system function, h(t), inside of it. Although this diagram appears overly simplified, we shall see that this representation of a system is really quite useful.

Like other functions, the input signal, the output signal, and the system functions can be continuous, discrete, or digital. Since most of us have an intuitive understanding of continuous functions, our description of convolution will use continuous signals and systems. Later we shall apply these same ideas to discrete signals and systems.

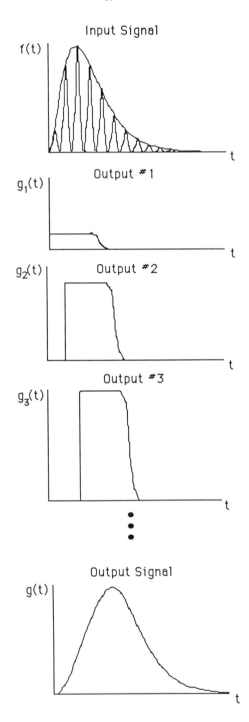

FIGURE 3.3.   Representation of an input as multiple boluses: the input signal, f(t), can be represented in terms of a large number of boluses (top panel). The outputs, $g_1(t)$, $g_2(t)$, $g_3(t)$, etc. are due to each of these boluses (middle panels). The actual output, g(t), is the sum of the individual outputs (bottom panel).

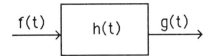

FIGURE 3.4. Diagrammatic representation of a system: a system is represented by a box with the system function, h(t), inside of it. The input to the system, f(t), is shown at the left of the box. The output from the system, g(t), is at the right of the box.

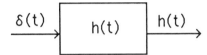

FIGURE 3.5. A system with a delta function as input: when the input function is a delta function, δ(t), then the output of the system is the system function, h(t).

The simplest input to consider is a **delta function.** Recall from Chapter 2 that a delta function is infinite at time 0 and zero at all other times, and that it has an area equal to one. The delta function is the mathematical equivalent of an idealized bolus. The output of a system in response to an input signal which is a delta function is by definition the system function, h(t). Figure 3.5 shows a delta function input producing an output equal to the system function.

An example of convolution using an input signal composed of two delta functions is shown in Figure 3.6. The input signal, f(t), consists of two delta functions where the first delta function has been scaled by one-half. Mathematically,

$$f(t) = \frac{1}{2} \cdot \delta(t) + \delta(t - \tau) \tag{3.1}$$

where τ is the time at which the second delta function occurs. The output of the system will be two system functions. The first system function is scaled by one-half, and the second system function is shifted by τ units. The two portions of the output are shown in the second and third panels of Figure 3.6. The sum of the two output functions is shown in the fourth panel of Figure 3.6. Mathematically,

$$g(t) = \frac{1}{2} \cdot h(t) + h(t - \tau) \tag{3.2}$$

A. BASIS FUNCTIONS

In Figure 3.3, the signal, f(t) was divided into a large number of boluses. Imagine that f(t) is divided into more and more, narrower and narrower boluses. In the limit, f(t), can be represented as the sum of an infinite number of shifted and scaled delta functions. The value of the signal gives the scaling factor at each offset. Figure 3.7 shows a signal which is made up from several delta functions. Mathematically this can be written:

$$f(t) = \int_{-\infty}^{+\infty} f(\tau) \cdot \delta(t - \tau) \, d\tau \tag{3.3}$$

f(t) is the sum of an infinite number of delta functions, one delta function for each position, τ. The scaling factor for the delta function is the value of the function, f(·), at

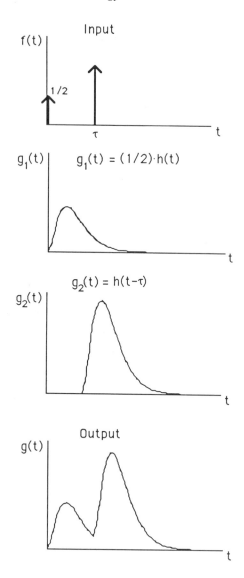

FIGURE 3.6. Output from two delta functions as input: the input signal, f(t), consists of two delta functions (top panel). The first delta function is one-half the size of the second delta function. The first delta function occurs at time, 0, and the second delta function occurs at time, τ. The output due to the first delta function is $^1/_2 \cdot$ h(t) (second panel). The output due to the second delta function is h(t − τ) (third panel). The output, g(t), is the sum of the two middle panels (bottom panel).

position τ, f(τ). f(τ) is the same signal as f(t) except for the change of the independent variable; however, conceptually it is quite different. Within the integral, f(τ) represents a number, a scaling factor. The various δ(t − τ) are functions, functions with only one nonzero value, but functions, none the less. The factors, f(τ), scale the functions, δ(t − τ). The sum of all of these scaled delta functions is the signal, f(t).

It may seem that we have derived an incredibly complicated method for describing an initially simple concept, a function. However, this description of the input signal will help us in understanding the action of a system on a signal. Furthermore, this technique for describing a signal in terms of a set of functions is a very basic technique which will be used throughout the book. A set of functions used to describe a signal are called **basis functions.** The basis functions are chosen so that they make it easy to understand some

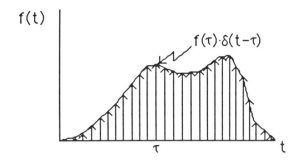

FIGURE 3.7. Representation of a signal with delta functions: the signal, f(t), can be represented by an infinite set of delta functions. A few of these delta functions are shown in this figure. The delta function at time τ is scaled by $f(\tau)$.

process. In this case, the basis functions are shifted delta functions, which make it easy to understand how a system effects an input signal.

B. CONVOLUTION INTEGRAL

With this representation of f(t) it will be easy to determine the output of a system. We can consider each portion of the input separately. The input signal at time τ is $f(\tau) \cdot \delta(t - \tau)$. Mathematically, $f(\tau)$ represents a single value, the value of $f(\cdot)$ at time τ, and $\delta(t - \tau)$ represents a function with one nonzero value. The output of the system to this input will be a shifted and scaled version of $h(\cdot)$, $f(\tau) \cdot h(t - \tau)$. The response of the system to f(t) will be the sum of the responses to the input at each time.

$$g(t) = \int_{-\infty}^{+\infty} f(\tau) \cdot h(t - \tau) \, d\tau \tag{3.4}$$

This integral is called the **convolution integral**. It gives us a formula for calculating the output of a system to any input so long as we know the system function (the output of a system to a delta function). The ability to calculate the output for any input is really quite remarkable, and it is the reason that the system function is so valuable. It is the reason that we have given the output in response to a delta function a special name, the system function, and have used it to represent the system.

Equation 3.4 is the mathematical representation of the process shown in Figure 3.3. The input signal is divided into an infinite number of shifted and scaled delta functions. The output is the sum of the response of the system to each of these inputs. It is the sum of an infinite number of shifted and scaled system functions.

C. EQUIVALENCE OF THE INPUT SIGNAL AND THE SYSTEM FUNCTION

Although the input signal and the system function represent very different concepts, it turns out that they have equivalent roles mathematically. We can show this quite simply by substitution of the variable of integration. The reader may wish to skip the following section on the first reading.

We shall substitute a new variable, τ', in the convolution integral (Equation 3.4) where,

$$\tau' = t - \tau \tag{3.5}$$

Therefore,

$$\tau = t - \tau' \tag{3.6}$$

and

$$d\tau = dt - d\tau' \tag{3.7}$$

Although t is a variable outside the integral, t is fixed within the convolution integral. Therefore, dt is equal to zero in the integral and

$$d\tau = 0 - d\tau' = -d\tau' \tag{3.8}$$

Substituting τ' for τ in the convolution integral gives:

$$g(t) = -\int_{+\infty}^{-\infty} f(t - \tau') \cdot h(\tau') \, d\tau' \tag{3.9}$$

Notice that the limits of integration are from plus infinity to minus infinity since τ and τ' are of opposite signs. Switching the limits of integration changes the sign of an integral (see Equation 2.19):

$$g(t) = \int_{-\infty}^{+\infty} f(t - \tau') \cdot h(\tau') \, d\tau' \tag{3.10}$$

Equation 3.10 is identical to the convolution integral (Equation 3.4) except that the roles of the system function and the input signal have been exchanged. Therefore, the system function and the input signal are equivalent. Because of the symmetrical roles of the input signal and the system function, convolution can be written as a binary operation. The asterisk symbol, *, is used to indicate convolution of two functions.

$$g(t) = f(t) * h(t) \tag{3.11}$$

With some fancy mathematical foot work we have shown that the input signal and the system function are equivalent. Exactly what this relation means may not be obvious at this point. Later we shall find that this relation is important for understanding what information about a system can be obtained from various types of input signals. It will also mean that two common problems — deconvolution and deblurring — are equivalent.

Although the * notation allows the convolution operation to be written quite simply, it is important to remember that this operation is really very complex. Other operations on functions which we have encountered are much simpler in the sense that the output at any time is dependent only on the input at that time. By contrast, the output of a convolution may depend upon all of the values of both the input signal and the system function. This complex nature of the convolution operation is apparent from the convolution integral, but not from the short-hand notation. Thus, we must remember that just by using this short hand notation, we have not mastered the complexity of convolution.

D. TWO-DIMENSIONAL CONVOLUTION

Most of the applications of interest to a radiologist involve two-dimensional convolution of images. All of the chapters in Part IV except for the first chapter will deal with two-dimensional convolution. Most image processing problems use or can be described using two-dimensional convolution. Two-dimensional convolution is very similar to one-dimensional convolution, so that to a large extent we can just extend what we have learned from one dimension to two dimensions.

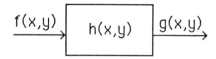

FIGURE 3.8. Diagrammatic representation of a two-dimensional system: a two-dimensional system is represented in the same fashion as a one-dimensional system except that the input signal, f(x,y), the output signal, g(x,y), and the system function, h(x,y) are all two-dimensional functions.

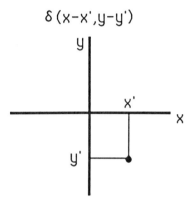

FIGURE 3.9. Two dimensional delta function: a two-dimensional delta function, $\delta(x - x', y - y')$, has a single nonzero value at position x',y'.

Convolution in two dimensions can be written symbolically by substituting two-dimensional signals for one-dimensional signals:

$$g(x,y) = f(x,y) * h(x,y) \tag{3.12}$$

Figure 3.8 shows a two-dimensional system using the same block diagram that was used for one-dimensional systems except that the input and output signals and the system function are two-dimensional. It is easy to substitute two-dimensional signals for one-dimensional signals, but obtaining an intuitive meaning of what this equation and this diagram means is more difficult.

By analogy to the one-dimensional case, we can imagine that the input image is composed of an infinite number of delta functions — one delta function for each point, x',y', in the input. The two-dimensional delta function is written:

$$\delta(x - x', y - y') \tag{3.13}$$

This delta function has only one nonzero point at x',y' (Figure 3.9).

The input at each point will give rise to a scaled and shifted system function in the output. The system function will be scaled by the value of the input, f(x',y'), and shifted by an amount x',y':

$$f(x',y') \cdot h(x - x', y - y') \tag{3.14}$$

The outputs due to each point in the input must be added together to give the total output:

$$g(x,y) = \int_{-\infty}^{+\infty} \int_{-\infty}^{+\infty} f(x',y') \cdot h(x - x', y - y') \, dx'dy' \tag{3.15}$$

The integration is a two-dimensional integration — over both the x' and y' directions.

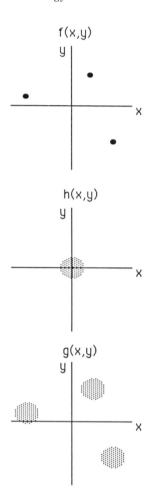

FIGURE 3.10.   Two dimensional convolution: f(x,y) is a simple input signal, which consists of three points (top panel). The system function, h(x,y), is a circle (middle panel). The output signal, g(x,y), consists of three circles (bottom panel).

The basic idea of convolution is the same in one, two, or any number of dimensions. For each point in the input there will be a scaled, shifted version of the system function in the output. All of these scaled and shifted system functions must then be added together. Convolution always involves shifting, scaling, and adding.

Figure 3.10 shows an example of two-dimensional convolution. The input signal, f(x,y), is very simple. It consists of an image with just three nonzero points. The system function, h(x,y), is a circle located at the origin. The output consists of three circles — one circle centered at each point in the input. For each point in the input, there is a scaled shifted system function in the output. In this simple example each point in the input was equal to one, so that all of the output circles have the same value. In a more realistic example, the intensities of the input and output signals and the system function would be different for different points in the images.

III. EXAMPLES OF CONVOLUTION

A. LUNG TIME ACTIVITY CURVE

As an example of convolution, consider the transit of radioactivity through the lungs after intravenous injection of a radiopharmaceutical. We can measure the time activity curve in a region of interest corresponding to the lungs with a gamma camera positioned over the chest. The system function is the time activity curve which would be obtained if a bolus of activity is injected into the superior vena cava. The input signal is the actual time activity curve in the superior vena cava after an intravenous injection. The output signal is the time activity curve over the lungs after an intravenous injection.

We can easily measure the input signal by placing a region of interest over the superior vena cava. We can measure the output signal from a region of interest over the lungs. The system function can be measured if the bolus of activity reaches the superior vena cava intact. However, after an antecubital injection, the bolus may be split between the cephalic and basilic veins. The input signal at the superior vena cava may look like that shown in Figure 3.2. We are interested in estimating the system function, but the output signal is not a good representation of the system function in this case. In Chapter 28, we shall describe a method (deconvolution) for obtaining a system function given the input and output signals.

This example is instructive in that the system which we have defined is not what one intuitively thinks of as a system. Instead, there are two signals where one signal, the output, depends upon the other signal, the input. The dependence between these two signals is defined to be the system. We could just as easily have taken the time activity curve in the aorta as the output signal and define a system which included the other system as a subsystem. However, with this method we are not concerned with the internal details of the system, only with the response of the system to a bolus input. One of the powerful aspects of using convolution to describe systems is that we do not need to know about the internal workings of the system in order to understand how it will affect an input signal.

B. X-RAY CASSETTE

As an example of two-dimensional convolution consider the production of an image using an X-ray cassette. When X-rays strike the screen in a cassette the screen produces a flash of light. Each X-ray photon gives rise to a number of light photons, and the light photons expose the film. The flash of light from each X-ray exposes the film in a small circle surrounding the location of the incoming X-ray. The resolution of the resulting image is affected by the size of this circle.

In terms of convolution, we can consider the two-dimensional distribution of X-rays as the input signal. The intensity of the X-rays contains a latent image. The image recorded on the film is the output signal. The spot of light produced when an X-ray strikes a cassette is the system function. For each point in the input signal, a spot of light proportional to the intensity of the X-rays at that point is produced (similar to Figure 3.10). The system function is shifted to the position of the input point and scaled by the value of the input. The output image is the sum of a spot of light for each input position. Again notice that the convolution operation involves shifting, scaling, and adding the system function.

The result of the cassette is to blur the latent image in the X-ray. We can improve the quality of the image by deconvolution or deblurring the output signal for the system function. This application is different from the previous application in that the goal is to obtain the input signal instead of the system function. However, since we know that the system function and the input signal are mathematically identical, we can predict that the deconvolution and the deblurring methods will be the same for both applications.

C. AUDIO AMPLIFIER

An audio amplifier is not a system which has direct application in radiology. However, we shall use our intuition about audio amplifiers to provide us with important insights in Part II. The input signal to an audio amplifier is a voltage from a device such as a compact disc. The output signal is the current which is sent to the speakers. The system function of the amplifier is the output when a brief voltage is applied to the input. The input voltage at each point in time will result in a output which is a scaled system function shifted to the time of the input. Just like the other systems which we have described, the output signal is the sum of all of these shifted scaled system functions.

We usually do not think of an amplifier in terms of its effect on an input voltage. Rather, we think of an amplifier in terms of its effect on the musical tones which are sent to it. The second part of the book will deal extensively with a frequency description of signals and systems. Our ears present our mind with frequency data, tones. Thus, we naturally think of audio signals in terms of frequencies. By contrast, our eyes present our mind with spatial data. Spatial frequencies seem quite foreign to us. When describing images in terms of frequencies, we shall find it useful to be able to appeal to the natural intuition about frequencies provided by hearing.

D. RADIOACTIVE DECAY

Radioactive decay is not a system which is usually described by convolution. Many of the properties of radioactive decay are best understood in terms of differential equations (see Chapter 7). However, one feature of radioactive decay which is difficult to understand using differential equations is why the daughter activity is greater than the parent activity in transient equilibrium. We shall see that this is an intuitive result when thinking about decay in terms of convolution.

In transient equilibrium, a parent isotope, A, decays to a daughter isotope, B, which in turn decays to isotope C.

$$A \rightarrow B \rightarrow C \tag{3.16}$$

We can define a system where the input signal, $f(t)$, represents the radioactivity of the parent, A, and the output signal, $g(t)$, represents the radioactivity of the daughter, B. The input signal, the radioactivity of A, produces isotope B which can then decay. The system function is the decay curve of B.

In order to gain an understanding of the relationship of the output signal to the input signal, we shall need to consider the convolution integral from a slightly different perspective. The convolution integral, Equation 3.4, is given by:

$$g(t) = \int_{-\infty}^{+\infty} f(\tau) \cdot h(t - \tau) \, d\tau \tag{3.17}$$

In the integral, $h(\cdot)$ is a function of τ, and t is a fixed parameter. $h(t - \tau)$ is a time reversed version of $h(\tau)$ which has been shifted by an amount t. Figure 3.11 shows the exponential, $h(\tau)$, and the time reversed, shifted function $h(t - \tau)$.

Figure 3.12 shows $f(\tau)$ and $h(t - \tau)$ for one value of t. The output value, $g(t)$, at this value of t is just the sum of the product of these two functions. The output is the average of the input values weighted for the time reversed function $h(t - \tau)$. The output at any other time can be obtained in the same manner by shifting $h(t - \tau)$ to another time, t.

The output at any time, t, is due not only to the input at time, t, but also to the previous inputs. The system introduces a delay between the production of isotope B and its decay. The daughter activity is a weighted average of the previous activity of A. In the case of transient equilibrium, the previous activities of the parent, A, are greater than the parent activity at time, t. Thus, the activity of the daughter, B, will be greater than that of the parent. The relationship between the daughter and parent activity is often obscure using the differential equation approach, but is easily understood using the convolution model.

Figure 3.12 is important since it shows another way of understanding convolution. Some

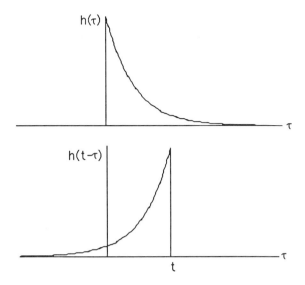

FIGURE 3.11. Shifted and time reversed function: h(τ) is an exponentially decaying signal (top panel). h(t − τ) is shifted by an amount, t, and time reversed (bottom panel).

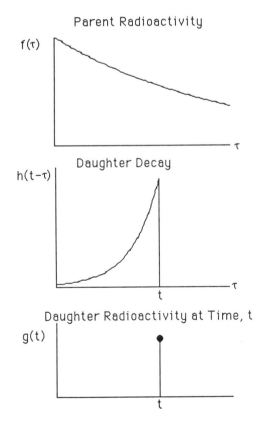

FIGURE 3.12. Radioactive decay. f(τ) is the radioactivity of a parent isotope (top panel). h(t − τ) is the shifted and time reversed system function which represents the decay of the daughter isotope. The output signal, g(t), is the radioactivity of the daughter, which is the convolution of the input from the parent with the decay of the daughter. The activity at time, t, is the integral of the product of parent activity and the daughter decay (bottom panel).

texts present convolution from this perspective. We have emphasized convolution in terms of shift, scale, and add, since this viewpoint is most natural to the radiologic applications for which we shall use convolution. Convolution is a difficult concept to grasp, and the best understanding of convolution comes from being able to view it from several perspectives.

IV. SUMMARY

Convolution is a complicated mathematical operation for combining two signals. The major use of convolution in this book will be to model one- and two-dimensional systems. In this chapter we have described a system by its output in response to a delta function input. This output is called the system function. The convolution integral (Equation 3.5) represents the output of a system in terms of a sum of shifted and scaled system functions where the scaling factors are given by the input. Convolution can be summarized as shift, scale, and add.

We have already indicated two uses of the convolution model. First, deconvolution will allow us to calculate the system function from the input and output signals or equivalently to calculate the input signal from the output signal and system function. Second, in the case of radioactive decay the description in terms of convolution provided insight into understanding a property of the system.

In this chapter we have boldly assumed that the output of a system can be derived from the sum of shifted and scaled inputs. In the next chapter, we shall determine what mathematical properties a system must follow in order for this approach to be valid.

V. FURTHER READING

The description of systems in terms of convolution is called linear systems analysis. There are several good books which deal with linear systems analysis. The topics covered in this chapter are also covered in Chapter 3 of the book by Oppenheim et al.[1] and Chapter 3 of the book by Bracewell.[2] Other references which describe convolution include Chapter 2 of the book by Gabel and Roberts,[3] Chapter 4 of the book by Liu and Liu,[4] and Chapter 4 of the book by Cooper and McGillem.[5] Two-dimensional convolution is described in Section 1.2.4 of the book by Dudgeon and Mersereau.[6]

REFERENCES

1. **Oppenheim, A. V., Willsky, A. S., and Young, I. T.,** *Signals and Systems,* Prentice Hall, Englewood Cliffs, NJ, 1983.
2. **Bracewell, R. N.,** *The Fourier Transform and Its Applications,* McGraw-Hill, New York, 1978.
3. **Gabel, R. A. and Roberts, R. A.,** *Signals and Linear Systems,* John Wiley & Sons, New York, 1973.
4. **Liu, C. L. and Liu, J. W. S.,** *Linear Systems Analysis,* McGraw-Hill, New York, 1975.
5. **Cooper, G. R. and McGillem, C. D.,** *Methods of Signal and System Analysis,* Holt, Rinehart & Winston, New York, 1967.
6. **Dudgeon, D. E. and Mersereau, R. M.,** *Multidimensional Digital Signal Processing,* Prentice-Hall, Englewood Cliffs, NJ, 1984.

Chapter 4

SYSTEMS

In the last chapter we used the concept of a system without exactly defining a system. The systems in the last chapter could all be described by convolution. However, not all systems can be defined by convolution. Therefore, we need to develop a more general description of systems.

The concept of a system in the first part of this chapter may appear at first to be different from the concept of a system as we used it in the last chapter, but toward the end of this chapter 'he similarity will become apparent. We shall learn that systems which are linear and time invariant can be described by convolution. Understanding the properties which distinguish different types of systems will enable us to better understand which types of systems are of interest in radiology.

I. MATHEMATICAL DESCRIPTION OF A SYSTEM

In its most general form, a system takes an input signal and transforms it into an output signal. Figure 4.1 shows an input signal, $f(t)$, going through a system, H, to produce an output signal, $g(t)$. Mathematically,

$$g(t) = H\{f(t)\} \tag{4.1}$$

The system, $H\{\cdot\}$, operates on the input signal in some as yet undefined fashion to produce the output. The braces are used to indicate that $H\{\cdot\}$ is a system. This notation is different from the function notation:

$$g(t) = h(f(t)) \tag{4.2}$$

which means that $g(t)$ is equal to a function $h(\cdot)$ of the input signal.

The mathematical notation $H\{\cdot\}$ and $h(\cdot)$ are very similar; however, we shall use these two notations to mean quite different operations. A function, such as $h(\cdot)$, operates on a single value of the input to produce an output value. A system, $H\{\cdot\}$, may operate on any or all of the input values to produce a single output value. In mathematical texts a system is sometimes called a **functional.** A system or functional is much more complicated than a function.

II. EXAMPLES OF SYSTEMS

Some systems are very simple, for example:

$$H\{f(t)\} = f(t) \tag{4.3}$$

This system produces as its output exactly the same signal as its input. It is an identity system. Another simple system is:

$$H\{f(t)\} = f(t - t_0) \tag{4.4}$$

This system delays the output signal by an amount t_0. Figure 4.2 shows this simple system. For both these simple systems, the output can be calculated from a single point in the input.

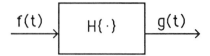

FIGURE 4.1.   Diagram of a system: this figure shows the diagram of a generalized system, H{·}. The system transforms an input signal, f(t), into an output signal, g(t).

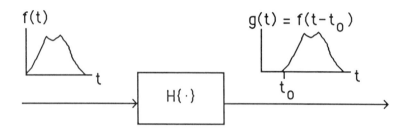

FIGURE 4.2.   Example of a system: the system, H{·}, delays the input signal, f(t), by an amount, t_0. The output signal, g(t), is equal to f(t − t_0).

A slightly more complicated system is:

$$H\{f(t)\} = a \cdot f(t - 8.2) + b \cdot \sin(f(t)) + 6 \tag{4.5}$$

In this example each point in the output depends on two input values.

In the last chapter we described systems which could be defined by convolution (see Equation 3.4):

$$H\{f(t)\} = \int_{-\infty}^{+\infty} f(\tau) \cdot h(t - \tau) \, d\tau \tag{4.6}$$

In this more complex case each output point may depend upon any of the points in the input. Similarly, a large number examples of systems involving different combinations of input values could be defined.

III. PROPERTIES OF SYSTEMS

It is useful to categorize systems in terms of mathematical properties which they follow, since the models which can be used to describe a system depend upon which properties they exhibit. The convolution model, described in the last chapter, assumes that systems be linear and time invariant. The differential equations model, described in Chapter 7, and the linear algebra model, described in Chapter 9, assume that systems are linear.

A. LINEARITY
One of the most important properties that a system can have is linearity. Linearity actually is defined in terms of two other properties — scaling and additivity. The **scaling** property can be defined as follows:

$$H\{a \cdot f(t)\} = a \cdot f(t) \tag{4.7}$$

The scaling property states that if the input signal is made larger or smaller, then the output becomes larger or smaller by the same factor.

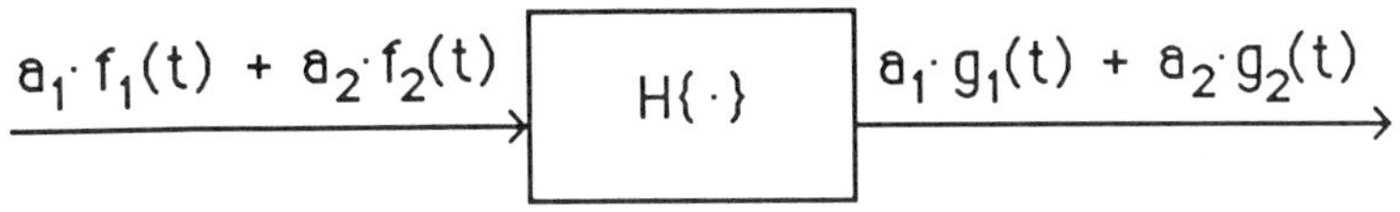

$$a_1 \cdot f_1(t) + a_2 \cdot f_2(t) \longrightarrow \boxed{H\{\cdot\}} \longrightarrow a_1 \cdot g_1(t) + a_2 \cdot g_2(t)$$

FIGURE 4.3. Linearity: the output of a system, $H\{\cdot\}$, to inputs $f_1(t)$ and $f_2(t)$ is defined to be $g_1(t)$ and $g_2(t)$, respectively. If the system is linear, then the output to a linear combination of the inputs is the same linear combination of the outputs.

In order to better understand the scaling property, let us examine a system which does not have this property. The output of the following system is the square of its input:

$$H\{f(t)\} = (f(t))^2 \qquad (4.8)$$

When the input to the system is scaled by a factor, a, the output is scaled by a factor a^2:

$$H\{a \cdot f(t)\} = a^2 \cdot f^2(t) \qquad (4.9)$$

Any system which involve powers or roots of the input will not obey the scaling property.

The second property which is a part of linearity is the **summing** property. The summing property can be expressed mathematically as:

$$H\{f_1(t) + f_2(t)\} = H\{f_1(t)\} + H\{f_2(t)\} \qquad (4.10)$$

This property means that the response of a system to the sum of two signals is the sum of the response to each signal. The output of the system in response to a signal is independent of other signals which may be going through it at the same time.

An example of a system which does not have the summing property is:

$$H\{f(t)\} = f(t) + 5 \qquad (4.11)$$

The result of applying this system to the sum of two signals is not equal to the sum of the responses to each signal separately:

$$H\{f_1(t) + f_2(t)\} = f_1(t) + f_2(t) + 5 \neq H\{f_1(t)\} + H\{f_2(t)\}$$

$$= f_1(t) + f_2(t) + 10 \qquad (4.12)$$

The **linearity** property (the scaling property plus the summing property) can be expressed mathematically as:

$$H\{a_1 \cdot f_1(t) + a_2 \cdot f_2(t)\} = a_1 \cdot H\{f_1(t)\} + a_2 \cdot H\{f_2(t)\} \qquad (4.13)$$

This property is shown diagrammatically in Figure 4.3. Linear systems are much simpler than nonlinear systems since the output of a system due to any portion of the input can be determined from a knowledge of how that portion goes through the system without regard to the rest of the system. We can divide the input signal into a set of signals and derive the output of the system from consideration of each portion separately.

Almost all real systems are nonlinear. For a very large input, real systems burn up or break down. However, many real systems have a region over which they are linear. For example, an audio amplifier is usually linear over the normal range of inputs. If the input becomes too large, the amplifier will introduce distortions in the sound. If the input is large enough, the amplifier will burn out. Modeling an audio amplifier as a linear system is still useful as long as we remember that the real amplifier will behave like the model only for a range of possible inputs.

B. LINEARIZABLE SYSTEMS

There are many systems which are not linear, but which can be made linear using some mathematical transformation. For example, consider the attenuation of X-rays as a function of the thickness of a tissue. We can define a system where the input signal is the thickness of a tissue as a function of position, $f(x)$. The output signal is the X-ray intensity as a function of position, $g(x)$. The system can be written mathematically as:

$$H\{f(t)\} = I_0 \cdot e^{-\mu f(x)} \tag{4.14}$$

where μ is the linear attenuation coefficient and I_0 is the intensity of the beam before it enters the tissue.

This system is not linear. However the system can be made linear by using the logarithm of the intensity instead of the intensity itself. We can define a new system as:

$$H'\{f(x)\} = -\ln(H\{f(x)\})/I_0 = \mu \cdot f(x) \tag{4.15}$$

This new system is a very simple linear system where the output is directly proportional to the thickness of the tissue.

In computed tomography, this linearization operation is performed on the raw projection data as the first step in data processing. The logarithm of the intensity makes the projection data proportional to the sum of the linear attenuation coefficients. However, in a real case like computed tomography, the problem is never quite this simple. It turns out that beam hardening adds another small nonlinearity to the problem. In early computed tomographic scanners this nonlinearity was ignored. Later, other corrections were made in order to linearize the data for this effect as well.

Another example of a nonlinear system is the response of film to light. Film exposure is proportional to the logarithm of the light intensity. Therefore, to linearize this system we can take the exponential of the exposure as the output signal. However, even this modified system will show nonlinearities for very low and very high exposures. In order for this model to be applicable, we must restrict the range of exposures to the linear portion of the film response curve.

Although almost all real systems are nonlinear, almost all mathematical models of systems are linear. The reason that linear models are used so extensively is that they are much easier to work with than nonlinear models. Using linear models to model systems which have nonlinearities is not as great a compromise as one would initially think. Many systems are linear over the range of input values which are encountered in real situations. Many other systems can be made to be roughly linear by using some sort of a transformation of their input or output.

C. TIME INVARIANCE

Another important property which a system can have is **time invariance.** Time invariance means that the system does not change over time. The input signal and the output signal are functions of time, but the operation of the system should not change as a function of time. For systems which refer to spatial dimensions, time invariance is called **shift invariance.** Except for the independent variable being used, time invariance and shift invariance are exactly the same property.

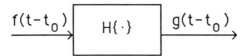

FIGURE 4.4. Time invariance: if a system, H{·}, is time invariant, then the response of the system to a shifted input, f(t − t₀), is a shifted output signal, g(t − t₀).

Time invariance can be stated mathematically as:

$$g(t - t_0) = H\{f(t - t_0)\} \tag{4.16}$$

In other words, if the input signal, f(t), is shifted in time by an amount, t_0, then the output signal is shifted by the same amount of time. Irrespective of the time which the input occurs, exactly the same output signal is obtained, except for the shift in time. This property is shown diagrammatically in Figure 4.4.

There are many types of systems which are not time invariant. For example, a system with an output equal to the input plus a delta function at time zero is not time invariant:

$$H\{f(t)\} = f(t) + \delta(t) \tag{4.17}$$

If the input is shifted in time, the delta function in the output is still at time zero. Systems which have an output which is not caused by an input are not time invariant. Furthermore, any system which is changing over time will not be time invariant. If someone is adjusting the volume on an audioamplifier, the output of the system will depend not only on the input, but also on the position of the volume knob.

Many real systems are not time or space invariant. All imaging systems are not space invariant since their field of view is of limited extent. If the input image is shifted out of the view of the imaging system, then no output image is produced. Thus, the output image depends upon the position of the input image with respect to the imaging system. However, with the field of view of an imaging system, a linear model can often be used. In fact, the major goal of this book is to explain linear methods for describing imaging systems.

IV. LINEAR, TIME INVARIANT SYSTEMS

If a system is linear and time invariant, we can describe the system by convolution. We shall now derive the convolution integral by applying the linear and time invariant properties. Understanding what each of these properties means in terms of calculating the response of a system to an input will help us to better understand what a system is.

In the last chapter we found it useful to divide up the input signal as an infinite sum of delta functions (see Equation 3.3):

$$f(t) = \int_{-\infty}^{+\infty} f(\tau) \cdot \delta(t - \tau) \, d\tau \tag{4.18}$$

The delta functions are a set of basis functions. f(τ) are a set of scale factors for the basis functions. The output of the system in response to f(t) can be written:

$$H\{f(t)\} = H\left\{ \int_{-\infty}^{+\infty} f(\tau) \cdot \delta(t - \tau) \, d\tau \right\} \tag{4.19}$$

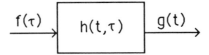

FIGURE 4.5.   Linear system function: the system function of a linear system can be given by a two-dimensional function, h(t,τ). The input signal is f(τ), and the output signal is g(t).

The summing property of linear systems, Equation 4.10, means that each portion of the input signal can be considered separately. The output will be the sum of the outputs from each portion of the input signal. Therefore the summing property means that the output of the system in response to f(t) is equal to the sum of the responses to the responses from each point in the input:

$$H\{f(t)\} = \int_{-\infty}^{+\infty} H\{f(\tau) \cdot \delta(t - \tau)\} \, d\tau \tag{4.20}$$

The scaling property of linear systems, Equation 4.7, means that the output of a system in response to f(γ) times an input is equal to f(γ) times the response to that input. Mathematically,

$$H\{f(t)\} = \int_{-\infty}^{+\infty} f(\tau) \cdot H\{\delta(t - \tau)\} \, d\tau \tag{4.21}$$

Thus, linearity allows us to calculate the response of a system to f(t) in terms of the response of the system to shifted delta functions.

If we knew the response of the system to a delta function at each time $H\{\delta(t - \tau)\}$, then we could determine the output of the system to any signal, f(t). We can define a two-dimensional function, h(t,τ), which gives the response of the system as a function of t to a delta function input at time τ.

$$h(t,\tau) = H\{\delta(t - \tau)\} \tag{4.21b}$$

We shall call this function the **linear system function**. We can rewrite Equation 4.19 as:

$$H\{f(t)\} = \int_{-\infty}^{+\infty} f(\tau) \cdot h(t,\tau) \, d\tau \tag{4.22}$$

This equation describes the response of a linear system to an input signal. We shall come back to this equation in Chapter 9 (Linear Algebra Description of Systems). The linear algebra model for systems is equivalent to this formation. The linear system function is shown diagrammatically in Figure 4.5.

Figure 4.6 shows an example of calculating the output of a system to a simple input. The input consists of three delta functions at times 1, 2, and 3. The three responses, h(t,1), h(t,2), and h(t,3), to the three portions of this input may be completely different in appearance. Thus, although Equation 4.22 looks similar to the convolution integral, the two-dimensional system function, h(t,τ), makes this system much more complex.

Now let us see what time invariance means in terms of our description of a system. The output of a linear system to a delta function at time τ is h(t,τ). If the system is time invariant, then this output must be equal to the output of the system to a delta function at time zero shifted by τ, h(t − τ, 0).

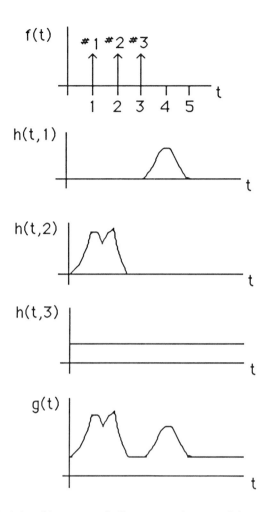

FIGURE 4.6. Calculation of the response of a linear system: the top panel shows a simple input signal, f(t), which consists of just three delta functions at times 1, 2, and 3. The middle three panels show the responses to each of the delta functions, h(t,1), h(t,2), and h(t,3). Because the system is linear, the output, g(t), can be calculated as the sum of the three responses. The output is shown in the bottom panel.

$$h(t,\tau) = h(t - \tau, 0) \qquad (4.23)$$

The left hand side of this equation is the response of the system to a delta function at time, τ. The right hand side of Equation 4.23 is the response to a delta function at time zero, shifted by τ.

Because of shift invariance we can write $h(t,\tau)$ as $h(t - \tau, 0)$ for any value of τ. Instead of the two-dimensional system function $h(t,\tau)$, we can define a one-dimensional system function, $h(t)$.

$$h(t - \tau) = h(t - \tau, 0) \qquad (4.24)$$

We shall call this one-dimensional function the **linear, time invariant system function.**

We can rewrite the response of a system to an input (Equation 4.22) as

$$g(t) = H\{f(t)\} = \int_{-\infty}^{+\infty} f(\tau) \cdot h(t - \tau) \, d\tau \qquad (4.25)$$

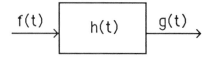

FIGURE 4.7.   Linear, time invariant system: the system function for a linear, time invariant system can be given by a one-dimensional function, h(t). The input signal is f(t), and the output signal is g(t).

This equation is the convolution integral, Equation 3.4. What we have shown is that any linear, time invariant system can be described by convolution. The linearity allowed us to consider each portion of the input separately. The time invariance allowed us to use a one-dimensional system function in place of the two-dimensional system function. A linear, time invariant system is down diagrammatically in Figure 4.7.

The approaches in the last chapter and in this chapter have been quite similar. We developed a method of describing systems using the response of the system to an impulse. The difference between the two chapters really has to do with mathematical rigor. In the last chapter we assumed that the systems were linear and time invariant without stating these properties. Very few readers would notice this omission, since the concepts of linearity and time invariance are really quite natural. In this chapter we have emphasized the assumptions which we need to make about a system in order to use convolution to describe the system.

V. SYSTEM COMPLEXITY

The most general form of a system is given by equation 4.1:

$$g(t) = H\{f(t)\} \tag{4.26}$$

All this equation says is that for each input f(t) there is some output g(t). This model really tells us nothing about the system. Knowing the output for any input or any set of inputs tells us nothing about what the output will be for a different input, even if the new input is nearly identical to one for which we know the output.

The lack of knowledge about the system represented by Equation 4.26 means that the system function for this most general form of a system is very complex. For each input f(t) there may be a different output, g(t). The number of possible inputs is enormous. There are an infinite number of points in f(t). Mathematically we could write the system function as $h(t,f(\tau))$. The second term, $f(\tau)$, actually represents an infinite number of independent variables. In other words, the system function is an infinite-dimensional function!

By restricting the system to be a linear system, we greatly reduce the complexity of the system function. In Equation 4.22, the linear system function is given by a two-dimensional function, $h(t,\tau)$. This system function gives the response of the system to delta functions at all possible times, τ. The linearity property changes the system function from an indefinite-dimensional function to a two-dimensional function. Linearity makes the description of a system tractable. This explains the great preference for systems that are linear.

By restricting the system to be both linear and time invariant, we further reduce the complexity of the system function. The system function for a linear, time invariant function is given in Equation 4.25 by a one-dimensional function, h(t). This system function gives the response of the system to a single delta function located at time zero. Addition of time invariance changes the system function from a two-dimensional function to a one-dimensional function. Description of even complicated linear, time invariant systems is reasonably easy. This explains the preference for systems that are both linear and time invariant.

When possible it is best from a computational standpoint to use a linear, time invariant model of a system. When a system is not time invariant, then it is best to use a linear model, even when some effort must be expended in order to linearize the system. In general nonlinear systems are not tractable. There are some special cases when nonlinear models can be used, but these are few and far between.

VI. SUMMARY

Description of systems is the major task in Part I of the book. This chapter has formalized the notion of a system. It began by listing the properties which could be used to characterize a system. Two properties were very important — linearity and time invariance. The linear property transforms the description of a system into a tractable problem. Description of linear systems will be the goal of Chapter 9.

Time invariance further simplifies systems. Linear, time invariant systems can be described by convolution. The system function of a linear, time invariant system is one dimensional. Linear, time invariant systems were described in the last chapter, but the linearity and the time invariance were not explicitly stated. The next chapter will deal with an important method of describing systems, eigenfunctions. We shall learn that another important property of linear, time invariant systems is that their eigenfunctions are a very special group of signals.

VII. FURTHER READING

The concepts of linearity and time invariance are discussed in almost all books on linear systems theory. The reader is referred to the references at the end of the last chapter.

Chapter 5

EIGENFUNCTIONS

In the last two chapters we have described the concept of a system. In the subsequent chapters in this part of the book we shall introduce other models of systems. In this chapter we shall try to develop an understanding of systems in terms of a special class of input signals called eigenfunctions. Eigenfunction is a partial translation of the German word, "eigenfunktion". The root, "eigen", means characteristic. We shall find that the eigenfunctions are signals which can be used to characterize the behavior of a system. The eigenfunctions of a system tell us about the system. An understanding of eigenfunctions will provide a further understanding of systems.

In this chapter, we shall show that the exponential functions are eigenfunctions of all linear, time invariant systems. In the next chapter, we shall show how to represent sinusoidal signals using exponential functions. One of the major goals of Part II is to develop a method, the Fourier transform, to characterize a system by its response to sinusoidal input signals. This characterization is an eigenfunction representation. Developing an understanding of eigenfunctions will help not only in understanding the Fourier transform method in Part II, but also in understanding image reconstruction in Part IV.

I. DEFINITION OF EIGENFUNCTIONS

An **eigenfunction** of a system is an input signal which results in an output signal which is in the same form as the input signal. For signals which are eigenfunctions of a system, the shape of the output is identical to the shape of the input signal. The system may multiply the eigenfunction by a constant; however, the output signal will otherwise be the same as the input.

Mathematically, this relation can be expressed as:

$$g(t) = H\{f(t)\} = \lambda \cdot f(t) \tag{5.1}$$

where $f(t)$ is the input, $H\{\cdot\}$ is the system, $g(t)$ is the output, and λ is a constant. The constant, λ, is called the **eigenvalue** for the eigenfunction. Generally speaking, the eigenfunctions of a system are a very limited set of signals. Of all of the possible input signals, very few will satisfy Equation 5.1.

II. EXAMPLES OF EIGENFUNCTIONS

A. AUDIO AMPLIFIER

Let us consider the response of an audio amplifier to a pure tone. Suppose that a pure middle C is the input. The output of the audio amplifier will be a pure middle C increased in intensity compared to the input. Thus, a pure tone is an eigenfunction of an audio amplifier. A pure tone can be modeled as a cosine wave. Later we shall show that sine and cosine waves are eigenfunctions of all linear, time invariant systems.

Figure 5.1 diagrammatically shows the operation of a system on an eigenfunction. The inputs signal, $f(t)$, is a sinusoid. The output signal is the same sinusoidal function decreased in amplitude. The effect of the system is to scale the input, but the system does not change its form.

The amplification or scaling factor of a system for an eigenfunction is given a special name, the eigenvalue. For each eigenfunction of a system there is an eigenvalue which gives the amount that the system amplifies the eigenfunction. The eigenvalues may be different

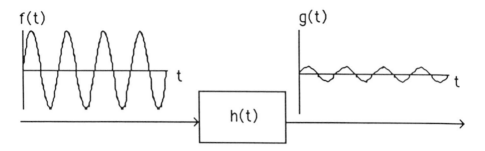

FIGURE 5.1.   Response of a system to eigenfunction: the input signal, f(t), is a sinusoid. The sinusoidal input is an eigenfunction of the linear, time invariant system, h(t). The output signal, g(t), is the same sinusoidal signal.

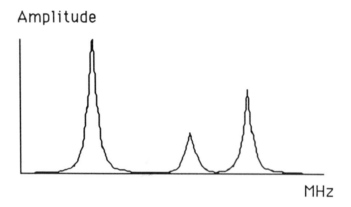

FIGURE 5.2.   Nuclear magnetic resonance spectrum: the nuclear magnetic resonance spectrum gives the response of a sample to a radio frequency input as a function of frequency.

for different eigenfunctions. In the case of an audio amplifier, low and high frequency tones are typically amplified less than the middle frequencies. The eigenvalues of these eigenfunctions will be less than the eigenvalues for the middle tones. For very high frequency tones, the eigenvalues will be zero. Very high frequencies cannot pass through the amplifier; they are stopped by the amplifier.

We hear sounds in terms of frequencies. We hear the eigenfunctions of audio amplifiers. Our eyes see in terms of the spatial positions. Later, we shall learn that the eigenfunctions of many imaging devices are spatial sinusoids. Thus, our hearing gives us a natural understanding of eigenfunctions of audio amplifiers, while our eyes do not give us a natural understanding of the eigenfunctions of imaging devices. One of the goals of Part II will be to develop an understanding of the eigenfunctions of imaging systems.

B. NUCLEAR MAGNETIC RESONANCE SPECTROSCOPY

In nuclear magnetic resonance spectroscopy, the response of a sample in an intense magnetic field to a radio frequency input is determined as a function of the frequency of the input signal. The frequency at which a nucleus in the sample responds to the input signal depends upon the chemical environment of a nucleus. The spectrum is the amplitude of the output signal as a function of the frequency of a sinusoidal input. Figure 5.2 shows a **nuclear magnetic resonance spectrum.** The abscissa is the frequency, and the ordinate is the amplitude of the response.

There are two methods of determining the spectrum — continuous wave nuclear magnetic

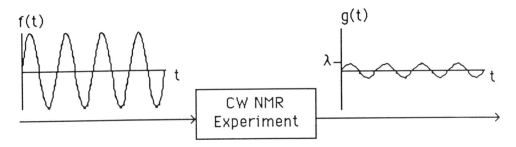

FIGURE 5.3. Continuous wave nuclear magnetic resonance: the input signal for a continuous wave (CW) magnetic resonance (NMR) experiment is a pure sinusoid, f(t). The output from the sample is a pure sinusoid of the same frequency, g(t). The scale factor, λ, is equal to the magnitude of the spectrum for this frequency.

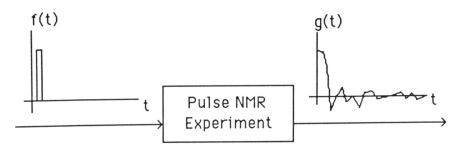

FIGURE 5.4. Pulsed nuclear magnetic resonance: the input signal for a pulsed nuclear magnetic resonance (NMR) experiment is a brief pulse, f(t). The output is the free induction decay, g(t). Notice that the input and output signals are very different.

resonance and plused nuclear magnetic resonance. For continuous wave nuclear magnetic resonance, the input signal is a sinusoid of a specific frequency. The output is also a sinusoid of the same frequency. Therefore, sinusoidally varying signals are eigenfunctions of nuclear magnetic resonance spectroscopy; sinusoids are the characteristic signals for the nuclear magnetic resonance experiment.

Figure 5.3 shows a continuous wave nuclear magnetic resonance experiment. The input signal, f(t), is a pure sinusoid. The output, g(t), is that same sinusoid scaled by a factor λ, the eigenvalue for the eigenfunction, f(t). The spectrum is equal to the eigenvalues for the eigenfunction of different frequencies. The continuous wave nuclear magnetic resonance experiment is similar to a pure tone input to an amplifier.

In order to measure the spectrum, the frequency of the input is varied slowly, and the amplitude of the output is determined as a function of frequency. The spectrum, as shown in Figure 5.2, is a graph of the eigenvalues of the system for eigenfunctions of different frequencies. The nuclear magnetic resonance system is characterized by the eigenvalues for a special set of input signals, the eigenfunctions.

Pulsed nuclear magnetic resonance spectroscopy uses a brief pulse of radio frequency as the input signal (Figure 5.4). The brief pulse is composed of equal amounts of all of the frequencies in the spectrum. The output signal, called the **free induction decay,** is very complicated. A typical free induction decay is shown in Figure 5.4. Unlike the continuous wave example, the input and output signals are of entirely different forms. A pulse is not an eigenfunction of the nuclear magnetic resonance system; it is not a characteristic signal for this system.

In the form shown in Figure 5.4, the free induction decay is not useful for characterization of the nuclear magnetic resonance system. It is difficult to obtain any information about the system by looking at the free induction decay. However, later we shall learn that the Fourier transform of the free induction decay is equal to the spectrum. In order to characterize the system, the free induction decay is transformed into a representation in terms of the eigen-functions of the system.

The purpose of the nuclear magnetic resonance experiment is to obtain an eigenfunction description of the system, since this description allows us to characterize and understand the nuclear magnetic resonance system. Although the continuous wave experiment allows us to collect data directly in terms of the eigenfunctions of the system, it turns out that the pulsed experiment is much more efficient for collection of data since each pulse provides measurement of all of the eigenfunctions simultaneously. Thus, most nuclear magnetic resonance spectroscopy is performed using the pulse technique followed by a Fourier trans-formation of the output signal.

C. EIGENVECTORS

In Chapter 9 we shall use vectors to represent signals and matrices to represent systems. We shall find that for each matrix there is a set of vectors, called eigenvectors, which are analogous to eigenfunctions. The eigenvectors will be useful for characterizing the matrices.

One of the major advantages of the vector, matrix description is that it provides geometric interpretations of various properties of systems. In Chapter 9 we shall learn that the eigen-vectors define the directions along which a system operates. The description of the operation of the matrix is often very simple if it is in terms of these special directions. Because of the analogy between vectors and signals, we shall say that the eigenfunctions of a system are signals along which the system operates. The system operates in the "direction" of these signals. But more of this later.

III. EIGENFUNCTIONS AS BASIS FUNCTIONS

One of the major advantages of linear systems is that the effect of a linear system on each portion of an input can be considered separately (see Chapter 4, Systems). It is often possible to represent an input signal as combinations of the eigenfunctions of a system. The response of a linear system to a linear combination of eigenfunctions can be calculated in terms of the response to each eigenfunction separately. Since the response to each portion of the input is easily calculated, the response to the entire input may be easily calculated.

For example, let us consider a linear system which has two eigenfunctions, $f_1(t)$ and $f_2(t)$. We can produce a set of functions which are linear combinations of these two eigen-functions:

$$f(t) = a_1 \cdot f_1(t) + a_2 \cdot f_2(t) \qquad (5.2)$$

Since the system is linear we know that the output will be:

$$g(t) = H\{f(t)\} = a_1 \cdot H\{f_1(t)\} + a_2 \cdot H\{f_2(t)\} \qquad (5.3)$$

Let us suppose that the eigenvalues corresponding to these two eigenfunctions are λ_1 and λ_2, respectively. The output of the system in response to each of these eigenfunctions will be the corresponding eigenvalue times the eigenfunction. Thus, the output will be:

$$g(t) = a_1 \cdot \lambda_1 \cdot f_1(t) + a_2 \cdot \lambda_2 \cdot f_2(t) \qquad (5.4)$$

Figure 5.5 shows an example of a signal which is the combination of two eigenfunctions. The eigenvalue for the first eigenfunction is one — this signal passes through the system unchanged. The eigenvalue for the second eigenfunction is zero — this signal does not pass

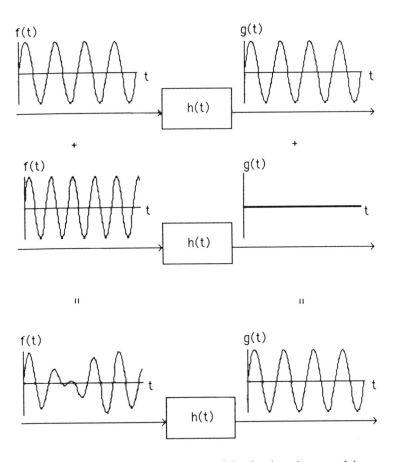

FIGURE 5.5. Response of a system to a sum of eigenfunctions: the top panel shows the response of a system, h(t), to an eigenfunction. The eigenvalue for this eigenfunction is one. The output is equal to the input. The second panel shows the response of the same system to another eigenfunction. The eigenvalue for this eigenfunction is zero. The system stops this eigenfunction. The bottom panel shows the response of the system to a signal which is the sum of these two eigenfunctions. The output is the sum of the outputs in the top two panels.

through the system. Since the system is linear, we can consider the effect of the system on each component of the signal separately. The output is equal to the first eigenfunction.

This example shows another feature of eigenfunction representation. The operation of the system on the whole signal is complicated and not easily understood. When the signal is expressed in terms of its eigenfunctions, the operation of the system is easily described — it passes one component and stops the other component. We shall find that the eigenfunctions make it easy to describe the operation of the system.

Calculating the output of a linear system to an input which is a combination of eigenfunctions is exceptionally simple. The calculation only involves scaling the eigenfunctions by their eigenvalues. Thus, for input signals which can be expressed as a combination of eigenfunctions, calculation of the output of a linear system is much simpler than calculating the output in general.

For linear, time invariant systems we now have two methods for calculating the output to a signal. The first method is convolution, a relatively complicated and difficult method. If the input can be expressed as a combination of eigenfunctions, then we have a much easier method — multiplication of the components by their eigenvalues. The complicated method, convolution, can be replaced by a simple method, multiplication. This idea of mapping a complicated problem into a simple method will be the theme of Part II (Transformations).

The value of this second method of calculating the output will depend upon whether linear combinations of eigenfunctions can be used to represent an interesting set of input signals, and if it is easy to transform an input signal into a representation in terms of the eigenfunctions of a system. It turns out that the eigenfunctions of linear, time invariant systems can be used to represent all naturally occurring signals. Part II of the book deals with methods for transforming signals into combinations of the eigenfunctions of linear, time invariant systems. These transformations are easier to calculate than convolution. Thus, the use of eigenfunctions for linear, time invariant systems is both practical and efficient.

IV. THE EIGENFUNCTIONS OF LINEAR, TIME INVARIANT SYSTEMS

The eigenfunctions of linear, time invariant systems are the exponential functions. In order to prove this fact we need to show that an exponential input signal will result in an output which is the same exponential except possibly for a change in scale. In the following derivation we shall show that all exponential functions are an eigenfunction of any linear, time invariant system. The reader may skip the following section without loss of continuity.

The output from a system with an exponential input can be written:

$$g(t) = H\{f(t)\} = H\{e^{st}\} \tag{5.5}$$

We can then determine some of the properties of $g(t)$ without actually knowing anything about the system, $H\{\cdot\}$, except for the fact that it is a linear and time invariant. Let us shift the input and then take advantage of the shift invariant property:

$$g(t + \tau) = H\{f(t + \tau)\} = H\{e^{s(t+\tau)}\} = H\{e^{st} \cdot e^{s\tau}\} \tag{5.6}$$

In this equation, we have shifted the input and output by an amount of time, τ. In the last equality we have used a property of exponents (see Table 2.3) to rewrite the input in terms of a product of exponentials.

The first exponential, e^{st}, is just $f(t)$; therefore, we can write:

$$g(t + \tau) = H\{f(t) \cdot e^{s\tau}\} \tag{5.7}$$

In this example, τ is a single number, the amount of shift, not a variable. Therefore, $e^{s\tau}$, is a constant. Since $e^{s\tau}$ is a constant, we can take advantage of the linearity property of $H\{\cdot\}$ to write:

$$g(t + \tau) = e^{s\tau} \cdot H\{f(t)\} \tag{5.8}$$

We can further simplify the relation using Equation 5.5:

$$g(t + \tau) = e^{s\tau} \cdot g(t) \tag{5.9}$$

Now we can do a trick which is reasonably common in these types of derivations. We can consider $g(\cdot)$ as a function of the constant, τ. If we consider the point in time where t is equal to zero we can rewrite Equation 5.9 as:

$$g(\tau) = g(0) \cdot e^{s\tau} \tag{5.10}$$

Furthermore, we recognize that $e^{s\tau}$ is equal to the input function with independent variable, τ:

$$g(\tau) = g(0) \cdot f(\tau) \tag{5.11}$$

In other words the output signal is equal to a scale factor, $g(0)$, times the input signal.

What we have shown in Equation 5.11 is that exponential input signals are eigenfunctions of all linear, time invariant systems. The eigenvalues for these eigenfunctions are equal to the output at time zero.

One value of finding the eigenfunctions of a system is that input signals defined in terms of the eigenfunctions provide a simple method of finding the output (see Equation 5.4). It may at first seem that exponentials are not a very useful set of functions. However, in the next chapter, we shall learn that sine and cosine functions can be written in terms of imaginary exponentials. The derivation above is completely valid for an imaginary value of the constant, s. In Chapter 15 (Fourier Transforms) we shall learn that all reasonably well behaved signals can be represented in terms of these imaginary exponentials.

The value of linear, time invariant system models may now begin to be apparent. The eigenfunctions of a linear, time invariant system are a class of functions (the exponentials) which can be used to describe all naturally occurring signals. Part II of this book will deal with an efficient mechanism, the fast Fourier transform, of transforming a signal into a description in terms of imaginary exponentials. With this eigenfunction description of the input signal, it is simple to calculate the output. Transformation of the input signal into a description in terms of eigenfunctions allows us to transform the complicated description of the system in terms of convolution into a simple description in terms of multiplication.

V. SUMMARY

Although this chapter is very short, it is very important. The eigenfunctions are a very special set of input signals. The operation of a system of these signals is very simple. The system operates along the direction of these signals. The eigenfunctions are the characteristic signals of a system.

The operation of a system can be characterized by the response of the system to a set of eigenfunctions. In a particular problem such as nuclear magnetic resonance spectroscopy, a description of the system in terms of eigenfunctions is often logical in terms of the physical details of the system.

Furthermore, the eigenfunctions are useful practically. Given the response of a system to a set of eigenfunctions, then it is efficient to calculate the response of the system to any linear combination of eigenfunctions.

The concept of eigenfunctions will be used extensively in this book. It will be especially important in understanding the transform methods used in Part II. In Part IV, the idea of an eigenfunction representation of signals will be central to understanding systems which produce images and to understanding how images are reconstructed.

VI. FURTHER READING

Eigenfunctions are described to some extent in most of the books which describe convolution, referenced at the end of Chapter 3. Eigenfunctions are also described in the Chapter 7 (Differential Equations) and in Chapter 9 (Linear Algebra Model of Systems). The references at the end of these chapters also provide more information about eigenfunctions.

Chapter 6

COMPLEX NUMBERS

Few radiologists are familiar with the use of complex numbers. However, complex numbers greatly facilitate the expression of several mathematical concepts. For example, sinusoidal functions are much easier to work with using complex exponentials than using the sine and cosine function themselves. Wave functions, such as ultrasound waves, are more easily expressed using complex exponentials. For these reasons engineers rarely use sine and cosine functions, but rather use complex exponentials.

The main reason for introducing complex exponentials in this book is in order to describe the Fourier transform, Chapters 14 to 16. Fourier transforms can be expressed in terms of sine and cosine functions; however, there are two problems with this approach. First, the notation is much more cumbersome to work with. Second, many of the properties of the Fourier transform are difficult to understand with this notation. With the complex exponential notation, these relations are more easily understood. Although working through this chapter may be a little painful for some readers, there will be considerable benefit in terms of understanding the concepts presented in the rest of the book.

I. NUMBER SYSTEMS

A. OTHER NUMBER SYSTEMS

In order to understand the complex number system, we shall consider some number systems which are more familiar. The following is a list of progressively more complicated number systems — nonzero positive integers, positive integers, integers, rational numbers, real numbers, and complex numbers. Each of these number systems includes more elements than the previous number system. As the number systems become more complicated, it is possible to perform more mathematical operations. In fact we can motivate the need for more complicated number systems based on the desire to perform various mathematical operations.

A very simple operation is counting. The counting operation can be performed with the simplest of these number systems, nonzero, positive integers. However, a problem arises if we find that there are no elements to be counted. To allow the possibility of no elements, zero must be added to the number system to give us the positive integers.

Addition can be performed with the positive integers. The sum of any two positive integers is also a positive integer. But the opposite operation subtraction presents a problem when a larger integer is subtracted from a smaller integer. We can overcome this problem by adding the negative numbers to give us the integers.

Multiplication can be performed with the integers. The product of any two integers is also an integer. But the opposite operation division presents a problem when the dividend is not a multiple of the divisor. We can overcome this problem by adding numbers which are the ratio of two integers to the number system. Numbers which can be expressed as the ratio of two integers are called the rational numbers.

The square of any rational number is a rational number. But the opposite operation, taking the square root of a positive rational number may result in a number which is not in the rational number system. For example, the square root of two is not a rational number. We can overcome this problem by adding the irrational numbers. The rational numbers plus the irrational numbers give the real number system.

B. COMPLEX NUMBER SYSTEM

With the real number system there is still an operation which cannot be performed. The square of all real numbers is positive; therefore, there is no square foot for a negative number.

Mathematicians overcome this problem by addition of the imaginary numbers. Imaginary numbers are real numbers multiplied by the square root of minus one. The square root of a negative real number is an imaginary number. An imaginary number plus a real number produces a complex number.

If y is a real number, then an imaginary number which is equal in magnitude to y is written:

$$i \cdot y \tag{6.1}$$

where i is equal to the square root of minus one:

$$i = \sqrt{-1} \tag{6.2}$$

A complex number consists of a real and an imaginary part. A complex number may be written:

$$z = x + i \cdot y \tag{6.3}$$

where x is the real part of z and $i \cdot y$ is the imaginary part of z. A complex number consists of two numbers, one representing the real part and one representing the imaginary part.

At first glance, it appears to be very artificial to introduce imaginary numbers, defined as a real number times the square root of minus one. However, it turns out mathematically that the properties of this awkward appearing number system are in fact quite natural. We can perform a large number of operations on complex numbers and the result is still a complex number. Unlike the other number systems for which some operation produced a result which was not a part of the number system, the complex numbers do not have this problem. The mathematicians like to say that the complex numbers are closed with respect to these operations.

C. APPLICATIONS OF COMPLEX NUMBERS

It is certainly pleasing for mathematicians that the complex numbers provide a closed number system with respect to the operations of arithmetic; however, the reader might ask, do complex numbers mean anything in terms of the world? For each of the other number systems, it is easy to conceive of an application which uses the numbers. Even the irrational numbers come from a real world problem, surveying. The hypotenuse of a right triangle is equal to the square root of the sum of the squares of the sides. If the sides are each length 1, then the hypotenuse is $\sqrt{2}$. Thus, even the irrational numbers are needed for reasonably common applications.

The applications of complex numbers to real-world problems are considerably less well-known to the average person. Below, we shall find that any well behaved function can be represented as the scaled sum of a sine and cosine function. The sine and cosine functions are awkward to use. It is necessary to remember several complex trigonometric relations and the notation is cumbersome. An imaginary exponential can be used to express the same sinusoidal function much more naturally — at least more naturally for the electrical engineer.

Complex numbers are integral to the most common mathematical description of quantum mechanics. The physical observables in quantum mechanics are always real numbers; however, the underlying description is formulated in terms of complex numbers. The underlying probability distributions in quantum mechanics require the complex number description. In a sense, the complex numbers are not only a mathematical convenience, but also a natural representation — at least natural to the physicist.

In radiology, complex numbers are used to describe the nuclear magnetic resonance signal. Modern nuclear magnetic resonance detectors are able to measure the signal intensity

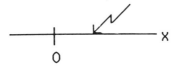

FIGURE 6.1. Real number line: the set of real numbers can be represented by the points on a line. Any particular number (arrow) is a point on that line.

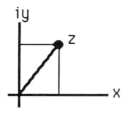

FIGURE 6.2. Complex plane: the set of complex numbers can be represented by the points in a plane. The abscissa gives the real part, x, of the complex number. The ordinate gives the imaginary part, i · y, of the complex number. The complex number, z, is the point in the plane with real part, x, and imaginary part, i · y.

in two perpendicular dimensions. The intensity in these two dimensions gives the real and imaginary component of complex signal.

The effects of a tissue on the ultrasound wave is two-fold. The wave may be attenuated by the tissue, and the phase of the wave may be altered. The most compact method of expressing these two effects is to use a complex impedance, where the real part defines the attenuation and the imaginary part defines the phase shift (see below).

Thus, complex numbers are needed mathematically in order to be able to take the square root of negative numbers. Complex numbers also come up in real-world applications, including radiological applications.

II. COMPLEX NUMBER REPRESENTATIONS

There are several different representations of complex numbers. The different representations each give a different insight into what a complex number means. Let us start with the graphical representation of a complex number. A line is often used to represent a set of real numbers. A single real number is a point on the line (see Figure 6.1). A complex number consists of a real number and an imaginary number. We can think of the set of complex numbers as a plane. A single complex number is a point in the complex plane (Figure 6.2). The x axis gives the real component, the y axis gives the imaginary component.

The most common method of writing a complex number was given above:

$$z = x + i \cdot y \qquad (6.4)$$

In the physics literature i is used to represent $\sqrt{-1}$. Since the symbol, i, is used for current, in the electrical engineering the symbol, j, is used to represent $\sqrt{-1}$. Although the general approach in this book will be most similar to the engineering approach, we have chosen to use the symbol i since it seems to be somewhat more common in the radiological literature.

Another way of writing the complex number is:

$$z = (x,y) \qquad (6.5)$$

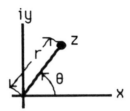

FIGURE 6.3.   Polar representation of complex numbers: the complex number can be represented by the rectilinear coordinates, x,i · y, or the polar coordinates, r,θ. The polar coordinates represent the distance of the number from the origin, r, and the angle with respect to the x axis, θ.

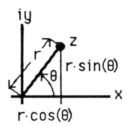

FIGURE 6.4.   Polar to rectilinear conversion: the relationship between the polar and the rectilinear coordinates can be determined from trigonometry. The x value is equal to r · cos(θ). The y value is equal to r · sin(θ).

where x is the real part of the number, and y is the magnitude of the imaginary part of the number. This method of writing the complex number emphasizes that it is a single entity with two components. It also emphasizes the concept that a complex number is equivalent in complexity to a pair of real numbers.

Complex numbers can also be expressed in **polar notation.** Let us consider again the graphical representation of a complex number. Above we equated the real and imaginary components with the x and y axis of a plane. Instead of using a rectilinear coordinate system to describe the point on the complex plane, we could use a polar coordinate system. The polar coordinate system represents a point by two numbers. One number, usually called r, represents the distance from the origin. The other number, usually called θ, represents the angle between the x axis and a line from the origin to the point (see Figure 6.3). In polar notation:

$$z = (r, \theta) \tag{6.6}$$

r is called the magnitude of the complex number and θ is called the phase of the complex number.

It is possible to convert between the x,y notation and the r, θ notation. The conversion that is used is the conversion from rectilinear to polar coordinates. From Figure 6.4 it can be seen that the trigonometric relationships are:

$$x = r \cdot \cos(\theta)$$
$$y = r \cdot \sin(\theta) \tag{6.7}$$

and:

$$r = (x^2 + y^2)^{1/2}$$
$$\theta = \tan(y/x) \tag{6.8}$$

III. OPERATIONS ON COMPLEX NUMBERS

Operations performed on complex numbers are more complicated than operations performed on real numbers since a complex number has two parts. The complex number representation using i is the most useful for figuring out how to perform most operations on complex numbers. The operations are performed using the usual real number operation and then the real and imaginary parts are collected. One somewhat tricky feature is that the result may include powers of i. If one remembers that i^2 is equal to -1, then the powers of i are easily calculated:

$$i^3 = i^2 \cdot i = -1 \cdot i = -i \tag{6.9}$$

$$i^4 = i^2 \cdot i^2 = -1 \cdot -1 = 1 \tag{6.10}$$

As an example of a typical operation let us try to add two complex numbers:

$$z_1 + z_2 = x_1 + i \cdot y_1 + x_2 + i \cdot y_2 \tag{6.11}$$

Collecting the real and imaginary terms:

$$z_1 + z_2 = (x_1 + x_2) + i \cdot (y_1 + y_2) \tag{6.12}$$

Thus, adding complex numbers is performed by adding their real and imaginary parts separately. We could equally express addition using the (x,y) notation:

$$z_1 + z_2 = (x_1, y_1) + (x_2, y_2) = (x_1 + x_2, y_1 + y_2) \tag{6.13}$$

This notation emphasizes that the real and imaginary parts add separately.

Multiplying complex numbers is more complicated, but the $x + iy$ notation will again help us determine what to do:

$$z_1 \cdot z_2 = (x_1 + i \cdot y_1) \cdot (x_2 + i \cdot y_2) \tag{6.14}$$

$$z_1 \cdot z_2 = x_1 \cdot x_2 + x_1 \cdot i \cdot y_2 + i \cdot y_1 \cdot x_2 + i \cdot y_1 \cdot i \cdot y_2 \tag{6.15}$$

The last term is equal to $i^2 \cdot y_1 y_2$ which is $-y_1 y_2$. Grouping the real and imaginary terms:

$$z_1 \cdot z_2 = (x_1 \cdot x_2 - y_1 \cdot y_2) + i \cdot (x_1 \cdot y_2 + y_1 \cdot x_2) \tag{6.16}$$

Notice that for multiplication both the real and imaginary parts of the multiplicand contribute to both the real and imaginary parts of the result. Thus, complex multiplication is more difficult than complex addition.

A much more difficult problem is complex division. We shall have to use a trick to perform complex division. The trick is to multiply the numerator and denominator by a number similar to the denominator except that the imaginary part is negative:

$$\frac{z_1}{z_2} = \frac{x_1 + i \cdot y_1}{x_2 + i \cdot y_2} = \frac{x_1 + i \cdot y_1}{x_2 + i \cdot y_2} \cdot \frac{x_2 - i \cdot y_2}{x_2 - i \cdot y_2} \tag{6.17}$$

Working out the algebra yields:

$$\frac{z_1}{z_2} = \frac{x_1 \cdot x_2 - i \cdot x_1 \cdot y_2 + i \cdot y_1 \cdot x_2 + y_1 \cdot y_2}{x_2^2 + y_2^2} \tag{6.18}$$

The trick has made the denominator a real number. Collecting the real and imaginary parts:

$$\frac{z_1}{z_2} = \frac{x_1 \cdot x_2 + y_1 \cdot y_2}{x_2^2 + y_2^2} + i \cdot \frac{x_2 \cdot y_1 - x_1 \cdot y_2}{x_2^2 + y_2^2} \tag{6.19}$$

Like complex multiplication, complex division yields a result where both the real and imaginary parts have contributions from both the real and imaginary parts of the divisor and dividend.

Other operations on complex numbers can be figured out in a similar fashion. First the numbers are expressed in the $x + i \cdot y$ form. Then the calculation is performed as if the numbers were real numbers. Any powers of i are reduced appropriately. Finally, the real and imaginary terms are collected. Using this algorithm, it is reasonably straight forward to perform any operation on complex numbers.

A. COMPLEX CONJUGATE

In order to perform division we took advantage of a trick — We multiplied the numerator and the denominator by a number similar to the denominator, but with a negative imaginary part. When working with complex numbers, this is a fairly common trick. A number which is made up of the same real part, but the negative imaginary part of another number is called a **complex conjugate**. The asterisk symbol as a superscript is used to indicate a complex conjugate. Thus, if:

$$z = x + i \cdot y \tag{6.20}$$

then:

$$z^* = x - i \cdot y \tag{6.21}$$

One of the uses of the complex conjugate is to calculate the magnitude of a complex number. For example,

$$z \cdot z^* = (x + i \cdot y) \cdot (x - i \cdot y) = x^2 + y^2 = r^2 \tag{6.22}$$

The last equality is given above by Equation 6.8. Thus, a number multiplied by its complex conjugate is equal to the square of the magnitude of the number. Since the magnitude of a complex number can be considered to be an extension of the absolute value of a real number, it is often written using the absolute value notation, $|z|$. The square of the magnitude is often written, $|z|^2$.

B. COMPLEX EXPONENTIAL

One of the major reasons for introducing complex numbers is so that we can use the complex exponential notation for sinusoidal functions. A complex exponential is an exponential function with a complex exponent:

$$e^z \tag{6.23}$$

where z represents a complex number. The meaning of a complex exponent is not at all obvious. However, let us see if we can understand its meaning using the properties of exponentials given in Table 2.3.

The exponent of the complex exponential can be written in terms of its real and imaginary parts:

$$e^z = e^{x+i\theta} = e^x \cdot e^{i\theta} \tag{6.24}$$

The symbol θ has been used instead of y for the imaginary part of the exponent. The reason for this change in symbols will become apparent shortly.

The first factor in Equation 6.24, e^x, is just a real number. The exponential of x. We already have a good understanding of this factor.

The second factor in Equation 6.24, $e^{i\theta}$, is much more complicated. Recall that the power series expansion of e^x was given in Chapter 2 (see Table 2.5). We can define $e^{i\theta}$ in terms of that same power series.

$$e^{i\theta} = 1 + i \cdot \theta + i^2 \cdot \theta^2/2! + i^3 \cdot \theta^3/3! + i^4 \cdot \theta^4/4! + i^5 \cdot \theta^5/5! \ldots \tag{6.25}$$

$$e^{i\theta} = 1 + i \cdot \theta - \theta^2/2! - i \cdot \theta^3/3! + \theta^4/4! + i \cdot \theta^5/5! \ldots \tag{6.26}$$

Collecting the real and imaginary part of Equation 6.26

$$e^{i\theta} = (1 - \theta^2/2! + \theta^4/4! + \ldots) + i \cdot (\theta - \theta^3/3! + \theta^5/5! + \ldots) \tag{6.27}$$

The real part of Equation 6.27 is the power series expansion for the cosine function; the imaginary part is the power series expansion for the sine function (see Table 2.5). Therefore we may write:

$$e^{i\theta} = \cos(\theta) + i \cdot \sin(\theta) \tag{6.28}$$

This relationship is known as **Euler's equation.**

Thus, $e^{i\theta}$ has a real part which is equal to the cosine function and an imaginary part which is equal to the sine function. Figure 6.5 shows a graphical representation of $e^{i\theta}$ where the real and imaginary parts of the function are shown on different axes. For some readers this figure may be reminiscent of electromagnetic radiation. In fact the complex exponentials are often used to describe electromagnetic radiation for this reason.

Equation 6.7 gives the formula for conversion from polar notation. Notice that this equation shows that the real part is equal to the cosine of the phase and the imaginary part is equal to the sine of the phase. This is the same relationship as given above. Therefore, we can identify θ as the phase of the complex number $e^{i\theta}$. In fact that is why we have used the same symbol θ for both the phase and the imaginary part of the exponent.

The negative portion of the cosine function is a mirror image of the positive portion. A function with this property is called an even function. Mathematically,

$$\cos(-\theta) = \cos(\theta) \tag{6.29}$$

The negative portion of the sine function is an up-side-down mirror image of the positive portion. A function with this property is called an odd function. Mathematically,

$$\sin(-\theta) = -\sin(\theta) \tag{6.30}$$

From these properties we can derive the value of $e^{-i\theta}$.

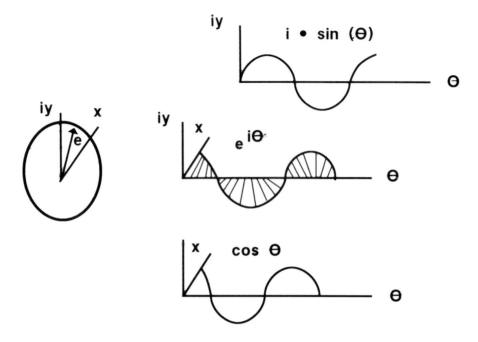

FIGURE 6.5. Imaginary exponential: the imaginary exponential, $e^{i\theta}$, can be shown with a three-dimensional graph. The real axis, x, goes into the page. The imaginary axis, $i \cdot y$, points up. The θ axis points to the right. As θ increases, the imaginary exponential circles around the θ axis at a distance of one from the axis. The projection of this function on the $i \cdot y, \theta$ plane is a sine function. The projection of this function on the x,θ plane is a cosine function. The projection of this function on the x,$i \cdot y$ plane is a circle.

$$e^{-i\theta} = \cos(-\theta) + i \cdot \sin(-\theta) = \cos(\theta) - i \cdot \sin(\theta) \qquad (6.31)$$

Let us try to determine the value of $e^{-i\theta}$ from the power series expansion:

$$e^{-i\theta} = 1 - i \cdot \theta + i^2 \cdot \theta^2/2! - i^3 \cdot \theta^3/3! + i^4 \cdot \theta^4/4! - i^5 \cdot \theta^5/5! \ldots \qquad (6.32)$$

Collecting the real and imaginary terms gives:

$$e^{-i\theta} = (1 - \theta^2/2! + \theta^4/4! + \ldots) - i \cdot (\theta - \theta^3/3! + \theta^5/5! + \ldots) \qquad (6.33)$$

Therefore:

$$e^{-i\theta} = \cos(\theta) - i \cdot \sin(\theta) \qquad (6.34)$$

Thus, with this more formal derivation we have obtained the same relation as in Equation 6.29.

Since $e^{-i\theta}$ has the same real part as $e^{i\theta}$ and minus the imaginary part of $e^{i\theta}$, it is the complex conjugate of $e^{i\theta}$. The magnitude of $e^{i\theta}$ is the square root of $e^{i\theta}$ times its complex conjugate $e^{-i\theta}$ (see Equation 6.22):

$$e^{i\theta} \cdot e^{-i\theta} = e^{i(\theta - \theta)} = e^0 = 1 \qquad (6.35)$$

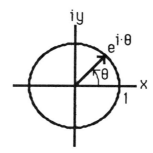

FIGURE 6.6. Imaginary exponential: the imaginary exponential, $e^{i\theta}$, shown on the x,i · y plane. This figure is similar to the left hand side of Figure 6.5, but viewed from a different angle.

The magnitude $e^{i\theta}$ is therefore equal to one. By the same argument, the magnitude of any exponential with a pure imaginary exponent must be equal to one.

Since the magnitude of $e^{i\theta}$ is equal to one, the magnitude of e^z must be equal to e^x. Thus, the complex exponential is quite remarkable. The real part of the exponential gives the magnitude of the number and the imaginary part gives the phase of the number.

Figure 6.6 shows a representation of $e^{i\theta}$ on the complex plane. The value of $e^{i\theta}$ will always lie on a circle which is a distance one from the origin. As θ increases from zero the value moves counter clockwise around the unit circle. The real part follows the cosine function and the imaginary part is the sine function.

The notation Re( ) is used to indicate an operator which takes the real part of a complex number. The notation Im( ) is used to indicate an operator which takes the imaginary part of a complex number and returns it as a real number. Thus,

$$Re(x + i \cdot y) = x \tag{6.36}$$

$$Im(x + i \cdot y) = y \tag{6.37}$$

Using these operators we have the relationships:

$$\cos(\theta) = Re(e^{i\theta}) \tag{6.38}$$

$$\sin(\theta) = Im(e^{i\theta}) \tag{6.39}$$

It is possible to calculate the value of $e^{i\theta}$ using Euler's equation. For example consider θ equal to 0, $\pi/2$, π, $3\pi/2$, and 2π:

$$e^{i0} = \cos(0) + i \cdot \sin(0) = 1 \tag{6.40}$$

$$e^{i\pi/2} = \cos(\pi/2) + i \cdot \sin(\pi/2) = i \tag{6.41}$$

$$e^{i\pi} = \cos(\pi) + i \cdot \sin(\pi) = -1 \tag{6.42}$$

$$e^{i3\pi/2} = \cos(3\pi/2) + i \cdot \sin(3\pi/2) = -i \tag{6.43}$$

$$e^{i2\pi} = \cos(2\pi) + i \cdot \sin(2\pi) = 1 \tag{6.44}$$

These values are the values every 90° around the unit circle in the complex plane.

Since the cosine and the sine are periodic functions, the value of e^{i0} and $e^{i2\pi}$ are both one. For any multiple of 2π, the imaginary exponential is equal to one:

$$e^{i2\pi n} = 1 \tag{6.45}$$

where n is an integer. More generally it can be seen from Figure 6.6 that the imaginary exponential is a periodic function with period of 2π.

IV. USES OF THE COMPLEX EXPONENTIAL

A. TRIGONOMETRIC RELATIONSHIPS

Euler's equation (Equation 6.28) expresses the imaginary exponential function in terms of the sine and cosine functions. Using Euler's equations and Equation 6.34 we can express the sine and cosine functions in terms of imaginary exponential functions.

$$e^{i\theta} + e^{-i\theta} = \cos(\theta) + i \cdot \sin(\theta) + \cos(\theta) - i \cdot \sin(\theta)$$
$$= 2 \cdot \cos(\theta) \tag{6.46}$$

Therefore,

$$\cos(\theta) = 1/2 \cdot (e^{i\theta} + e^{-i\theta}) \tag{6.47}$$

Similarly, we can derive the relation:

$$\sin(\theta) = 1/2i \cdot (e^{i\theta} - e^{-i\theta}) \tag{6.48}$$

Thus, using these relations we can convert from trigonometric to imaginary exponential notation.

It is often easier to use the exponential notation to work out trigonometric relationships. For example, consider:

$$\cos^2(\theta) + \sin^2(\theta) = (1/_2 \cdot (e^{i\theta} + e^{-i\theta}))^2 + (1/2i \cdot (e^{i\theta} - e^{-i\theta}))^2$$
$$= 1/_4 \cdot (e^{i2\theta} + 2 \cdot e^{i(\theta - \theta)} + e^{-i2\theta})$$
$$- 1/_4 \cdot (e^{i2\theta} - 2 \cdot e^{i(\theta - \theta)} + e^{-i2\theta})$$
$$= 1/_4 \cdot (e^{i2\theta} + 2 + e^{-i2\theta} - e^{i2\theta} + 2 - e^{-i2\theta})$$
$$= 1/_4 \cdot (4)$$
$$= 1 \tag{6.49}$$

Thus we are able to prove this well-known relationship using simple algebraic operations and the imaginary exponential.

B. MATHEMATICAL OPERATIONS

The imaginary exponential provides another notation which can be used to write a complex number. For any complex number, z, which has a magnitude, r, and a phase, θ, we can write:

$$z = r \cdot e^{i\theta} \tag{6.50}$$

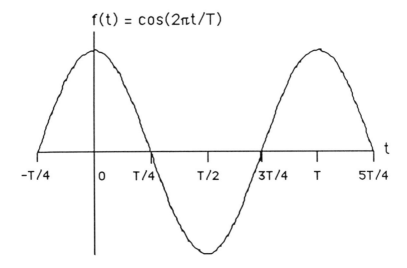

FIGURE 6.7.   Cosine function with period T: the cosine function $\cos(2\pi t/T)$ has a period equal to T. The values of the function repeat every time t increases by T.

Notice that we have switched gears with regard to notation. We are now using z as the symbol for a complex number, not for an exponent, and we are using r as the symbol for the magnitude, not e^x. This method of writing the polar form of a complex number is useful for performing some mathematical operations.

For example, it is easier to perform multiplication with this notation:

$$z_1 \cdot z_2 = r_1 \cdot e^{i\theta_1} \cdot r_2 \cdot e^{i\theta_2}$$

$$= r_1 \cdot r_2 \cdot e^{i\theta_1} \cdot e^{i\theta_2}$$

$$= r_1 \cdot r_2 \cdot e^{i(\theta_1 + \theta_2)} \tag{6.51}$$

And similarly division can be easily performed:

$$z_1/z_2 = r_1/r_2 \cdot e^{i(\theta_1 - \theta_2)} \tag{6.52}$$

However, this notation makes addition and subtraction very difficult. Therefore, it is not used for most calculations.

C. SINUSOIDAL FUNCTIONS

The cosine function is one of the sinusoidal functions. Using the cosine notation:

$$f(t) = \cos(2\pi \cdot t/T) \tag{6.53}$$

where t is the independent variable and T is a constant. The cosine function is shown in Figure 6.7. The cosine function goes through one period as t goes from zero to T. Therefore, T is called the period of f(t). The period of f(t) has a simple relation to the **frequency**, ν:

$$\nu = 1/T \tag{6.54}$$

The frequency is given in Hertz, which is defined as cycles per second. As the period of the cosine function increases the frequency decreases.

$$f(t) = \cos(\omega t - \tfrac{1}{2}\pi)$$

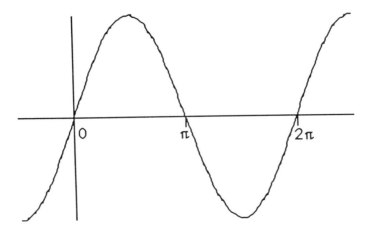

FIGURE 6.8.   Cosine function shifted by $^1/_2\pi$: a cosine function shifted by one quarter of its period, $^1/_2\pi$, is equal to a sine function.

We can rewrite Equation 6.53 using the frequency, v:

$$f(t) \; = \; \cos(2\pi \cdot v \cdot t) \tag{6.55}$$

The argument for the cosine function, $2\pi \cdot v$, is somewhat complicated. To simplify the notation, the cosine function is often written in terms of angular frequency, ω. The **angular frequency** is defined as:

$$\omega \; = \; 2\pi \cdot v \tag{6.56}$$

Therefore,

$$f(t) \; = \; \cos(\omega \cdot t) \tag{6.57}$$

The angular frequency, ω, is simpler to use than the frequency, v, in this case, since it gets rid of the 2π. In other cases, it is more complicated. We have chosen to use ω in this book, but this choice is reasonably arbitrary.

The angular frequency, ω, can be understood in terms of a point traveling in a circle which is distance one from the origin (Figure 6.6). The cosine function is equal to the projection of this point on the x axis. In one revolution, the point traverses a distance of 2π. The rate of change of the angle between a line from the point to the origin and the x axis is given by ω. The units of the angle are radians, the units of ω are radians per second.

We shall derive three formats for expressing sinusoidal functions. Real sinusoids other than the cosine function can be expressed as a shifted cosine function. If a cosine is shifted to the left by an amount θ/ω.

$$f(t - \theta/\omega) \; = \; \cos(\omega t - \theta) \tag{6.58}$$

Figure 6.8 shows a cosine wave shifted to the left by a quarter of a period:

$$\theta \; = \; {}^1/_2\pi \tag{6.59}$$

As can easily be seen, a cosine function shifted to the left by $^1/_2\pi$ is a sine function.

We have chosen to write the shift as θ/ω so that θ is the phase of the cosine function. We can derive an expression for a shifted cosine function in terms of a sum of a cosine function and a sine function using a two angle formula from trigonometry.

The complex exponential expression for the cosine can be used to derive the two angle formula for $\cos(\omega t - \theta)$.

$$\cos(\omega t - \theta) = \tfrac{1}{2} \cdot [e^{i(\omega t - \theta)} + e^{-i(\omega t - \theta)}]$$

$$= \tfrac{1}{2} \cdot [e^{-i\theta} \cdot e^{i\omega t} + e^{i\theta} \cdot e^{-i\omega t}] \qquad (6.60)$$

Now we can use Euler's equation 6.28, to expand $e^{i\theta}$:

$$\cos(\omega t - \theta) = \tfrac{1}{2} \cdot [(\cos(\theta) - i \cdot \sin(\theta)) \cdot e^{i\omega t}$$

$$+ (\cos(\theta) + i \cdot \sin(\theta)) \cdot e^{-i\omega t}] \qquad (6.61)$$

Rearranging the terms gives:

$$\cos(\omega t - \theta) = \cos(\theta) \cdot [\tfrac{1}{2} \cdot (e^{i\omega t} + e^{-i\omega t})]$$

$$+ \sin(\theta) \cdot [\tfrac{1}{2} \cdot (e^{i\omega t} - e^{-i\omega t})] \qquad (6.62)$$

The factors in the brackets are the imaginary exponential expressions for the cosine and the sine functions. Therefore,

$$\cos(\omega t - \theta) = \cos(\theta) \cdot \cos(\omega t) + \sin(\theta) \cdot \sin(\omega t) \qquad (6.63)$$

Equation 6.63 is a standard two-angle formula from trigonometry; however, it also provides insight into sinusoidal functions. Equation 6.58 represented a sinusoidal function with an arbitrary phase, θ, as a shifted cosine function. Equation 6.63 shows that we can also express any sinusoidal function as the weighted sum of a sine and a cosine function. The weighting factors are related to the phase of the sinusoid, θ.

We can express the sinusoidal function in Equation 6.58 using the imaginary exponential:

$$f(\omega t - \theta) = \text{Re}[e^{i(\omega t - \theta)}] \qquad (6.64)$$

This form expresses the general sinusoidal function as a shift of the function $e^{i\omega t}$ to the left by an amount θ. We can also write:

$$f(\omega t - \theta) = \text{Re}[e^{-i\theta} \cdot e^{i\omega t}] \qquad (6.65)$$

In this format, the sinusoidal function is $e^{i\omega t}$ and the phase shift is seen to be a complex number, $e^{-i\theta}$. This form is equivalent to Equation 6.63. The real part of $e^{-i\theta}$, $\cos(\theta)$, picks out the real part of $e^{i\omega t}$, $\cos(\omega t)$. The imaginary part of $e^{-i\theta}$, $-i \cdot \sin(\theta)$, picks out the imaginary part of $e^{i\omega t}$, $i \cdot \sin(\omega t)$.

We have three methods of writing any real sinusoidal function. Equation 6.58 expresses the sinusoid as a shifted cosine function. Equation 6.63 expresses the sinusoid as a linear combination of a cosine and a sine function. Equation 6.65 expresses the sinusoid as the real part of an imaginary exponential with a complex scale factor. The complex scale factor from Equation 6.65 gives the linear combination in Equation 6.63, and the linear combination in Equation 6.63 is related to the shifted cosine by the two angle formula.

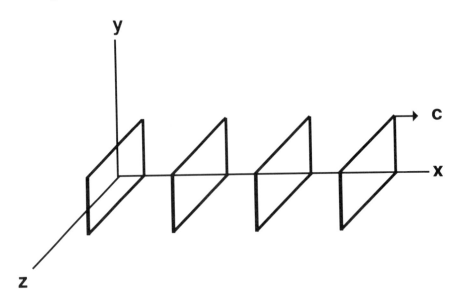

FIGURE 6.9.   Plane wave: a plane wave varies in intensity along one of its axes, x, but does not vary along the other two, y and z. All the planes parallel to the y,z plane have constant intensity.

D. PLANE WAVES

A plane wave is a three-dimensional signal which has a sinusoidal variation of one dimension. The intensity of the wave is not a function of the other two dimensions. These two dimensions represent planes perpendicular to the wave. The center portion of an ultrasound beam can be considered to be a plane wave. The compression and rarefaction of the ultrasound wave occur in the axial direction. For at least the center portion of the beam, there is no change of intensity in the transverse direction.

Figure 6.9 shows a plane wave. The intensity of the plane wave varies along the x axis. There is no variation along the y and the z axes.

The equation of a plane wave can be written in terms of the cosine function:

$$f(x,y,z) = \cos(2\pi \cdot x/\lambda) \tag{6.66}$$

The plane wave is a sinusoidal function of x. The function goes through one oscillation as x goes from zero to λ. The wave length, the distance covered by one oscillation, is λ. Writing the function as $f(x,y,z)$ emphasizes that the plane wave is a three-dimensional function. However, since there is no variation in the function with respect to y and z, it is simpler to write:

$$f(x) = \cos(2\pi \cdot x/\lambda) \tag{6.67}$$

In exponential notation:

$$f(x) = \mathrm{Re}(e^{i2\pi x/\lambda}) \tag{6.68}$$

In analogy to the relationship between the period, T, and the angular frequency, ω, a value called a **wave number** is often defined as $2\pi/\lambda$. The wave number is a spatial frequency. It is often given by the symbol k. Later we shall use k as a spatial frequency variable.

We have developed a representation for a plane wave which could be used to represent an ultrasound wave. But so far the wave is not moving. The next task is to consider how to express the change in the wave due to motion. In other words we need a function, f(x,t), which is a function not only of position, but also of time.

Let us assume that the plane wave is moving to the left at a speed, c. In an amount of time, t, the wave will have moved to the left by a distance equal to ct. The effect of the motion of the wave is the same as a shift to the left. We can express this mathematically as:

$$f(x,t) = f(x - ct) = Re(e^{i2\pi(x - ct)/\lambda}) \tag{6.69}$$

The amount of time that it will take for the wave to move the distance of one wave length will be:

$$T = \lambda/c \tag{6.70}$$

At a fixed point in the tissue the wave will appear to be passing at an angular frequency of:

$$\omega = 2\pi \cdot \nu = 2\pi/T = 2\pi \cdot c/\lambda \tag{6.71}$$

Thus we can rewrite Equation 6.69 as:

$$f(x,t) = Re(e^{i(2\pi x/\lambda - \omega t)}) \tag{6.72}$$

$$f(x,t) = Re(e^{i2\pi x/\lambda} \cdot e^{-i\omega t}) \tag{6.73}$$

At a fixed point, for example $x = 0$, the wave equation is:

$$f(0,t) = Re(e^{-i\omega t}) \tag{6.74}$$

Namely, the variation in intensity of the wave is just a cosine function. The minus sign is due to the fact that the wave is passing over the point of observation. This is equivalent to traveling backwards on a cosine function. At any other fixed point, x_0:

$$f(x_0,t) = Re(e^{i2\pi x_0/\lambda} \cdot e^{-i\omega t}) \tag{6.75}$$

$e^{i2\pi x_0/\lambda}$ is a complex number. Therefore, at any fixed point, x_0, we can consider that $f(x_0,t)$ is a cosine function which is shifted by an amount given by this complex number.

At any fixed time, t_0, we can write the wave equation as:

$$f(x,t_0) = Re(e^{-i\omega t_0} \cdot e^{i2\pi x/\lambda}) \tag{6.76}$$

$e^{-i\omega t_0}$ is a complex number. Therefore, at any fixed time, t_0, we can consider that $f(x,t_0)$ is a plane wave which is shifted by an amount given by this complex number.

Thus the plane wave equation (Equation 6.72) provides a great deal of information. It tells us about a plane wave both in terms of how it is distributed in space and how it moves in time. We can consider the plane wave either from the stand point of a fixed point in space or a fixed time. In either case the effect of the fixed variable is a phase shift. This compact notation helps make these relationships more obvious.

E. TISSUE IMPEDANCE TO ULTRASOUND

The effect of tissue on an ultrasound beam is due to two effects — attention and phase shift. The attenuation of the ultrasound is similar to X-ray attenuation and to radioactive decay (see Chapter 7, Differential Equations). The attenuation will decrease the intensity of the ultrasound beam as a function of depth in the tissue. We can write the attenuation mathematically as:

$$e^{-\mu x} \tag{6.77}$$

The phase shift of the beam will also increase as a function of distance. We can write the phase shift as an imaginary exponential:

$$e^{i\theta x} \tag{6.78}$$

We can combine these two factors:

$$e^{-\mu x} \cdot e^{i\theta x} = e^{(-\mu + i\theta)x} = e^{zx} \tag{6.79}$$

where z is a complex number:

$$z = -\mu + i \cdot \theta \tag{6.80}$$

z is called the impedance. The impedance gives the effect of both the attenuation and the phase shift.

We can combine the impedance with the wave equation to give us the complete equation for the ultrasound beam:

$$f(x,t) = Re(e^{zx} \cdot e^{i(2\pi x/\lambda - i\omega t)}) \tag{6.81}$$

The first factor gives the effects of the impedance and the second factor gives us the plane wave. Using complex notation, Equation 6.81 is able to provide a great deal of information. It includes attenuation, phase shift, the shape of the plane wave in space, and the change of the plane wave in time. This example is one reason that engineers find complex numbers so useful.

V. FUNCTIONS OF A COMPLEX VARIABLE

So far we have only been using complex numbers as values for the dependent variable. It is possible to have a function with a complex independent variable, $f(z)$. Such a function assigns a value to the dependent variable, f, for each value of the complex independent variable, z. Such a function is more complicated than a function of a real variable. The single variable, z, represents any value in the complex plane. Thus a function of a complex variable, $f(z)$, is equivalent to a function of two real variables, $f(x,y)$. $f(z)$ assigns a value to each combination of its real and imaginary parts.

A function of the complex variable can have a value in any number system. The function could give a real number or it could give a complex number. If $f(z)$ is a **complex valued function**, then each point in the complex plane, $f(z)$, gives a complex number. A complex valued function is like two real valued functions. For example we could write:

$$f(z) = f_r(x,y) + i \cdot f_i(x,y) \tag{6.82}$$

where the complex valued function of a complex variable has been written in terms of two real valued functions of two real variables. Thus, the simple notation $f(z)$ may hide a considerable amount of complexity.

An example of a complex valued function of a real variable is the ultrasound attenuation as a function of depth:

$$f(x) = e^{zx} = e^{(-\mu + i\theta)x} \tag{6.83}$$

An example of a complex valued function of a complex variable is the exponential function:

$$f(z) = e^{sz} \tag{6.84}$$

where s may or may not be a complex number.

A. ANALYTIC FUNCTIONS

There is a class of complex functions of a complex variable called the **analytic functions**. This class of functions is defined in terms of the relation between the real and imaginary parts of the functions. These relationships, called the **Cauchy-Riemann Equations**, can be written in terms of two partial differential equations. An understanding of analytic functions is well beyond the scope of this book; however, there are some properties of analytic functions which shed light on the Fourier transform relations described in Part II.

Analytic functions are interesting for several reasons. Roughly speaking, all functions which have physical meaning are analytic. Thus the only functions of interest to us are the set of analytic functions. Functions which are not analytic are generally only of interest to mathematicians. Requiring a function to be analytic greatly restricts the function.

It turns out that the value of an analytic function for any point in the complex plane can be calculated from knowledge of the values of the function along a single line in the plane. For example, if the values of an analytic function are known for all real values of the independent variable, then the value of the function for all values of an independent variable can be calculated. Similarly, if the values of an analytic function are known for all imaginary values of the independent variable, the value of the function can be calculated for all values of the independent variable.

Analytic functions are complex functions of a complex variable. As such, one would think that they would have a complexity equal to a function of two real variables. However, the ability to calculate the value of the function at any point from knowledge of the value along a line means that analytic functions have a complexity which is similar to functions of a single real variable.

In Part II we shall see that the Fourier Transform of a function is determined from the values of the function along a single line in the complex plane. The reason that all the information about the function can be obtained from this one line is that the Fourier Transform is restricted to analytic functions.

B. DERIVATIVES OF COMPLEX FUNCTIONS OF COMPLEX VARIABLES

Taking derivatives of complex functions can become tricky. To give some flavor to these problems we shall derive one result which will be needed later on. Let us define a complex function, $f(z)$:

$$f(z) = f_r(z) + i \cdot f_i(z) \tag{6.85}$$

where $f_r(z)$ is the real part of the function and $f_i(z)$ is the imaginary part of the function.

The magnitude of the function is given by:

$$|f(z)|^2 = f_r^2(z) + f_i^2(z) \tag{6.86}$$

The magnitude is a real number. The derivative of the magnitude is given by:

$$d|f(z)|^2/dz = 2 \cdot f_r(z) \cdot df_r(z)/dz + 2 \cdot f_i(z) \cdot df_i(z)/dz \qquad (6.87)$$

Consider f(z) times the derivative of the complex conjugate of f(z):

$$f(z) \cdot df^*(z)/dz = [f_r(z) + i \cdot f_i(z)] \cdot [df_r(z)/dz - i \cdot df_i(z)/dz] \qquad (6.88)$$

Multiplying and collecting the real and imaginary terms yield:

$$f(z) \cdot df^*(z)/dz = [f_r(z) \cdot df_r(z)/dz + f_i(z) \cdot df_i(z)/dz]$$
$$+ i \cdot [f_i(z) \cdot df_r(z)/dz - f_r(z) \cdot df_i(z)/dz] \qquad (6.89)$$

Equation 6.87 is twice the real part of Equation 6.89.

If $f(z) \cdot df^*(z)/dz$ is zero then both the real and imaginary parts of Equation 6.89 must be zero. Therefore,

$$f(z) \cdot df^*(z)/dz = 0 \qquad (6.90)$$

implies that

$$d|f(z)|^2/dz = 0 \qquad (6.91)$$

This relation will be useful later.

VI. EIGENFUNCTIONS OF LINEAR, TIME INVARIANT SYSTEMS

In Chapter 5, we found that exponentials were the eigenfunctions of linear, time invariant systems. The arguments in Chapter 5 were stated in terms of real exponentials; however, the argument is the same for complex exponentials. Therefore, the eigenfunctions of a linear, time invariant system are:

$$f(t) = e^{st} = e^{(r+i\omega)t} = e^{rt} \cdot e^{i\omega t} \qquad (6.92)$$

We have used s instead of z for the complex exponential factor in order to be compatible with the most common variable used for the Laplace transform.

If we consider values of s for which ω is zero, then:

$$f(t) = e^{rt} \qquad (6.93)$$

Functions of this type are typical real exponentials. If r is positive, the f(t) is an increasing exponential. If r is negative, the f(t) is a decaying exponential. Values of s for which r is zero give:

$$f(t) = e^{i\omega t} \qquad (6.94)$$

Functions of this type are sinusoidal functions. These functions are used for the Fourier transform.

In the more general case, where neither r nor ω is zero, f(t) is an exponentially decaying or increasing sinusoidal function. An example of a decaying sinusoidal function is shown in Figure 6.10. These functions are used for the Laplace transform.

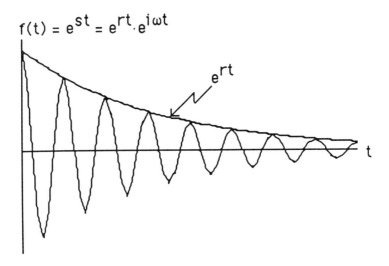

FIGURE 6.10. Complex exponential: the complex exponential, $e^{(r+i\omega)t}$, has a sinusoidal variation determined by the imaginary part of the exponential, $e^{i\omega t}$, which is modified by the real part of the exponential, e^{rt}. The result is a sinusoid that either increases or decreases with time.

VII. SUMMARY

The complex numbers are foreign to most radiologists; however, we have seen that they are a very useful mathematical tool. They are a simple method for describing sinusoids. Equation 6.81 gave a compact method for modeling several features of the plane waves used in ultrasound imaging. Most important in this book is that the complex exponentials provide us with an understanding of the eigenfunctions of linear, time invariant systems. Complex exponential notation will provide us with an important tool for understanding the transform techniques presented in Part II.

VIII. FURTHER READING

The complex number system and operations on complex numbers are discussed in a wide variety of mathematical texts. An advanced treatment of functions of a complex independent variable can be found in Chapter 10 of the book by Hildebrand.[1] This treatment is particularly relevant to the use of complex numbers in this book. Several important topics which have been omitted are covered. The reader interested in a deep understanding of Fourier transforms, is particularly recommended to investigate the properties of analytic functions.

Use of imaginary exponentials in place of sinusoidal functions is standard in most engineering texts. Medical ultrasound texts do not use complex exponentials. However, this type of treatment is typical of more general purpose acoustic texts.

REFERENCE

1. **Hildebrand, F. B.,** *Advanced Calculus for Applications,* Prentice-Hall, Inc., Englewood Cliffs, NJ, 1962.

Chapter 7

DIFFERENTIAL EQUATIONS

Differential equations are used extensively in physics. The laws of physics can often be expressed compactly using the differential equation notation. Part of the reason that differential equations are so useful in physics is that the laws of physics are relatively simple and very exact. Unlike physics, most of the relationships in biology are complex and inexact. Therefore, while differential equations are used to describe the basic physics of radiology, they are not useful for describing the complex imaging data.

Although we shall not use differential equations for solving image processing problems, we shall use differential equations as a method for better understanding the concept of a system. The mathematical methods used with differential equations are different from the mathematics in the rest of the book. However, the basic concept of a system operating on an input signal to produce an output signal is exactly the same. Studying the differential equations model of systems should help separate the underlying ideas associated with the concept of a system from the particular model which is used to describe a system.

The differential equation model is particularly useful for understanding two properties of systems — resonance and state. **Resonance,** the enhancement in the response of a system to a periodic input at a particular frequency, is a feature of many of the simple systems described by differential equations. The **state** of a system describes the information stored in the system. The state of a system is also useful for understanding how a system remembers signals, and how the system function is related to the state of the system.

This chapter will start with two simple examples of systems which can be described by differential equations — radioactive decay and a mass on a spring. Although a mass on a spring may not appear to be relevant to radiology, it exhibits resonance, a fundamental property of nuclear magnetic resonance. These two simple examples will highlight several of the properties of differential equations which are important for understanding systems. The second part of the chapter will describe these properties more fully.

Since differential equations are used infrequently in radiologic image processing, we shall present a very superficial discussion of the mathematics of differential equations. This chapter may provide some useful insights into systems for those readers who already have some intuition about differential equations. Those readers who have never studied differential equations may wish to skip this chapter. This chapter can be omitted without loss of continuity.

I. DEFINITION OF A DIFFERENTIAL EQUATION

A differential equation gives a relationship between an input signal, $f(t)$, an output signal, $g(t)$, and the derivatives of $f(t)$ and $g(t)$. In its most general form, a differential equation can include powers, roots, and all sorts of special functions. For example, the following complicated equation is a differential equation:

$$g^5(t) \cdot dg(t)/dt + e^{g(t)} + \sin(g(t)) = df(t)/dt \qquad (7.1)$$

Differential equations which are of interest to us will be of a much more limited type. They will include only the input signal, the output signal, and their derivatives. We shall exclude all powers and special functions such as the sine and exponential functions. We can write the general expression for differential equations of this type as:

$$\sum_i a_i \cdot d^i g(t)/dt^i = \sum_i b_i \cdot d^i f(t)/dt^i \qquad (7.2)$$

where the summation symbol Σ means a sum of terms with respect to i (see Chapter 2, Basic Concepts). $d^i f(t)/dt^i$ is the ith derivative of the function f(t) with respect to the independent variable t. For i equal to 0, $d^i f(t)/dt^i$ is f(t); for i equal to 1, $d^i f(t)/dt^i$ is df(t)/dt; for i equal to 2, $d^i f(t)/dt^i$ is $d^2 f(t)/dt^2$, etc. Equations of this form are called **linear differential equations with constant coefficients.** The values a_i and b_i are the constant coefficients.

Other models of systems presented in this book describe the input and output signals over all time. The differential equation model is quite different. Equation 7.2 describes the relation of the input and output at a single time, t, for example at time zero. However, rather than just giving the input and output values at time, t, the differential equation also describes the derivatives of the signals at time, t. The derivatives tell how fast the value of the signal is changing. The differential equation model tells exactly how the system is changing at a single point in time. We are then able to calculate what will happen over time. The differential equation model is a derivative model while the other models are integral models.

For the mathematically inclined reader, this view point may be reminiscent of the Taylor series expansion of a function described in Chapter 2. The Taylor series expansion of a function gives a description of the signal in terms of the function and its derivatives at a point. The Taylor series expansion can be used to calculate the value of a function in a region around a point in terms of the value of the derivatives of the function at a point. The differential equation model of a system is similar to a Taylor series expansion in that it can be used to calculate the behavior of a system in terms of the derivatives of the input and output at a point.

II. EXAMPLES OF SYSTEMS DESCRIBED BY DIFFERENTIAL EQUATIONS

A. RADIOACTIVE DECAY

Differential equations are used in radiology in those areas where radiology and physics intersect. For example, a natural application of differential equations is radioactive decay. The physical law of decay says that the rate of decay is directly proportional to the number of radioactive atoms present, i.e., a constant fraction of isotopes decays in each time interval. Mathematically, we can express this relation:

$$dg(t)/dt = -\lambda \cdot g(t) \tag{7.3}$$

The rate of change of the isotope, dg(t)/dt, is proportional to the amount of substance present, g(t). The minus sign is because the substance is decreasing with time.

Using the standard form, given by equation 7.2, the decay equation is written:

$$dg(t)/dt + \lambda \cdot g(t) = 0 \tag{7.4}$$

This equation is an example of why differential equations are so useful for physics. The equation exactly expresses the basic physical principle, that the rate of change of the isotope is proportional to the amount of isotope. In Chapter 3, radioactive decay was described in terms of a system function. That model was more cumbersome, and it did relate as directly to the underlying physics.

The solution of differential equations is a subject beyond the scope of this book. Suffice it to say that often the method used is to guess the form of the answer and then to prove that the answer is correct by substituting it back into the equation. With much experience, and with several rules of thumb, a mathematician is often able to guess the right form for the answer.

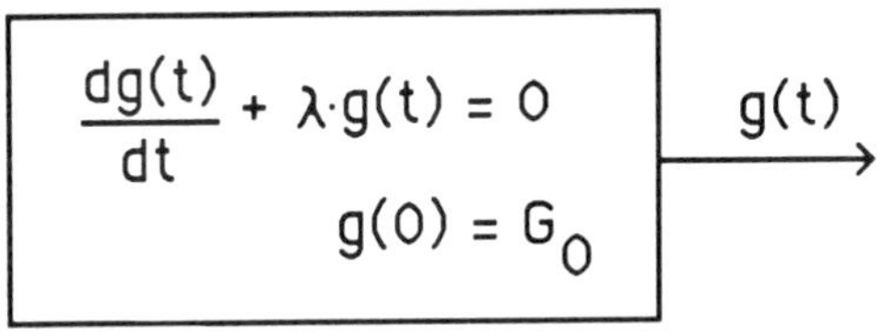

$$\frac{dg(t)}{dt} + \lambda \cdot g(t) = 0 \qquad g(t)$$

$$g(0) = G_0$$

FIGURE 7.1. Radioactive decay: the output signal, g(t), is the amount of radioisotope remaining. The system is defined by the decay differential equation and the amount of isotope present at time zero, G_0.

The usual way to solve the decay equation (Equation 7.3) is to use integration. However, to demonstrate the more typical method of solving more complicated differential equations, let us use the educated guess method, applied to the equation in the form given in Equation 7.4. We can guess that the solution:

$$g(t) = G_0 \cdot e^{-\lambda t} \tag{7.5}$$

where G_0 is a constant. At time zero g(0) is equal to G_0. Thus we can identify this constant as the activity at time zero. We can show that this is the correct solution by substituting back in Equation 7.4:

$$G_0 \cdot (-\lambda) \cdot e^{-\lambda t} + \lambda \cdot G_0 \cdot e^{-\lambda t} = 0 \tag{7.6}$$

Thus, Equation 7.5 gives a correct solution to the differential (Equation 7.4). Below, this solution to the decay system is referred to as the natural solution.

We can show the radioactive decay system symbolically (Figure 7.1). The box represents the radioactive isotope system. The output from the box is the amount of isotope, g(t), which is present. Equation 7.4 describes how g(t) will change in time. G_0 is the amount of daughter isotope present at time zero, g(0).

Now suppose that there is a parent nucleus which decays to the daughter nucleus, g(t). The change in the amount of the daughter, dg(t)/dt, will be due to both the decay of the daughter, and the decay of the parent. Decay of the daughter will decrease the amount of daughter, while decay of the parent will increase the amount of the daughter. We shall use f(t) to indicate the amount of daughter produced by the parent decay.

$$dg(t)/dt = -\lambda \cdot g(t) + f(t) \tag{7.7}$$

In standard form:

$$dg(t)/dt + \lambda \cdot g(t) = f(t) \tag{7.8}$$

This is an example of a system expressed by a differential equation. The input signal is new isotope due to the decay of the parent, f(t). The output signal is the amount of daughter isotope, g(t). We shall define the system function, h(t), as the exponential decay of the daughter. The exponential decay of the daughter is modified by the input due to decay of the parent.

Let us assume that the decay constant of the parent isotope is λ'. Then the input due to the decay of the parent will be:

$$f(t) = e^{-\lambda' t} \tag{7.9}$$

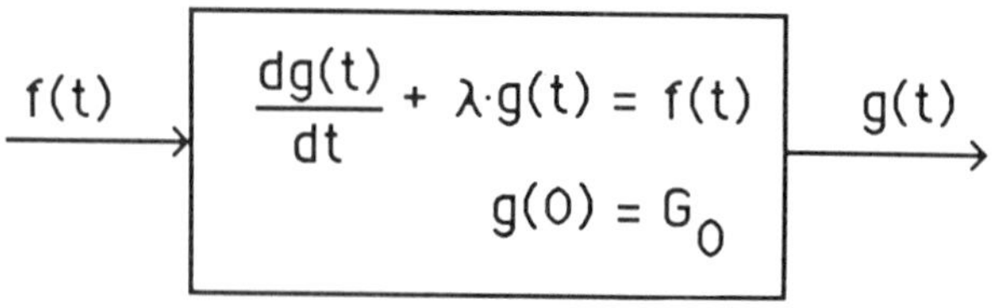

FIGURE 7.2.   Parent-daughter radioactive decay: the input to the system, f(t), is the amount of daughter isotope produced by decay of the parent. The output of the system, g(t), is the amount of daughter radioisotope. The system is defined by the decay differential equation and the amount of isotope present at time zero, G_0.

where we have assumed for simplicity that F_0 is one. The differential equation for the parent/daughter system is:

$$dg(t)/dt + \lambda \cdot g(t) = e^{-\lambda' t} \tag{7.10}$$

Again let us solve this equation by guessing the solution:

$$g(t) = a \cdot e^{-\lambda' t} \tag{7.11}$$

substituting into Equation 7.10 we get:

$$-\lambda' \cdot a \cdot e^{-\lambda' t} + \lambda \cdot a \cdot e^{-\lambda' t} = e^{-\lambda' t} \tag{7.12}$$

We can simplify this equation by dividing through by $e^{-\lambda' t}$:

$$-\lambda' \cdot a + \lambda \cdot a = 1 \tag{7.13}$$

Therefore:

$$a = 1/(\lambda - \lambda') \tag{7.14}$$

We have shown by substitution that the output signal given in Equation 7.11 is a valid solution of the parent daughter system if the constant, a, is given by Equation 7.14. a, the amplitude of the output signal, is inversely related to the difference between the two decay constants. Notice that the output signal decays with a decay constant equal to the decay constant of the parent isotope.

The output signal, g(t), is equal to the input signal, f(t), times the scale factor, a. Therefore, an input signal of the form given by Equation 7.9 is an eigenfunction of the decay system (see Equation 5.1). The eigenvalue is the constant a. Any exponential function of the form given by Equation 7.9 is an eigenfunction of this system.

The natural solution (Equation 7.5) can be added to the solution given in Equation 7.11:

$$g(t) = G_0 \cdot e^{-\lambda t} + 1/(\lambda - \lambda') \cdot e^{-\lambda' t} \tag{7.15}$$

The reader can show by substitution in Equation 7.10, that Equation 7.15 is another valid solution to the parent-daughter problem. Selecting the correct solution for a particular situation requires an additional constraint, the amount of daughter present at time zero, G_0.

Figure 7.2 shows the parent-daughter system diagrammatically. The input to the system is f(t), the output is g(t), and the relationship between the input and the output is given by Equation 7.8. The initial amount of daughter isotope present is G_0.

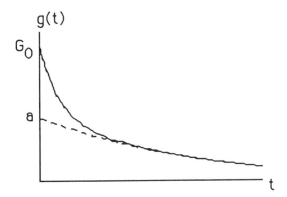

FIGURE 7.3. Radioactive decay: this graph shows a possible output from the system diagrammed in Figure 7.2. Initially there is an excess of daughter isotope which decays away rapidly with the daughter decay constant. At equilibrium, the daughter isotope decreases with the slower parent decay constant.

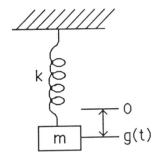

FIGURE 7.4. Mass on a spring: a mass which weighs, m, is suspended from a spring which has a spring constant, k. The position of the mass as a function of time, g(t), is the distance between the center of the mass and the zero point. The zero point is defined to be the position where the mass would hang if it were not moving.

Figure 7.3 shows a possible solution to the parent-daughter decay problem. We assume that the daughter has a shorter half-life, i.e., a larger decay constant. Initially there is an excess amount of daughter present. This daughter activity decays rapidly with decay constant, λ. Eventually, all of the parent-daughter system comes into equilibrium. At equilibrium the amount of daughter decreases according to the decay constant of the parent, λ'.

In Chapter 3, we described the parent to daughter decay problem using convolution. That model was useful since it explained why the daughter activity was greater than the parent activity — the system introduces a delay between the decay of the parent and the decay of the daughter. The same result can be derived from Equation 7.14, but the differential equation model provides less insight. However, the differential equation model is useful since it most clearly expresses the underlying physics. Using both models together provides one with the best overall understanding of radioactive decay.

B. MASS ON A SPRING

One of the most frequently used examples of a system described by differential equations is a mass on a spring. This problem might seem to be of little relevance to the radiologist; however, this problem shares similarities with nuclear magnetic resonance. Understanding this problem will shed some light on the basic principle of resonance.

Hook's law of the spring says that the force exerted by a spring is related directly to the stretch of the spring (Figure 7.4):

$$F = -k \cdot g(t) \qquad (7.16)$$

where k is called the spring constant, and where $g(t)$ represents the position of the mass as a function of time. The position where the spring is neither stretched or compressed is defined to be $g(t) = 0$. The greater the stretch, the greater the force exerted by the spring.

Newton's second law states that force is equal to mass times acceleration:

$$F = m \cdot d^2g(t)/dt^2 \qquad (7.17)$$

where we have written the acceleration as the second time derivative of the position of the mass.

Combining these two laws gives:

$$m \cdot d^2g(t)/dt^2 + k \cdot g(t) = 0 \qquad (7.18)$$

Hook's law combined with Newton's second law allows us to write a differential equation (Equation 7.18) which defines the motion of a mass on a spring. Notice how these very basic laws of physics are well expressed by this differential equation.

We shall use the same process to solve the equation that we used for the decay system. Let us guess that the answer is of the form:

$$g(t) = a \cdot e^{bt} \qquad (7.19)$$

If we substitute this answer into Equation 7.18 we get:

$$m \cdot a \cdot b^2 \cdot e^{bt} + k \cdot a \cdot e^{bt} = 0 \qquad (7.20)$$

We can divide this equation by $a \cdot e^{bt}$ to obtain:

$$m \cdot b^2 + k = 0 \qquad (7.21)$$

$$b^2 = -k/m \qquad (7.22)$$

$$b = +/- i \cdot (k/m)^{1/2} \qquad (7.23)$$

where we have used i to represent the square root of -1 (see Chapter 6, Complex Numbers).

The $+/-$ sign in Equation 7.23 indicates that there are two square roots, one which is positive and one which is negative. We can substitute these values for b into Equation 7.18 to get two solutions to the mass on the spring problem. If we combine the solutions, then we can write the general solution as:

$$g(t) = a_1 \cdot e^{+i(k/m)^{1/2}t} + a_2 \cdot e^{-i(k/m)^{1/2}t} \qquad (7.24)$$

Recall from the last chapter that complex exponentials represent sinusoidal motion. Thus, the solution to the mass on a spring problem is sinusoidal motion of the mass. Equation 7.24 is the natural solution for the mass on a spring problem. The natural frequency of motion is $(k/m)^{1/2}/2\pi$. The frequency will increase as the spring gets stiffer (increased k) and decrease as the mass gets heavier.

The general solution (Equation 7.24) to the differential equation (Equation 7.18) has left us with two unknowns, a_1 and a_2. In order to determine the actual motion of a particular instance, we must know more than just the physics of motion. We need to know some

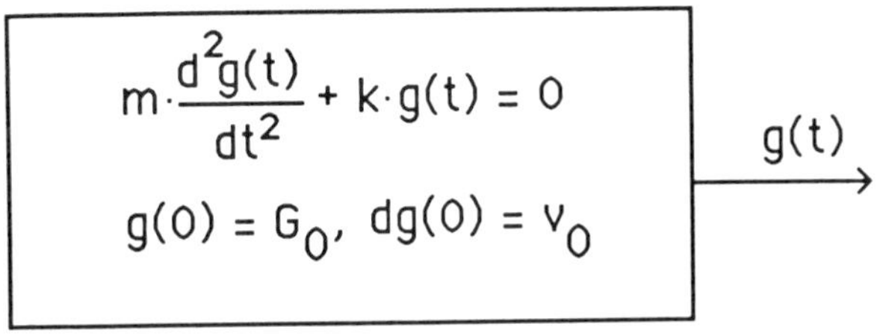

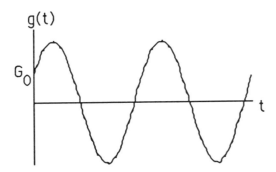

$$m \cdot \frac{d^2 g(t)}{dt^2} + k \cdot g(t) = 0$$

$$g(0) = G_0, \quad dg(0) = v_0$$

$g(t)$

FIGURE 7.5.   Mass on a spring: this figure is a diagrammatic representation of the problem shown in Figure 7.4. The output, g(t), is the position of the mass. The system is defined by the differential equation and the initial position and velocity of the mass.

FIGURE 7.6.   Mass on a spring: an example of a solution to the mass on a spring problem shown diagrammatically in Figure 7.5. The mass moves up and down with time in a sinusoidal motion. G_0 is the initial position of the mass.

additional constraints which determine the state the system is in at some point. For example, if we know the position and the velocity of the mass at time zero, we could solve for these two unknown parameters. Additional knowledge about the system at time zero is known as initial conditions (see below).

Figure 7.5 shows the mass on a spring system diagrammatically. The output of the system is the position of the mass, g(t). The system is defined by equation 7.18. The initial position of the mass, g(0), is G_0. The initial velocity of the mass, dg(0)/dt is v_0. A possible solution to Equation 7.18 is shown in Figure 7.6. The position of the mass, g(t), varies sinusoidally with time.

Now let us consider a more complicated situation. Rather than just letting the mass oscillate at its natural frequency, let us apply an external force to the mass. We can call this external force, f(t). The motion of the spring given by Newton's law will be equal to the sum of the two forces — the force due to the spring and the applied force. The differential equation for this problem is:

$$m \cdot d^2g(t)/dt^2 + k \cdot g(t) = f(t) \qquad (7.25)$$

We show the mass on a spring problem diagrammatically in Figure 7.7. The input force is f(t). The output signal, the position of the mass, is g(t). The system is described by Equation 7.25. The initial state of the system is given by g(0) and dg(0)/dt.

Let us see what happens when we apply a sinusoidal force at some angular frequency, c:

$$f(t) = e^{ict} \qquad (7.26)$$

(Recall from Chapter 6 that angular frequency, c, is equal to frequency, $c/2\pi$.)

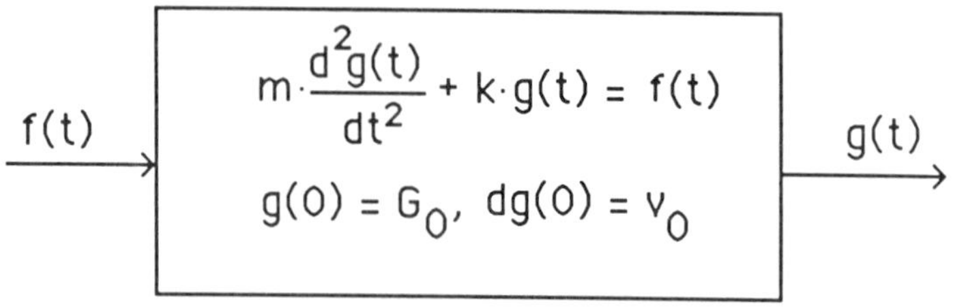

$$m \cdot \frac{d^2 g(t)}{dt^2} + k \cdot g(t) = f(t)$$

$f(t)$ →

$$g(0) = G_0, \quad dg(0) = v_0$$

→ $g(t)$

FIGURE 7.7.   Mass on a spring with an imposed force: the input signal, f(t), is the externally applied force on the mass. The output signal, g(t), is the position of the mass. The system is described by the differential equation and the initial position and velocity of the mass.

Note: f(t) as defined is a complex function and therefore it is not physically realizable. To be physically correct we could define f(t) to be the real part of complex exponential $Re(e^{ict})$. However, this distinction is not important to the problem and the extra notation would obscure comprehension.

We might imagine that since we are applying a periodic force at angular frequency, c, then the mass is likely to move at the same angular frequency. Let us guess that the solution to the differential equation will be:

$$g(t) = a \cdot e^{ict} \tag{7.27}$$

Substituting this solution into Equation 7.25:

$$-m \cdot a \cdot c^2 \cdot e^{ict} + k \cdot a \cdot e^{ict} = e^{ict} \tag{7.28}$$

Again we can divide through by e^{ict} and then solve for a:

$$a = 1/(k - mc^2) \tag{7.29}$$

The output signal, g(t), is equal to the input signal, f(t), times a constant, a. Therefore sinusoidal signals of the form given by Equation 7.26 are eigenfunctions of the mass on a spring problem. When the applied force has an angular frequency equal to the natural angular frequency of the system, $c = (k/m)^{1/2}$, then:

$$a = 1/(k - k) = 1/0 = \infty \tag{7.30}$$

In other words if we push the mass at the natural frequency of the system, then the amplitude of the output signal is infinite!

The relationship between a, the amplitude of the motion of the mass, and c, the angular frequency of the applied force is shown in Figure 7.8. The mass on a spring system demonstrates the property of resonance, an amplification of the output signal for certain frequency input signals. The frequency with the maximum amplification is called the resonance frequency. Notice that in this example the resonance frequency is equal to the natural frequency of the system.

Obviously in a real system some effect will limit the oscillation of the mass on the spring. However, the idea is that if we push the mass at the resonant frequency, the amplitude of the output oscillation will build up until the spring will no longer function as an ideal spring. As the applied force moves away from the resonant frequency, the amplitude of the output oscillation will rapidly decrease to more closely follow the applied signal.

The mass on a spring is not particularly relevant to radiologic applications; however, it has shown us several important characteristics of the differential equation model of systems.

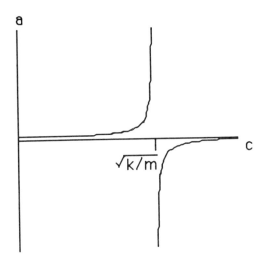

FIGURE 7.8.   Mass on a spring: the amplitude of the output of the system diagrammed in Figure 7.7 as a function of the input angular frequency. The amplitude of the motion of the mass is given by a. As the angular frequency of the input force approaches $\sqrt{(k/m)}$, the output amplitude approaches infinity. The negative amplitude for frequencies greater than the resonant frequency indicates that the motion lags behind the rapidly changing force.

The model allows us to express the physical principles involved in an exact fashion. In order to have a complete solution we must add some initial conditions which tell us about the state of the system. An input signal which is near in frequency to the natural frequency of the spring will result in resonance, amplification of the output signal.

III. ADDITIONAL CONSTRAINTS

In the examples, the differential equations did not fully define the outputs. Instead it was necessary to include a set of additional constraints. The purpose of the additional constraints was to describe the state of the system. In the case of the parent-daughter decay problem, the additional constraint defines how much daughter isotope was present at time zero. In the case of the mass on a spring, the additional constraints define where the mass is positioned and whether it is oscillating before the external force is applied. The differential equation tells about the relationship between the input and output signal; the additional constraints tell those additional facts about the state of the system which are necessary to determine the output of the system.

In our diagrammatic representation of these systems, we have included not only the differential equation, but also the initial condition. We have done this to emphasize that a complete description of a system includes both the differential equation and the additional constraints.

If the set of additional constraints on the system is given in terms of the values of the output signal and the derivatives of the output signal at time zero, then the constraints are called **initial conditions.** Often, the initial condition is that the output and all of the derivatives of the output are zero at time zero. In this case the system is said to initially be at rest.

One way to think about initial conditions is that they summarize the previous inputs to the system, the history of the system. The output of the system is due to the previous, current, and future input to the system. The initial conditions summarize all the information about the history of the system which is needed in order to determine the output of the system from the current and future input.

The additional constraints on the system need not be given at time zero. Instead, constraints on the output can be given at any time or any combination of times. If the constraints are given at the beginning and the end of the time interval of interest, then they are called **boundary conditions.** A good example of a system for which boundary conditions are appropriate is a violin string. The constraints for this system are that the position of the violin string at either end is fixed.

The clear separation of the model of the system, as defined by the differential equation, from the state of a particular system, as defined by the additional constraints, is very convenient for physics problems. The laws of physics are embodied in the differential equations while the particulars of a problem are given by the additional constraints. This distinction is much less useful in image processing problems, but the idea of the state of a system is a valuable concept.

IV. PROPERTIES OF LINEAR DIFFERENTIAL EQUATIONS WITH CONSTANT COEFFICIENTS

This section will deal with linear differential equations with constant coefficients where the additional constraints are specified as initial conditions. The general equation for the set of linear differential equations with constant coefficients, given in Equation 7.2 is repeated here:

$$\Sigma \; a_i \cdot d^i g(t)/dt^i \; = \; \Sigma \; b_i \cdot d^i f(t)/dt^i \tag{7.31}$$

where we assume that the summation is with respect to the variable, i. The initial conditions will generally be given as the values of $g(t)$ and its derivatives at time equal to zero.

The two problems described above — radioactive decay and a mass on a spring — are examples of linear differential equations with constant coefficients. These examples have already introduced many of the properties of this type of differential equation. In this section we shall describe these properties more formally.

A. LINEAR, TIME INVARIANT SYSTEMS

Since the differentiation operation is a linear operation, we can write:

$$d^i(a_1 \cdot f_1(t) \; + \; a_2 \cdot f_2(t))/dt^i \; = \; a_1 \cdot d^i f_1(t)/dt^i \; + \; a_2 \cdot d^i f_2(t)/dt^i \tag{7.32}$$

Therefore, the terms in Equation 7.31 are linear. The differentiation operation is also time invariant — the derivative of a shifted function is identical to a shifted derivative of the function. Thus, linear differential equations with constant coefficients have linear, time invariant terms.

Even though the terms in equation 7.31 are linear and time invariant, the systems which they represent are not necessarily linear and time invariant. In order to make the systems linear and time invariant, the initial conditions must also be properly specified.

An example of a system which is not linear is the parent-daughter decay system with daughter activity present at time zero. The daughter isotope will produce an output which we can call $g_0(t)$. An input from the parent, $f_1(t)$, will produce an output which has two parts — one part due to the daughter present at time zero, and the other due to the input:

$$g_0(t) \; + \; g_1(t) \tag{7.33}$$

A different input, $f_2(t)$, will produce an output:

$$g_0(t) \; + \; g_2(t) \tag{7.34}$$

The sum of these two outputs is:

$$2 \cdot g_0(t) + g_1(t) + g_2(t) \qquad (7.35)$$

However, the output produced by $f_1(t) + f_2(t)$ is:

$$g_0(t) + g_1(t) + g_2(t) \qquad (7.36)$$

Thus, the output from a linear combination of inputs is not the same as the linear combination of the outputs from each of the inputs separately.

We can generalize this result. If a system has any output which is not due to an input, then the system cannot be a linear, time invariant system. (This result was previously derived in Chapter 4.) In order for a differential equation to represent a linear, time invariant system, we must not only specify the form of the differential equation, but we must also define the additional constraints. The additional constraints must be defined so that if there is no input, the system produces no output. The system must be at rest at time zero.

B. NATURAL AND FORCED SOLUTIONS

The solutions to a differential equation when the input is zero are called the **natural solutions.** A differential equation with no input is called a homogeneous differential equation, and the natural solutions are also called **homogeneous solutions.** These solutions represent outputs for which there is no input, outputs determined by the initial state of the system. For linear, time invariant systems, there will be no contribution to the output from the natural solutions. However, we are still interested in the natural solutions, since they tell us a great deal about the system.

The solution to a differential equation which is due to the input is called the **forced solution** or **nonhomogeneous solution.** For linear, time invariant systems, the output is equal to the forced solution. If the input, $f(t)$, is zero, then the forced solution must also be zero.

In the parent-daughter isotope decay example, the daughter isotope present at time zero gives the natural solution. The supply of isotope from the parent is the forced solution. In the mass on a spring problem, oscillation due to initial motion and position of the mass is the natural solution. Motion due to an applied force is the forced solution.

If there is more than one natural solution to a linear differential equation, then any linear combination of the natural solutions is also a solution. For two natural solutions $g_1(t)$ and $g_2(t)$:

$$\Sigma \; d^i g_1(t)/dt^i = 0 \qquad (7.37)$$

$$\Sigma \; d^i g_2(t)/dt^i = 0 \qquad (7.38)$$

Therefore:

$$\Sigma \; d^i(a_1 \cdot g_1(t) + a_2 \cdot g_2(t))/dt^i = a_1 \cdot \Sigma \; d^i g_1(t)/dt^i + a_2 \cdot \Sigma \; d^i g_2(t)/dt^i$$

$$= 0 \qquad (7.39)$$

The particular linear combination of natural solutions used for an individual problem is determined by the initial conditions. For example, the solution of the mass on a spring problem involved a linear combination of natural solutions; see Equation 7.24. The initial conditions determine the actual combination of the sinusoidal functions.

There is a single forced solution for a differential equation. This forced solution is the output of the system due to the particular input signal. For linear differential equations, the natural solution is added to the forced solution to obtain the complete solution. Adding the natural solution to the forced solution does not change the differential equation since the natural solution just adds zero to both sides of the equation.

In the case of the parent-daughter decay, the contribution of the natural solution becomes very small with time. After a period of time almost all of the daughter is due to the forced solution, the decay of the parent to the daughter. In similar problems, the natural solution is sometimes called the **transient solution,** and the forced solution is called the **equilibrium solution.** These terms make sense for certain problems, but they are less relevant to other problems.

Consider the case where the input to a system is nonzero for times less than zero, but the input is zero for times greater than zero. The system can be modeled as a homogeneous differential equation, i.e., $f(t) = 0$. The input up to time zero will determine the initial conditions, the state of the system. By definition the output of the system must be a linear combination of the natural solutions.

The only output signal in the absence of input are the natural solutions. In other words, the natural solutions of a system are the only signals that the system can remember. The only way the system can respond to previous input is as a combination of the natural solutions.

C. EIGENFUNCTIONS

The eigenfunctions of a differential equation are signals which pass through the system unchanged except possibly for a change in scale (see Chapter 5, Eigenfunctions). Mathematically, the eigenfunctions of a differential equation are solutions for which:

$$g(t) = a \cdot f(t) \tag{7.40}$$

Linear differential equations with constant coefficients which are initially at rest are linear, time invariant systems. Therefore, from Chapter 5 we know that complex exponentials are eigenfunctions for these differential equations. The two examples in this chapter are in the form of linear differential equations with constant coefficients. In the first example, we found that exponential input signals were eigenfunctions of the decay system. In the second example, we found that imaginary exponentials were eigenfunctions of the mass on a spring problem. With zero initial conditions, both of these systems are linear, time invariant systems; therefore, more generally, all complex exponentials will be eigenfunctions of both of these systems.

In Chapter 5 we found that a system could be characterized by the eigenvalues for a set of eigenfunctions. Figure 7.8 shows the eigenvalues of the imaginary exponential eigenfunctions for the mass on a spring problem. These eigenvalues give us an easy method for understanding how the system operates on sinusoidal inputs, and inputs which are linear combinations of sinusoidal functions. The eigenvalues characterize the system.

The eigenvalues provide a method for calculating the output of a system in response to a signal which is a linear combination of the eigenfunctions. In Chapter 5, we indicated that this method was computationally faster than convolution. Eigenfunctions are less useful for calculation of the output in the case of differential equations, since it is usually simpler to use the differential equation itself to calculate the output. The reason that this is true is not because differential equations are computationally more simple than convolution, but rather because differential equations are typically used to describe very simple systems.

D. RESONANCE

In the case of the mass on a spring, we saw that for sinusoidal inputs with frequencies near the natural frequency of the spring there was a very large output. For an input which was at the natural frequency of the system, the output was infinite, or at least that is what the simplistic model predicted. This type of behavior, where certain types of inputs result in very large outputs is called resonance. We can define **resonance** as the enhancement in the output of a system to a periodic input which occurs for frequencies near the resonance frequency.

A radiological example of resonance is found in continuous wave, nuclear magnetic resonance spectroscopy. For excitation pulses very near to the resonance frequency of a nucleus in the sample, an output signal is produced. For other excitation frequencies, only noise is produced. Figure 7.8, which shows the resonance behavior of the mass on a spring, is similar to an NMR spectrum shown in Figure 5.2, except that the spectrum has several resonances. The spectrum is from a system which is more complicated than the mass on a spring; however, it is still quite a simple system.

In the case of the mass on a spring, the resonance frequency is equal to the frequency of the natural solution. Although the resonance frequencies of a system need not be equivalent to the frequencies of the natural solutions, they are typically related. Resonance is due to a build-up of the input signal by the system. In order to build-up, the signal must be stored in the system. The natural solutions represent signals that can be remembered by and stored in a system. Resonant signals must be able to interact with the natural solutions so that energy can be stored in the system.

E. SYSTEM FUNCTION

The system function is the response of a system to a delta function input signal. Except for time zero, the input is zero. Therefore, except for time zero, the output of a system represented by a linear differential equation with constant coefficients which is initially at rest must be a linear combination of the natural solutions, *vide supra*. **For times greater than zero, the system function, h(t), is a linear combination of the natural solutions of the homogeneous differential equation.**

Since the natural solutions are solutions which the system can remember, it makes sense that the system function must be composed of these signals. The differential equation model gives us insight into the relationship between the memory of the system, the natural solutions, and the system function.

From the discussion, it would seem that the right hand side of Equation 7.2 has little to do with defining the system. In the simple examples which we have used, this is in fact true. However, the right hand side can include any number of derivatives of the input signal. Although the left hand side of Equation 7.2 determines the natural solutions and the system function must be a linear combination of these natural solutions, it is the right hand side of the equation which determines how the natural solutions are combined. Thus, the system function depends on both the left- and right-hand sides of the equation as one would expect.

In Part II of the book, we shall learn how to represent the system function in terms of its Fourier transform. The correspondence between linear differential equations with constant coefficient and the system function can be most exactly stated in terms of the Fourier transform of the system function. Linear differential equations with constant coefficients correspond to systems which have Fourier transforms which are the ratio of rational functions. In Chapter 16, we shall learn what this means.

F. STATE

In our discussion, we have been using differential equations in two ways. With initial conditions equal to zero, the differential equations are a model of linear, time invariant systems. The input starting at time zero results in an output also starting at time zero. On the other hand, a system with input prior to zero can be modeled using differential equations by nonzero initial conditions. The input determines the state of the system at time zero, where the state is defined by the initial conditions.

This second way of using the differential equation model is very useful for understanding the concept of the state of a system. We could give the initial conditions at any point in time, not just zero, and these conditions would define the state of the system at that time. Independent of the model, it is useful to conceptualize the state of a system. The state of the system is what it remembers about the input up to the current point in time.

One way of defining the state of the system is in terms of the initial conditions. It is also useful to define the state in terms of the future output. If there is no input after some point in time, then the output after that time will be a linear combination of the natural solutions (shifted to that point in time). The state of the system can be defined by this linear combination. The scaling factors in the linear combination determine the output due to the previous input. The system can only remember signals in the form of the natural solutions. The state of the system determines how much of each of the natural solutions will be in the output.

The state of the system ties the previous input to the subsequent output. The previous input determines the state of the system, and the state of the system determines the contribution of each of the natural functions to the subsequent output.

The idea of a state often has physical meaning in terms of the system being described. For the radioactive decay problem, the state is the amount of daughter isotope present at any point in time. For the mass on a spring, the state is the position and the velocity of the mass at any point in time. The output of these systems due to the previous input can be determined from the state through the laws of physics.

In complicated radiological problems, there is often not any easy way describing the physical state of the system. But the idea that the state ties the previous input to future output is still useful. The output due to the state must be a linear combination of the natural functions, since the system can only remember signals which are in the form of the natural functions.

V. SUMMARY

Our treatment of differential equations is considerably different from the usual presentation of differential equations. Most presentations are designed to show how to solve physics problems with differential equations. Our purpose was to show that differential equations can be used to describe systems. The differential equations model of systems is different from other models which we describe in that it describes the system at one point. The other models are integral models describing the system over time.

In addition to the differential equation, it was necessary to give additional constraints in order to completely define a system. These additional constraints are analogous to the constants of integration when converting from a derivative to an integral. The additional constraints are used to define the state of the system. The state of the system can be viewed as the memory of the system of prior inputs. Since the system can only remember the natural solutions to the differential equation, the system function must be a linear combination of the natural solutions.

The idea of resonance comes naturally from the differential equations model. The resonant signals of a system are related to the natural solutions of the differential equation. Inputs which interact with the natural motions of the system can store energy in the system. Inputs which interact with the natural motions of a system result in larger outputs than inputs which cannot interact with the system.

Differential equations are most often used to describe simple systems, systems for which there are a small number of natural signals. The basic physics of radiology often deals with these types of simple systems. However, the emphasis in this book is on image processing. Image processing usually involves more complex systems and therefore, the differential equation model of systems will rarely be used in the rest of the book. We choose to present the differential equation model since understanding the differential equation model provides a better understanding of systems in general.

VI. FURTHER READING

There are a large number of books which deal with differential equations, for example;[1,2,3] however, they do not discuss differential equations from the point of view taken in this book. In this book we are not interested in differential equations for their own sake, but rather for how they illuminate general properties of systems.

The relation between differential equations and system models is covered in many engineering texts. Generally, the presentation is at a somewhat more advanced level than in this book; for example, see Chapter 3 of the book by Oppenheim and Willsky.[4] In mathematical texts, the Laplace transform (described in Chapter 20) is used as a method for solution of differential equations with initial conditions.

Our treatment of the eigenfunctions is quite atypical. Generally, eigenfunctions are not discussed in the context of initial value problems (problems with the additional constraints given as initial values). Eigenfunctions provide a realtively small amount of insight about these differential equations, and they are not useful for solving problems. Eigenfunctions are most useful in understanding how the differential equations model relates to other system models.

Eigenfunctions are very important in understanding boundary value problems (problems with the additional constraints given as boundary values). A particular class of boundary value problems, called Strum, Liouville problems, are related to the transform methods described in Part II. We have not included this material since it tends to have a more mathematical flavor; however, the interested reader may find that Chapter 5 of the book by Hildebrand[1] adds to the understanding of Part II.

The concept of resonance is essential to nuclear magnetic resonance imaging, and it is discussed in many sources on this subject. Linear system analysis is used extensively in circuit analysis, and the reader is referred to the book by Siebert[5] for an understanding of resonance from the perspective of circuit analysis.

A state model of systems uses a group of parameters to define the state of the system. The output at any point in time can be calculated from these parameters. The model determines how the parameters change with time. Since this model is most useful when the number of parameters is small, it is not particularly useful for complex radiological problems. However, it is a useful model for understanding the concept of the state of a system. The interested reader will find a good description of this model in Chapter 3 of the book by Gabel and Roberts,[6] or Chapter 3 of the book by Liu and Liu.[7] The state of the system is very important in an area of linear system analysis called control theory.

REFERENCES

1. **Hildebrand, F. B.,** *Advanced Calculus for Applications,* Prentice-Hall, Inc., Englewood Cliffs, NJ, 1962.
2. **Arfken, G.,** *Mathematical Methods for Physicists,* Academic Press, Orlando, FL, 1985.
3. **Birkhoff, G. and Rota, G-C.,** *Ordinary Differential Equations,* Blaisdell Publishing Co., Waltham, MA, 1962.
4. **Oppenheim, A. V. and Willsky, A. S.,** *Signals and Systems,* Prentice-Hall, Englewood Cliffs, NJ, 1983.
5. **Siebert, W. Mc. C.,** *Circuits, Signals, and Systems,* The MIT Press, Cambridge, MA, 1986.
6. **Gabel, R. A. and Roberts, R. A.,** *Signals and Linear Systems,* John Wiley & Sons, New York, 1973.
7. **Liu, C. L. and Liu, J. W. S.,** *Linear Systems Analysis,* McGraw-Hill, New York, 1975.

Chapter 8

LINEAR ALGEBRA

The methods of linear algebra are most often used to solve sets of simultaneous linear equations. For example, the computed tomography problem is often described as a large set of simultaneous linear equations. Each of the measurements represent the sum of the attenuation coefficients of the elements through which the X-ray beam passes. The reconstruction of a cross-sectional image can be performed by solution of this very large set of simultaneous linear equations.

In this chapter we shall show how matrix algebra can be used to describe the simultaneous linear equation problem. We shall only very briefly describe the usual methods of solving simultaneous linear equations. We shall spend the bulk of the chapter on describing the techniques of matrix algebra. In Part IV, we shall come back to linear algebra as a method for image reconstruction, but we shall find that solution of a very large set of simultaneous equations requires special techniques.

While the solution of simultaneous linear equations is a common motivation for studying linear algebra, our main use of linear algebra will be as a method for describing linear systems. In the next chapter, we shall show the analogy between a vector and a signal, and between a matrix and a system. The product of a vector and a matrix is another vector which is analogous to the output of the system.

Matrix algebra ties the concept of a system to the idea of vector spaces. Vector spaces give a geometrical insight into the operation of systems. The concept of vector subspaces will help to explain why some signals pass through a system and other signals do not. In Part II, we shall see that the Fourier transformation operations are analogous to a multidimensional rotation of a vector. But, more of this later. The task at hand is to obtain some understanding of elementary linear algebra methods.

I. SOLUTION OF SIMULTANEOUS LINEAR EQUATIONS

Simultaneous linear equations arise naturally in several radiologic applications. For example, when a gamma scintillation well counter is used to measure the radioactivity of two separate isotopes, two energy windows are used. The windows are selected so that one isotope contributes most heavily to one window, and the other isotope to the other window. However, in general each of the isotopes will contribute some counts to each of the windows.

This problem can be expressed mathematically using two linear equations in two unknowns:

$$g_1 = h_{11} \cdot f_1 + h_{12} \cdot f_2$$
$$g_2 = h_{21} \cdot f_1 + h_{22} \cdot f_2 \tag{8.1}$$

g_2 and g_2 are the counts in window 1 and 2, respectively. The unknown quantities, f_1 and f_2, represent the counts from isotope 1 and isotope 2. The factors, h_{11} etc., represent the efficiencies in each of the windows for each of the isotopes.

Typically, in linear algebra texts the simultaneous equations are written the other way around — with the gs on the right and the fs on the left. We have chosen to write the equations in this form so that they will be analogous to the form used for linear systems (Equation 4.1):

$$g(t) = H\{f(t)\} \tag{8.2}$$

Let us suppose that the well counter system has a sensitivity of 2 for isotope 1 in window 1, $h_{11} = 2$, and a sensitivity of 1 for isotope 2 in window 1, $h_{11} = 1$, and a sensitivity of 1 for isotope 1 in window 2, $h_{21} = 1$, and a sensitivity of 2 for isotope 2 in window 2, $h_{22} = 2$. Suppose that we measured 250 counts in window 1, $g_1 = 250$, and 200 counts in window 2, $g_2 = 200$. Then the equations would be:

$$250 = 2f_1 + f_2$$
$$200 = f_1 + 2f_2 \tag{8.3}$$

These equations can be cast in a different form without changing the solution by dividing the first equation by the coefficient of the first term, 2.

$$125 = f_1 + 0.5f_2$$
$$200 = f_1 + 2f_2 \tag{8.4}$$

We can again modify the form of the equations without changing the solution by subtracting the first equation from the second equation.

$$125 = f_1 + 0.5f_2$$
$$75 = 1.5f_2 \tag{8.5}$$

In this form, the equations can be solved simply. The second equation gives $f_2 = 50$. Substituting this value in the first equation gives $f_1 = 100$.

It may seem that the method we have used to solve this simple set of equations was very tedious. However, the method which we followed can be applied to any set of simultaneous linear equations to obtain the exact solution. This method is known as Gaussian elimination; in each successive equation one more variable is eliminated by this procedure until there is an equation with just one variable. The solution proceeds back up the set of equations by substitution.

So long as the number of variables equals the number of equations and the equations all represent different relationships among the variables, then the equations can be solved exactly with this procedure. If there are fewer equations than unknowns or if some of the equations give the same information, then there is a family of possible solutions. Such a set of linear equations is said to be **under determined.** In order to pick one solution from the family of solutions, more information must be provided. if there are more unique equations than unknowns, then there will be no solution. Such a set of equations is said to be **over determined,** the set of equations is called **inconsistent.**

The details of the solution of a set of simultaneous linear equations is discussed extensively in any linear algebra text. However, the solution of a set of simultaneous linear equations rapidly becomes unwieldy as the number of equations becomes large. This is exactly the case in which we are most interested in radiology. Exact solution techniques must be replaced by approximate solution methods. Since we are most interested in these approximate methods, we shall not emphasize the exact solution techniques.

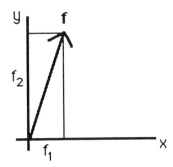

FIGURE 8.1.   Geometrical representation of a vector: the geometrical representation of a two-dimensional vector, **f**, is a line from the origin to the point (f_1, f_2). f_1 is the x component of the vector and f_2 is the y component of the vector.

II. VECTOR AND MATRIX NOTATION

Writing down a set of simultaneous linear equations in two or three unknowns is a simple task. For example, a set of three equations in three unknowns can be written:

$$g_1 = h_{11} \cdot f_1 + h_{12} \cdot f_2 + h_{13} \cdot f_3$$

$$g_2 = h_{21} \cdot f_1 + h_{22} \cdot f_2 + h_{23} \cdot f_3$$

$$g_3 = h_{31} \cdot f_1 + h_{32} \cdot f_2 + h_{33} \cdot f_3 \tag{8.6}$$

When the number of unknowns becomes large, it is quite difficult to write the equations; therefore, a more compact notation is needed.

We can indicate a set of three unknowns in Equation 8.6 by a vector with three components.

$$\mathbf{f} = \begin{pmatrix} f_1 \\ f_2 \\ f_3 \end{pmatrix} \tag{8.7}$$

The boldface notation, **f**, indicates that **f** is a vector. It stands for the three components f_1, f_2, and f_3. Similarly, we can define a vector, **g**, which stands for the data values in Equation 8.6.

$$\mathbf{g} = \begin{pmatrix} g_1 \\ g_2 \\ g_3 \end{pmatrix} \tag{8.8}$$

Two and three component vectors have natural geometrical interpretations. They can be used to represent the points in a plane or a volume. Figure 8.1 shows a two-dimensional vector, **f**. The tail of the vector is at the origin of the coordinate system. In linear algebra, we always place the tail of the vector at the origin. The head of the vector is at the point f_1, f_2, where f_1 is the x coordinate of the vector and f_2 is the y component of the vector. Similarly, we can imagine a three-dimensional vector as defining a point in a volume. For vectors with more than three components, there is no geometrical analog; however, we shall frequently appeal to the two- and three-dimensional case to provide geometrical insight into vector problems.

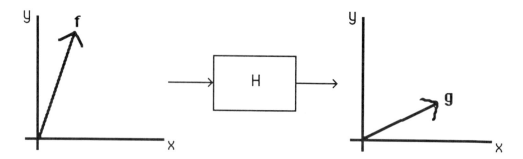

FIGURE 8.2.   Operation of a matrix on a vector: on the left is a vector, **f**. The effect of the matrix, H, on the vector is to produce a new vector, **g**.

We can represent the set of nine coefficients in Equation 8.6 by a matrix of values:

$$H = \begin{pmatrix} h_{11} & h_{12} & h_{13} \\ h_{21} & h_{22} & h_{23} \\ h_{31} & h_{32} & h_{33} \end{pmatrix} \tag{8.9}$$

The set of nine coefficients representing the coefficients of the three equations in three unknowns is represented by the single captial letter, H. The convention in linear algebra is to indicate single values by small letters, vectors by bold face letters, and matrices by captial letters. Below we shall see that a vector can be thought of as a matrix with one column. However, since vectors are conceptually different from matrices, it is useful to have a separate notation.

In the next chapter we shall see that the vector and matrix notation can be applied to the description of a linear system. The vector of unknowns, **f**, is analogous to an input signal, f[n]; the vector of known values, **g**, is analogous to the output signal, g[n]; and the matrix of coefficients, H, is analogous to the linear system H{·}. In the computed tomography problem, **f** or f[n] corresponds to the unknown attenuation coefficients; **g** or g[n] corresponds to the measured values; and H or H {·} corresponds describes how the computed tomographic system collects data.

Geometrically, the operation of H is to transform one vector, **f**, into another vector, **g**. Figure 8.2 shows the operation of the matrix H on vector **f** to produce vector **g**. Below we shall explain this operation mathematically.

Both a matrix and an image are two-dimensional arrays of numbers, and often in radiology an image is referred to as a matrix. However, in this book **an image is not a matrix.** An image is a two-dimensional signal. Later, we shall show how an image can be represented by a vector. A matrix will be used to represent an imaging system.

There are some special terms used when working with matrices. The **dimension** of a matrix is the number of rows and columns of the matrix. A matrix with three rows and four columns has a dimension of 3 by 4. A matrix with the same number of rows and columns is called a **square matrix.** The elements of a matrix with the same row and column number are called the **diagonal** of the matrix. For example, the underlined numbers in the following matrix are the diagonal elements:

$$\begin{array}{cccc} \underline{0} & 1 & 5 & 3 \\ 7 & \underline{4} & 8 & 2 \\ 0 & 6 & \underline{1} & 5 \end{array} \tag{8.10}$$

The elements of a matrix, H, are given with subscripts where the first subscript is the row and the second subscript is the column. h_{ij} is the element in the ith row and the jth column. We also will use the notation:

$$H = (h_{ij}) \tag{8.11}$$

where (h_{ij}) is shorthand for the matrix with all the elements, h_{11}, h_{12}, etc.

Before we can complete the description of simultaneous linear equations using matrix notation we need to take an excursion into the definition of vector spaces and into the operations which can be performed with matrices. After this excursion, we shall return to complete our description of simultaneous linear equations.

III. OPERATIONS WITH MATRICES

A. MATRIX ADDITION

Some of the operations which can be performed on matrices are defined in an intuitive way. For example, **matrix addition** is defined as adding the components of the two matrices:

$$A + B = \begin{pmatrix} a_{11} & a_{12} \\ a_{21} & a_{22} \end{pmatrix} + \begin{pmatrix} b_{11} & b_{12} \\ b_{21} & b_{22} \end{pmatrix} = \begin{pmatrix} a_{11} + b_{11} & a_{12} + b_{12} \\ a_{21} + b_{21} & a_{22} + b_{22} \end{pmatrix} \tag{8.12}$$

In the shorthand notation we can write this as:

$$(a_{ij}) + (b_{ij}) = (a_{ij} + b_{ij}) \tag{8.13}$$

B. SCALAR MULTIPLICATION

Multiplication of a number, x, times a matrix is defined as multiplication of the number times each element of the matrix:

$$x \cdot A = \begin{pmatrix} x \cdot a_{11} & x \cdot a_{12} \\ x \cdot a_{21} & x \cdot a_{22} \end{pmatrix} \tag{8.14}$$

Or in the shorthand notation:

$$x \cdot (a_{ij}) = (x \cdot a_{ij}) \tag{8.15}$$

A number, x, is called a **scalar** to emphasize the distinction between a single number and a group of numbers like a vector or a matrix. Multiplication of a matrix times a number is called **scalar multiplication.**

C. MATRIX MULTIPLICATION

Unlike addition and scalar multiplication, **matrix multiplication** is defined in quite an unusual fashion. The reason for this definition will become clear below as we see how matrix multiplication can be used for simultaneous linear equation. The value of each element of the product matrix is defined as the sum of the products of the elements of a row of the first matrix times the elements of the column of the second matrix. For example, multiplication of two 2 by 2 matrices is given by:

$$A \cdot B = \begin{pmatrix} a_{11} \cdot b_{11} + a_{12} \cdot b_{21} & a_{11} \cdot b_{12} + a_{12} \cdot b_{22} \\ a_{21} \cdot b_{11} + a_{22} \cdot b_{21} & a_{21} \cdot b_{12} + a_{21} \cdot b_{22} \end{pmatrix} \tag{8.16}$$

Since this operation may be a bit unfamiliar to the reader, we can show it in a different way. The underlined row and column of matrices A and B give rise to the underlined value in the product matrix C:

$$\begin{pmatrix} \underline{a_{11}} & a_{12} \\ a_{21} & a_{22} \end{pmatrix} \cdot \begin{pmatrix} b_{11} & \underline{b_{12}} \\ b_{21} & \underline{b_{22}} \end{pmatrix} = \begin{pmatrix} c_{11} & \underline{c_{12}} \\ c_{21} & c_{22} \end{pmatrix} \tag{8.17}$$

We can write a general equation for matrices of any dimension using our shorthand notation:

$$(c_{ij}) = \left(\sum_k a_{ik} \cdot b_{kj} \right) \tag{8.18}$$

where the summation is over the index, k. Each element c_{ij} of the product matrix is the sum of the elements of the ith row of A times the jth column of B.

In order to multiply two matrices, the number of columns of the first matrix must be equal to the number of rows of the second matrix. However, the matrices do not have to be square matrices. The product matrix will have a number of rows equal to the number of rows in the first matrix and a number of columns equal to the number of columns in the second matrix. If the first matrix does not have a number of columns equal to the rows of the second matrix, then the operation of matrix multiplication is not defined.

D. ASSOCIATIVE AND COMMUTATIVE PROPERTIES

When three matrices are multiplied together, for example, A · H · B, the order of multiplication does not matter. Operations which have this property are said to be **associative**. We can prove that matrix multiplication is associative using the definition given in Equation 8.18.

$$A \cdot (H \cdot B) = A \cdot \left(\sum_k h_{mk} \cdot b_{kj} \right) = \left[\sum_m a_{im} \cdot \left(\sum_k h_{mk} \cdot b_{kj} \right) \right]$$

$$= \left[\sum_m \sum_k (a_{im} \cdot h_{mk} \cdot b_{kj}) \right] = \left[\sum_k \left(\sum_m a_{im} \cdot h_{mk} \right) \cdot b_{kj} \right] = (A \cdot H) \cdot B \tag{8.19}$$

The key step in this derivation, switching the order of the summation operations, takes advantage of the fact that scalar addition is associative. Since the order in which multiplication takes place is not important, multiplication of three matrices is often written without parentheses.

$$A \cdot (H \cdot B) = A \cdot H \cdot B = (A \cdot H) \cdot B \tag{8.20}$$

Another important property which most common operations have is the **commutative** property. The commutative property states that the order of the factors is not important. Matrix multiplication is not commutative:

$$A \cdot B \neq B \cdot A \tag{8.21}$$

Matrix A multiplied times matrix B does not in general produce the same result as matrix B multiplied time matrix A. To see this mathematically we can again use definition Equation 8.18

$$A \cdot B = \left(\sum_k a_{ik} \cdot b_{kj} \right) \neq \left(\sum_k b_{ik} \cdot a_{kj} \right) = B \cdot A \tag{8.22}$$

Entirely different elements contribute to the two sums. If the matrices are not square matrices, then matrix multiplication may be defined for only one of the two products.

E. MULTIPLICATION OF A MATRIX TIMES A VECTOR
A special case of matrix multiplication is multiplication of a matrix by a vector. In this case we can consider the vector to be a matrix with a single column. The product of a matrix times a vector is:

$$\begin{pmatrix} g_1 \\ g_2 \end{pmatrix} = \begin{pmatrix} h_{11} & h_{12} \\ h_{21} & h_{22} \end{pmatrix} \cdot \begin{pmatrix} f_1 \\ f_2 \end{pmatrix} = \begin{pmatrix} h_{11} \cdot f_1 + h_{12} \cdot f_2 \\ h_{21} \cdot f_1 + h_{22} \cdot f_2 \end{pmatrix} \tag{8.23}$$

Since the number of columns of the second factor is one the number of columns of the product is one — namely the product is a vector. In shorthand notation we can write the general equation for the product of a matrix and a vector:

$$\mathbf{g} = \mathbf{H} \cdot \mathbf{f} = \left(\sum_k h_{ik} \cdot f_k \right) \tag{8.24}$$

F. IMAGE ARITHMETIC
Image processing systems often have image processing operations. Images are two-dimensional arrays of numbers like matrices. The **image addition** operation is identical to the matrix addition operation. However, **image multiplication** is different from matrix multiplication. The product image in image multiplication is the product of the corresponding elements of the input images. While image and matrix addition are the same operation, image multiplication is entirely different from matrix multiplication. Since it is common in radiology to think of image and matrices interchangeably, it is important not to confuse these two operations.

IV. SIMULTANEOUS LINEAR EQUATIONS IN MATRIX NOTATION

The definition of matrix multiplication is complicated; however, the payoff is that we can now write down a set of linear equations very simply. Equation 8.1 becomes:

$$\mathbf{g} = \mathbf{H} \cdot \mathbf{f} \tag{8.25}$$

Using matrix multiplication, we can express a complicated set of simultaneous linear equations with a very simple notation. However, it is important to remember that although the notation is simple, the operation is still complicated. The complexity has simply been hidden in the matrix multiplication sysmbol, "·".

We now have an efficient method of writing a set of simultaneous linear equations. We shall leave this problem for the time being so that we can develop more of the mathematical properties of matrices which we shall need later in the book. These properties will allow us to introduce the important concept of a vector space, and subsequently the concepts of projection and orthogonality. These two concepts will help provide geometrical insight into the relationships between signals.

V. MORE OPERATIONS WITH MATRICES

A. MATRIX INVERSE
In order to define the inverse of a matrix, we must first introduce a special square matrix, I, which is defined as having ones along the diagonal and zeros off the diagonal.

$$I = \begin{pmatrix} 1 & 0 & 0 \\ 0 & 1 & 0 \\ 0 & 0 & 1 \end{pmatrix} \tag{8.26}$$

This matrix is called the **identity matrix**. The nonzero elements of the identity matrix have the same row and column number.

$$i_{ij} = \begin{cases} 1 & \text{if } i = j \\ 0 & \text{if } i \neq j \end{cases} \tag{8.27}$$

The name comes from the fact that multiplication of any matrix by the appropriate size identity matrix results in a product matrix which is identical to the initial matrix.

$$H \cdot I = (\Sigma \, h_{ik} \cdot i_{kj}) \tag{8.28}$$

The only nonzero i_{kj} are the elements for which $k = j$; therefore,

$$H \cdot I = (h_{ij} \cdot 1) = (h_{ij}) = H \tag{8.29}$$

The identity matrix is "like" the number, 1, for scalar multiplication. For scalar multiplication, the inverse is defined as a number which multiplied times the original number yields 1.

$$x^{-1} \cdot x = 1 \tag{8.30}$$

x^{-1} is the inverse of x. In analogy to this definition, the inverse matrix which we shall call H^{-1} is defined by:

$$H^{-1} \cdot H = I \tag{8.31}$$

The inverse matrix times the original matrix is the identity matrix. The notation for the inverse matrix, H^{-1}, can be confusing. Although it is some respects analogous to a reciprocal, it is not a reciprocal:

$$H^{-1} \neq 1/H \tag{8.32}$$

In fact $1/H$ has no meaning in linear algebra.

In scalar multiplication, there is an inverse for every number except 0. The equation

$$y \cdot x = 1 \tag{8.33}$$

can be solved as

$$y = 1/x = x^{-1} \tag{8.34}$$

for every number, x, except $x = 0$. All other numbers have an inverse. By analogy, the matrix equation

$$B \cdot A = I \tag{8.35}$$

can be solved

$$B = A^{-1} \tag{8.36}$$

However, matrix multiplication is different from scalar multiplication in that there are a large number of matrices which do not have inverses. These matrices are called **singular**. Singular matrices have a "zero like" property.

If we have a set of simultaneous linear equations:

$$\mathbf{g} = H \cdot \mathbf{f} \tag{8.37}$$

then the solution is calculated:

$$H^{-1} \cdot \mathbf{g} = H^{-1} \cdot H \cdot \mathbf{f} = I \cdot \mathbf{f} = \mathbf{f} \tag{8.38}$$

It would seem that we have come across a wonderful way to solve simultaneous linear equations. If H^{-1} exists, then it gives us an easy method of solution for the unknown $\mathbf{f}$. Most linear algebra texts discuss the calculation of H^{-1} at length. However, calculation of H^{-1} is very difficult and fraught with errors for matrices with large dimensions. Even more important, for most radiological applications H is singular — H^{-1} does not exist. Therefore, we shall not discuss the calculation of H^{-1}. The idea of an inverse matrix will be important to us conceptually, but not practically.

B. TRANSPOSE OF A MATRIX

An operation called the **transpose** is performed by switching the rows and the columns of a matrix. The rows and columns are switched as if there were a mirror along the diagonal of the matrix. The capital letter, T, as a superscript is used to indicate the transpose operation. For example, if

$$A = \begin{pmatrix} a_{11} & a_{12} & a_{13} \\ a_{21} & a_{22} & a_{23} \end{pmatrix} \tag{8.39}$$

then

$$A^T = \begin{pmatrix} a_{11} & a_{21} \\ a_{12} & a_{22} \\ a_{13} & a_{23} \end{pmatrix} \tag{8.40}$$

Using the shorthand notation:

$$(a_{ij})^T = (a_{ji}) \tag{8.41}$$

The transpose operation switches the indexes in the subscript.

A special case of the transpose operation is the transpose of a vector:

$$\mathbf{f}^T = (f_1 \quad f_2 \quad f_3) \tag{8.42}$$

The transpose of a vector is sometimes called a **row vector**. Some texts allow a vector, $\mathbf{f}$, to represent either a column vector or a row vector. We shall only define vectors as column vectors. When we wish to indicate a row vector we shall use the transpose notation, $\mathbf{f}^T$.

The transpose of the product of two matrices results in an unusual result:

$$(A \cdot B)^T = B^T \cdot A^T \tag{8.43}$$

In order to prove this relationship, we need to expand this expression with Equation 8.18.

$$(A \cdot B)^T = \left(\sum_k a_{ik} \cdot b_{kj}\right)^T = \left(\sum_k a_{ki} \cdot b_{jk}\right) = \left(\sum_k b_{jk} \cdot a_{ki}\right) = B^T \cdot A^T \tag{8.44}$$

In order to see what all this fancy footwork with the subscripts means, let us consider an example.

$$A \cdot B = C \tag{8.45}$$

In this example, the element in the first row and third column of the product, c_{13}, comes from the first row of A times the third column of B.

$$\begin{pmatrix} \underline{a_{11}} & \underline{a_{12}} & \underline{a_{13}} \\ a_{21} & a_{22} & a_{23} \\ a_{31} & a_{32} & a_{33} \end{pmatrix} \cdot \begin{pmatrix} b_{11} & b_{12} & \underline{b_{13}} \\ b_{21} & b_{22} & \underline{b_{23}} \\ b_{31} & b_{32} & \underline{b_{33}} \end{pmatrix} = \begin{pmatrix} c_{11} & c_{12} & \underline{c_{13}} \\ c_{21} & c_{22} & c_{23} \\ c_{31} & c_{32} & c_{33} \end{pmatrix} \tag{8.46}$$

The underlined row of A times the underlined column of B results in the underlined element of C. Now consider

$$B^T \cdot A^T = C^T \tag{8.47}$$

Again the corresponding elements are underlined.

$$\begin{pmatrix} b_{11} & b_{21} & b_{31} \\ b_{12} & b_{22} & b_{32} \\ \underline{b_{13}} & \underline{b_{23}} & \underline{b_{33}} \end{pmatrix} \cdot \begin{pmatrix} \underline{a_{11}} & a_{21} & a_{31} \\ \underline{a_{12}} & a_{22} & a_{32} \\ \underline{a_{13}} & a_{31} & a_{33} \end{pmatrix} = \begin{matrix} c_{11} & c_{21} & c_{31} \\ c_{12} & c_{22} & c_{32} \\ \underline{c_{13}} & c_{23} & c_{33} \end{matrix} \tag{8.48}$$

Element c_{13} is the same for both of these products. Similarly, all of the elements, c_{ij} will be the same. Thus,

$$(A \cdot B)^T = B^T \cdot A^T \tag{8.49}$$

C. VECTOR MULTIPLICATION

Vector multiplication is a simplified version of matrix multiplication. The multiplication of two vectors **h** and **f** can be written using the transpose notation:

$$\mathbf{h}^T \cdot \mathbf{f} \tag{8.50}$$

The number of columns of $\mathbf{h}^T$ must be the same as the number of rows of **f** — namely, the vectors must have the same number of components. The product will have one row (the number of rows of $\mathbf{h}^T$) and one column (the number of columns of **f**) — namely, the output will be a single number, a scalar. For two-dimensional vectors:

$$\mathbf{h}^T \cdot \mathbf{f} = h_1 \cdot g_1 + h_2 \cdot g_2 \tag{8.51}$$

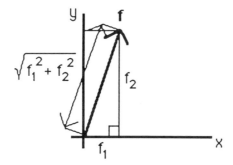

FIGURE 8.3. Length of a vector: a two-dimensional vector, **f**, has components, f_1 and f_2. The length of the vector given by the Pythagorean theorem is the square root of the sum of the squares of the two sides.

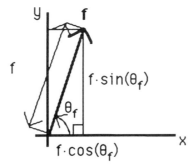

FIGURE 8.4. Vector **f**: the angle between the x axis and the vector, **f**, is defined to be θ_f. The components of the vector are $f \cdot \cos(\theta_f)$ and $f \cdot \sin(\theta_f)$, where f is the length of **f**.

Figure 8.3 shows a two-dimensional vector. The **length of a vector**, given by the Pythagorean theorem, is the square root of the sum of the squares of its sides. We shall use the symbol, f, with no bold face to indicate the length of the vector, **f**. The length of the vector is:

$$f = \sqrt{(f_1^2 + f_2^2)} \tag{8.52}$$

Using Equation 8.51 we can see that this value is equal to:

$$f = \sqrt{(\mathbf{f}^T \cdot \mathbf{f})} \tag{8.53}$$

Thus, the square root of a two-dimensional vector multiplied by itself gives the length of the vector. Similarly, the square root of a three-dimensional vector multiplied by itself gives the length of the vector. For vectors with more than three dimensions, there is no geometrical meaning for length. However, by definition Equation 8.53 is taken as the definition of length in linear algebra for a vector with any number of components.

A vectors, **f**, is shown in Figure 8.4. We can define the angle that this vector makes with the x axis as θ_f. The components of the vector are:

$$\mathbf{f} = \begin{pmatrix} f \cdot \cos(\theta_f) \\ f \cdot \sin(\theta_f) \end{pmatrix} \tag{8.54}$$

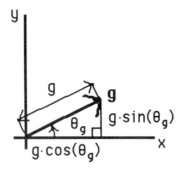

FIGURE 8.5.   Vector **g**: the angle between the x axis and the vector, **g**, is defined to be θ_g. The components of the vector are $g \cdot \cos(\theta_g)$ and $g \cdot \sin(\theta_g)$, where g is the length of **g**.

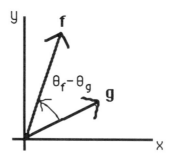

FIGURE 8.6.   Angle between two vectors: the angle between **f** and **g** is $\theta_f - \theta_g$.

Figure 8.5 shows a second vector, **g**, with components:

$$\mathbf{g} = \begin{pmatrix} g \cdot \cos(\theta_g) \\ g \cdot \sin(\theta_g) \end{pmatrix} \tag{8.55}$$

We have used f and g as the lengths of **f** and **g** respectively.
   The **product of two vectors** is given by:

$$\mathbf{f}^T \cdot \mathbf{g} = f_1 \cdot g_1 + f_2 \cdot g_2 \tag{8.56}$$

Using Equations 8.54 and 8.55 we can express this product as

$$\mathbf{f}^T \cdot \mathbf{g} = f \cdot \cos(\theta_f) \cdot g \cdot \cos(\theta_g) + f \cdot \sin(\theta_f) \cdot g \cdot \sin(\theta_g)$$
$$= f \cdot g \cdot [\cos(\theta_f) \cdot \cos(\theta_g) + \sin(\theta_f) \cdot \sin(\theta_g)] \tag{8.57}$$

The factor in brackets can be shown to be equal to $\cos(\theta_f - \theta_g)$ (see Chapter 6, Complex Numbers). Therefore,

$$\mathbf{f}^T \cdot \mathbf{g} = f \cdot g \cdot \cos(\theta_f - \theta_g) \tag{8.58}$$

Figure 8.6 shows **f**, **g**, and the angle between the vectors, $\theta_f - \theta_g$.
   When two vectors are lined up (θ_f is equal to θ_g), then their product is the product of their lengths:

$$\mathbf{f}^T \cdot \mathbf{g} = f \cdot g \cdot \cos(0) = f \cdot g \tag{8.59}$$

When they are at right angles (separated by $\pi/2$) to each other, then the product is zero:

$$\mathbf{f}^T \cdot \mathbf{g} = f \cdot g \cdot \cos(\pi/2) = f \cdot g \cdot 0 = 0 \qquad (8.60)$$

Thus, the product of two vectors is "like" the product of their lengths with an additional factor which determines how well lined up they are. When they are colinear, then the product is equal to the product of the lengths. When they are perfectly misaligned, at right angles to each other, then the product is zero.

Like the other geometrical insights, it is not possible to attach any meaning to the angle between two vectors in vector spaces with more than three dimensions. However, we can still use the vector product defined by Equation 8.56. In Chapter 10, (Random Variables and Stochastic Processes) we shall introduce the concept of correlation. Loosely speaking, correlation is how much the two signals are alike. Mathematically, the correlation is very similar to vector multiplication. Both operations result in a product which has a factor for how much the two factors are lined up or alike. We shall use the geometrical insight from vector multiplication to help us understand the correlation operation.

VI. VECTOR SPACE

We shall now introduce the concept of a **vector space** and subspaces which can be contained in a vector space. The idea of a vector space is actually quite abstract; however, again our geometrical insight will help to make it more understandable. Understanding vector spaces will allow us to understand the concepts of projection and orthogonality. These concepts are important not only in linear algebra, but also in understanding systems in general.

For a two-dimensional vector it is natural to think of the two components as the x and y axes of a plane. A two-dimensional vector, $\mathbf{f}$, could be used to represent a point in the plane (Figure 8.1). Similarly, a three-dimensional vector could be used to represent a point in a volume. A plane is a vector space for a two-dimensional vector and a volume is the vector space of a three-dimensional vector. A vector space is the set of all of the possible vectors.

Since a vector can have any number of components, we need to extend the definition of a vector space to include an arbitrary number of dimensions. Our geometrical intuition fails us for vectors spaces larger than three dimensions, since there are only three spatial dimensions. However, there are certainly common situations where multidimensional vector spaces arise.

A. EXAMPLES OF VECTOR SPACES

The most obvious example of a four-dimensional vector space is three spatial dimensions and a time dimension. A vector in this four-dimensional space gives both a physical position and a time. A point in this vector space defines a position and a time.

Nuclear magnetic resonance imaging gives us another example of a four-dimensional space — three spatial dimensions and one dimension representing chemical shift. A vector in this space defines not only a position, but also a particular chemical shift at that position.

There are several other possible vector spaces which make sense in nuclear magnetic resonance imaging — a four-dimensional space with two spatial dimensions, a chemical shift dimension, and a time dimension; a five-dimensional space with three spatial dimensions, a chemical shift dimension, and a time dimension; a six-dimensional space with three spatial dimensions and three velocity dimensions; etc.

B. COMPLEXITY OF A VECTOR SPACE VERSUS A SIGNAL

Working with multidimensional vector spaces may at first seem to be much more

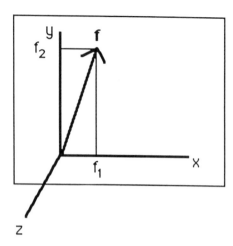

FIGURE 8.7. x,y plane in the x,y,z volume: the x,y plane is a subspace in the volume defined by the x,y,z axes. A vector, **f**, in this subspace has components, f_1, f_2, and 0. The component along the z axis is zero for all vectors in the x,y plane.

complicated than working with functions. However, they are actually of the same complexity. A discrete function, f[n], has a value for each point n, while a vector **f** represents only a single point, albeit in a multidimensional space. The components of the vector along the various dimensions are analogous to the values of the functions at different points, n. Each value, f[n], corresponds to one component of the vector, f_i.

A function is complicated since it represents a large number of values, but it is simple since there is only one dimension; a vector is complicated since it represents a large number of components, but it is simple since it represents a single point. Since a discrete function or a vector can be used to represent the same entity, their overall complexity is equivalent.

C. VECTOR SUBSPACE

The geometrical equivalent of a one-dimensional space is a line; the equivalent of a two-dimensional space is a plane; and the equivalent of a three-dimensional space is a volume. A volume can contain a plane or a line; a plane can contain a line. A space which is contained within another space is called a subspace. The subspace must have a dimension which is less than or equal to the space which contains it. All of the points and all of the lines in a plane are also part of a volume which contains the plane, but there are points and lines in the volume which are not in the plane.

If we imagine a three-dimensional coordinate system with axes, x, y, and z, then a vector in this space has three components corresponding to these three axes. The x,y plane is a two-dimensional subspace of this three-dimensional space. We could still represent vectors in the x,y plane using a three-component vector, but the last component of all of the vectors would be zero (Figure 8.7). It may seem like a waste of effort to use a three-component vector when one component is always zero. But, this notation lets us express the idea that the two-dimensional subspace is embedded in a three-dimensional space.

The x,y plane is only one of an infinite number of planes in the three-dimensional space. Were we to choose a plane which was not aligned with two of the original axes, then all three components of the vector could be nonzero (Figure 8.8). The three components would, however, be constrained so that they would define a vector in the two-dimensional plane. Thus, even though the vectors have three components, they would lie in a two-dimensional subspace. In Part II we shall learn how to rotate the coordinate system. It is always possible to rotate the coordinates so that a two-dimensional subspace is represented by a vector with only two nonzero components.

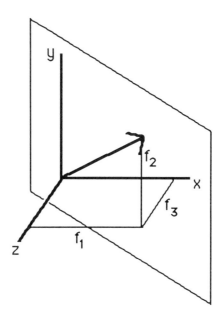

FIGURE 8.8. Planar subspace in a volume: a vector, **f**, in a plane which is not aligned with the x,y plane may have three nonzero components, f_1, f_2, and f_3.

It is possible to imagine planes which do not pass through the origin of the coordinate system. However, we have defined vectors with their tails starting at the origin. Since the zero vector will always be the origin by definition, the zero vector is always included in every subspace. Therefore, all of the planes will pass through the origin.

The operations which we have defined such as scalar multiplication, vector addition, matrix multiplication, etc., result in vectors that are in the same subspace as the starting vectors. If we start with a vector in a plane, there are all sorts of operations which we can perform which result in vectors which are still contained in that plane. Mathematicians like to say that the space is **closed** with respect to these operations. A subspace which is not aligned with the original coordinate axes is still closed with respect to vector operations in the subspace. If we start with vectors in some space, then operations on those vectors will not let us get out of the space.

D. PROJECTION

In a two-dimensional coordinate system a vector, **f**, is represented by a line from the origin to a point, (f_1, f_2). A vector is shown in figure 8.1. The first component of the vector, corresponding to the x coordinate, is the point on the x axis which is closest to the end of the vector. A line from the x coordinate to the end of the vector forms a right angle with the x axis. The x coordinate is called the projection of the vector on the x axis. Similarly, the y coordinate is the projection of the vector on the y axis.

A vector of length, 1, is called a unit vector. If we take a unit vector aligned with the x axis, $\mathbf{d}_1$, and multiply it times **f**, we get:

$$(1 \quad 0) \cdot \begin{pmatrix} f_1 \\ f_2 \end{pmatrix} = 1 \cdot f_1 + 0 \cdot f_2 = f_1 \tag{8.61}$$

These vectors are shown in Figure 8.9. Therefore, vector multiplication with a unit vector is a method of determining the projection of a vector along an axis. This operation may seem to be a complex way of coming up with f_1, which we already know is the first component

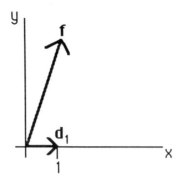

FIGURE 8.9.   Unit vector: the vector, **f**, and the unit vector, $\mathbf{d}_1$, are shown. The unit vector, $\mathbf{d}_1$, has length one and it is aligned along the x axis.

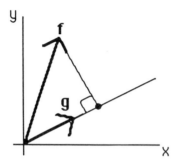

FIGURE 8.10.   Projection of **f** along **g**: the projection of the vector, **f**, along a line colinear with the vector, **g**, is the point closest to **f** along that line. A line from **f** to the projection of **f** along **g** forms a right angle with the line.

of **f**. But the advantage of this procedure is that we can use it to determine the projection of **f** along any line not just the x axis.

Figure 8.10 shows the projection of a vector, **f**, onto a line in the direction of **g**. The projection of **f** onto this line is the point on the line which is the closest to **f**. In order to calculate the projection we need to have a unit vector in the direction of **g**. We can easily produce this vector by dividing **g** by its length, g:

$$\mathbf{d}_g = \mathbf{g}/g \qquad (8.62)$$

Therefore, the projection of **f** onto **g** can be calculated as:

$$\mathbf{f}^T \cdot \mathbf{g}/g = f \cdot g \cdot \cos(\theta_f - \theta_g)/g = f \cdot \cos(\theta_f - \theta_g) \qquad (8.63)$$

The projection of **f** on **g** is the length of **f** times the cosine of the angle between **f** and **g**.

The concept of the projection of a vector along a line translates immediately to a multidimensional vector space. The projection of a vector along an axis is the value of the corresponding component. The projection of a vector along another vector can still be calculated as:

$$\mathbf{f}^T \cdot \mathbf{g}/g \qquad (8.64)$$

However, in a multidimensional vector space another operation also becomes possible — projection of a vector onto a subspace. For example, in a three-dimensional space we

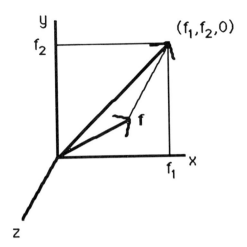

FIGURE 8.11.   Projection of a vector onto a subspace: the projection of a vector, **f**, with components, (f_1, f_2, f_3) onto the subspace which is the x,y plane is just a vector with components, $(f_1, f_2, 0)$.

can visualize the projection of a vector onto the x,y plane. The projection is the point on the plane which is closest to the vector (Figure 8.11). We can calculate the projection by calculating the projection on the x and y axes separately and then making a vector in the x,y plane which is made up from these two components. In this simple case the projection is a vector from the origin to the point $(f_1, f_2, 0)$.

The term projection is used in computed tomography to describe the data collection process. The computed tomography system is more complicated than the simple projection operation we have described, but it relies on the simple projection operation. A transverse section is two dimensional, but the data are collected in a one-dimensional subspace. The point at which a datum from the cross section is recorded is the projection of the location of the datum on the collection array. The datum itself is not ''projected'' in the sense used in this chapter. Rather, the position of the datum is projection onto the collection subspace.

E. ORTHOGONALITY

Two vectors are said to be orthogonal if their product is zero. In two dimensions we have already seen that the product of two vectors is zero if the vectors are at right angles to one another. The same is true in three dimensions. Although we have no geometrical intuition, the same idea can be extended to a multidimensional vector space. Orthogonality is a term which means:

$$\mathbf{f}^T \cdot \mathbf{g} = 0 \qquad (8.65)$$

The geometrical analog of orthongonality is perpendicularity (Figure 8.12).

The concept of orthogonality is sometimes applied to subspaces. If **f** is a vector in one subspace and **g** is a vector in another subspace, then the two subspaces are said to be orthogonal if the product of **f** and **g** is zero for all vectors. Orthogonal subspaces have no components in common except for the zero vector.

The concept of orthogonality turns out to be very important not only for linear algebra, but also for the other model of systems. For discrete signals, orthogonality is defined as:

$$\Sigma f[n] \cdot g[n] = 0 \qquad (8.66)$$

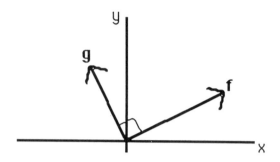

FIGURE 8.12. Orthogonal vectors: orthogonal vectors, **f**, and **g**, are vectors at right angles to each other.

For continuous signals, orthogonality is defined as:

$$\int_{-\infty}^{+\infty} f(t) \cdot g(t) \, dt = 0 \tag{8.67}$$

But what does it mean to say that two signals are orthogonal? Much of the intuition about orthogonality comes from the linear algebra model of systems. Orthogonal signals or vectors are not at all alike. They are ''perpendicular'' to each other. Above we stated the projection of a vector is related to correlation. Two signals which are orthogonal to each other have a projection which is zero; therefore, they are uncorrelated. The idea of orthogonality will come up repeatedly in the rest of the book. The geometric intuition about perpendicular vectors will help in understanding this important concept.

VII. SUMMARY

This chapter has covered many of the basic concepts of linear algebra. We have introduced vector and matrix notation and seen how they can be used to efficiently write down a set of simultaneous linear equations. We have introduced a large number of mathematical operations which can be performed on vectors and matrices.

Several of the concepts of linear algebra are important for understanding signals. The idea of projection or correlation of two signals will provide a useful insight in understanding the transform operations in Part II. The concept of orthogonality of signals provides a useful insight for basis signals. However, the most important use of linear algebra is described in the next chapter — definition of linear systems with matrix and vector notation.

VIII. FURTHER READING

A highly recommended book for those who wish to obtain a more detailed understanding of the methods of linear algebra is the book by Strang.[1] Our description of linear algebra is similar to the exposition in that book, except that our presentation is considerably less mathematically rigorous. Chapter 1 describes many of the basic operations with matrices and vectors. Chapter 1 of that book also describes the Gaussian elimination method of solving simultaneous linear equations in detail. Chapter 2 explains the important concept of a vector space from a more mathematically rigorous point of view. Chapter 3 describes the projection operation; however, the reader might wish to read Chapters 9 and 10 of this book before reading further about projection.

REFERENCE

1. **Strang, G.**, *Linear Algebra and its Applications,* Academic Press, New York, 1980.

Chapter 9

LINEAR ALGEBRA DESCRIPTION OF SYSTEMS

In the last chapter we introduced some of the basic concepts of linear algebra. In this chapter we shall see how the methods of linear algebra can be used to describe systems. The convolution model, described in Chapter 3, is the most common method of describing linear, time invariant systems. The linear algebra model, described in this chapter, is the most common method of describing linear systems, which are not time invariant.

We shall introduce the concept of basis vectors as a method of defining a vector space. We shall see that selection of the right basis vectors will provide an understanding of which signals pass through a system and which signals are stopped by a system. The idea of basis vectors will also be important in Part II when we describe rotations. The rotation of a vector space provides an understanding of transform operations. We shall come back to the linear algebra model in Part IV in order to solve the problem of single photon emission computed tomography.

I. LINEAR ALGEBRA MODEL OF A SYSTEM

In the linear algebra model of systems, vectors are used to represent the input and the output signals, and matrices are used to represent systems. A vector, $\mathbf{f}$, is equivalent to the input signal f[n], and the vector, $\mathbf{g}$, is equivalent to the output signal g[n]. The matrix, H, is equivalent to the system H $\{\cdot\}$. The operation of a linear system on a signal can be written mathematically:

$$\mathbf{g} = H \cdot \mathbf{f} \tag{9.1}$$

This relationship is shown diagrammatically in Figure 9.1.

This linear algebra notation is the same notation that was used to define a set of simultaneous linear equations in the last chapter. The input vector, $\mathbf{f}$, is analogous to the unknowns of the simultaneous linear equations. The output vector, $\mathbf{g}$, is analogous to the measured quantities. And the system, H, is analogous to the coefficients in the equations.

Let us expand Equation 9.1 using Equation 8.24, the equation describing the multiplication of a vector and a matrix:

$$g_i = \sum_j h_{ij} \cdot f_j \tag{9.2}$$

Each coefficient in the output vector is a linear combination of all of the input values. In Chapter 4 (Systems) we defined a linear system using continuous signals with the Equation 4.22:

$$g(t) = \int_{-\infty}^{+\infty} h(t,\tau) \cdot f(\tau) \, d\tau \tag{9.3}$$

Equation 9.2 is the discrete analog of Equation 9.3. The h_{ik} are analogous to the two-dimensional function h(t,τ). Thus, we can see that the linear algebra description of a system is the same as our previous definition of a linear system except that continuous signals and systems have been replaced by discrete signals and systems.

Equation 9.3 represents signals from $-\infty$ to ∞, i.e. signals over all time. So far we have considered vectors and matrices which are finite in dimension. It is possible to extend our description of vectors and matrices to include an infinite number of dimensions. In fact

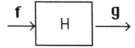

FIGURE 9.1.   The linear algebra model of a system: this figure shows a diagrammatic representation of a system in terms of a linear algebra model. H is a matrix representing the system. **f** is a vector representing the input signal. **g** is a vector representing the output signal.

in much of what follows we shall implicitly imply that the dimensions are infinite. However, in any real radiological problem, the signals will necessarily be finite. Since from a practical standpoint we only need finite signals, we shall ignore the mathematical fine points of the distinctions between finite and infinite dimensional vector spaces.

A. COMPARISON BETWEEN LINEAR AND LINEAR, TIME INVARIANT MODELS

Discrete convolution is a method of describing linear, time invariant systems. Discrete convolution can be written:

$$g(n) = \sum_{k} h[n - k] \cdot f[n] \qquad (9.4)$$

In order to see how discrete convolution relates to linear systems, let us recast this equation in terms of a matrix equation:

$$\begin{pmatrix} g[1] \\ g[2] \\ g[3] \\ \cdot \end{pmatrix} = \begin{pmatrix} h[1] & h[2] & h[3] & \ldots \\ 0 & h[1] & h[2] & \ldots \\ 0 & 0 & h[1] & \ldots \\ \cdot & \cdot & \cdot & \cdot \end{pmatrix} \cdot \begin{pmatrix} f[1] \\ f[2] \\ f[3] \\ \cdot \end{pmatrix} \qquad (9.5)$$

Notice that the rows of H take on a very special format. They are the values of h[n] shifted appropriately. Thus for an N by N matrix, H, the N^2 values in the matrix are given by the N values in the system function h[n].

The convolution method of describing a system is much more limited than the matrix method. The convolution method uses only N values to describe the system, while the matrix method has N^2 values. The difference between the two representations is due to the shift invariant property. The matrix description does not assume shift invariance. If the elements of **f** are shifted up or down, the output, **g**, will not in general be a shifted version of the original output.

In Chapter 4, we discovered this same fact, that shift invariance greatly simplified the description of a system. However, that argument was made in terms of continuous signals and convolution. Here we made the argument in terms of discrete signals and matrix multiplication.

Recall from Chapter 4, that many systems are not shift invariant. Almost all imaging systems are not shift invariant since the imaging system only records objects in the field of view. If the input signal moves out of the field of view, there is no output signal. In Chapter 4, we noted that it is still possible to use a linear, shift invariant model with many systems as long as we restrict the input signal to be contained in the field of view.

The major advantage of the linear algebra approach over the linear systems approach is that it can be used to describe systems which are not shift invariant. The major disadvantage is that the calculations are consequently much more time consuming. When possible it is better to use the convolution model; however, if the system is not shift invariant and if it cannot be made shift invariant, then the linear algebra model must be used.

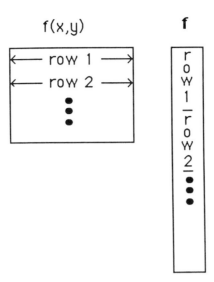

FIGURE 9.2. Representation of an image by a vector: the two-dimensional figure, f(x,y), can be represented by the one-dimensional vector, **f**, by assigning the successive rows of f(x,y) to sequential position in the vector.

Computed tomography is an example of a system for which a linear, shift invariant model can be used (see Chapter 31). The nonshift invariant effects, such as beam hardening, are relatively small so that they can be handled by using corrections. Single photon emission tomography, Chapter 33, is an example of a system where the linear model should be used. The shift invariances due to attenuation are too great to be easily corrected for.

B. TWO-DIMENSIONAL SIGNALS

The linear algebra description of a system uses vectors, which are one dimensional, as input and output signals. Yet images are two-dimensional signals, images. One might hope that there was some generalization of the linear algebra methods which allows the use of multi-dimensional input signals. Unfortunately, there is no such generalization.

Instead, what is usually done to overcome this incompatibility is to define an algorithm for placing the values from the image into a vector. Figure 9.2 shows a typical method of making a one-dimensional vector from an image. This algorithm can be used to transform an input image into a vector and it can be reversed to transform the output vector back into an image.

Although it is possible to describe a method which will allow a two or even a higher dimensional signal to be converted to a vector, the fact that the input signal must always be a vector is a major limitation of the linear systems model. A vector is not a very natural method for describing a two-dimensional signal, and the algorithms which must be used are consequently more complicated than for models which treat two-dimensional signals naturally.

Notice also that the size of the input vector and the matrix are enormous for picture processing operations. A 256 by 256 image has 65,536 elements, and therefore, the input and output vecotrs will have 65,536 components. The system is described by a 65,536 by 65,536 matrix — 4,294,967,296 elements! It is easy to appreciate why we shall need to describe special solution techniques for the computed tomography problem in Part IV.

II. BASIS VECTORS

In order to better understand the description of a system in terms of the methods of

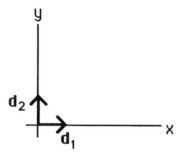

FIGURE 9.3.   Basis vectors for a two-dimensional coordinate system: $\mathbf{d}_1$ and $\mathbf{d}_2$ are orthonormal vectors along the x and y axes, respectively.

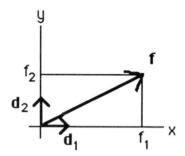

FIGURE 9.4.   Projections along a set of basis vectors: the projection of the vector, $\mathbf{f}$, along the direction of the basis vector, $\mathbf{d}_1$, is the first component of $\mathbf{f}$, f_1. The projection of $\mathbf{f}$ along the direction of the basis vector, $\mathbf{d}_2$, is the second component of $\mathbf{f}$, f_2.

linear algebra, we need to consider in greater detail the definition of a vector space. In the last chapter we defined a vector space in terms of intuitive geometrical concepts. We can obtain a deeper understanding of vector spaces by showing how a vector space can be defined in terms of a set of basis vectors. Basis vectors will not only help in understanding the operation of systems on signals, but also it will be important in Part II when we introduce the concept of rotation.

A set of basis vectors are vectors which can be used to define other vectors. The canonical set of basis vectors are unit vectors along the directions of the coordinate axis. We can define these vectors as:

$$
\begin{aligned}
\mathbf{d}_1^T &= (1 \quad 0 \quad 0 \quad ...) \\
\mathbf{d}_2^T &= (0 \quad 1 \quad 0 \quad ...) \\
\mathbf{d}_3^T &= (0 \quad 0 \quad 1 \quad ...) \\
... &= \cdot \quad \cdot \quad \cdot
\end{aligned}
\tag{9.6}
$$

Figure 9.3 shows the unit vectors for a two-dimensional vector space. $\mathbf{d}_1$ and $\mathbf{d}_2$ are unit vectors along the x and y axes, respectively.

Figure 9.4 is a geometric representation of a two-dimensional vector, $\mathbf{f}$. Again the basis vectors, $\mathbf{d}_1$ and $\mathbf{d}_2$, are unit vectors along the x and y axis of the coordinate system. The components of $\mathbf{f}$, f_1 and f_2, are the projections of $\mathbf{f}$ on the x and y axes. Figure 9.5 shows that the vector $\mathbf{f}$ can be constructed as the sum of two vectors, $f_1 \cdot \mathbf{d}_1$ and $f_2 \cdot \mathbf{d}_2$, which are scaled basis vectors. Obviously, any vector in this two-dimensional vector space can be constructed in a similar manner as a linear combination of the basis set, $\mathbf{d}_1$ and $\mathbf{d}_2$.

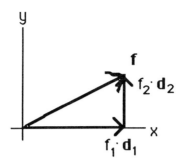

FIGURE 9.5. Construction of a vector using basis vectors: any vector, **f**, in the plane can be constructed using the basis vectors $\mathbf{d}_1$ and $\mathbf{d}_2$. The first component of **f** is f_1, times the basis vector, $\mathbf{d}_1$, and the second component of **f** is f_2, times the basis vector, $\mathbf{d}_2$.

In a vector space of any dimension a vector can be expressed as a linear combination of the canonical set of basis vectors:

$$\mathbf{f} = f_1 \cdot \mathbf{d}_1 + f_2 \cdot \mathbf{d}_2 + f_3 \cdot \mathbf{d}_3 + \ldots \tag{9.7}$$

The factors, f_1, are just the components of the vector along each of the directions $\mathbf{d}_1$.

The unit vectors, $\mathbf{d}_1$, $\mathbf{d}_2$ . . . , are a **basis** for the vector space. The word basis means that any vector in the vector space can be expressed as a linear sum of this vector set. The number of basis vectors is equal to the dimension, N, of the vector space. Using a weighted sum of these N vectors it is possible to construct every vector in the entire vector space.

This particular set of basis vectors has a number of useful properties. All of the basis vectors have length of one.

$$\mathbf{d}_i^T \cdot \mathbf{d}_i = 1 \tag{9.8}$$

Vectors of length one are called unit vectors. All of the basis vectors are orthogonal.

$$\mathbf{d}_i^T \cdot \mathbf{d}_j = 0 \qquad \text{if} \qquad i \neq j \tag{9.9}$$

Vectors which are orthogonal and of unit length are called **orthonormal** vectors.

Describing one vector in terms of the sum of a set of other vectors may seem like an unnecessary complication. However, this procedure should remind the reader of the description of a function in terms of shifted delta functions in Chapters 3 and 4. Remember that we defined a signal, f(t), as a sum of weighted and shifted delta functions, Equation 3.3:

$$f(t) = \int_{-\infty}^{+\infty} f(\tau) \cdot \delta(t - \tau) \, d\tau \tag{9.10}$$

The weighting factors for the delta functions were the values of f(·).

Description of f(t) in terms of the shifted delta functions is analogous to defining **f** in terms of the basis vectors, $\mathbf{d}_1$. Recall that the use of the delta function description made determination of the operation of a system on a signal particularly simple. We shall also find that description of a vector in terms of the proper basis will make understanding the operation of a system much more simple.

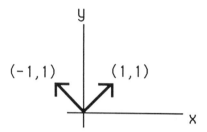

FIGURE 9.6.   A set of orthogonal basis vectors: the two vectors $(1\ 1)^T$ and $(-1\ 1)^T$ form a set of basis vectors for the x,y plane. In addition they are orthogonal to each other.

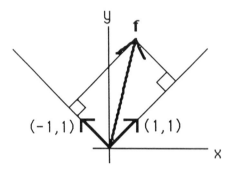

FIGURE 9.7.   Projection of a vector on a basis: the projections of **f** on the basis vectors from Figure 9.6 are shown by the lighter lines.

A.   DEFINITION OF A VECTOR SPACE IN TERMS OF A SET OF BASIS VECTORS

In the last chapter we introduced the concept of a vector space. We relied heavily on the geometrical intuition of two- and three-dimensional vector spaces in order to define vector spaces of any dimensions. A more mathematically rigorous approach is to define a set of basis vectors and then define a vector space as the set of all possible vectors which are linear combinations of the basis vectors.

The basis vectors, $\mathbf{d}_1, \mathbf{d}_2$ . . . are very special. They each have only a single nonzero value and that value is one. This set of basis vectors is very convenient since it corresponds exactly to our method of writing the components of a vector. Therefore, we can determine the weighting terms for this basis by inspection. There is, however, another point of view. Rather than saying that this basis set is determined by the way we have written the components of a vector, we could say that the method we have used to write the components of a vector is determined by this basis vector set.

It is possible to use some other set of vectors as a basis. For example, for a two-dimensional space, we could use the vectors:

$$\begin{pmatrix} 1 \\ 1 \end{pmatrix} \quad \text{and} \quad \begin{pmatrix} -1 \\ 1 \end{pmatrix} \tag{9.11}$$

These vectors are shown in Figure 9.6. This basis set is similar to the canonical basis except that the direction of the vectors has been rotated by $\pi/4$ and the length of the vectors is $\sqrt{2}$. Any vector in the plane can be made up from a linear combination of these two vectors. Figure 9.7 shows a vector, **f**, which is defined in terms of a linear combination of these vectors. The components of **f** are the projections of **f** along each of the basis vectors divided by $\sqrt{2}$.

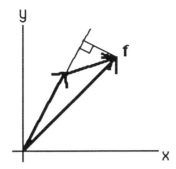

FIGURE 9.8. Nonorthogonal basis vectors: any vector, **f**, in the x,y plane may be constructed from any two noncolinear vectors which have been scaled appropriately. However, when the vectors are not orthogonal, the projection of **f** along the direction of the vectors will not give the scaling factor.

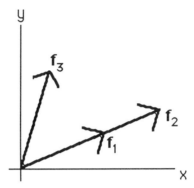

FIGURE 9.9. Vector spaces and basis vectors: each of the vectors, $\mathbf{f}_1$, $\mathbf{f}_2$, and $\mathbf{f}_3$, by itself defines a one-dimensional vector space. $\mathbf{f}_1$ and $\mathbf{f}_2$ taken together still only define a one-dimensional space, since they are not linearly independent vectors. Either $\mathbf{f}_1$ and $\mathbf{f}_3$, or $\mathbf{f}_2$ and $\mathbf{f}_3$ can be used as the basis of the x,y plane.

More generally, any vector in a plane can be made up from a linear combination any two vectors so long as the two vectors are not colinear. Basis vectors need not be orthogonal, and they need not be of length one. Of course it is useful if the basis vectors have these properties. Figure 9.8 shows an example of a vector which is made up as a sum to two other vectors. Notice that when the basis vectors are not orthogonal, then the components are not simply projections.

Given any set of vectors, we can define a vector space as the set of vectors which can be constructed as a linear combination of those vectors. The dimension of the vector space will be less than or equal to the number of vectors. Again let us use our geometrical intuition. Let us say that we have three vectors which each have three components. If the three vectors are all colinear, then the vector space which they define is one dimensional. If the three vectors lie in a single plane, then the vector space is two dimensional. If there is no plane which contains the three vectors, then the vector space is three dimensional.

Figure 9.9 shows three vectors, $\mathbf{f}_1$, $\mathbf{f}_2$, and $\mathbf{f}_3$. $\mathbf{f}_1$ and $\mathbf{f}_2$ are colinear; therefore, the vector space defined by these two vectors is a one-dimensional vector space, a line. Either combination $\mathbf{f}_1$ and $\mathbf{f}_3$, or $\mathbf{f}_2$ and $\mathbf{f}_3$ will define a vector space which is a plane. If all three vectors are used, then the vector space will still be a plane.

Although a vector space can be defined in terms of a set of basis vectors, it is important to understand the difference between the vector space and the basis vectors. In particular, two different sets of basis vectors may define the same vector space.

B. LINEAR INDEPENDENCE

The concept of **linear independence** will allow us to extend the idea of colinearity to any number of dimensions. Two vectors, f_1 and f_2, are said to be linearly dependent if there are numbers a_1 and a_2 such that:

$$a_1 \cdot f_1 + a_2 \cdot f_2 = 0 \qquad (9.12)$$

If this equation can be solved, the f_2 is just a multiple of f_1. The two vectors are colinear. If there are no numbers a_1 and a_2 which solve this equation, then the two vectors point in different directions.

Figure 9.9 shows three vectors, f_1, f_2, and f_3. f_1 and f_2 are linearly dependent since they point in the same direction. f_3 is linearly independent of f_1, and f_3 is linearly independent of f_2, since f_3 points in a different direction.

Let us extend the idea of linear independence to three dimensions. Three vectors are linearly dependent if there are numbers a_i such that:

$$a_1 \cdot f_1 + a_2 \cdot f_2 + a_3 \cdot f_3 = 0 \qquad (9.13)$$

If this equation can be solved, then f_3 can be written in terms of a linear combination of f_1 and f_2. For example, if f_1 is a vector along the x axis and f_2 is a vector along the y axis, then any vector in the x,y plane can be written as a linear combination of f_1 and f_2. If f_3 is in the x,y plane then the vectors are linearly dependent. If f_3 has a component in the z direction, then the vectors are linearly independent.

We can extend the idea of linear independence to any number of vectors:

$$\sum_i a_i \cdot f_i = 0 \qquad (9.14)$$

If there is no set of numbers a_i which will solve this equation, then the set of vectors f_i are linearly independent. We have no geometrical insight for more than three vectors, but again we shall extend our three-dimensional insight to larger dimensional vector spaces.

Now let us return to the definition of a vector space in terms of an arbitrary set of vectors. If the vectors are all linearly independent, then no vector can be defined in terms of the remaining vectors. All of the vectors point in "different directions". The **dimension of the vector space** defined by these vectors is equal to the number of vectors in the set. If the vectors are not linearly independent, then some of the vectors can be defined as linear combinations of other vectors. In this case some of the vectors could be discarded without decreasing the dimension of the vector space. The vector space will have a dimension which is equal to the number of vectors in the largest set of linearly independent vectors.

C. EXAMPLES OF VECTOR SPACES

Although the idea of a vector space, and the idea of a set of basis vectors defining a vector space may seem very abstract, in real problems, the set of basis vectors is defined very naturally. For example, in nuclear magnetic resonance imaging a natural basis set would be unit vectors corresponding to each of the spatial dimensions, d_x, d_y, d_z, and a unit vector corresponding to the intensity of the signal coming from this point d_I. This basis vector set would define a four-dimensional vector space. A vector, f, in this vector space could be written in terms of its components or in terms of a linear combination of the basis vectors.

$$f^T = (x \quad y \quad z \quad I)$$
$$= x \cdot d_x + y \cdot d_y + z \cdot d_z + I \cdot d_I \qquad (9.15)$$

If we were also interested in chemical shift and flow, we could add a unit vector corresponding to chemical shift and three unit vectors which correspond to flow in each of the three dimensions. These eight vectors would then define an eight dimensional vector space. The first three components of a vector in this eight-dimensional vector space, could represent the x, y, and z position of a point. The next component could give a particular chemical shift. The next three components could define a velcoity in a particular direction. The last component would give the intensity of the signal arising from nuclei at this particular position, chemical shift, and velocity.

III. SIGNALS WHICH PASS THROUGH A SYSTEM

Definition of a vector space in terms of a set of basis vectors will help to explain the class of signals which pass through a linear system. Some signals will pass through a system, H, and some signals will be stopped by the system. In order to understand which signals will pass through H and which signals will be stopped by H, we shall need to take an excursion into some of the mathematics associated with matrices.

An important number associated with any matrix is the **rank,** r, of the matrix. If we think of a matrix as representing a set of simultaneous linear equations, the rank is the number of independent equations.

Independent equations give unique relationships between the knowns and the unknowns. A dependent equation gives a relationship which could be derived from other equations. For example, consider the two equations:

$$g_1 = 3f_1 + f_2$$
$$g_2 = 6f_1 + 2f_2 \tag{9.16}$$

The unknowns in the second equation are two times the value of the unknowns in the first equation. Therefore, these two equations are not independent. g_1 and g_2 are just two measurements of the same relationship. A matrix given by the coefficients of this set of equations would have a rank of one.

In the following discussion it is useful to consider a matrix as a set of vectors. We can view a matrix, H, as a set of column vectors $\mathbf{h}_j$:

$$H = (\mathbf{h}_j) = (\mathbf{h}_1 \quad \mathbf{h}_2 \quad \mathbf{h}_3) = \begin{pmatrix} | & | & | \\ h_{i1} & h_{i2} & h_{i3} \\ | & | & | \end{pmatrix} \tag{9.17}$$

Alternately, we can think of a matrix as a collection of row vectors h_i^T:

$$H = (\mathbf{h}_i^T) = \begin{pmatrix} \mathbf{h}_1^T \\ \mathbf{h}_2^T \\ \mathbf{h}_3^T \end{pmatrix} = \begin{pmatrix} -h_{1j}- \\ -h_{2j}- \\ -h_{3j}- \end{pmatrix} \tag{9.18}$$

A. VECTOR SPACES ASSOCIATED WITH A MATRIX

The set of simultaneous linear equations represented by the matrix, H, can be rewritten in terms of $\mathbf{h}_j$, the columns of H:

$$\mathbf{g} = H \cdot \mathbf{f} = \left(\sum_j h_{ij} \cdot f_j \right) = \sum_j f_j \cdot \mathbf{h}_j \tag{9.19}$$

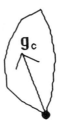

FIGURE 9.10.   Artistic representation of a vector space: since it is not possible to draw a multidimensional vector space, we shall represent a vector space as a blob. The point on the bottom of the blob is used to indicate the position of the origin. The vector $\mathbf{g}_c$ is a vector in this vector space.

where we have written the summation in terms of the column vectors $\mathbf{h}_j$. Expanding the summation gives:

$$\mathbf{g} = f_1 \cdot \mathbf{h}_1 + f_2 \cdot \mathbf{h}_2 + f_3 \cdot \mathbf{h}_3 + \ldots \qquad (9.20)$$

The f_i are the scalars which are the components of the vector $\mathbf{f}$, and the $\mathbf{h}_j$ are vectors which are the columns of H. This equation says that $\mathbf{g}$ is a linear combination of the columns of H. We can define a vector space which is made up from all of linear combinations of the vectors which are the columns of H. This vector space is called the **column space** of H. Equation 9.20 says that $\mathbf{g}$ must be in the column space of H.

For this discussion we shall emphasize that $\mathbf{g}$ is in the column space of H, by writing it as $\mathbf{g}_c$. It is not possible to draw a picture of a multi-dimensional vector space, so we need an abstract method of representing the column space of H. In Figure 9.10 we have chosen to represent this multi-dimensional space as a blob with a point indicating the zero vector.

The columns of H do not all need to be independent vectors. If they were all independent, then the dimension of the vector space made of the columns of H will be equal to the number of columns, n. Otherwise, the vector space will have a dimension less than n. It can be shown[1] that the dimension of the column space of H is equal to the rank of H.

The rows of H also represent vectors. We can also define a vector space made from the rows of H. This vector space is called the **row space** of H. It can be shown[1] that the row space and the column space of H have the same dimension. Thus, the dimension of these two vector spaces and the rank of H are all equal to the same number.

Another important space associated with H is the null space of H. We can define the null space of H with use of the equation:

$$H \cdot \mathbf{f} = \mathbf{0} \qquad (9.21)$$

where $\mathbf{0}$ is the zero vector, a vector with all zero components. Clearly, one possible solution for this equation is for the vector $\mathbf{f}$ to be equal to $\mathbf{0}$. However, for some systems, there are other vectors which satisfy this equation. If there are other vectors which satisfy the equation, then the matrix is said to be **singular** (see Chapter 8). The **null space** of H is defined as all those vectors which satisfy this equation. In terms of systems, signals which satisfy this equation do not pass through the system. They are stopped by the system.

From Equation 9.18, we can rewrite Equation 9.21 with an equation for each row of H, $\mathbf{h}_i^T$:

$$\mathbf{h}_i^T \cdot \mathbf{f} = 0 \qquad (9.22)$$

In other words, vectors in the null space of H are orthogonal to all of the rows of H. This implies that all vectors in the null space of H are orthogonal to all vectors in the row space

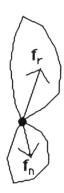

FIGURE 9.11. Row space and null space of H: the row space and the null space of H are shown as two blobs. $\mathbf{f}_r$ is a vector in the row space of H and $\mathbf{f}_n$ is a vector in the null space of H.

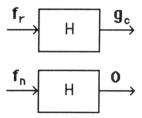

FIGURE 9.12. Signals which pass through H: any input vector, $\mathbf{f}$, can be divided into two parts — $\mathbf{f}_r$, the projection of $\mathbf{f}$ on the row space of H, and $\mathbf{f}_n$, the projection of $\mathbf{f}$ on the null space of H. $\mathbf{f}_r$ pass through H to produce the output vector, $\mathbf{g}_c$. $\mathbf{f}_n$ is stopped by H; the output is the zero vector, $\mathbf{0}$.

of H. This result is very interesting in terms of systems. Signals which are in the row space of H, pass through H; signals which are not in the row space of H are stopped by H.

We can divide the input signal $\mathbf{f}$ into two components — the portion in the row space of H, $\mathbf{f}_r$, and the portion in the null space of H, $\mathbf{f}_n$:

$$\mathbf{f} = \mathbf{f}_r + \mathbf{f}_n \tag{9.23}$$

The two spaces are orthogonal — the only vector they have in common is the zero vector. Figure 9.11 shows these relationships artistically. The two orthogonal spaces, the row space and the null space are shown as blobs. They share in common one point, the zero vector. Figure 9.12 shows the operation of H as a system using block diagrams. $\mathbf{f}_r$ goes through H to produce $\mathbf{g}_c$. $\mathbf{f}_n$ is stopped by H. Figure 9.13 shows this same relationship with the vector spaces represented as blobs. The portion of f which is in the row space of H, $\mathbf{f}_r$, gives rise to the output vector, $\mathbf{g}_c$. The other portion of $\mathbf{f}$, which is in the null space of H, $\mathbf{f}_n$, gives rise to the zero vector.

If there are two signals, $\mathbf{f}$ and $\mathbf{f}'$, which give the same output signal $\mathbf{g}_c$, then:

$$H \cdot (\mathbf{f} - \mathbf{f}') = H \cdot \mathbf{f} - H \cdot \mathbf{f}' = \mathbf{g}_c - \mathbf{g}_c = \mathbf{0} \tag{9.24}$$

Thus, the difference between any two vectors which give rise to the same output vector is in the null space of H. What Equation 9.24 means is that any two vectors which give rise to the same output are different only in terms of the subspace of vectors which do not pass through H. Thus, for each vector, $\mathbf{f}_r$, in the row space of H, there is one and only one output vector. We have already shown that the output vector, $\mathbf{g}_c$, is in the column space of H.

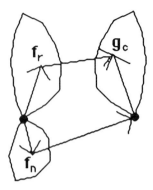

FIGURE 9.13. The effect of a system: a system, H, maps the portion of **f** in its row space, **f**$_r$, into the output vector **g**$_c$. The other portion, **f**$_n$, is mapped into the zero vector, **0**.

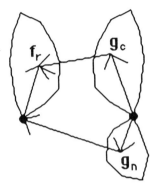

FIGURE 9.14. The effect of the pseudoinverse of a system: the pseudoinverse of a system maps, **g**$_c$, the portion of a vector, **g**, which is in the column space of H into **f**$_r$. The other portion of **g**, **g**$_n$, is mapped into the zero vector.

Thus, there is a one-to-one relation between input vectors in the row space of H and output vectors in the column space of H.

Since there is a one-to-one relationship between input vectors in the row space of H and output vectors in the column space of H, it is possible to construct an inverse relationship for these spaces. This inverse relationship is called the **pseudoinverse** of H. The pseudoinverse is whimsically written as, H^+. The pseudoinverse takes vectors from the column space of H and transforms them into the row space of H. There are techniques for calculating the pseudoinverse; however, we are more interested in the concept of a pseudoinverse than in its implementation. Therefore, we shall not discuss these techniques.

The input vectors, **g**$_c$, for the pseudoinverse, H^+, are the output vectors of H. Therefore, the column space of the pseudoinverse is the same space as the row space of H or the column space of H^T. The column space of H^T and H^+ are the same; however, the column vectors are different. Although H^T and the pseudoinverse have some similarities, the reader should be aware that they are different matrices.

There may be vectors, **g**, which are not in the column space of H. By definition the pseudoinverse, H^+, maps these vectors into the zero vector, **0**. In other words the vectors which are not a part of the column space of H form the null space of the pseudoinverse. This space is also called the **left null space** of H. We shall call these vectors, **g**$_n$. Like the input vectors, **f**, the output vectors, **g**, are divided into to parts, **g**$_c$ and **g**$_n$. Figure 9.14 shows

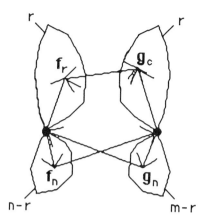

FIGURE 9.15. Vector spaces associated with a matrix: this diagram shows the vector spaces associated with a matrix and its pseudoinverse. $\mathbf{f}_r$ is a vector in the r dimensional row space, where r is the rank of the matrix. $\mathbf{f}_n$ is a vector in the n − r dimensional null space of the matrix. $\mathbf{g}_c$ is a vector in the r dimensional column space of the matrix. $\mathbf{g}_n$ is a vector in the m − r dimensional null space of the pseudoinverse of the matrix.

the operation of the pseudoinverse diagrammatically. The portion of $\mathbf{g}$ which is in the column space of H, $\mathbf{g}_c$, is mapped into $\mathbf{f}_r$. The other portion of $\mathbf{g}$, $\mathbf{g}_n$ is mapped into $\mathbf{0}$.

The input vectors have a number of dimensions, n, equal to the columns of H. The column space of H is equal to r, the rank of the matrix. Since vectors in the null space of H are orthogonal to the column space of H, the dimension of the null space is n − r. Output vectors have a number of dimensions, m, equal to the rows of H. The row space of H is also equal to r, the rank of the matrix. The dimension of the null space of the pseudoinverse, H^+, of H is m − r. Figure 9.15 attempts to summarize all of these realtionships graphically.

In linear algebra texts it is common to refer to a system, H, as a **mapping** from the row space to the column space. The row space is called the **domain** of the mapping, and the column space is called the **range** of the mapping.

B. EXAMPLES OF THE VECTOR SPACES ASSOCIATED WITH MATRICES

Let us consider a very simple system:

$$H = \begin{pmatrix} 1 & 0 & 0 \\ 0 & 1 & 0 \\ 0 & 0 & 0 \end{pmatrix} \tag{9.25}$$

This system takes a three-dimensional input vector and zeroes the third component. Figure 9.16 shows the action of this system in terms of an x,y,z coordinate system. A basis for the row space of H is given by the first two rows of H, $\mathbf{d}_1$ and $\mathbf{d}_2$, respectively. The row space of H includes all vectors in the x,y plane. Thus, $\mathbf{f}_r$ is the projection of $\mathbf{f}$ on the x,y plane.

The output, $\mathbf{g}_c$, will be in the column space of H. A basis of the column space is given by the first two columns of H. In this very special case, the column space is the same as the row space. For any vector in the row space of H plane, the output will be the same vector in the x,y plane.

Any vector in the one-dimensional space along the z axis will give an output of $\mathbf{0}$. Therefore, $\mathbf{d}_3$ is a basis of the null space of H. For any input vector $\mathbf{f}$, the projection of $\mathbf{f}$ along the x,y plane, $\mathbf{f}_r$, will pass through the system, H, while the projection along the z axis, $\mathbf{f}_n$, will be stopped by the system.

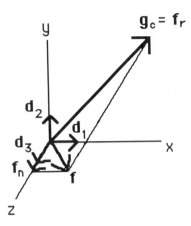

FIGURE 9.16.   Effect of A matrix which projects a vector on the x,y plane: this figure shows the effect of the matrix given by Equation 9.25. This matrix zeroes the z component of a vector. d_1 and d_2 are a basis for the row space of the matrix. The output vector, g_c, is equal to the projection of f on the x,y plane. d_3 is a basis for the null space of the matrix. The projection of f on the null space of the matrix is f_n.

In this special case, the pseudoinverse of this system, H^+, is equal to the same matrix, H. The null space of the pseudoinverse is all vectors, g_n, along the z axis. The projection of g on the x,y plane, g_c, passes through the pseudoinverse to produce, f_r, while the projection of g on the z axis, g_n, is stopped by the pseudoinverse.

As a second example, consider the system:

$$H = \begin{pmatrix} 1 & 0 & 0 \\ 0 & 0 & 1 \\ 0 & 0 & 0 \end{pmatrix} \qquad (9.26)$$

This system switches the third component of f to the second component of g, passes the first component through unchanged, and zeros the last component of g:

$$g = (f_1 \quad f_3 \quad 0)^T \qquad (9.27)$$

Like the system given by Equation 9.25, this system is very simple. The y component of the vector is stopped by the system, and the z component of the vector is flipped to the y axis.

The output vectors are in the column space of H, which is the x,y plane. The input vectors are in the row space of H, which is the x,z plane. The null space of H is the y axis, and the left null space of H is the z axis. The component of f which is in the x,z plane is mapped by H into g which is in the x,y plane.

A more radiological example is limited angle tomography in nuclear medicine. In limited angle tomography, a cross section is viewed from some but not all angles around the cross section. Due to this incomplete sampling, the vector space associated with the data has fewer dimensions than the vector space associated with the cross section. Some of the information about the cross section is mapped to the data, but some of the information is not. The cross section can not be exactly reconstructed since some components from the cross-sectional space are not mapped to the data space. These components are stopped by the data collection process.

IV. EIGENVECTORS OF A LINEAR SYSTEM

In Chapter 5 the eigenfunctions of a system were defined as signals which pass through a system without changing their form except possibly for a change in magnitude (Equation 5.1):

$$g(t) = H\{f(t)\} = \lambda \cdot f(t) \tag{9.28}$$

where λ is called the eigenvalue. Analogously we can define the **eigenvectors** of a matrix as those input vectors which go through the systems represented by the matrix without changing except possibly for a change in magnitude:

$$\mathbf{g} = H \cdot \mathbf{f} = \lambda \cdot \mathbf{f} \tag{9.29}$$

where λ is the **eigenvalue** for the eigenvectors, $\mathbf{f}$.

If we have a vector which is a linear combination of the eigenvectors of matrix, then the product of the matrix times the signal is particularly easy to calculate. It is just the same linear combination of the eigenvectors with each eigenvector multiplied times its eigenvalue. In Chapter 5, we noted that this property is one of the great values of the eigenvector description of systems.

In order to better understand eigenvectors, let us consider a simple example:

$$H = \begin{pmatrix} 2 & 0 \\ 0 & 1 \end{pmatrix} \tag{9.30}$$

This simple system multiplies the first component of a vector by two and the second component of the vector by one. A set of eigenvectors of this matrix is $\mathbf{d}_1$ and $\mathbf{d}_2$ since

$$H \cdot \mathbf{d}_1 = 2 \cdot \mathbf{d}_1 \tag{9.31}$$

and

$$H \cdot \mathbf{d}_2 = 1 \cdot \mathbf{d}_2 \tag{9.32}$$

The eigenvalues are 2 and 1, respectively. Vectors in other directions are not eigenvectors.

$$\begin{pmatrix} 2 & 0 \\ 0 & 1 \end{pmatrix} \cdot \begin{pmatrix} 1 \\ 1 \end{pmatrix} = \begin{pmatrix} 2 \\ 1 \end{pmatrix} \tag{9.33}$$

The output vector, $(2\ 1)^T$ is not a multiple of the input vector, $(1\ 1)^T$.

Let us consider a slightly more complicated matrix:

$$H = \begin{pmatrix} 1.8 & .4 \\ .4 & 1.2 \end{pmatrix} \tag{9.34}$$

The eigenvectors of this matrix are $(2\ 1)^T$ and $(-1\ 2)^T$. We can prove this by multiplication:

$$\begin{pmatrix} 1.8 & .4 \\ .4 & 1.2 \end{pmatrix} \cdot \begin{pmatrix} 2 \\ 1 \end{pmatrix} = \begin{pmatrix} 4 \\ 2 \end{pmatrix} = 2 \cdot \begin{pmatrix} 2 \\ 1 \end{pmatrix} \tag{9.35}$$

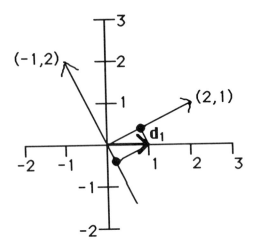

FIGURE 9.17.   Projection of $\mathbf{d}_1$ on the eigenvectors of H: this figure shows the projection of the unit vector along the x axis, $\mathbf{d}_1$, on the vectors $(2\ 1)^T$ and $(-1\ 2)^T$.

and

$$\begin{pmatrix} 1.8 & .4 \\ .4 & 1.2 \end{pmatrix} \cdot \begin{pmatrix} -1 \\ 2 \end{pmatrix} = \begin{pmatrix} -1 \\ 2 \end{pmatrix} \tag{9.36}$$

The eigenvalues are 2 and 1, respectfully.

Other vectors, such as $\mathbf{d}_1$, change direction when they pass through the matrix:

$$\begin{pmatrix} 1.8 & .4 \\ .4 & 1.2 \end{pmatrix} \cdot \begin{pmatrix} 1 \\ 0 \end{pmatrix} = \begin{pmatrix} 1.8 \\ .4 \end{pmatrix} \tag{9.37}$$

Figure 9.17 shows the projection of $\mathbf{d}_1$ on the eigenvectors of this matrix.

Equation 5.4 gave a simple method of calculating the effect of a system on functions which could be expressed as linear combinations of eigenfunctions of a system. If $\mathbf{f}$ is a vector which can be written as a linear combination of the eigenvectors, $\mathbf{f}_1$ and $\mathbf{f}_2$, of a system:

$$\mathbf{f} = a_1 \cdot \mathbf{f}_1 + a_2 \cdot \mathbf{f}_2 \tag{9.38}$$

Then Equation 5.4 can be rewritten in terms of vectors:

$$\mathbf{g} = a_1 \cdot \lambda_1 \cdot \mathbf{f}_1 + a_2 \cdot \lambda_2 \cdot \mathbf{f}_2 \tag{9.39}$$

where λ_1 is the eigenvalue of $\mathbf{f}_1$, and λ_2 is the eigenvalue of $\mathbf{f}_2$.

For example, $\mathbf{d}_1$ can be written in terms of the eigenvectors of the matrix given by Equation 9.34:

$$\mathbf{d}_1 = \begin{pmatrix} 1 \\ 0 \end{pmatrix} = .4 \cdot \begin{pmatrix} 2 \\ 1 \end{pmatrix} + .2 \cdot \begin{pmatrix} -1 \\ 2 \end{pmatrix} \tag{9.40}$$

This representation can be used to calculate the output, $H \cdot \mathbf{d}_1$:

$$.8 \cdot \begin{pmatrix} 2 \\ 1 \end{pmatrix} - .2 \cdot \begin{pmatrix} -1 \\ 2 \end{pmatrix} = \begin{pmatrix} 1.8 \\ .4 \end{pmatrix} \tag{9.41}$$

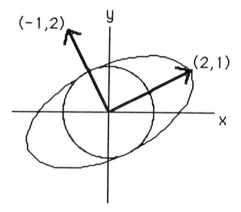

FIGURE 9.18.   The effect of the system given by Equation 9.34: the circle is used to represent a whole set of input vectors for the system given by Equation 9.34. The set of output vectors which result by applying this system is shown by the ellipse. The effect of this system is to multiply the projection of the input vector which is along the major axis of the ellipse by two and to multiply the projection of the input vector which is along the minor axis of the ellipse by one.

where .8 is equal to .4 times the eigenvalue, 2, of the first eigenvectors and .2 is equal to .2 times the eigenvalue, 1, of the second eigenvectors. This result is the same result which we obtained by matrix multiplication in Equation 9.37. In this simple case, calculation of the output from a linear combination of the eigenvectors is not easier than from the matrix multiplication. However, with a large matrix, this process would be much simpler.

The operation of the matrix given by Equation 9.34 is shown graphically in Figure 9.18. For input vectors which lie around the unit circle (a circle with radius equal to one), the output vectors lie along an ellipse. The eigenvectors are in the directions of the major and minor axes of the ellipse.

The eigenvectors and eigenvalues tell us a great deal about this matrix. The portion of the input vector which lies along the major axis $(2\ 1)^T$ is multiplied by 2 and the portion which lies along the minor axis $(-1\ 2)^T$ is unchanged. The eigenvectors characterize this system. The directions of the eigenvectors are the directions in which the system operates. Other directions are not characteristic of the system, rather the system operates on them in proportion to the projections along the eigenvectors.

The matrix given in Equation 9.30 would be the same as that given in Equation 9.34 if the x and y axes were rotated to the vectors $(2\ 1)^T$ and $(-1\ 2)^T$. We shall describe rotation of vector spaces in Chapter 19. In that chapter, we shall learn that the operation of a Fourier transform is analogous to a rotation. The Fourier transform rotates the coordinate axes to a set of axes which are eigenvalues of the system. Since these are the directions along which the system operates, it is simpler to calculate the results of the operation of the system and to understand the system in this eigenvector coordinate system. But more of this later.

All of the vectors which are linear combinations of the eigenvectors define a vector space. For any vector in this vector space we have a simple method of calculating the effect of a system on a signal. In the case of linear, time invariant systems we have stated that transposing a signal into a description in terms of its eigenfunctions can be done efficiently with the fast Fourier transform. Unfortunately, there is no efficient method of transforming a signal into a description in terms of the eigenvectors of a linear system. Furthermore, the eigenvector space may not include all of the interesting input vectors. Thus, although the eigenvectors of a matrix provide us with some useful insights, they do not in general lead to efficient methods of solving radiological problems.

V. SUMMARY

In this chapter we have shown that linear algebra can be used as a model for describing the action of a system on a signal. The linear algebra model relies on the fact that the system is linear, but does not require that it be time invariant. Because it does not impose the time invariant restriction on the system it can be used to model a much wider class of systems. However, the price paid is that calculations are much more difficult.

Two simple methods of calculating the output of a system appeared briefly — the inverse matrix and eigenvectors. Unfortunately, neither of these methods is of much use for radiological problems. We shall see in Part III that approximate methods must be used.

The important concept of a vector space was considered more deeply in this chapter, and the vector spaces associated with a matrix were introduced. From these vector spaces we were able to understand that certain portions of a signal get through systems and other portions are stopped by a system. If we wish to make a measurement with a system, then it is important that the data in which we are interested are in the row space of the system and not in the null space. If the data are in the null space, then none of the data which we collect will be of any use.

VI. FURTHER READING

As for the last chapter, the major reference for this chapter is the book by Strang.[1] The defintion of a vector space in terms of a set of basis vectors is described in Chapter 2 of that book. The vector spaces associated with a matrix are also described in Chapter 2. There is a considerably more detailed description of the eigenvectors of a matrix in Chapter 5. A more advanced book by the same author[2] discusses the use of matrices to represent systems at greater length.

REFERENCES

1. **Strang, G.,** *Linear Algebra and Its Applications,* Academic Press, New York, 1980.
2. **Strang, G.,** *Introduction to Applied Mathematics,* Wellesley-Cambridge Press, Wellesley, MA, 1986.

Chapter 10

RANDOM VARIABLES

We have described three different models which can be used to describe a system — convolution, differential equations, and linear algebra. However, so far we have not considered the effects of noise on systems. In all radiologic applications the signals which we measure will have measurement noise. Therefore, if these models are to be of use to us we shall have to consider what happens when the signals are not exact, but rather have noise added to them.

In the next three chapters, we shall introduce some of the basic concepts of the statistical description of signals. There are several important concepts which will be introduced, but in addition much of this material is basic mathematics which will be of use later. In Part III we shall see how noisy signals pass through systems. In Part IV we shall solve several radiological problems involving noisy signals.

I. PROBABILITY DENSITY FUNCTION

If we make a number of measurements of a quantity, we shall find that each measurement results in a slightly different value. If the measurement technique is good, then the values will tend to be close together. If the measurement is less good, then the values will be more spread out. We can describe this experiment by defining a **probability density function,** p(f), which is the probability that the value, f, will be obtained on each trial. Figure 10.1 shows an example of a probability density function. A value of three is the most likely value; however, other values close to three also occur fairly commonly. Values farther from three occur less frequently.

The probability of obtaining some value is obviously equal to one. Therefore, the area under any probability density function must be one:

$$\int_{-\infty}^{+\infty} p(f) \, df = 1 \qquad (10.1)$$

A typical example of an experiment which can be described by a probability density function is counting a radioactive sample. Each time the sample is counted, a different value may be obtained. It is possible to derive the shape of the probability density function for radioactive decay; it is a Poisson distribution. Determination of the shape of probability density functions come from probability theory. In this book we shall not discuss probability theory. The references at the end of the chapter all include discussions of probability theory.

The probability density function is an abstract concept, which is used to model real situations. We can estimate the probability density function by obtaining a large number of experiments and seeing how frequently each value occurs. However, the probability density function obtained from some sample of values is just an estimate. The assumption which is made by having a statistical model of the experiment is that there is a ''true'' probability density function. It is important to retain the distinction between the ''true'' model of the system and the estimates obtained from a set of sample values.

If we know the probability density function for an experiment, we know a great deal about what to expect from the experiment. We know for example that certain outcomes are exceedingly unlikely. We know other values are quite likely. The probability density function provides *a priori* information about an experiment. In radiological application we usually do not know the probability density function, but we often know something about it, e.g., estimates of the mean and standard deviation. The basic reason for having a statistical model

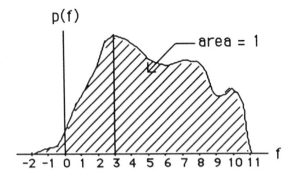

FIGURE 10.1.   Probability density function: this figure shows an example of a probability density function. The probability, p(f), of obtaining the value, f, for each experiment represented by random variable, *f*, is shown in graphical form. The most likely value is three. The area under all probability density functions is equal to one.

of an experiment is that this *a priori* information helps us to evaluate a particular experimental outcome.

II. RANDOM VARIABLES

In simple situations, the probability density function can be used to describe everything which we need to know about an experiment. However, when we are interested in describing a complex experiment, it is awkward to use the probability density notation. Therefore, we shall introduce a concept called a **random variable.** We shall use italics to indicate a random variable, e.g., *f. f* is a shorthand notation to indicate that in an experiment the values, f, will be obtained with a frequency given by a probability density function, p(f). A random variable is considerably more complicated than a simple variable since it implies an underlying probability density function, p(f).

A few words about notation may be in order. We shall use the nonitalics letters such as, f, to indicate the values which the random variable, *f*, can assume. Thus the probability density function for the random variable *f* is $p_f(f)$, where the independent variable, f, is the possible outcome values for the experiment represented by the random variable, *f*. The subscript, *f*, on p is used to indicate that $p_f(f)$ is the probability density function for *f*. When there is no confusion about which random variable is being referenced, we shall abbreviate $p_f(f)$ as p(f).

A. SUM OF TWO RANDOM VARIABLES

The value of defining a random variable is that more complicated experiments can be easily expressed. For example, we can write:

$$g = f + n \qquad (10.2)$$

to indicate that an experiment *g* consists of adding the results of two random variables *f* and *n*. For example, *f* might represent the value of an attenuation coefficient in a region of interest in a computer tomography examination. *n* could represent the measurement noise. The measured value, *g*, is the sum of the attenuation coefficient and the noise.

Using a random variable, *f*, to represent the attenuation coefficient implies that we have some *a priori* knowledge about what value to expect. We also have an *a priori* model of the measurement noise. The model of the experiment given by equation 10.2 allows us to combine our medical knowledge about the expected value of the attenuation coefficient with our radiological knowledge about the noise in the measurement process to determine the expected value of the measurement.

Equation 10.2 expresses how the individual samples from the two random variables are combined by the experiment — they add. However, it does not express how the probability density functions are combined. The probability density function for g, $p(g)$, is not a simple addition of $p(f)$ and $p(n)$. A particular value, g, of g can be produced by any combination of values for f and n which add up to g.

If on a particular experiment we obtain a value for n which is n, then if the value for f is equal to g $-$ n, the value for g will be:

$$n + (g - n) = g \qquad (10.3)$$

The likelihood of getting value n for n and g $-$ n for f is $p_n(n) \cdot p_f(g - n)$. To determine the probability of getting the value g for g we can integrate over all of the possible values of n:

$$p_g(g) = \int_{-\infty}^{+\infty} p_f(g - n) \cdot p_n(n) \, dn \qquad (10.4)$$

This relation is shown in Figure 10.2.

Equation 10.4 is identical to the convolution integral, Equation 3.4. The probability density function of the sum of two random variables is the convolution of the probability density functions of these variables. The simple equation:

$$g = f + n \qquad (10.5)$$

hides the fact that the probability density functions are combined in a very complicated way. We have defined random variables so that we can easily define how the various factors contribute to an experimental result. However, it is important to remember that this simple notation stands for a much more complex operation.

Figure 10.3 shows three probability density functions, $p(f)$, $p(n)$, and $p(g)$. The probability density function for f, $p(f)$ provides the *a priori* radiological knowledge about the measurement. Suppose that we know that only the values from zero to one are possible, but we do not know which of these values is most likely. This knowledge can be modeled as a probability density function where all values from zero to one are equally likely. The probability density function, $p(n)$, contains our *a priori* information about the measurement noise. We have assumed that the noise is Gaussian with a standard deviation of one. The probability density function, $p(g)$, is a model of the experiment which combines the two sources of *a priori* information.

B. MEAN

The probability density function of a random variable contains all of the information about the random variable. However, in real situations we hardly ever know or even have an estimate of the probability density function. Instead we often deal with parameters which describe it, such as the mean and the variance. We shall define the **mean** as:

$$m_f = E\{f\} = \int_{-\infty}^{+\infty} f \cdot p(f) \, df \qquad (10.6)$$

When there is no confusion about which random variable is being referred to we shall use m instead of m_f.

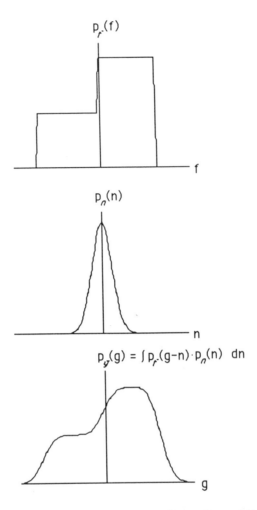

FIGURE 10.2.   Probability density function for the sum of two random variables: the top panel shows the probability density function, $p_f(f)$, for random variable, f. The second panel shows the probability density function, $p_n(n)$, for a second random variable, n. The bottom panel shows the probability density function, $p_g(g)$, for a random variable, g, which is the sum of f and n. $p_g(g)$ is equal to the convolution of the probability density functions for f and n.

Equation 10.6 states that the mean is the sum of the possible values, f, of the random variable, *f*, times the probability of obtaining that values, p(f). The mean is the "center of mass" of the probability density function. The mean is also called the expected value of *f*, and the operator E{·} is called the **expectation operator**. Finally, the mean is also called the **first moment** of the random variable. The mean is a **first order statistic** since it involves only the first power of the random variable.

In this book we shall be concerned with continuous probability distributions; however, in the case where there are a limited number of equally likely outcomes of an experiment, the mean is defined as:

$$m = \sum_i f_i/N \qquad (10.7)$$

where f_i are the outcomes and N is the size of the population. Equation 10.7 is the discrete analog of Equation 10.6, where the probability of each outcome is 1/N.

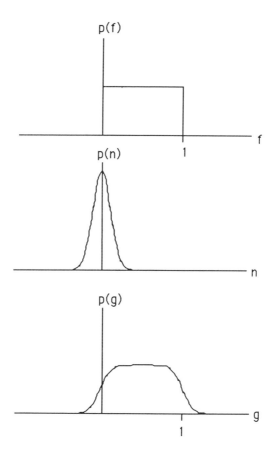

FIGURE 10.3. Radiological measurement: the top panel shows the probability density function, $p_f(f)$, for a radiological variable. The model states that we have *a priori* medical knowledge that this variable is uniformly distributed between 0 and 1. The second panel shows the probability density function, $p_n(n)$, for the measurement noise. The *a priori* knowledge about the noise is that the noise is zero mean with a standard deviation of one. The bottom panel shows the probability density function, $p_g(g)$, for the measurement. It is equal to the convolution of $p_f(f)$ and $p_n(n)$.

There is an important distinction between the "true" mean of the probability density function and the mean of a sample of values obtained experimentally. It is the difference between the model of the experiment and the experimental data. However, the equation for the sample mean is the same as the equation for the true mean:

$$\mu = \sum_i f_i / N \qquad (10.8)$$

where f_i are the sample values which are obtained. In this case N is equal to the size of the sample, not the size of the population. The symbol μ is used to distinguish the sample mean from the "true" mean, m.

C. SOME COMMENTS ABOUT THE EXPECTATION OPERATOR

Values which are known exactly are called **deterministic**, whereas values which are associated with noise are called statistical. The expectation operator, $E\{\cdot\}$, transforms a statistical entity, f, into a deterministic entity, the mean value of the probability density function. Thus, it is an operator which connects our statistical model to our deterministic models. Deterministic quantities are not affected by the expectation operator:

$$E\{a\} = \int_{-\infty}^{+\infty} a \cdot p(f) \, df = a \cdot \int_{-\infty}^{+\infty} p(f) \, df = a \cdot 1 = a \qquad (10.9)$$

and:

$$E\{a \cdot f\} = \int_{-\infty}^{+\infty} a \cdot f \cdot p(f) \, df = a \cdot \int_{-\infty}^{+\infty} f \cdot p(f) \, df = a \cdot E\{f\} \qquad (10.10)$$

If the expectation operator is applied twice, $E\{E\{f\}\}$, the result of the first application is a deterministic quantity; therefore, the second operator has no effect. Thus,

$$E\{E\{f\}\} = E\{f\} \qquad (10.11)$$

D. VARIANCE

Another valuable parameter in describing a probability density function is the variability or the dispersion of the function. The **variance** is a parameter which is related to the variability of the probability density function:

$$\sigma_f^2 = E\{|f - m|^2\} \qquad (10.12)$$

where m is the mean of f. We shall refer to $f - m$ as the deviation from the mean of the random variable, or more simply the **deviation**. It is the variation of the random variable about the mean value. The variance, which is the mean of the square of the deviation, is sometimes called the mean square deviation.

The deviation can be both positive and negative; however, the square of the deviation must always be positive. Therefore, the variance is always positive. When there is no confusion about which random variable is being considered, we shall us σ^2 instead of σ_f^2. The variance is called a **second order statistic** since it involves the square or second power of the random variable.

We have used the square of the magnitude $|\cdot|^2$ instead of a simple square to allow for f to be a complex random variable. Recall from Equation 6.22 that the square of the magnitude of a complex number can be written:

$$|f|^2 = f \cdot f* \qquad (10.13)$$

where $f*$ is the complex conjugate of f (see Chapter 6). Often f will be a real number, and then, $|f|^2$ is the same as f^2.

For a random process with a finite number of equally likely outcomes, the variance is defined as:

$$\sigma_f^2 = \sum_i |f_i - m|^2/N \qquad (10.14)$$

The variance is the average of the square of the deviation of the outcomes from the mean.

In the case of the variance, the sample variance is defined by a slightly different equation than the "true" variance:

$$s^2 = \sum_i |f_i - \mu|^2/(N - 1) \qquad (10.15)$$

TABLE 10.1
Population and Sample Statistics

	Mean	Variance
Population	$m = \sum_i f_i/N$	$\sigma^2 = \sum_i |f_i - m|^2/N$
Sample	$\mu = \sum_i f_i/N$	$s^2 = \sum_i |f_i - \mu|^2/N - 1$

where μ is the sample mean. It is the sum of the square of the deviations of the sample values from the smaple mean divided by $N - 1$. N is replaced by $N - 1$ since one of the degrees of freedom is used up to calculate the sample mean. The sample variance, with $N - 1$ in the denominator, gives an unbiased estimate of the variance. The symbol, s^2, is used in place of σ^2 to indicate that s^2 is the variance of a sample not the "true" variance. The true mean and variance and the sample mean and variance are shown in Table 10.1.

E. SECOND MOMENT

A parameter closely related to the variance is the second moment, R_f, of the probability density function. The **second moment** is defined as:

$$R_f = E\{|f|^2\} \tag{10.16}$$

When there is no confusion about which random variable is being considered, we shall use R in place of R_f. The variance is a measure of the variability of f with respect to the mean; the second moment is a measure of the variability of f with respect to zero. The second moment, like the variance, is a second order statistic.

The relation of the second moment to the variance can be shown by expanding Equation 10.12:

$$\sigma^2 = E\{|f - m|^2\}$$
$$= E\{|f|^2\} - E\{f \cdot m^*\} - E\{m \cdot f^*\} + E\{|m|^2\} \tag{10.17}$$

Using Equations 10.10 and 10.6 on the second and third terms and Equation 10.9 on the fourth term:

$$\sigma^2 = E\{|f|^2\} - 2 \cdot |m|^2 + |m|^2 = E\{|f|^2\} - |m|^2 \tag{10.18}$$

$$\sigma^2 = R - |m|^2 \tag{10.19}$$

The variance is equal to the second moment minus the square of the mean.

F. STANDARD DEVIATION

The variance gives the dispersion of a signal in terms of the square of the deviation. However, it is often desirable to compare the dispersion of a signal with the signal itself. Therefore, the **standard deviation** is defined as the square root of the variance:

$$\sigma = \sqrt{\sigma^2} \tag{10.20}$$

The standard deviation is of the same dimensions as the signal so that we can compare it directly with the signal. Figure 10.4 shows a probability density function with its mean and standard deviation.

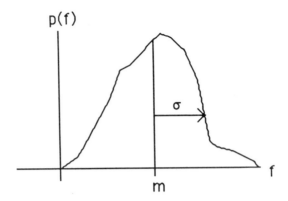

FIGURE 10.4.   Probability density function: this figure shows a probability density function, p(f). The mean of the probability density function is given by m, and the standard deviation is given by σ.

In biostatistics, the standard deviation is used more commonly than the variance, and the reader is likely much more at home with the standard deviation than the variance. However, in signal processing, the variance is often easier to work with than the standard deviation.

G. POWER AND ENERGY

In signal analysis, the term **power** is often applied to the square of a signal, f(t). The origin of the term power comes from physics. There are several branches of physics where the product of two variables gives power, for example, in mechanics, force and velocity; in electrical circuits, voltage and current; in electromagnetism, the electric field and the magnetic field; and in ultrasound, excess pressure and particle motion.

Under certain circumstances, these two variables are related by an impedance. In that case, power is equal to the square of the first variable divided by the impedance. Since the impedance is just a constant, the power is proportional to the square of the amplitude of the signal. By analogy in signal processing we define the power as the square of the signal.

$$\text{power} = |f(t)|^2 \tag{10.21}$$

We shall also apply the term power to the square of the amplitude of a random variable. The average power of a random variable is given by the second moment:

$$\text{average power} = R = E\{|f|^2\} \tag{10.22}$$

The average power of the deviation of f is given by the variance:

$$\text{average power of deviation} = \sigma^2 = E\{|f - m|^2\} \tag{10.23}$$

In physics, **energy** is defined to be the integral of power over time. Again by analogy, we shall define the integral of square of the amplitude of a function as the energy in the signal.

$$\text{energy} = \int_{-\infty}^{+\infty} |f(t)|^2 \, dt \tag{10.24}$$

In the case of a discrete signal, the analogous definition is:

$$\text{energy} = \sum_i |f_i|^2 \tag{10.25}$$

For a vector, **f**, the analogous definition is the vector product:

$$\text{energy} = \mathbf{f}^T \cdot \mathbf{f} \tag{10.26}$$

Thus, the energy in a signal is analogous to the product of a vector with itself.

In order to consider energy in the context of random variables, we need to consider a set of N samples of a random variable, f. The samples will be labeled f_i where i takes on the values one to N. The average energy in this set of samples is the sum of the average powers:

$$\sum_i E\{|f_i|^2\} = \sum_i R = N \cdot R \tag{10.27}$$

where R is the second moment, given by Equation 10.16. The average energy in the deviation from the mean is analogous to $N \cdot \sigma^2$.

The terms power and energy are used frequently in signal processing because of the analogies with the physical principles. We shall find that like energy in physics, the energy in a signal is often conserved. One of the reasons that the second order statistics are so useful is because of this fact. Below we shall show the analogy between energy and the square of the length of a vector. But more of this later.

III. TWO RANDOM VARIABLES

We shall often be interested in the joint properties of two random variables, f and g. The most complete description of the two variables is given by a two-dimensional probability density function p(f,g). This function gives the probability of simultaneously obtaining an outcome value of f, for random variable f, and a value of g for random variable g. We shall present a very selected list of the statistics of two random variables.

A. CORRELATION OF DEVIATIONS

One of the most frequent questions which arises about two random variables is how they are related. A parameter which is used to assess the relationship between random variables is the **correlation of their deviations**. The correlation of the deviations of two random variables is defined to be:

$$\sigma_{fg}^2 = E\{[f - m_f] \cdot [g - m_g]^*\} \tag{10.28}$$

The definition includes the complex conjugate of the deviation of the second variable. We shall include the possibility of having complex variables without going into an explanation of what this implies. The correlation shows how similar the variation from the mean is for the two variables.

We have used the same symbol, σ^2, for correlation and for variance with different subscripts since the equation definition of these quantities is similar. The correlation of the deviation of a random variable with itself, σ_{ff}^2, is equal to the variance, σ_f^2. The correlation, like the variance, is called a second order statistic since it is derived from the product of two random variables. Again we shall use the concepts of power and energy with the second order statistics. The correlation of the deviations of two variables is equal to the **mutal or cross power** of their variability.

TABLE 10.2
Second Order Statistics

	wrt Mean	wrt Zero
One random variable	$\sigma_f = E\{|f - m_f|^2\}$	$R_f = E\{|f|^2\}$
Two random variables	$\sigma_{fg} = E\{|f - m_f| \cdot |g - m_g|^*\}$	$R_{fg} = E\{|f \cdot g^*|\}$

The correlation between variables as defined in Equation 10.28 will depend upon the power in the deviations of each of the variables. As we shall see below, this is often useful. However, at times we are interested in how similar the random variables are independent of the power of their deviations. The **correlation coefficient** is defined with a normalization for the power of the deviation of the random variables.

$$r = E\{[f - m_f] \cdot [g - m_g]^*\}/\sqrt{(E\{|f - m_f|^2 \cdot E\{|g - m_g|^2\})}} \tag{10.29}$$

$$r = \sigma_{fg}^2/\sqrt{(\sigma_f^2 \cdot \sigma_g^2)} \tag{10.30}$$

The correlation coefficient will take on values from 1, perfectly correlated, to -1, perfectly correlated in opposite directions. If the random variables have no relation to each other, r will be zero.

B. CORRELATION

For a single random variable, the variance gives the power of the deviation of the random variable with respect to the mean, and the second moment gives the power in the random variable with respect to zero. For two random variables, σ_{fg}^2 gives the correlation, or mutual power, of the deviations of the two variables. And as one might expect, we define the **correlation** of two random variables to be:

$$R_{fg} = E\{f \cdot g^*\} \tag{10.31}$$

The same symbol is used for the correlation between random variables and for the second moment, since the definitions are similar. The correlation of a random vaiable with itself, R_{ff}, is equal to the second moment, R_f. The second moment gives the power of a random variable. The correlation gives the **mutual or cross power** in two random variables. The second order statistics for one and two random variables are shown in Table 10.2.

The correlation of two random variables and the correlation of their deviations are related in a fashion which is similar to the second moment and the variance:

$$\sigma_{fg}^2 = E\{(f - m_f) \cdot (g - m_g)^*\}$$

$$= E\{f \cdot g^*\} - E\{f \cdot m_g^*\} - E\{m_f \cdot g^*\} + E\{m_f \cdot m_g^*\} \tag{10.32}$$

The means are deterministic quantities, so the last three terms may be further simplified using Equations 10.6, 10.9, and 10.10:

$$\sigma_{fg}^2 = R_{fg} - m_f \cdot m_g^* - m_f \cdot m_g^* + m_f \cdot m_g^*$$

$$= R_{fg} - m_f \cdot m_g^* \tag{10.33}$$

C. INDEPENDENT, ORTHOGONAL, AND UNCORRELATED VARIABLES

There are three important types of relations between two random variables — independence, orthogonality, and uncorrelatedness. The two variables are said to be **statistically independent** if:

$$p(f,g) = p(f) \cdot p(g) \tag{10.34}$$

In other words, they are statistically independent if the probability of simultaneously obtaining values, f and g, is equal to the product of the probabilities of getting each of them separately.

In many cases of interest the two random variables will not be independent. For example, if f is a random variable which is determined by whether a patient smokes and g is a random variable which is determined by whether a patient has lung cancer, then f and g will not be independent. The probability that a patient smokes and has lung cancer is not equal to the chance that a patient smokes times the chance that a patient has lung cancer.

Two random variables are called **orthogonal** if:

$$R_{fg} = 0 \tag{10.35}$$

The mutual power between f and g is zero. The definition of the correlation between random variables (Equation 10.31) is analogous to the equation for a vector product Equation 8.51. Orthogonal random variables are analogous to orthogonal vectors — they are completely unaligned, at right angles to each other. The same term, orthogonal, is used to indicate the similarity between the random variable description and the vector description.

We say that two random variables are **uncorrelated** if:

$$E(f \cdot g^*) = E(f) \cdot E\{g^*\} \tag{10.36}$$

Or equivalently:

$$R_{fg} = m_f \cdot m_g^* \tag{10.37}$$

From Equation 10.33, it can be seen that this is equivalent to:

$$\sigma_{fg}^2 = 0 \tag{10.38}$$

Uncorrelated random variables have orthogonal deviations. Uncorrelated means that the deviation of one random variable is not related to the deviation of another random variable.

We can show that if two random variables are independent, then they are uncorrelated.

$$R_{fg} = E\{f \cdot g^*) = \int_{-\infty}^{+\infty} \int_{-\infty}^{+\infty} f \cdot g^* \cdot p(f,g) \, dfdg \tag{10.39}$$

Since p(f,g) is equal to p(f)·p(g) we can separate the terms:

$$R_{fg} = \int_{-\infty}^{+\infty} f \cdot p(f) \, df \cdot \int_{-\infty}^{+\infty} g^* \cdot p(g) \, dg = m_f \cdot m_g^* \tag{10.40}$$

However, uncorrelated does not imply independent. Uncorrelated relates only to second order statistics, not to the whole probability density function. Independent is stronger than uncorrelated.

D. SUM OF TWO UNCORRELATED RANDOM VARIABLES

At the beginning of the chapter we described a simple experiment where the measured value was the sum of two random variables:

$$g = f + n \tag{10.41}$$

In this section we shall determine the mean and the variance of the g. Because of the linearity of the expectation operator the mean is relatively simple:

$$E\{g\} = E\{f + n\} = E\{f\} + E\{n\} \tag{10.42}$$

Thus:

$$m_{f+n} = m_f + m_n \tag{10.43}$$

The derivation of a formula for the variance is more difficult and it requires the assumption that the random variables are uncorrelated.

$$
\begin{aligned}
\sigma_g^2 &= E\{|g - m_g|^2\} = E\{|g|^2\} - E\{|m_g|^2\} \\
&= E\{|f + n|^2\} - |E\{f + n\}|^2 \\
&= E\{|f|^2\} + E\{f \cdot n^* + f^* \cdot n\} \\
&\quad - |m_f|^2 - m_f \cdot m_n^* - m_f^* \cdot m_n - |m_n|^2
\end{aligned}
\tag{10.44}
$$

If f and n are uncorrelated, then $-m_f \cdot m_n^* - m_f^* \cdot m_n$ is equal to $-E\{f \cdot n + f^* \cdot n\}$; therefore:

$$
\begin{aligned}
\sigma_g^2 &= E\{|f|^2\} + E\{f \cdot n^* + f^* \cdot n\} \\
&\quad - |m_f|^2 - E\{f \cdot n^* + f^* \cdot n\} - |m_n|^2 \\
&= E\{|f - m_f|^2\} + E\{|n - m_n|^2\} \\
&= \sigma_f^2 + \sigma_n^2
\end{aligned}
\tag{10.45}
$$

Thus, if two random variables are uncorrelated, the variance of their sum is the sum of their variances — the variances add:

$$\sigma_{f+n}^2 = \sigma_f^2 + \sigma_n^2 \tag{10.46}$$

However, the standard deviations do not add simply:

$$\sigma_{f+n} = \sqrt{(\sigma_f^2 + \sigma_n^2)} \tag{10.47}$$

This is one of the reasons why the variance not the standard deviation is the most useful measure of dispersion.

Equations 10.43 and 10.45 are quite remarkable. Recall that at the beginning of the chapter we showed that the probability density function of the sum of two random variables was very complicated — it was the convolution of the two probability density functions. However, if the random variables are uncorrelated, the mean and the variance are simple sums. The statistics of the probability density functions are much easier to work with than the probability density functions themselves! This fact is one of the values of the statistical description of random processes.

Let us return to the example at the beginning of the chapter, the measurement of the computed tomography number in a region of interest. Recall that we modeled this experiment with the equation:

$$g = f + n \tag{10.48}$$

where g was the measured value; f represented the biological variability; and n represented the measurement noise. Let us suppose that from a number of measurements that we find that the variance of the measurement, s_g^2, is 1000 square CT units. (Note that this is the variance of a sample, not the "true" variance, σ.) From a series of phantom experiments we might find that s_n^2 is 100 square CT units. Then we would know that the variability in the measured value was predominantly due to biological variability.

By contrast let us assume that s_g^2 is 200 square CT units and the s_n^2 is again 100 square CT units. From equation 10.45 we know that s_f^2 is 100 square CT units. In this case the biological variability and the measurement variability contribute equally to the measurement variability. We cannot use the measurement variability to reflect the biological variability. However, our model has allowed us to estimate the biological variability using a very simple relationship. In comparing this result with the data itself, the standard deviation, 10 CT units, would be most useful.

IV. RANDOM VECTORS

We can expand our discussion from two random variables to many random variables. With many random variables we could imagine all sorts of interesting combinations; however, it turns out that the most useful parameters are still the first and second order statistics which we have already covered. Consequently, this section will be very short.

When we have multiple random variables, it will often be useful to use vector notation. Thus, the random vector, $\boldsymbol{f}$, with three components, stands for three random variables, f_1, f_2, and f_3. The boldface indicates a vector quantity and the italics indicates a random quantity. On a deeper level random vectors are a discrete analog of stochastic processes, but more of this in the next chapter.

A. ENERGY AND LENGTH

We can use the concept of a random vector to get a geometrical understanding of second order statistics. Figure 10.5 shows two-dimensional vector space. $\boldsymbol{f}$ is a random vector with components, f_1 and f_2, along the x and y axes. The square of the length of $\boldsymbol{f}$ is given by the Pythagorean theorem:

$$f^2 = f_1^2 + f_2^2 \tag{10.49}$$

where the nonboldface, f, stands for the length of $\boldsymbol{f}$.

We can think of $\boldsymbol{f}$ as a set of random variables. The concept that the components are geometrically orthogonal is equivalent to the idea that the set of random variables is statistically orthogonal. The second moment of the sum of random variables, the average energy, is equal to the sum of the second moments of the component random variables.

$$R_f = R_{f_1} + R_{f_2} \tag{10.50}$$

The second moment is identical to the square of the length of the vector $\boldsymbol{f}$, Equation 8.51.

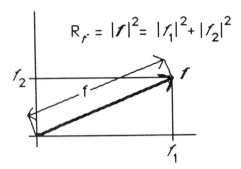

FIGURE 10.5. Random vector: the components of the random vector, f, are the two random variables, f_1 and f_2. If f_1 and f_2 are orthogonal, then the second moment of the sum of the random variables is equal to the square length of f, $|f|^2$.

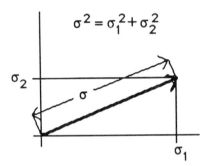

FIGURE 10.6. Sum of standard deviations: the length of a vector, σ, which has components σ_1 and σ_2, is equal to the standard deviation of the sum of two random variables with standard deviations σ_1 and σ_2.

Rather than considering the energy in a set of random variables, we could consider the energy in the deviations of the random variables. The relationships derived for the second moment will then apply to the variances. Figure 10.6 shows the variance of the sum and of two random variables. The variance of the sum is analogous to the square of the length of the vector.

The standard deviation is analogous to the length of the vector. Adding uncorrelated random variables (with orthogonal deviations) is like adding orthogonal vectors. The lengths of the component vectors are analogous to the standard deviations of the component random variables. The length of the sum of the vectors is analogous to the standard deviation of the sum of the random variables.

In Chapter 12 we shall describe the least mean square error criterion. One heuristic for choosing to minimize the square of the error is that it is like the variance of the sum of errors. It is the energy of the errors. Therefore by minimizing the square of the error, the energy in the errors is minimized.

The correlation of two random variables is similar to the cross product of two vectors, $f^T \cdot g/N$, where we have divided the product by the number of components, N. Recall in Chapter 8, that the product of two vectors is like the product of their lengths with a factor for how well "lined up" the vectors are. Similarly, the correlation of two random variables has a factor for how well "lined up" the random vectors are.

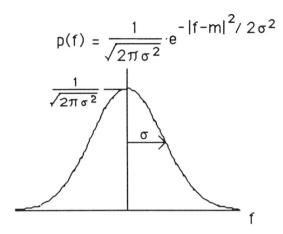

FIGURE 10.7. Normal distribution: the probability density function of a normal distribution with mean equal to zero and standard deviation equal to σ.

V. NORMALLY DISTRIBUTED RANDOM VARIABLES

Normally distributed random variables have a probability density function which is given by:

$$p(f) = 1/\sqrt{(2\pi \cdot \sigma^2)} \cdot e^{-|f-m|^2/2\cdot\sigma^2} \tag{10.51}$$

The first factor is a constant which normalizes the probability density function so that the total area is equal to one. The second factor is the exponential of the square of the distance from the mean. The normal distribution is a function of two parameters, m and σ. We have used symbols for the mean and the standard deviation since it turns out that these parameters are equal to the mean and standard deviation of this probability density function.

A normal probability density function is shown in Figure 10.7. About 68% of the area of the curve occurs within one standard deviation of the mean and about 95% of the area is within two standard deviations of the mean.

Above we have shown that means and variances of random variables are often much easier to work with than the probability density functions themselves. If the random variables are normally distributed, then the mean and the variance determine the probability density functions. Thus, the assumption that a random variable is normally distributed buys a great deal of simplicity.

The reader is probably very familiar with the common assumption that statistical entities follow a normal distribution, but he may not know why the normal distribution is used so commonly. There are really two reasons. First, as we have shown, the normal distribution is very easy to work with. It has just two parameters, the mean and the standard deviation. If we know these two parameters we know everything about the random variable. Thus in our discussion about random variables we have discussed only the mean and the variance. Furthermore, as we shall see, the normal assumption will simplify many other calculations.

The second reason that the normal distribution is used so frequently is that it is encountered frequently in nature. There is a theorem called the **central limit theorem** which states that any random variable which is the sum of a number of other random variables will tend toward a normal distribution as the number of underlying distributions increases. In fact, if only a few random variables are added together, the distribution of the sum rapidly approaches a normal distribution. The errors in almost all biological experiments come from a myriad of sources. Thus, the outcomes are frequently normally distributed.

VI. SUMMARY

The most important concept introduced in this chapter is the random variable. We shall find that having a method of simply describing an experiment will be very useful, especially when we wish to describe more complicated experimental models. We have introduced many statistics which can be used to describe random variables. Although this material is somewhat tedious to go through, it provides the vocabulary which we shall need to consider more interesting problems.

We shall use the concepts of power and energy throughout the rest of the book. If these concepts still seem a bit vague to the reader, it may be useful to review that part of this chapter. Particularly useful is the geometrical analogy between the square of the length and the energy in a signal.

VII. FURTHER READING

The theory of random variables are dependent upon probability theory. We introduced the idea of a probability density function and have given one example, the normal distribution. However, the interested reader might wish to explore probability theory in much greater depth.[1]

We have been very superficial in our description of the mathematical basis of random variables. A more rigorous approach relies on an underlying probability space. The reader who is interested in a more theoretical derivation is referred to the book by Davenport.[2] A more advance treatment is found in the excellent book by Papoulis.[3]

REFERENCES

1. **Drake, A. W.**, *Fundamentals of Applied Probability Theory,* McGraw-Hill, New York, 1967.
2. **Davenport, W. B.**, *Random Processes,* McGraw-Hill, New York, 1970.
3. **Papoulis, A.**, *Probability, Random Variables, and Stochastic Processes,* McGraw-Hill, New York, 1965.

Chapter 11

STOCHASTIC PROCESSES

In the last chapter, the concept of a random variable was introduced. Random variables are used to model experiments which have an outcome which is a single value. This chapter will generalize the concept of a random variable to a random signal or **stochastic process**. Stochastic processes are used to model experiments which have an outcome which is a signal. This chapter will introduce some basic statistics associated with a stochastic process. The statistics of a stochastic process provide *a priori* information about the type of signals which are obtained on each experiment.

In Part III, we shall combine the linear systems model with the stochastic process model to show how stochastic processes pass through systems. In Part IV, where radiologic applications are described, stochastic processes will be used for two purposes. Some of our medical knowledge about the cross-sectional objects which are imaged by tomographic systems can be captured by using a stochastic process model. Some of our technical knowledge about the detector can be captured by using a stochastic process model of the detector noise. Understanding the models of the cross-sectional objects and the detector noise and understanding how these signals pass through the radiological imaging systems will be important in understanding reconstruction.

I. PROBABILITY DENSITY FUNCTION

The concept of a stochastic process, $f(t)$, is considerably more complicated than the concept of a random variable, f. Each experiment represented by a random variable, f, produces a single value, f. Each experiment represented by the stochastic process, $f(t)$, produces an entire signal, f(t). The notation used for stochastic processes in this book is similar to that used for random variables; a stochastic process is represented by an italicized function, $f(t)$, and a single value of the stochastic process is represented by the nonitalicized, f(t).

We can define a probability density function for a stochastic process as p(f(t)). In other words for every possible signal f(t), the probability density function p(f(t)) gives the probability that the signal f(t) will be the outcome of the stochastic process.

At first glance it appears that extension from random variables to stochastic processes is quite simple; however, we need to consider what p(f(t)) means. The "independent variable", f(t), is a signal. It is equivalent to an infinite set of independent variables. p($\cdot$) gives a probability for every possible combination of values at every possible combination of times.

Obviously, this generalization of the probability density function is too complex to be of any value. We shall need to find a useful description of some features of the probability density function in terms of a small set of parameters. From the discussion of random variables, the reader might suspect that first and second order statistics will be the most useful.

Although the primary definition of a stochastic process is as a set of random signals, we can consider the stochastic process from a different point of view — as a collection of random variables at different points in time. We can write f_1 to indicate a random variable which is equal to the values of a random process at some specific time $f(t_1)$. We can define a probability density function, $p(t_1;f_1)$, for this random variables as a function of the time, t_1, and the value, f_1, of the random variable at that time. $p(t_1;f_1)$ gives the probability that the stochastic process will take on the value, f_1, at time t_1. This two-dimensional probability density function gives the first order statistics of the stochastic process.

Two random variables, f_1 and f_2, which represent the values of the stochastic process at different points in time, t_1 and t_2 may not be independent of each other. Therefore, a description of these two random variables requires a joint probability density function, $p(t_1,t_2;f_1,f_2)$. The joint probability density function gives the probability of obtaining values f_1 and f_2 for any possible combination of times, t_1 and t_2. The four-dimensional joint probability density function, $p(t_1,t_2;f_1,f_2)$, gives the second order statistics of the stochastic process.

More generally a stochastic process can be defined by a joint probability density function, $p(t_1,t_2, \ldots ;f_1,f_2, \ldots)$, where the "t"'s are a set of points in time and the "f"'s are the values of the random variables at these times. A complete description of the stochastic process requires an infinite number of time variables and an infinite number of value variables so that this description is no simpler than the random signal description. However, the advantage of considering a stochastic process as a set of random variables is that the first and second order statistics can be obtained from the relatively simple, four-dimensional probability density $p(t_1,t_2;f_1,f_2)$.

We have described two different methods of describing a stochastic process — as a random signal and as an infinite set of random variables. These two methods are both useful for understanding a stochastic process and each will be useful in certain circumstances. The random signal method is more descriptive of the experimental processes. For each experiment we get an entire signal. The random variable method will be more useful in developing the statistics which we shall use to describe a random process.

II. EXAMPLES OF STOCHASTIC PROCESSES

Before continuing with the abstract discussion of the properties of stochastic processes, let us consider some examples of stochastic processes. We can define a stochastic process whose outcomes are liver spleen scans. For each experiment, one signal, a liver spleen scan, is produced. The sequential outcomes of the stochastic process are all different; however, they all come from the same class of signals, liver spleen scans. The stochastic process model provides information about the statistics of the biological variability in liver spleen scans.

Now let us try to understand how this model of liver spleen scans can be useful to us. The various points in a single liver spleen scan are not independent. If all but one point in the liver spleen scan are known, then the remaining point can be predicted with a high degree of accuracy. The various points in the signal are correlated; they contain mutual information. The fact that the signal represents a liver spleen scan provides a considerable amount of *a priori* information about the signal. The value of using this stochastic process model is that some of this *a priori* information can be captured in the statistical properties of the stochastic process.

In the case of real liver spleen scans, the difference between the various outcomes is determined by two factors, interpatient variability and the Poisson counting noise. We shall see that it is frequently useful to model radiological images as the sum of two stochastic processes, one representing the biological variability and the second representing the noise.

$$p(x,y) = f(x,y) + n(x,y) \tag{11.1}$$

$p(x,y)$ is the measured signal, $f(x,y)$ is the biological image, and $n(x,y)$ is the measurement noise. The statistics of $f(x,y)$ contain the *a priori* biological information, and the statistics of $n(x,y)$ contain the *a priori* information about how noise arises in the measurement process.

Figure 11.1 shows this model of the imaging process diagrammatically. Noise is added to the input to produce the output signal. In the case of Poisson noise, the noise is equal to

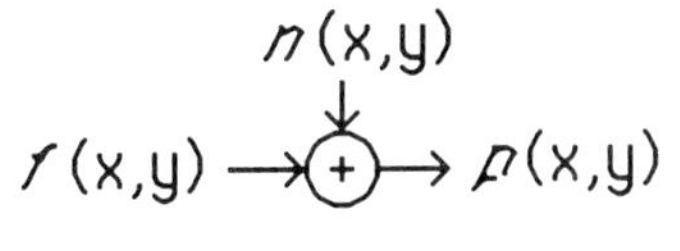

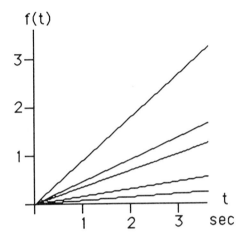

FIGURE 11.1. Image collection model: this figure shows a diagrammatic representation of a model for image data collection. The object is represented by a stochastic process, $f(x,y)$; the detector noise is represented by another stochastic process, $n(x,y)$; and the data, $p(x,y)$ is a stochastic process which is the sum of $f(x,y)$ and $n(x,y)$.

FIGURE 11.2. Outcomes of a stochastic process: the lines in the graph represent various outcome signals for a stochastic process, $f(t)$. The stochastic process, $f(t)$, represents the position of a ball which is kicked at a velocity between 0 and 1 m/sec.

the square root of the signal. This additive noise model is therefore not strictly correct. However, in almost all real radiological problems we shall use this model since we shall see that it simplifies the calculations.

The liver spleen scan points out several interesting features of stochastic processes of interest in Radiology. If we know that the signal will be a liver spleen scan, we have a great deal of *a priori* information about what the signal and the noise will look like. We shall find that by combining this information with the information obtained from a particular scan, we can make a better prediction of the "true" liver spleen scan by selectively reducing the noise (see Chapter 26, Wiener Filtering).

But we are not yet ready for complex radiological problems; rather let us consider a much simpler example of a stochastic process. Imagine that we have a ball on a frictionless surface. On each experiment we kick the ball such that the ball moves away at a speed from 0 to 1 m/sec. The probability of all velocities between 0 and 1 is equally likely. We define the stochastic process to be the position of the ball as a function of time.

Figure 11.2 shows some of the possible outcomes of this stochastic process. The position, $f(t)$, is the value of the particular sample of the stochastic process. All of the outcomes are straight lines. The various outcomes differ only in slope. This is a very simple stochastic process, with very little variability between samples; however, it will show us some features of stochastic processes.

Let us consider the first order probability density function, $p(t_1;f_1)$. If the ball were kicked with a velocity of 1 m/sec, then at time, t_1, the ball will be at position, $1 \cdot t_1$. If the ball started with velocity 0 m/sec, then at time t_1, the ball will be at position $0 \cdot t_1$. Since all velocities between 0 and 1 are equally likely, all of the positions between 0 and t_1 will be equally likely. Outside of this range the probability will be zero. Figure 11.3 shows the

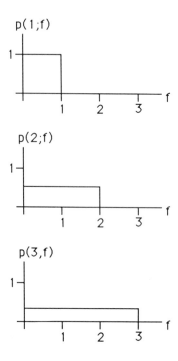

FIGURE 11.3.   Probability density function: this graph shows the probability density function, $p(t_1; f_1)$, for the stochastic process shown in Figure 11.2 at three points in time, 1 sec, 2 sec, and 3 sec. At 1 sec, positions between 0 and 1 m are equally likely. At 2 sec, positions between 0 and 2 m are equally likely. And, at 3 sec, positions between 0 and 3 m are equally likely. Since the area under the probability density function must be equal to one, the height of the graph decreases as it becomes wider.

probability density function for three values of time. As time progresses the function widens, we have less information about the position of the ball. Since the area under any probability density function must be equal to one, as it widens, it must also decrease in height.

Suppose that we know the value of a sample of the stochastic process at time 1 sec. Since the outcomes are all straight lines that go through the origin, we can determine the value of the signal at all points in time. In this simple case, the entire signal can be determined from a single value.

The second order probability density function for this stochastic process will also be very simple. The random variables at different nonzero times are exactly correlated with each other. Therefore, the joint probability density function, $p(t_1,t_2;f_1,f_2)$, will be equal to one for

$$f_2 = f_1 \cdot t_2/t_1 \tag{11.2}$$

And it will be zero for all other values of f_2. We have derived this probability density function from the properties of the stochastic process; however, we could equally as well derive the properties of the stochastic process from this probability density function.

The random variable at time zero is also quite unusual. The value zero occurs with probability equal to one, and all other values have a probability zero. Thus at time zero there is no variability in the position of the ball.

This example is exceedingly simple. We could model this experiment with a single random variable, the speed of the ball. However, the more complicated model shows how the values at various points in time may be correlated with each other, and how the probability density function can be used to provide information about the process.

TABLE 11.1
Stochastic Process Statistics

Mean	$m_f(t) = E\{f(t)\}$
Autocorrelation	$R_f(t_1,t_2) = E\{f(t_1) \cdot f^*(t_2)\}$
Crosscorrelation	$R_{fg}(t_1,t_2) = E\{f(t_1) \cdot g^*(t_2)\}$

III. MEAN

One important parameter used to describe a stochastic process is the **mean**. In general, the mean of a stochastic process will be a function of time (Table 11.1). The mean is defined as:

$$m_f(t) = E\{f(t)\} = \int_{-\infty}^{+\infty} f(t) \cdot p(t;f) \, df \qquad (11.3)$$

where $p(t;f)$ is the first order probability density function, $p(t_1;f_1)$, for the stochastic process. When there is no confusion about which stochastic process is being referenced, we shall use $m(t)$ instead of $m_f(t)$. In our simple example of the ball on a frictionless surface, the mean value will be:

$$m(t) = t/2 \qquad (11.4)$$

The mean of the process, $m(t)$, is a function of time as are the individual outcomes signals, $f(t)$. However, it is important to distinguish between this statistical property of the stochastic process and the actual outcome signals. The mean is deterministic; it does not change. The mean can be equal to one of the outcomes of the stochastic process; however, it is also possible that the mean is different from all of the possible outcomes of the stochastic process.

IV. AUTOCORRELATION

The autocorrelation function compares two points in a stochastic process. It is defined as:

$$R_f(t_1,t_2) = E\{f(t_1) \cdot f^*(t_2)\}$$

$$= \int_{-\infty}^{+\infty} f_1 \cdot f_2^* \cdot p(t_1,t_2;f_1,f_2) \, df_1 df_2 \qquad (11.5)$$

We have used the same symbol, R, for the second moment, the correlation of a random variable, and the autocorrelation of a stochastic process since all of these functions are defined in a similar way. They are all second order statistics. When no confusion exists we shall use $R(t_1,t_2)$ without the subscript instead of $R_f(t_1,t_2)$.

The autocorrelation of a stochastic process is the correlation of the two random variables, f_1 and f_2, from the stochastic process. The autocorrelation gives the mutual power of these random variables. The autocorrelation of a stochastic process is much more complicated than a simple correlation, since it gives the correlation between any point in the stochastic process with any other point. Rather than being a single number, it is a two-dimensional function.

TABLE 11.2
Stationarity

$$m(t) = m$$
$$R(t_1,t_2) = R(\tau)$$

V. CROSSCORRELATION

The crosscorrelation between two stochastic processes, $f(t)$ and $g(t)$, is defined as:

$$R_{fg}(t_1,t_2) = E\{f(t_1) \cdot g^*(t_2)\}$$

$$= \int_{-\infty}^{+\infty} f_1 \cdot g_2^* \cdot p(t_1,t_2;f_1,g_2) \, df_1 dg_2 \qquad 11.6$$

The crosscorrelation gives the relationship between two different stochastic processes at two different times. The crosscorrelation of a stochastic process with itself, $R_{ff}(t_1,t_2)$, is equal to the autocorrelation, $R_f(t_1,t_2)$.

The crosscorrelation gives the mutual power between two different stochastic processes as a function of time. Again the crosscorrelation is a two-dimensional function. We shall find that it provides very useful information about the relationships between two stochastic processes.

VI. STATIONARITY

In Chapter 4, we found that the description of a system was made considerably simpler if the system was time invariant. In terms of stochastic processes, a similar property is called stationarity. Stationarity means that the statistical properties of the process do not vary with time. The signals from the stochastic process will vary, but not the statistical properties (Table 11.2).

If a process is stationary, the mean cannot vary with time. Therefore we can write:

$$m(t) = m \qquad (11.7)$$

This equation implies that the mean is a constant.

Let us consider the autocorrelation function $R(t_1,t_2)$. Let us define a variable which is the difference in time between the two points, t_1 and t_2:

$$\tau = t_2 - t_1 \qquad (11.8)$$

The autocorrelation process can be written:

$$R(t_1,t_2) = R(t_1, t_1 + \tau) \qquad (11.9)$$

If the process is stationary, then the autocorrelation function will not change with a shift in time. Therefore if we shift the time variables by an amount, t_1, we get:

$$R(t_1,t_2) = R(0,\tau) = R(\tau) \qquad (11.10)$$

where we define $R(\tau)$ to be shorthand abbreviation for $R(0,\tau)$.

Stationarity is a very powerful property. It transforms the two-dimensional autocorrelation function into a one-dimensional function. The independent variable is the difference in time between the two points being considered. In exactly the same fashion we can define a stationary crosscorrelation function, $R_{fg}(\tau)$.

The stationary cross correlation function can be written in terms of the expectation operator:

$$R_{fg}(\tau) = E\{f(t) \cdot g*(t + \tau)\} \tag{11.11}$$

Let us define t' by:

$$t' = t + \tau \tag{11.12}$$

Using this change variable:

$$R_{fg}(\tau) = E\{f(t) \cdot g*(t + \tau)\} = E\{f(t' - \tau) \cdot g*(t')\} = R_{gf}^*(-\tau) \tag{11.13}$$

By substituting $f(t)$ for $g(t)$, we can derive:

$$R_f(\tau) = R_f^*(-\tau) \tag{11.14}$$

Functions with the property given by Equation 11.14 are called conjugate symmetric functions.

There are two types of stationarity which are usually defined, strict sense stationarity and wide sense stationarity. We have already defined **strict sense stationarity** — none of the statistical properties of the stochastic process can change in time. **Wide sense stationarity** is less restrictive than strict sense stationarity; it only requires that the first and second order statistics be stationary. Mathematically, we can define wide sense stationarity as:

$$m(t) = m \tag{11.15}$$

$$R(t_1, t_2) = R(\tau) \tag{11.16}$$

Strict sense stationarity implies wide sense stationarity. But the converse is not in general true. It is possible for a wide sense stationary process to have higher order moments which vary with time. We shall largely ignore this important distinction between strict and wide sense stationarity, since this distinction is not often important in radiological problems. Furthermore, since first and second order statistics completely define Gaussian stochastic processes, wide sense stationarity does imply strict sense stationarity for Gaussian processes.

Since stationarity greatly simplifies problems involving stochastic processes, we shall use it frequently. However, almost all radiological problems are not stationary. Radiologic images have boundaries. At the boundaries, the signals go to zero or some other fixed value. Obviously, the statistics of the stochastic process must change at the boundary. The reader may recall that the same problem was true of time invariance. In both cases, the approach is not to discard these important properties, but rather to recognize the limits of our model. We may say that the signal is stationary within certain boundaries.

Radiologic images are almost always centered in the field of view of the imaging device. Therefore, the true statistics will reflect this fact. If we model these images as stationary stochastic process, it is not possible to make use of this *a priori* information.

VII. ERGODICITY

A very frequent situation is to wish to calculate the statistics of a stochastic process from a single sample of a process. In general, it is not possible to calculate the statistics of a stochastic process from a single sample. However, if the stochastic process has the same statistics with regard to the different outcomes as it does in time, then the statistics can be determined from a single sample.

Stochastic processes which have the same statistics as a function of outcome and of time are called ergodic. Although ergodicity would seem to be a very special property, it turns out that many stochastic processes of interest in radiology have this property.

If a process is ergodic, then the statistics can be calculated from time averages instead of outcome averages. Thus the autocorrelation function could be calculated as:

$$R(\tau) = \int_{-\infty}^{+\infty} f(t) \cdot f^*(t + \tau) \, dt \qquad (11.17)$$

The value of the autocorrelation function at $\tau = 0$, $R(0)$, is equal to the energy in the signal:

$$R(0) = \int_{-\infty}^{+\infty} f^*(t) \cdot f(t) \, dt \qquad (11.18)$$

It can be shown that the magnitude of the autocorrelation function at zero, $R(0)$, is the maximum of the autocorrelation function. $f(t)$ correlates at least as well with itself as with a shifted version of itself.

VIII. POISSON PROCESS

A stochastic process which occurs frequently in Radiology is the Poisson process. An example of an experiment which can be modeled with the Poisson process is counting a radioactive sample. The values obtained on successive experiments will have a probability density function described by the Poisson distribution. The key feature of this experiment is that the decay of each radioactive atom is independent of all other atoms. The Poisson process is used to model experiments which consist of a sequence of discrete independent events.

If the discrete independent events which make up the Poisson process occur at a rate given by w, then the probability of obtaining a number of events equal to f in a period of time, Δt, is given by the probability density function, $p(f)$:

$$p(f) = e^{-w\Delta t} \cdot (w \cdot \Delta t)^f / f! \qquad (11.19)$$

where f! is the factorial of f defined in Equation 2.47. Note that there is a single parameter which describes this probability density function, $w \cdot \Delta t$. $w \cdot \Delta t$ is the rate of occurrence of events, w, times the sampling interval, Δt. It can be shown that the mean of this probability density function is $w \cdot \Delta t$ and the variance is also equal to $w \cdot \Delta t$.

The Poisson distribution is quite remarkable. It is even simpler than the normal distribution. The normal distribution is defined by two parameters, the mean and the variance. The Poisson distribution is defined by only one parameter which is both the mean and the variance. In a counting experiment if $w \cdot \Delta t$ is equal to N counts, then N is both the mean and the variance. If N counts are obtained, then an estimate of the standard deviation is given by $\sqrt{N}$.

A sequence of measurements can be represented by a Poisson stochastic process, $f(t)$. The mean value of the process can be a function of time as in the case of a short-lived isotope; however, often the mean value does not change over the time of interest. If the process is stationary, ergodicity means that a sequence of measurements can be used to provide an estimate of the statistical variation of the process at a single time point.

A stochastic process which is related to the Poisson process is called the random telegraph signal. The random telegraph signal, $f(t)$, can take on only two values, e.g., -1 and 1. The signal switches back and forth between -1 and 1 at random times. The random switching is like the discrete independent events of the Poisson process. Rather than incrementing the value of the signal at each event, the random telegraph signal switches values.

The parameter, w, gives the rate at which the random telegraph signal switches values. A correlation time, τ_c, can be defined:

$$\tau_c = 1/2 \cdot w \qquad (11.20)$$

If we pick a point in time, then the average length of time before the signal switches values is related to τ_c. The correlation time tells how long the signal will be the same value.

It can be shown[1] that the telegraph signal has an autocorrelation function given by:

$$R(\tau) = e^{-|\tau|/\tau_c} \qquad (11.21)$$

The autocorrelation function decreases exponentially from a value of one at τ equal to zero in both the positive and the negative directions. The autocorrelation function, like the correlation time, tells how long the signal maintains the same value.

In nuclear magnetic resonance, one of the important parameters is the T_1, or spin lattice, relaxation time. (Lattice is a physical/chemical term which refers to the surrounding milieu.) The T_1 value determines the length of time it takes a nucleus to return to equilibrium after a perturbation. The T_1 value of a particular type of nucleus changes as a function of the magnetic field. These changes can be explained by understanding the relation between the frequency of precession of the nucleus and the frequency content of the changes in the magnetic field of the lattice.

In many cases the local magnetic field can be modeled as a random positive, negative fluctuation. Thus, the local field can be modeled as a random telegraph signal. The autocorrelation function which is the square of the field is proportional to the power in the field. In Part III, the Fourier transform of the autocorrelation function will be defined to be the power spectral density function, $S(\omega)$. The power spectral density function gives the power in the magnetic field as a function of frequency. Using these relations, the interaction of the local magnetic field with the nucleus can be understood in terms of the correlation time. The variation of T_1 as a function of the main magnetic field can be shown to be related to the correlation time τ_c.

The goal of this brief description is not to explain these complicated applications of stochastic processes, but rather to suggest that stochastic processes are important for understanding radiologic problems. Radioactive decay and nuclear magnetic resonance are only two examples of the many uses of these principles in radiology.

IX. SUMMARY

In this chapter the important concept of a stochastic process has been introduced. Stochastic processes combine the concept of statistical variation with the idea of a signal. They are statistical signals. Stochastic processes can be used to describe several types of signals in radiology. However, our major use of stochastic processes will be to describe images. Most of the signals describing the radiological images in Part IV will be modeled using stochastic processes.

The importance of first and second order statistics has been emphasized. The mean of a stochastic process gives the first order statistics. The autocorrelation gives the second order statistics for a single process, and the cross correlation gives the second order statistics for two processes.

Two important properties — stationarity and ergodicity — were described. Stationarity means that the statistics of the process do not change with time. Stationarity simplifies the description of the first and second order statistics of a process. Ergodicity means that the successive values of a single sample of a stochastic process have the same statistics as multiple samples of the stochastic process at the same time. This property is often used to estimate the statistics of a process from a single sample.

X. FURTHER READING

The description of stochastic processes has only briefly mentioned probability theory on which stochastic processes rely. The reader interested in a more complete description is referred to the book by Davenport.[2] A more advanced description is found in the book by Papoulis.[1] The book by Parzen[3] presents several examples of stochastic processes. Other books include References 4 and 5. The application of the autocorrelation function to understanding of the variations in T_1 should await the description of the power spectral density function in Chapter 24. This application is discussed in the books by Farrar and Becker[6] and Slichter.[7]

REFERENCES

1. **Papoulis, A.,** *Probability, Random Variables, and Stochastic Processes,* McGraw-Hill, New York, 1965.
2. **Davenport, W. B.,** *Probability and Random Processes: An Introduction for Applied Scientists and Engineers,* McGraw-Hill, New York, 1970.
3. **Parzen, E.,** *Stochastic Processes,* Holden-Day, San Francisco, 1962.
4. **Papoulis, A.,** *Signal Analysis,* McGraw-Hill, New York, 1977.
5. **Breiman, L.,** *Probability and Stochastic Processes: With a View Toward Applications,* Houghton Mifflin, Boston, MA, 1969.
6. **Farrar, T. C., and Becker, E. D.,** *Pulse and Fourier Transform NMR: Introduction to Theory and Methods,* Academic Press, New York, 1971.
7. **Slichter, C. P.,** *Principles of Magnetic Resonance,* Springer-Verlag, Berlin, 1978.

Chapter 12

LINEAR, LEAST MEAN SQUARE ESTIMATION

The major goal of this book is to develop methods for estimating a signal from measurements of that signal. For example, in computed tomography, the cross-sectional distribution of attenuation coefficients is estimated from a series of projection measurements. The major estimation technique which will be used is linear, least mean square estimation. The goal of this chapter will be to gain an understanding of simple applications of linear, least mean square estimation.

In Chapter 25 (Normal Equations) we shall apply linear, mean square estimation to linear systems. In Chapter 26 (Wiener Filtering) we shall apply linear, mean square estimation to linear, time invariant systems. Finally, in Part IV, we shall use linear, least mean square estimation to solve various reconstruction problems.

I. MODEL

The goal of this chapter is to estimate the mean value of some unknown quantity, f, from a series of noisy measurements which we shall call, p_j. The random variable notation can be used to describe this model of the measurement process:

$$p_j = a_j \cdot f + n_j \qquad (12.1))$$

The a_j are scale factors and n_j is the measurement noise. p_j is a random variable, since the measured values will vary from experiment to experiment.

Equation 12.1 can be written using random vector notation:

$$\boldsymbol{p} = \mathbf{a} \cdot f + \boldsymbol{n} \qquad (12.2)$$

Normally a scalar quantity such as f is written in front of a vector quantity such as $\mathbf{a}$, but we shall use $\mathbf{a} \cdot f$ to be consistent with later notation. Each component of the vector equation represents one measurement of f. Figure 12.1 shows a diagrammatic representation of this model, and Figure 12.2 shows a representation of this model in terms of the vector Equation, 12.2. We shall have more to say about the vector representation below.

This model could be applied to the problem of measurement of the T_1 of a tissue sample in an NMR spectrometer. Each measurement produces a separate result, p_j. Often the statistics of the noise are the same for each of the measurements. However, if a variety of pulse sequences are used, the statistics of the noise might be different for each of the measurements. In that case, the n_j could be different for each measurement. Similarly, if different methods were used for each measurement, then the scale factor, a_j, could be different for each experiment. Equation 12.1 allows us to model this quite complicated experiment.

We shall make a distinction between the words measurement and experiment. We shall refer to all of the measurements on a single tissue sample as one experiment. One experiment may involve many measured values of the unknown; however, only a single unknown tissue sample is measured. Multiple tissue samples will result in multiple experiments, where each experiment is divided into a series of measurements. The distinction between the measurements in an experiment and a sequence of experiments is somewhat artificial, but this distinction will be very important in understanding the differences between the different estimation models.

The statistical properties of the model deal with the different experiments, not with the individual measurements in a single experiment. The means and variances of the unknown and the noise are taken over a sequence of experiments. For each experiment, there is a

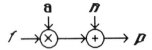

FIGURE 12.1.   Model of measurement process: the unknown is represented by a random variable, f. Multiple measurement of the unknown are modeled by the multiplication of f by the vector, **a**, followed by the addition of the measurement noise represented by a random vector, **n**. The multiple measurements are represented by a random vector, **p**.

$$p = a \cdot f + n$$

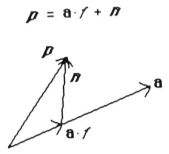

FIGURE 12.2.   Diagram of the measurement process: the random vector, **p**, represents multiple measurements of a random variable, f. The vector, **a**, is the set of scale factors used in the measurement. The random variable, f, is related to the measurement space by the model through these scale factors. The random variable, f, is shown in the measurement space as $\mathbf{a} \cdot f$. The measurement noise is represented by the vector, **n**. The measurement vector, **p**, is the sum of $\mathbf{a} \cdot f$ and **n**.

single outcome of each of the random variables, f, n_j, and p_j. The statistics of the model happens over a series of experiments.

In Equation 12.1 the different measurements are indicated by the subscript, j. The different experiments are indicated by the statistical model. Statistical variables which change from experiment to experiment are indicated by the italics. For each experiment, there is a single unknown, f; f does not have a subscript. Each measurement of the unknown is associated with a different scale factor, a_j, and a different noise, n_j; a_j and n_j both have subscripts. For different experiments, there are different outcomes of the unknown and different values for the noise; f and n_j are in italics. The scale factors do not change from experiment to experiment; a_j is not italicized.

Using a random variable, f, to model the unknown allows us to include *a priori* information about the statistics of the unknown in the problem. For example, we might know the mean and the variance of the T_1 values for samples from the population from which a tissue sample was taken. Using a statistical model of the unknown, f, allows us to model this type of information. If we have no *a priori* information about the unknown, then a more appropriate model would be to use a deterministic model of the unknown, f. The statistics of n_j allow us to model our *a priori* knowledge about the accuracy of the measurement process.

II. LINEAR ESTIMATION

If the measured quantities can be combined in any possible way to produce an estimate, then the problem of determining the best estimate is very difficult. If we restrict the problem to allow only linear combinations of the measurements, then the solution of the problem is much simpler. In this book we shall only consider linear estimates. The reader should be aware that this may mean that the solutions which we derive will be suboptimal; however,

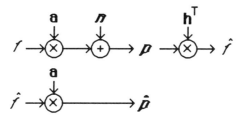

FIGURE 12.3. Model of linear estimation: as in Figure 12.1, the random vector, p, represents multiple measurements of the unknown, f. All linear estimates, $\hat{f}$, of the unknown, f, based on the data, p, can be represented as the vector product, $\mathbf{h}^T \cdot p$. The vector, $\mathbf{h}$, determines the linear estimate of the unknown from the data.

in many cases of interest in radiology linear estimates will be either the best or at least quite good estimates.

The general equation for a linear estimate, $\hat{f}$, of the unknown, f, from the measurements, p_i, is:

$$\hat{f} = \sum_i \mathbf{h}_i \cdot p_i \qquad (12.3)$$

namely, the estimate, $\hat{f}$, is a linear combination of the data values, p_i. The process of estimation amounts to finding the best set of factors, $\mathbf{h}_i$. In vector notation, this equation can be written:

$$\hat{f} = \mathbf{h}^T \cdot p \qquad (12.4)$$

p is a random vector, $\hat{f}$ is a random variable, and $\mathbf{h}$ is a deterministic vector. Figure 12.3 shows a diagrammatic representation of the measurement and estimation process.

In Part III, we shall be concerned with estimating a signal, f, from the measurement of another signal, p. The general equation for a linear estimate, $\hat{f}$, of the vector, f, from the data, p, is

$$\hat{f} = H \cdot p \qquad (12.5)$$

where the vectors $\hat{f}$ and p are random vectors and the matrix H is deterministic. Estimation amounts to determining the best matrix, H. This problem will be covered in Chapter 25 (Normal Equations).

If we assume that the random signals are stationary, then we can use a linear, time independent estimation. As the reader might expect, a linear, time independent estimate of $f(t)$ from $p(t)$ can be written as a convolution:

$$\hat{f}(t) = h(t)*p(t) \qquad (12.6)$$

$\hat{f}(t)$ and $p(t)$ are stochastic processes, and $h(t)$ is a deterministic signal. Estimation in this case amounts to determining the best signal, $h(t)$. This problem will be covered in Chapter 26 (Wiener Filtering). But more of this later.

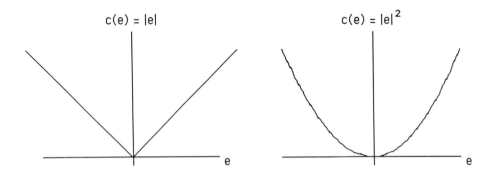

FIGURE 12.4.   Cost functions: the graph on the left shows a situation where the cost of making an error is equal to the magnitude of the error. The graph on the right shows a situation where the cost of making an error is equal to the square of the magnitude of the error. This cost function leads to the mean square error criterion which we shall use throughout the book.

III. LEAST MEAN SQUARE ERROR

In general there will be an error in the estimate. One method of defining the error is as the difference between the true value and the estimate:

$$e = f - \hat{f} \tag{12.7}$$

The error will be a random variable since it will vary from experiment to experiment. The goal of estimation is to minimize the error with regard to some criteria.

Often it is reasonable to assume that the cost of making an estimation error is related to the size of the error. In this case we can define a cost function, $c(e)$, which assigns a cost to each error value. The total cost of the estimate error is the sum of the cost of each error times the likelihood that the error will occur:

$$\int_{-\infty}^{+\infty} c(e) \cdot p(e) \, de = E\{c(e)\} \tag{12.8}$$

where $p(e)$ is the probability that the estimation error is equal to e. The total cost, the left hand side of Equation 12.8 is equal to the expected value of the cost function (see definition of the expected value, Equation 10.6).

As a part of the model of a system, we can select the cost function, $c(e)$. One possibility is to assign a cost equal to the magnitude of the error. That cost function is shown in the first graph in Figure 12.4. In that case the total cost is:

$$E\{c(e)\} = E\{|e|\} \tag{12.9}$$

This is a reasonable cost function; however, it tends to be somewhat hard to work with in practice. A cost function which turns out to give much simpler results is the square cost function shown in the second panel of Figure 12.4. In this case the total cost is:

$$E\{c(e)\} = E\{|e|^2\} \tag{12.10}$$

This cost is known as the mean square error since it is the mean value of the square of the error.

In this book, we shall be concerned almost exclusively with linear estimates which minimize the mean square error. The primary reason that we limit ourselves to linear, mean

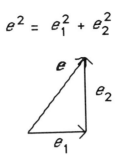

FIGURE 12.5. Orthogonal errors: often the errors in two measurements of an unknown are unrelated. The errors are orthogonal in the statistical sense. This situation is analogous to a vector e which has two components, e_1 and e_2, which are orthogonal in the geometric sense. The square of the length of e^2 is equal to the sum of the squares of the components, $e_1^2 + e_2^2$.

square estimates is that the results come out in a particularly simple fashion. Furthermore, in many radiological applications linear, mean square estimates are either optimal or close to optimal. However, the reader must remember that it is always possible that a nonlinear estimate using some other criteria could be more appropriate in certain circumstances. For example, maximum likelihood estimation has been successfully applied to many radiological problems.

We have selected the mean square error criteria because it turns out that it leads to very good results. But why is the mean square error criteria so good? This question cannot be answered in a mathematically pure sense; however, we can give some heuristic reasons why it works well. Minimizing the mean square error amounts to minimizing the energy in the error (see the discussion of energy in Chapter 10). By analogy between signal processing and physics, the energy in the error is a good thing to minimize.

If we consider the errors which are obtained from a set of measurements as a vector where each component of the vector is one of the measurements, then the square of the length is equal to the sum of the squares of the errors. Thus, minimizing the mean square error amounts to minimizing the length of the total error vector. Figure 12.5 shows an error vector with two components. The length of the vector, e, is the square root of the sum of the squares of the two components, e_1 and e_2.

For many types of estimation, if the measurements are independent and the noise has a mean of zero, then the errors can be shown to be orthogonal in the statistical sense:

$$E\{e_1 \cdot e_2\} = 0 \qquad (12.11)$$

This statistical orthogonality corresponds to the geometric assumption that the components of the error vector are at right angles. The squares of orthogonal errors, like orthogonal vectors are additive. Thus, our mean square error criteria is like assuming that the various experiments are unrelated.

IV. PROJECTION OF A VECTOR ONTO A SECOND VECTOR

The first problem which we shall consider is the linear, mean square estimation of a vector, $\mathbf{p}$, in terms of another vector, $\mathbf{a}$. This linear estimate can be written in the simple form:

$$\hat{\mathbf{p}} = \hat{f} \cdot \mathbf{a} \qquad (12.12)$$

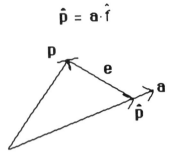

FIGURE 12.6.   Estimation of a vector by another vector: an estimate, $\hat{\mathbf{p}}$, of a vector, $\mathbf{p}$, in terms of another vector, $\mathbf{a}$, can be written as $\mathbf{a} \cdot \hat{f}$, where $\hat{f}$ is a scale factor. The error, $\mathbf{e}$, in the estimate is equal to $\mathbf{p} - \hat{\mathbf{p}}$.

The estimate, $\hat{\mathbf{p}}$, must be a multiple of the vector, $\mathbf{a}$. Estimation using this model amounts to determining the best scalar factor, $\hat{f}$.

This problem is shown in Figure 12.6. $\mathbf{p}$ is the vector which we wish to estimate. The estimate, $\hat{\mathbf{p}}$, is a multiple of the vector, $\mathbf{a}$; therefore, $\hat{\mathbf{p}}$ is in the same direction as $\mathbf{a}$. We can see that the problem of estimating $\mathbf{p}$ in terms of $\mathbf{a}$ amounts to picking the point along $\mathbf{a}$ which is closest to $\mathbf{p}$. We have already solved this same problem in Chapter 8, namely, $\hat{\mathbf{p}}$ is the projection of $\mathbf{p}$ on $\mathbf{a}$.

We can consider $\mathbf{p}$ to be like an experimental data value. The *a priori* information provided by the model of the experiment is that the true value lies along the direction of $\mathbf{a}$. Finding $\hat{\mathbf{p}}$, the point along $\mathbf{a}$ which is closest to $\mathbf{p}$, amounts to combining the experimental data, $\mathbf{p}$, with the *a priori* information that $\hat{\mathbf{p}}$ must be in the same direction as $\mathbf{a}$.

This problem has been set up as an estimation problem; however, it does not include any random variables or noise. If we were only interested in this problem, we would solve it as a problem in geometry; however, we are interested in a geometrical interpretation of the estimation problem, so we shall solve this simple problem using the estimation terminology. The real estimation problems described below will have features which are analogous to the projection problem.

One of the difficulties with understanding estimation problems is keeping straight what is being estimated and what assumptions are made about the model. Notice that we have used the symbol, $\mathbf{p}$, instead of $\mathbf{f}$ for the unknown quantity. And we have used $\hat{f}$ instead of h for the scale factor. The reason for choosing these symbols should become clearer as we progress through the various estimation problems. The part of the problem on which we are working is the second line in Figure 12.3. The reader is warned to make a special effort to keep track of the differences between each of the models which will be discussed.

We shall define an error vector:

$$\mathbf{e} = \mathbf{p} - \hat{\mathbf{p}} \qquad (12.13)$$

The error vector is the difference between the vector, $\mathbf{p}$, and the estimate, $\hat{\mathbf{p}}$. The square of the error vector is:

$$e^2 = \mathbf{e}^T \cdot \mathbf{e} \qquad (12.14)$$

e^2 defined in this way is the sum of the squares of the components of $\mathbf{e}$. Below we shall see that the components of $\mathbf{e}$ are analogous to the errors for each measurement. Thus, e^2/N, where N is equal to the number of components, is equal to the mean square error.

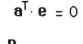

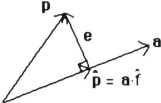

FIGURE 12.7. Linear, least mean square estimation as a projection: the orthogonality principle states that for linear, least mean square estimation, the error, **e**, should be orthogonal to the estimation space defined by the vector, **a**. Therefore, the estimate, $\hat{\mathbf{p}}$, of **p** is the projection of **p** on the vector **a**.

Minimization of e^2 is analogous to mean square error estimation. e^2 is the energy in the error; e^2/N is the average power of the error components.

The square of the error vector, e^2, was used in Chapter 8 to calculate the length, e, of **e**. Minimizing the square of the error, e^2, will also minimize the length of the error vector, e. From Figure 12.7 we have already determined the minimum mean square error estimate from geometrical considerations. The shortest vector, **e**, will occur when **e** is orthogonal to **a**. The orthogonality of **e** to **a** and the minimum mean square error are connected by the definition of the length in terms of the sum of the squares of the components.

Now that we have derived the solution geometrically, let us try to derive the same result algebraically. The minimum of e^2 will occur where the derivative with respect to $\hat{f}$ is equal to zero.

$$\partial(\mathbf{e}^T \cdot \mathbf{e})/\partial\hat{f} = 2 \cdot (\partial\mathbf{e}^T/\partial\hat{f}) \cdot \mathbf{e} = 0 \qquad (12.15)$$

The derivative of the error vector with respect to $\hat{f}$ can be expanded:

$$\partial\mathbf{e}^T/\partial\hat{f} = \partial(\mathbf{p}^T)/\partial\hat{f} - \partial(\hat{f} \cdot \mathbf{a}^T)/\partial\hat{f} = \mathbf{a}^T \qquad (12.16)$$

The vector, $\mathbf{p}^T$, is not a function of $\hat{f}$, so the first term is zero. Substituting back into Equation 12.15, we derive the very important result:

$$\mathbf{a}^T \cdot \mathbf{e} = 0 \qquad (12.17)$$

This equation states that the error vector must be perpendicular to the vector which we are using in the estimate.

We shall run into Equation 12.17 over and over again in linear, mean square estimation problems. It is an example of the **orthogonality principle**. The vector, **a**, defines a one-dimensional vector space of allowable estimates which we shall call the estimation space. Using the idea of an estimation space, we can state the orthogonality principle in a general form: **for linear, mean square estimation the error is orthogonal to the estimation space**.

Below we shall find the same relation for problems with random variables. In that case, the error and the estimators are orthogonal in the statistical sense. Orthogonality of the error and the estimators means that error and the estimators are uncorrelated. Since the error and the estimators are uncorrelated, all of the information about the estimate has been removed from the estimators. But more of this later.

The orthogonality principle can be expanded to obtain a relation between the cross product of the estimators with the data and the estimate:

$$\mathbf{a}^T \cdot \mathbf{e} = \mathbf{a}^T \cdot (\mathbf{p} - \hat{f} \cdot \mathbf{a}) = 0 \tag{12.18}$$

Thus,

$$\mathbf{a}^T \cdot \mathbf{p} = \mathbf{a}^T \cdot (\hat{f} \cdot \mathbf{a}) \tag{12.19}$$

The left hand side of this equation is the product of the estimator, $\mathbf{a}$, with the data. The right hand is the product of the estimator with the estimation. We can interpret this equation as saying that the correlation of the estimator and the data is equal to the correlation of the estimator and the estimate. **The mutual energy of the estimator and the data is equal to the mutual energy of the estimator and the estimate**.

Now let us solve equation 12.19 for the scalar factor, $\hat{f}$.

$$\hat{f} = \mathbf{a}^T \cdot \mathbf{p}/(\mathbf{a}^T \cdot \mathbf{a}) \tag{12.20}$$

The estimate, $\hat{\mathbf{p}}$, is given by $\hat{f} \cdot \mathbf{a}$:

$$\hat{\mathbf{p}} = \mathbf{a}^T \cdot \mathbf{p}/(\mathbf{a}^T \cdot \mathbf{a}) \cdot \mathbf{a} \tag{12.21}$$

The estimate is the projection of the vector $\mathbf{p}$ onto $\mathbf{a}$.

Let us summarize the results of this section:

Given:	Two vectors $\mathbf{p}$ and $\mathbf{a}$.	
Estimate:	$\hat{\mathbf{p}} = \hat{f} \cdot \mathbf{a}$	(12.22)
Error:	$\mathbf{e} = \mathbf{p} - \hat{\mathbf{p}}$	(12.23)
Orthogonality:	$\mathbf{a}^T \cdot \mathbf{e} = 0$	(12.24)
Solution:	$\hat{f} = \mathbf{a}^T \cdot \mathbf{p}/(\mathbf{a}^T \cdot \mathbf{a})$	(12.25)

The model states that the true value must lie in the direction of the vector $\mathbf{a}$. The best linear, least mean square estimate of the data vector, $\mathbf{p}$, in terms of the vector, $\mathbf{a}$, is the projection of $\mathbf{p}$ on $\mathbf{a}$. The estimate is the point along the line defined by $\mathbf{a}$ which is closest to $\mathbf{p}$. The error in the estimate is orthogonal to the estimation space. The estimation space, the set of allowable estimates is the *a priori* information provided by the model. The model shown in Figure 12.3 shows that in the absence of noise the data p lies along $\mathbf{a}$. The second line of the figure incorporates this *a priori* knowledge in the estimate.

V. LINEAR, MEAN SQUARE ESTIMATION FROM MULTIPLE MEASUREMENTS

So far, a number of preliminaries have been covered — the model of the system, the definition of linear estimation, the cost function for mean square estimation, and projection of a vector onto a second vector. Now we shall try our first real estimation problem. The model of the experiment has been described above. There are multiple, independent mea-

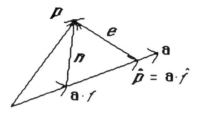

FIGURE 12.8. Linear estimation of the data: the model of the measurement process is the same as in Figure 12.2. In addition, the random vector, $\hat{p}$, is a linear estimate of p in the estimation space defined by the vector, $\mathbf{a}$. The model of the measurement and estimation processes requires the estimate to be in the form $\mathbf{a} \cdot \hat{f}$. This figure is similar to Figure 12.6 except for the change from a deterministic to a statistical model.

surements, p_j, of an unknown, f, where each measurement may be associated with a different scale factor, a_j, and a different amount of measurement noise, n_j.

The model was given in Equation 12.1:

$$p_j = a_j \cdot f + n_j \tag{12.26}$$

The model of the experiment was given in terms of random vectors in Equation 12.2:

$$p = \mathbf{a} \cdot f + n \tag{12.27}$$

where p and n are random vectors, f is the unknown random variable, and $\mathbf{a}$ is a deterministic vector.

Figure 12.1 shows a diagrammatic representation of the measurement process, and Figure 12.2 shows a vector representation. $\mathbf{a} \cdot f$ is a vector in the measurement space which represents the unknown quantity. Because of the model we have assumed the unknown must always lie along the direction of the vector, $\mathbf{a}$. The noise which is added in the measurement process is represented by the random vector, n. The actual measurement, p, is the sum of $\mathbf{a} \cdot f$ and n.

Linear estimation means that the estimate must be of the form given by Equations 12.3 or 12.4:

$$\hat{f} = \sum_j h_j \cdot p_j = \mathbf{h}^T \cdot p \tag{12.28}$$

where $\hat{f}$ is the estimate of f based on the measurements p_j. The estimation process amounts to finding the best values for the factors, h_j. In addition to defining the estimate, $\hat{f}$, we can also define a random vector, $\hat{p}$, which represents an estimate of the data values:

$$\hat{p} = \mathbf{a} \cdot \hat{f} \tag{12.29}$$

Figure 12.8 shows the estimate, $\hat{p}$, of the data, p. Because of the model, the estimate of the data must lie along $\mathbf{a}$. The estimation space consists of all the vectors in the one-dimensional space defined by $\mathbf{a} \cdot \hat{f}$.

Ultimately, we are most interested in estimating the quantity, f. However, it is often easier to estimate the data, p, than to estimate the unknown, f. To find the estimates, $\hat{p}$, it is first necessary to estimate, $\hat{f}$, so the reader may be a little confused about why these two estimates are different. The major difference is how the error is defined. We can define the error either as the difference between f and $\hat{f}$ or as the difference between p and $\hat{p}$. The first definition gives us an estimate of f; the second gives us an estimate of p.

These two different approaches, estimation of the unknown or estimation of the data, are both used in real problems. In Chapter 26, we shall see that Wiener Filtering is a method of estimating the unknown. Wiener filtering is a linear, time invariant estimation. The normal equations from linear algebra described in Chapter 25 solve the more difficult problem of linear estimation. However, they are based on the simpler problem of estimation of the data. In this section, we shall go over both approaches, but again the reader is warned to make a special effort to keep the various models straight.

VI. ESTIMATION OF THE DATA

In order to estimate the data, we shall define the error for each measurement as:

$$e_k = p_k - \hat{p}_k \tag{12.30}$$

Using vector notation:

$$e = p - \hat{p} \tag{12.31}$$

Mean square error estimation means that we wish to minimize the sum of the squares of the errors for each measurement:

$$E\{c(e)\} = E\left\{\sum_k e_k^2\right\} \tag{12.32}$$

The new feature in this problem as compared to the projection problem is the random variables. Because of these random variables we need to use the expected value, $E\{\cdot\}$, of the error.

A. ALGEBRAIC DERIVATION

Minimization of 12.32 with respect to the parameters, h_i, can be accomplished mathematically by setting the partial derivative of Equation 12.32 equal to zero:

$$\delta E\left\{\sum_k e_k^2\right\}/\delta h_i = E\left\{\sum_k 2 \cdot \delta e_k/\delta h_i \cdot e_k\right\} = 0 \tag{12.33}$$

The derivative can be expanded using Equations 12.30 and 12.28:

$$\delta e_k/\delta h_i = \delta\left(p_k - a_k \cdot \sum_j h_j \cdot p_j\right)/\delta h_i \tag{12.34}$$

The first term, p_k, is the measured value which does not depend on h_i; therefore, the derivative is zero. The second term is a summation. However, the only term in the summation which depends upon h_i is when j is equal to i. Therefore, Equation 12.33 can be simplified as:

$$E\left\{2 \cdot p_i \cdot \sum_k a_k \cdot e_k\right\} = 0 \tag{12.35}$$

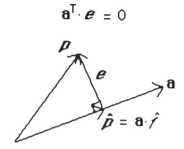

FIGURE 12.9.   Linear, least mean square estimation of the data: the orthogonality principle states that for linear, least mean square estimation, the error, e, must be orthogonal to the estimation space defined by the vector, $\mathbf{a}$. Therefore, the estimate, $\hat{p}$, is the projection of p onto the vector, $\mathbf{a}$. This figure is similar to Figure 12.7 except for the change to a statistical model.

Since Equation 12.35 must be true for any data value, p_i, the summation must be zero:

$$E\left\{ \sum_k a_k \cdot e_k \right\} = 0 \tag{12.36}$$

We can write this result using vector notation as:

$$E\{\mathbf{a}^T \cdot e\} = 0 \tag{12.37}$$

The expected value will be zero if the vector product within the expected value is zero:

$$\mathbf{a}^T \cdot e = 0 \tag{12.38}$$

Again we have encountered the orthogonality principle (Equation 12.38). The errors for the different measurements must be orthogonal to the scale factors. This solution is somewhat unusual since we have required that $\mathbf{a}^T$ be orthogonal to e for all experimental values p. Generally, we shall find that the orthogonality principle only holds on average instead of being true for each experiment.

B. GEOMETRIC DERIVATION

The result given in Equation 12.38 is exactly analogous to the result which we obtained for estimation of a vector, $\mathbf{p}$, in terms of another vector, $\mathbf{a}$. Figure 12.9 shows these relations graphically. Figure 12.9 is the same as Figure 12.7 except that the statistical quantities have been used instead of the deterministic quantities. The estimate, $\hat{p}$, must lie along the vector, $\mathbf{a}$, since it is defined to be $\mathbf{a} \cdot \hat{f}$. The error vector is orthogonal to $\mathbf{a}$, so $\hat{p}$ is the projection of p on $\mathbf{a}$.

Figure 12.9 shows how the measured information, p, is combined with the *a priori* information provided by the model. The model tells us that in the absence of noise, the measurements would be $\mathbf{a} \cdot f$. Thus, the "true" data must lie along $\mathbf{a}$. Our actual measurements, $\hat{p}$ do not lie along $\mathbf{a}$ due to the noise. The best linear, mean square estimate, $\hat{p}$, is the point along $\mathbf{a}$ which is closest to the data.

Figure 12.10 shows the noise vector, n, separated into two components — one component is along the vector $\mathbf{a}$, and the other component is perpendicular to $\mathbf{a}$. Our model states that the estimate of the data must lie along, $\mathbf{a}$. What has happened with the least mean square estimation is that this information is combined with the measurement, p. The portion of the noise which is inconsistent with the model, the noise perpendicular to $\mathbf{a}$, is removed by the

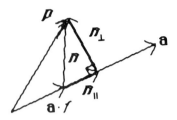

FIGURE 12.10.   Components of the measurement noise: the noise, n, can be divided into two components, $n_{\parallel}$ and $n_{\perp}$, with regard to the estimation space. The noise which is perpendicular to the estimation space is inconsistent with the model of the measurement process. The portion of the noise which is parallel to the estimation space is consistent with the model. The estimation process removes the perpendicular component of the noise, the noise which is inconsistent with the model. It does not affect the parallel component of the noise.

estimation. The portion of the noise which is consistent with the model, the noise along the direction of **a**, cannot be removed. Using the *a priori* information we are able to improve the accuracy of our estimate over the raw data by removing the inconsistent data.

Now we can use the orthogonality principle to solve for the factors **h**. Using equations 12.38 and 12.31:

$$\mathbf{a}^{\mathrm{T}} \cdot e = \mathbf{a}^{\mathrm{T}} \cdot p - \mathbf{a}^{\mathrm{T}} \cdot \mathbf{a} \cdot \hat{f} = 0 \qquad (12.39)$$

$$\hat{f} = \mathbf{a}^{\mathrm{T}} \cdot p / \mathbf{a}^{\mathrm{T}} \cdot \mathbf{a} \qquad (12.40)$$

Comparing equations 12.40 and 12.28 we see that:

$$\mathbf{h} = \mathbf{a}/(\mathbf{a}^{\mathrm{T}} \cdot \mathbf{a}) \qquad (12.41)$$

Thus, **h** is equal to **a** divided by the square of the length of **a**. We have not shown **h** in the diagrams since it is just a scaled version of **a**.

The estimate of the data is $\hat{f} \cdot \mathbf{a}$:

$$\hat{p} = (\mathbf{a}^{\mathrm{T}} \cdot p/(\mathbf{a}^{\mathrm{T}} \cdot \mathbf{a})) \cdot \mathbf{a} \qquad (12.42)$$

The result is very similar to the projection of a vector onto another vector. Since the answer does not use the statistic of f, we can restate Equation 12.27 using a deterministic model of the unknown:

$$p = \mathbf{a} \cdot \mathrm{f} + n \qquad (12.43)$$

We have used the random variable notation, f, during the derivation in order to be consistent with estimation of the unknown.

C. EXAMPLE OF ESTIMATION OF THE DATA

To understand this result, consider a very simple example where a_i is one for all i. In other words we have a sequence of measurements without any scale factors. Then Equation 12.40 reduces to:

$$\hat{f} = \sum_{k} p_k/N \qquad (12.44)$$

where N is the number of measurements. In other words after all this mathematical folderol, the answer is to average the measurements!

It is obvious that we could have come to this simple answer with much less work; however, the approach used is analogous to the approach which we shall use for the more difficult problems yet to come. Hopefully, the reader will be able to understand these problems better after having seen this simple problem.

Let us summarize the results of this section:

$$\text{Measurement:} \quad p = \mathbf{a} \cdot f + n \tag{12.45}$$

$$\text{Estimate:} \quad \hat{p} = \mathbf{a} \cdot \hat{f}, \quad \text{where} \quad \hat{f} = \mathbf{h}^T \cdot p \tag{12.46}$$

$$\text{Error:} \quad e = p - \hat{p} \tag{12.47}$$

$$\text{Orthogonality:} \quad \mathbf{a}^T \cdot e = 0 \tag{12.48}$$

$$\text{Solution:} \quad \mathbf{h} = \mathbf{a}/\mathbf{a}^T \cdot \mathbf{a}$$

$$\text{For } a_i = 1, \quad h_j = 1/N \tag{12.49}$$

The best estimate of the data, p, which is consistent with the *a priori* information provided by the model is the projection of p on $\mathbf{a}$. The information provided by the model is that without noise, the data would be $\mathbf{a} \cdot f$. Thus, the estimate must be of the form, $\mathbf{a} \cdot \hat{f}$. The best linear, least mean square estimate is the point in this estimation space which is closest to the data. In the simple case where all the scale factors are equal to one, the estimate is the average of the measurements.

D. WHAT IS WRONG WITH ESTIMATION OF THE DATA?

We have derived a linear, least mean square estimate of the data as we had set out to do. It would seem we have solved the problem. So the reader may be asking, "why isn't this the end of the chapter?" The problem is that we have not included any *a priori* information about f in the estimation. In problems for which there is no *a priori* information about f, then the estimate given above is the best linear, least mean square estimate. When there is some information about f, then we can obtain a better estimate by including that information.

An additional piece of *a priori* information which we may have is the second moments of f and n. The second moments of f and n are the average powers of the unknown and the noise. If the second moment of $\mathbf{a} \cdot f$ is small compared to that of n, then the data, p, is mostly composed of noise, i.e., the power in p is largely due to the power in n.

The previous figures in this chapter have all shown a single possible outcome of an experiment. They have not shown the statistical nature of the model. Figure 12.11 shows two possible outcomes for the case where the noise power is large with respect to the unknown. The data values, p, are predominant related to the noise, not to the unknown. The projection of p on $\mathbf{a}$ gives a very poor estimate of the unknown. Zero would be a better estimate of f than that obtained by projection of p on $\mathbf{a}$.

Figure 12.11 suggests that when the power in the noise is larger than the power in the signal, an estimate which is more "zero like" will be better than that obtained when the signal power is larger than the noise power. This observation suggests that the estimate should be scaled with some relationship to the power in the signal and the power in the noise. In the next section we shall derive an estimate which depends upon the relationship of the powers in the signal and the noise.

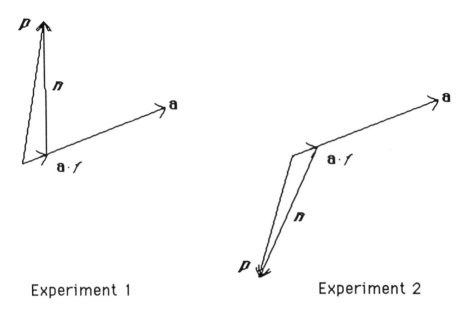

Experiment 1   Experiment 2

FIGURE 12.11.   Measurements with a large amount of noise: when the power in the noise, n, is large
with respect to the power in the signal, $\mathbf{a} \cdot \hat{f}$, then the data, p, predominantly represent the noise, not
the signal. This figure shows two experiments where there is a large amount of measurement noise. In
these two examples the projection of the data onto the estimation space defined by $\mathbf{a}$ would give poor
estimates of the unknown.

The reader may wonder why we are interested in trying to make an estimate when the
data are predominantly due to noise. When estimating a single unknown, it makes much
more sense to try to get better data. However, our goal in Part IV will be to estimate an
entire signal, $f(t)$. In that case the data about some aspects of the signal may be very good
and the data about other aspects of the signal may be very poor. In order to estimate the
entire signal, we shall need to estimate the aspects of the signal about which our information
is very poor. Thus, the situation diagrammed in Figure 12.11 will occur frequently.

VII. ESTIMATION OF THE UNKNOWN

The next problem which we shall consider is similar to the previous problem, but we
shall estimate the unknown, f, instead of the data p. The model of the measurement process
is the same as for the last problem except that we shall make use of the statistical properties
of the unknown:

$$p = \mathbf{a} \cdot f + n \tag{12.50}$$

The estimate is defined:

$$\hat{f} = \mathbf{h}^T \cdot p \tag{12.51}$$

The definition of the error is different than above:

$$e = f - \hat{f} \tag{12.52}$$

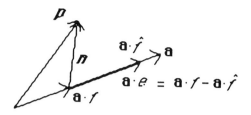

FIGURE 12.12.   Estimation of the unknown: the representation of the estimate of the unknown, **a** · $\hat{f}$, in the measurement space must lie along the direction of the vector, **a**. The representation of the error, **a** · e, must also lie along the direction of the vector, **a**. The orthogonality principle for estimation of the unknown cannot be diagrammed in the measurement space.

e is defined in terms of the unknown, not the data. e is a random variable, not a random vector since we are estimating a single unknown. We shall represent the estimate in the measurement space as:

$$\hat{p} = \mathbf{a} \cdot \hat{f} \qquad (12.53)$$

However, for this problem, $\hat{f}$, is being estimated, not $\hat{p}$. Figure 12.3 shows a diagrammatic representation of this estimation process.

A. UNKNOWN, MEASUREMENT, AND ESTIMATION SUBSPACES

In order to better understand the difference between estimation of the data and estimation of the unknown, it is useful to define various vector spaces associated with the estimation process. The unknown space, associated with the unknown, f, has one dimension. The measurement space, associated with the measurement, p, has a number of dimensions equal to the number of measurements.

The previous diagrams, such as Figure 12.8, have attempted to show the measurement space. The unknown space is related to the measurement space by the model through the vector, **a**. When estimating the data, the estimate, **a** · $\hat{f}$, must lie in the one-dimensional estimation space defined by the vector **a**. The estimation space must be a subspace of the measurement space. The diagrammatic representation of both the unknown space and the estimation space in Figure 12.8 are along the vector, **a**.

Figure 12.12 shows a diagrammatic representation of estimation of the unknown. The estimate, $\hat{f}$, must lie in the one-dimensional estimation space which is the same space as the unknown space. The unknown, f, and the estimate of the unknown, $\hat{f}$, are shown in the measurement space with the vectors, **a** · f and **a** · $\hat{f}$.

When estimating the data, the error, e, is a vector in the measurement space (Figure 12.8). When estimating the unknown, the error, e, is a scalar in the unknown space. The error, e, can be represented in the measurement space by multiplying equation 12.52 by **a**:

$$\mathbf{a} \cdot e = \mathbf{a} \cdot f - \mathbf{a} \cdot \hat{f} \qquad (12.54)$$

In Figure 12.12 we represent the scalar error, e, in the measurement space with the vector, **a** · e.

The major difference between the two models is that when estimating the unknown, the estimation space is a subspace of the measurement space. When estimating the data, the estimation space is a subspace of the unknown space (a subspace equal to the unknown space).

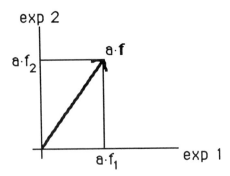

FIGURE 12.13.   Two outcomes for the unknown: the value of the unknown is diagrammed for two separate experiments. In the first experiment the "true" value of the unknown is a · f_1 and in the second experiment the value is a · f_2. These values represent the outcomes of two samples of the random variable, f. The vector, a · **f**, represents the possible experimental outcome of the random variable, f. The different components of a · **f** represent the statistical aspects of the random variable.

B. GEOMETRIC DERIVATION

In the previous derivation, orthogonality was true for each experimental outcome. The axes of the diagrams were different measurements of a single experiment. In the derivation which follows, the orthogonality will be true statistically. In order to obtain a geometric diagram of the orthogonality, we shall need to draw a diagram which shows the results of two experimental outcomes.

Since we cannot diagram a multi-dimensional space which shows both the different measurements and the different outcomes, we shall have to simplify the model to allow only a single measurement:

$$p = a \cdot f + n \tag{12.55}$$

The estimate involves scaling the single data value:

$$\hat{f} = h \cdot p \tag{12.56}$$

Figure 12.13 shows a diagram of a single measurement for two different experiments. The outcome for experiment 1 is a · f_1; the outcome for experiment 2 is a · f_2. At the risk of causing a great deal of confusion, we have defined a vector, a · **f**, which is a vector of the outcomes of the random variable, f, times the single scale factor, a. The vector, a · **f**, is not a random vector since it represents a set of discrete outcomes.

The space defined by the outcomes of the unknown, **f**, has a number of dimensions equal to the number of outcomes. The representation of these outcomes in the space defined by the outcomes of the measurements, a · **f**, is a vector. Similarly, a noise vector **n** consists of two outcomes from the random variable n; and a data vector, **p**, consists of the two outcomes for the measurement, p. Figure 12.14 shows a · **f**, **n**, and **p** for two experimental outcomes.

We can define a vector, a · $\hat{\mathbf{f}}$, which represents the outcomes of the estimate of $\hat{f}$. This vector is defined by the model to be:

$$a \cdot \hat{\mathbf{f}} = a \cdot h \cdot \mathbf{p} \tag{12.57}$$

Thus, the estimation outcome space must be the one-dimensional subspace of the measurement outcome space which is defined by the data vector, **p**. The error vector, **e**, represents

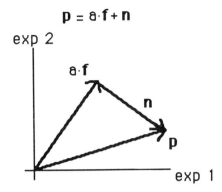

FIGURE 12.14. Two experimental outcomes: this diagram shows two outcomes of an experiment. For each experiment there is a single measurement of the unknown, f. The two samples of the unknown are represented by the vector, a · **f**. The two outcomes of the measurement noise are represented by the vector, **n**. The two outcomes of the measurement are represented by the vector **p**.

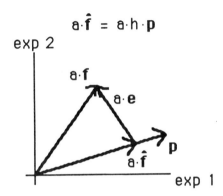

FIGURE 12.15. Outcome of linear estimation of the unknown: linear estimates of the unknown in terms of the data must be in the form, a · h · **p**. Therefore the estimate, a · $\hat{\mathbf{f}}$, must lie along the direction of the data **p**.

the outcomes of the random variable, e. Figure 12.15 shows the estimate, a · $\hat{\mathbf{f}}$, and the error vector a · **e** for a single measurement.

The reader who is not totally confused by the change in the model can probably guess the solution from Figure 12.15. The orthogonality principle will state that the error must be orthogonal to the estimation space, the space defined by the **p**. Figure 12.16 shows this result diagrammatically. The estimate is the projection of a · **f** on **p**. The error vector, **e**, is orthogonal to the data, **p**:

$$\mathbf{p}^T \cdot (a \cdot \mathbf{e}) = 0 \qquad (12.58)$$

The orthogonality principle has led to a result which is similar to the last problem — the estimate, $\hat{\mathbf{f}}$, is the projection of a · **f** on **p**. However, unlike the last problem this fact does not provide an algorithm for solution. We do not know the unknown, a · **f**; therefore, we cannot project it on **p** to derive the estimate. We must modify the result so that we can express, a · $\hat{\mathbf{f}}$, in terms of the data, **p**.

The orthogonality principle given in Equation 12.58 can be expanded:

$$\mathbf{p}^T \cdot (a \cdot \mathbf{f} - a \cdot \hat{\mathbf{f}}) = 0 \qquad (12.59)$$

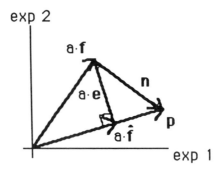

FIGURE 12.16.   Outcome of linear, least mean square estimation of the unknown: the orthogonality principle states that for linear, least mean square estimation of the unknown the error must be statistically orthogonal to the data. Diagrammatically, the error vector, a · **e**, must be geometrically orthogonal to the data vector, **p**. The estimate, a · $\hat{\mathbf{f}}$, is the projection of the unknown, a · **f**, onto the data, **p**.

Thus,

$$\mathbf{p}^T \cdot (a \cdot \hat{\mathbf{f}}) = \mathbf{p}^T \cdot (a \cdot \mathbf{f}) \qquad (12.60)$$

This equation can be interpreted as saying that the correlation between the data and the estimate is equal to the correlation between the data and the unknown. **The mutual energy between the data and the estimate is equal to the mutual energy between the data and the unknown.**

Multiplying both sides of Equation 12.60 by **p** gives:

$$(\mathbf{p} \cdot \mathbf{p}^T) \cdot (a \cdot \hat{\mathbf{f}}) = (\mathbf{p}^T \cdot (a \cdot \mathbf{f})) \cdot \mathbf{p} \qquad (12.61)$$

In Chapter 8, we used the notation p^2 for the square length of a vector, **p** · $\mathbf{p}^T$. Thus,

$$(a \cdot \hat{\mathbf{f}}) = (\mathbf{p}^T \cdot (a \cdot \mathbf{f}))/p^2 \cdot \mathbf{p} \qquad (12.62)$$

The estimate, a · $\hat{\mathbf{f}}$, is equal to the data, **p**, scaled by the ratio of the mutual energy in the data and the unknown to the energy in the data. We shall see this same result later in Chapter 26.

Often the unknown is orthogonal to the noise in the statistical sense. If $\mathbf{n}^T \cdot \mathbf{f}$ is equal to zero then:

$$\mathbf{p}^T \cdot (a \cdot \mathbf{f}) = (a \cdot \mathbf{f} + \mathbf{n})^T \cdot (a \cdot \mathbf{f}) = (a \cdot f)^2 \qquad (12.63)$$

where f is the length of **f**, and

$$p^2 = (a \cdot \mathbf{f} + \mathbf{n})^T \cdot (a \cdot \mathbf{f} + \mathbf{n}) = (a \cdot f)^2 + n^2 \qquad (12.64)$$

Therefore,

$$a \cdot \hat{\mathbf{f}} = (a \cdot f)^2/[(a \cdot f)^2 + n^2] \cdot \mathbf{p} \qquad (12.65)$$

When the noise is orthogonal to the unknown, the estimate is equal to the data scaled by the ratio of the energy in the unknown to the energy in the unknown plus the energy in the noise. This is a result which we shall encounter frequently.

C. ALGEBRAIC DERIVATION

Now that we have derived the orthogonality principle from a geometric argument, let us derive it algebraically. We shall follow the same procedure of minimizing the square of the error with regard to the parameters, h_i, that we used when estimating the data.

$$\partial E\{e^2\}/\partial h_i = E\{2 \cdot \partial e/\partial h_i \cdot e\} = 0, \quad \text{for all i} \qquad (12.66)$$

The derivative can be expanded:

$$\partial e/\partial h_i = \partial\left(f - \sum_j h_j \cdot p_j\right)/\partial h_i, \quad \text{for all i} \qquad (12.67)$$

The first term, f, the unknown, does not depend on h_i; therefore, the derivative is zero. The second term is a summation. However, the only term in the summation which depends upon h_i is when j is equal to i. Therefore, the derivative simplifies to:

$$\partial e/\partial h_i = p_i, \quad \text{for all i} \qquad (12.68)$$

Substituting Equation 12.68 into Equation 12.66 yields:

$$E\{p_i \cdot e\} = 0, \quad \text{for all i} \qquad (12.69)$$

This equation represents a set of equations, one equation for each value of i. In vector notation:

$$E\{p \cdot e\} = 0 \qquad (12.70)$$

This equation expresses the orthogonality principle in a statistical sense. The data random vector, p, is statistically orthogonal to the error, random variable e. Notice that each data value, p_i, is orthogonal to the error.

This orthogonality principle given in Equation 12.70 is considerably different than that given in Equation 12.38. In that case, the orthogonality was true inside the expectation operator; it was true for each experiment. The orthogonality in Equation 12.70 is true in a statistical sense. On average the product of the data and the error will be the zero vector. For any particular outcome the product will most likely not be zero.

The orthogonality principle tells us that the data and the error are uncorrelated. If the data and the error were correlated, then using this information, it would be possible to reduce the error. The estimation process removes all of the mutual information between the data and the error. The orthogonality principle means that all of the information in the data has been used in making the estimate. None of the information about the unknown is left in the error; only noise is left in the error.

The orthogonality principle can be used to solve for the factors **h**.

$$E\{p_i \cdot e\} = E\left\{p_i \cdot \left(f - \sum_j h_j \cdot p_j\right)\right\} = E\{p_i \cdot f\} - \sum_j h_j \cdot E\{p_i \cdot p_j\} = 0 \quad (12.71)$$

We can use the second moment notation (Equation 10.31) to rewrite this equation as:

$$\sum_j h_j \cdot R_{p_i p_j} = R_{p_i f}, \quad \text{for all i} \qquad (12.72)$$

Equation 12.72 represents a set of linear equations, one equation for each value of i. This set of equations can be solved in a particular case to determine the factors h_j. This set of equations shows the factors which determine the estimation parameters — the cross powers between the measurements and the cross power between the measurement and the signal. These factors will also be important in Chapter 26 (Wiener Filtering).

D. EXAMPLE OF ESTIMATION OF THE UNKNOWN

In order to understand this solution, let us consider a simple example. Let us assume that the scale factors are all equal to one, that the noise has a mean of zero, that the noise for different measurements is uncorrelated, and that the noise and the signal are uncorrelated. Mathematically,

$$a_i = 1, \quad \text{for all i} \tag{12.73}$$

$$E\{n_i\} = 0, \quad \text{for all i} \tag{12.74}$$

$$R_{n_i n_j} = E\{n_i \cdot n_j\} = 0, \quad \text{for } i \neq j \tag{12.75}$$

$$R_{nf} = E\{n_i \cdot f\} = 0 \tag{12.76}$$

From these conditions we can derive simpler expressions for the cross powers:

$$R_{p_i p_j} = E\{f + n_i) \cdot (f + n_j)\}$$

$$= R_f + R_{nf} + R_{fn} + R_{n_i n_j} = R_f \tag{12.77}$$

$$R_p = R_{p_i p_i} = E\{(f + n_i) \cdot (f + n_i)\}$$

$$= R_f + R_{n_i f} + R_{fn_i} + R_{n_i n_i} = R_f + R_{n_i} \tag{12.78}$$

$$R_{p_i f} = E\{f \cdot p_i\} = E\{f^2\} + E\{f \cdot n_i\} = R_f \tag{12.79}$$

In Equations 12.72, all of the terms in the summation on the left of the equal sign are equal to $h_j \cdot R_f$ except for the term where $i = j$; that term is equal to $h_i \cdot (R_f + R_n)$. Therefore, this equation can be rewritten as:

$$\sum_j h_j \cdot R_f + h_i \cdot R_n = R_f, \quad \text{for all i} \tag{12.80}$$

Each of these equations is identical; therefore, all of the factors, h_j, must be the same. Using this fact, we can further simplify this equation:

$$h_j \cdot (N \cdot R_f + R_n) = R_f \tag{12.81}$$

Solving for h_j:

$$h_j = 1/N \cdot R_f/(R_f + R_n/N) \tag{12.82}$$

The first factor, 1/N, gives the same result as in Equation 12.44. This factor averages the data values. In order to understand the second factor, we need to consider the power in the signal and the power in the noise. If we have two measurements, p_1 and p_2, where each measurement has the same power, then the power in the sum of the measurement is:

$$E\{(p_1 + p_2)^2\} = E\{p_1^2\} + E\{p_1 \cdot p_2\} + E\{p_2 \cdot p_1\} + E\{p_2^2\} \qquad (12.83)$$

If the measurements are perfectly correlated, then all of the second moments are equal. In this case the power in the sum is equal to four times the power in each of the measurements. If the measurements are independent, then the cross products are zero. In this case, the power in the sum is equal to only two times the power in the measurements.

By counting the terms, one can easily show that for three measurements, the power in the sum is nine times the power in each measurement if the measurements are perfectly correlated, but only three times the power if the measurements are independent. In general, the power in the sum of N terms is equal to N^2 if the terms are perfectly correlated, and N if the terms are independent.

The estimate, $\hat{f}$, is the sum of N terms with f and N terms with n. The power in $\hat{f}$ will include all combinations of these terms, but the cross terms with f and n are all zero (Equation 12.76), so we can consider the terms in f and in n separately. Since the terms in f are exactly correlated, the power due to these terms will be $N^2 \cdot R_f$. Since the terms in n are independent, the power due to these terms will be $N \cdot R_n$.

The solution given by Equation 12.44 for the case of estimating the data is similar to this solution where we have estimated the unknown. Recall in that case that the estimate was an average of the measurements. The two estimates differ by the factor, $N^2 \cdot R_f/(N^2 \cdot R_f + N \cdot R_n)$, where we have multiplied the numerator and denominator by N^2. This factor is the **power in the signal divided by the power in the signal plus the power in the noise**. We shall encounter this factor again in Chapter 26.

When the noise is small or the number of measurements are large, this factor is equal to one. Thus, when we are sure of the result, this factor does not affect the estimate. The estimate is a simple average. When the power in the noise is much larger than the power in the signal, then this factor goes to zero. In this case the measurements are almost completely noise, so the best estimate is zero. In between these extremes, this factor tries to scale the estimate down according to how much of the power is due to noise.

Let us summarize the results of this section:

Measurement: $\quad p = a \cdot f + n \quad .$ $\qquad\qquad\qquad\qquad\qquad$ (12.84)

Estimate: $\quad \hat{f} = h^T \cdot p$ $\qquad\qquad\qquad\qquad\qquad\qquad\qquad$ (12.85)

Error: $\quad e = f - \hat{f}$ $\qquad\qquad\qquad\qquad\qquad\qquad\qquad\qquad$ (12.86)

Orthogonality: $\quad E\{p \cdot e\} = 0$ $\qquad\qquad\qquad\qquad\qquad\qquad$ (12.87)

Solution: $\quad \sum_j h_j \cdot R_{p_i p_j} = R_{p_i f}, \qquad$ for all i $\qquad\qquad$ (12.88)

$\qquad$ For $a_i = 1$, $\quad E\{n_i\} = 0$, $\quad R_{n_i n_j} = 0$, $\quad$ and $\quad R_{n_i f} = 0$:

$$h_j = 1/N \cdot R_f/(R_f + R_n/N) \qquad (12.89)$$

In the measurement space (Figure 12.12) the estimate, $a \cdot \hat{f}$, must lie along the vector, **a**, as it did for the previous problem. If the power in the data is entirely due to the signal, then the estimate is the same as in the last example. If the power in the data is mostly due to noise, then the estimate is made more ''zero like''. The error is orthogonal to the data; the error and the data are completely uncorrelated. Thus, all of the information about the unknown is extracted from the data.

VIII. SUMMARY

This chapter has introduced linear, least mean square estimation of an unknown value from noisy measurements. We found that minimizing the mean square error is analogous to minimizing the energy in the error. Furthermore, we found that minimizing the mean square error is geometrically analogous to minimizing the length of the error. Although these two analogies provide heuristic reasons for choosing the least mean square error criteria, the major reason for its choice is that it leads to simple results.

In this chapter we have found a procedure for solving estimation problems. Linear, least mean square estimation leads to the orthogonality principle — the error in the estimate is orthogonal to the estimation space. The orthogonality principle can then be used to solve for the factors used in the estimation.

Two problems were solved in this chapter. They both involved estimation of an unknown, f, given measurements described by the equation:

$$p = \mathbf{a} \cdot f + n \tag{12.90}$$

In the first problem, the data, p, was estimated. The estimate was the projection of the data onto the estimation space, $\mathbf{a}$. This result is exactly analogous to estimation of a vector with another vector. In the simple case where $\mathbf{a}$ is equal to one, the estimate is a simple average. The *a priori* information from the model about the statistics of f was not used.

In the second problem, the unknown, f, was estimated. The orthogonality principle stated that the error is orthogonal to the data on average. All of the information about the unknown is removed from the data. In the simple case where $\mathbf{a}$ is equal to one, the noise is zero mean, and the noises from different measurements are uncorrelated, the estimate was an average weighted by the ratio of the power in the signal divided by the power in the signal plus the power in the noise.

In Part III, we shall develop two methods of estimating unknown signals in terms of noisy measurements. One method, the normal equations (Chapter 25), is analogous to the first problem. The second method, Wiener filtering (Chapter 26), is analogous to the second problem. The difference between those problems and the problems in this chapter is that a signal instead of a single value will be estimated.

IX. FURTHER READING

A good geometrical discussion of linear, mean square estimation of the data can be found in Chapter 3 of the book by Strang.[1] An algebraic description of this problem can be found in Section 7-4 of the book by Papoulis.[2] The treatment of estimation of the unknown in this chapter is a bit unusual. It is similar to the development of the Wierner filter except that a single unknown is estimated. The references at the end of Chapter 26 develop linear, mean square estimation for the Wiener filter.

REFERENCES

1. **Strang, G.,** *Linear Algebra and Its Applications,* Academic Press, New York, 1980.
2. **Papoulis, A.,** *Probability, Random Variables, and Stochastic Processes,* McGraw-Hill, New York, 1965.

Chapter 13

SUMMARY OF SYSTEM MODELS

The goal of Part I has been to introduce the concept of a system. A system operates on an input signal to produce an output signal. Part I has described several models which can be used to describe systems — convolution, matrix multiplication, differential equations, and stochastic processes. Including all of these models is useful since each model is most useful for explaining certain features of systems.

The primary goal of this book is to explain image reconstruction. It may seem that the discussion of system models in Part I is excessively detailed. However, in Part IV we shall see that the major task in understanding reconstruction is to clearly understand the model of the data collection process. This is one reason why we have spent so much time on system models.

Systems can be used to model all parts of radiologic imaging. Part I has shown examples of how systems can be used to model data collection. Part III will use systems to model filtering operations. And, Part IV will use systems to model image reconstruction. Furthermore, a single, complex system can be used to model the entire imaging process with subsystems representing data collection, image reconstruction, and image filtering.

Certain concepts have occurred frequently throughout Part I — representation of a signal in terms of a linear combination of basis signals; the relationship between the complexity of the model and the complexity of systems which can be represented by the model; that certain signals, the eigenfunctions, are characteristic of a system; the idea of the state of a system; the analogy between the physical concept of energy, the energy in a signal, and the square of the length of a vector; the analogy of mutual energy in two signals, the product of two vectors, and the statistical concept of correlation; and the analogy between geometric, signal, and statistical orthogonality. The purpose of this chapter is to bring together these similar ideas.

I. CLASSIFICATION OF SYSTEMS

Systems can be classified in terms of their properties. These properties are important because they determine which models can be used to describe a system. Systems can be classified as (1) continuous or discrete, (2) having memory or memoryless, (3) linear or nonlinear, (4) time invariant or nontime invariant, and (5) statistical or deterministic. Table 13.1 lists various types of models and indicates whether they can be used to model systems with various properties.

Continuous systems produce continuous output signals, $g(t)$, in response to continuous input signals, $f(t)$. **Discrete** systems produce discrete output signals, $g[n]$, in response to discrete input signals, $f[n]$. We shall predominantly use continuous models to describe the properties of systems. In practice almost all applications are represented in the computer by discrete models. In Chapter 23 we shall describe the relationships between continuous and discrete system models with particular attention to the artifact (aliasing) produced by representing a continuous system with a discrete model.

In Chapter 2, we reviewed the idea of a function, $f(t)$. A function assigns a value to the dependent variable, f, for each value of the independent variable, t. For a single valued function, there is only one value of f for each value of t. The value of the dependent variable can be calculated from a single value of the independent variable. The output, $g(t)$, of a system without memory depends upon only the value of the input at that same time, $f(t)$. A **memoryless** system can be defined by a function:

$$g(t) = h(f(t)) \tag{13.1}$$

TABLE 13.1
Properties of System Models

System function	Discrete continuous	Memory	Time invariant	Linear	Statistical
H{f(t)}	C,D	Y,N	Y,N	Y,N	N
h(t,τ)	C	Y,N	Y,N	Y	N
h[n,k]	D	Y,N	Y,N	Y	N
H	D	Y,N	Y,N	Y	N
h(t)	C	Y,N	Y	Y	N
h[n]	D	Y,N	Y	Y	N
h(f(t))	C	N	Y	Y,N	N
h[f[n]]	D	N	Y	Y,N	N
h	C,D	N	Y	Y	N

Similarly, for discrete systems:

$$g[n] = h[f[n]] \tag{13.2}$$

In Chapter 4, we introduced a more generalized concept of a system, H{·}, which includes systems with **memory**. In general, a system assigns an output signal, g(t), for each input signal, f(t):

$$g(t) = H\{f(t)\} \tag{13.3}$$

A system is diagrammed in Figure 4.1. Each point in the output signal may depend upon all of the points in the input signal, the system is able to remember the value of the input. We are using the term "memory" somewhat loosely to refer to both prior and future input. For image processing the concept of prior and future do not have meaning.

Systems may be classified as linear or nonlinear. **Nonlinear** systems are beyond the scope of this book. The most general model which we have presented is the **linear** system. All continuous, linear systems can be represented by Equation 4.22:

$$g(t) = \int_{-\infty}^{+\infty} f(\tau) \cdot f(t,\tau) \, d\tau \tag{13.4}$$

For discrete signals:

$$g[n] = \sum_{k} f[k] \cdot h[n,k] \tag{13.5}$$

Discrete signals can also be modeled by matrix multiplication (Equation 9.1):

$$\mathbf{g} = \mathbf{H} \cdot \mathbf{f} \tag{13.6}$$

The vector, **f**, represents the input signal; the vector, **g**, represents the output signal; and the matrix, H, represents the system. There is no continuous system model analogous to the vector-matrix model. For linear systems we shall generally use the vector-matrix model, since this linear algebra formulation expresses the properties of linear systems well.

Systems can be **time invariant** or **nontime invariant**. The matrix model can be used to represent both time invariant and nontime invariant systems. In Chapter 3, linear, time invariant systems were described by convolution (Equation 3.4):

$$g(t) = \int_{-\infty}^{+\infty} f(\tau) \cdot h(t - \tau) \, d\tau \qquad (13.7)$$

For discrete systems:

$$g[n] = \sum_k f[k] \cdot h[n - k] \qquad (13.8)$$

Although the systems which can be described by convolution are very limited, we shall find that convolution will find a broad application in radiology.

Both the input and output signals, and the systems themselves can be either **statistical** or **deterministic**. This book will only cover deterministic systems. We shall make considerable use of statistical signals in order to model both input signals and detector noise, but the systems through which these signals pass will always be deterministic. The same input will always lead to the same output.

II. REPRESENTATION OF SIGNALS IN TERMS OF BASIS FUNCTIONS

Throughout Part I, we have frequently represented one signal in terms of a linear combination of signals called basis functions. The convolution integral (Equation 3.4) can be viewed as a linear combination of a set of basis functions which are the shifted system functions, $h(t - \tau)$:

$$g(t) = \int_{-\infty}^{+\infty} f(\tau) \cdot h(t - \tau) \, d\tau \qquad (13.9)$$

The output signal, $g(t)$, is a linear combination of shifted system functions. The scale factors for the shifted system function are the values of the input signal, $f(\tau)$.

Similarly, the signal, $f(t)$, can be considered to be a linear combination of a set of basis functions which are a shifted delta function, $\delta(t - \tau)$ (Equation 3.3):

$$f(t) = \int_{-\infty}^{+\infty} f(\tau) \cdot \delta(t - \tau) \, d\tau \qquad (13.10)$$

Although this integral is a complicated way of writing the signal, $f(t)$, it emphasizes the similarity between the idea of a basis function description of a signal and the canonical representation of a signal as $f(t)$. It also suggests that the canonical basis set for the time domain representation is a set of shifted delta functions. Exactly what this last sentence means should become clearer in Part II.

Chapter 5 (Eigenfunctions) introduced the reason that basis functions are so useful to us. Some signals, the eigenfunctions, make description of a system particularly simple. Representation of a signal as linear combinations of the eigenfunctions of a system allows a simple description of the system. Developing this description is the goal of Part II of the book.

Representation of a signal as a linear combination of basis functions is analogous to representation of a vector as a linear combination of basis vectors. The shifted delta functions, $\delta(t - \tau)$, are analogous to the canonical basis vectors $\mathbf{d}_i$. A signal, $f(t)$, is analogous to a

TABLE 13.2
Complexity of System
Models

System function	Dimension
H{f(t)}	∞
h(t,τ)	2
h[n,k]	2
H	2
h(t)	1
h[n]	1
h(f(t))	0
h[f[n]]	0
h	0

vector, **f**, in an infinite dimensional vector space. A vector space defined by a set of basis vectors is analogous to representing a signal as a linear combination of a set of basis functions. The analogy between basis vectors and basis functions provides some geometrical intuition about basis functions.

III. COMPLEXITY OF SYSTEM MODELS

The complexity of the various system models is of importance in understanding why certain models can be used for systems of a particular type. Table 13.2 shows the various models and the complexity of the systems they can represent. The most general system, H{·}, is very complicated. Each different input signal, f(t), may produce any output signal, g(t). H{f(t)} is a functional; it is like an infinite dimensional function, but instead of a dependent variable there is a dependent signal. The infinite set of independent variables are the values of f(·) at all times. This infinite dimensional model of a system is obviously much too complex to be of any value.

The model of the system can be made much simpler by requiring the system to be linear. Continuous, linear systems can be represented with the integral given in Equation 13.4. The system function, h(t,τ), in this integral is two dimensional. A linear system can be completely described by specifying this function. Similarly, a matrix, H, can be used to completely specify a discrete linear system. The matrix, H, is a two-dimensional array of numbers analogous to the two-dimensional system function, h(t,τ). Linear systems, which require a two-dimensional description, are much less complicated than nonlinear systems, which in general require an infinite dimensional description.

Linear, time or shift invariant systems can be described by convolution (Equation 13.7). The system function for linear, time invariant systems, h(t), is a one-dimensional function. Time invariance simplifies the system function of a linear system from a two-dimensional function to a one-dimensional function. Although the systems which can be described by convolution are very limited, we shall find that convolution will find a broad application in radiology.

The differential equation description of systems describes the signals in terms of the relation of the derivatives of the input and output signals at a point in time. The other models describe the relationship in terms of integrals. Differential equations are generally used to describe very simple systems, systems that can be defined by a small number of parameters. The simple relationships in physics are often well expressed by differential equations. Although the physics of radiology makes extensive use of differential equations, the more complicated systems used for image formation are usually not conveniently described by differential equations.

Linear differential equations with constant coefficients can be written in the form given by Equation 7.2:

$$\sum_i a_i \cdot d^i g(t)/dt^i = \sum_i b_i \cdot d^i f(t)/dt^i \qquad (13.11)$$

If the initial conditions are selected properly, then systems of this form are linear and time invariant. In Part II, we shall learn that the Fourier transform of the system function is the ratio of a polynomial with coefficients equal to a_i and b_i.

Although reasonably complicated systems can be modeled using very high-order derivatives, more typically only first and second order derivatives are used. These types of systems are quite simple and the differential equations provide a simple description of these systems.

The most simple systems are memoryless systems. Nonlinear, memoryless systems can be represented by a function:

$$g(t) = h(f(t)) \qquad (13.12)$$

Linear, memoryless systems can be represented by a single value, h:

$$g(t) = h \cdot f(t) \qquad (13.13)$$

This simple system multiplies a signal times a constant. The most complicated model can be used to describe the most simple of systems. However, it is best to use the most simple model which is applicable to the system.

IV. EIGENFUNCTIONS

The eigenfunctions of a system are signals which pass through a system unchanged except possibly for a change in scale (Equation 5.1):

$$H\{f(t)\} = \lambda \cdot f(t) \qquad (13.14)$$

The eigenfunctions are also called the characteristic functions of a system since they can be used to characterize the system. A particularly simple description of a system can be obtained using the eigenvalues. The operation of a system on its eigenfunctions is typically much more simple than the operation of a system on other signals.

The operation of the system on input signals which are linear combinations of its eigenfunctions can be calculated from the eigenvalues. Thus, we could think of the eigenvalues as another system model. The description of the system requires only these eigenvalues. The usefulness of this model depends upon the set of input signals which can be described by the set of eigenfunctions. In Part II we shall see that for linear, time invariant systems, the eigenfunctions are the exponential functions, and that these functions can be used to represent all of the signals which are important in Radiology.

In linear algebra, the eigenvectors of a matrix are defined by a similar relationship (Equation 9.29):

$$H \cdot f = \lambda \cdot f \qquad (13.15)$$

The eigenvectors do not change direction when multiplied by a matrix; they are only scaled by the eigenvalue. The analogy between vectors and functions gives us a geometric interpretation of the eigenfunctions; they do not change "direction" as they pass through a system. The system operates along the "direction" of these signals.

In Chapter 9, we gave the example of a matrix which stretched vectors along the direction at 45° to the x axis, along the vector $(1\ 1)^T$ (see Figure 9.18). The two orthogonal vectors $(1\ 1)^T$ and $(-1\ 1)^T$ are eigenvectors of this system with eigenvalues of 2 and 1, respectively. Expressing a vector as a linear combination of these eigenvectors makes it easy to determine the effects of a system on a vector.

The mathematical simplicity of the eigenvector description is mirrored by a simplicity in understanding the system. When we described this sytem in words, we said that it stretches vectors along the direction of the vector $(1\ 1)^T$. It is easy to understand what the system does using this eigenvector description means. A description of the system in terms of the x and y components would require a paragraph, and after having read such a paragraph, one would likely not have any feel for what the system does. Thus, the eigenvector description is conceptually as well as mathematically simple.

V. STATE

A system with no memory can be represented by a function, $h(f(t))$. The value of the output at some point in time is due only to the value of the input at that one point in time. Most of the systems of interest in radiology are more complicated — the value of the output depends upon the input at several points in time. These systems have memory. The memory of a system for previous input is defined by the state of the system. The state of the system ties the previous input to the future output. In the differential equations model of systems, the state of the system can be defined by initial conditions.

The natural solutions of the differential equations were defined as the solutions when there is no input. The only signals which can be remembered by a system are linear combinations of the natural solutions. The state of the system can also be defined by the scale factors in this linear combination; the state is the amount of each of these natural solutions which is stored in the system.

The idea of the state of a system is most useful for simple systems which have a small number of natural solutions. The only part of the input signal which can be remembered by a system is the part which interacts with these natural solutions. The idea of the state of the system and of memory is less useful for complicated imaging systems. Furthermore, imaging systems may "remember" inputs in all directions, forward as well as backward in space. However, the basic concept that the output of a system at some point in time depends not only upon the input at that time, but also what the system remembers of inputs at other times is still useful.

VI. ENERGY, CORRELATION, ORTHOGONALITY, AND VECTOR PRODUCT

The related ideas of energy, correlation, orthogonality, and vector product have occurred repeatedly in Part I. The energy of a signal was defined in Equation 10.24:

$$\int_{-\infty}^{+\infty} f(t) \cdot f^*(t)\ dt \tag{13.16}$$

The definition of energy is analogous to the definition of energy in physics. In physics, energy is conserved. In Part II, we shall find that the energy of a signal is conserved by the Fourier transformation operation.

The energy between two signals is defined as:

$$\int_{-\infty}^{+\infty} f(t) \cdot g^*(t)\ dt \tag{13.17}$$

This mutual energy or correlation between two signals is analogous to the correlation between two random variables (Equation 11.6):

$$E\{f \cdot g^*\} = \int_{-\infty}^{+\infty} \int_{-\infty}^{+\infty} f \cdot g^* \cdot p_f(f) \cdot p_g^*(g) \, dfdg \qquad (13.18)$$

And to the vector product:

$$\mathbf{f}^T \cdot \mathbf{g} \qquad (13.19)$$

All of these operations yield a number which is related to how much the one signal or vector is related to the other signal or vector. Signals and vectors which are correlated are of a similar form or point in the same direction. Signals and vectors which are orthogonal are different in form or point at right angles to each other. The geometrical and statistical intuition should help the reader to understand the analogous signal processing operations.

VII. ESTIMATION

The last three chapters of Part I introduced the ideas of random variables, stochastic processes, and estimation. A random variable is used to represent experiments with statistical outcomes. The most important statistics are the first and second order statistics, the mean and the variance of the random variable. A stochastic process is used to represent experiments with outcomes which are random signals. Again the most important statistics are the first and second order statistics, the mean and the autocorrelation function. Stochastic processes will be important in modeling systems where the outcome is a random signal.

Chapter 12 introduced estimation from experimental samples of a random variable. Estimation of stochastic processes will be described in Part III. Real radiological problems have noise. In Part IV we shall model both the cross-sectional objects and the detector noise using stochastic processes. An important problem in Part IV, will be reconstruction of images from noisy samples. The ideas of estimation will need to be incorporated into the reconstruction problem.

The purpose of introducing the statistical model of data collection is to allow *a priori* information about the model to be included in deriving an estimate from the data. The *a priori* information provides constraints about the form of the estimate. The noise that is inconsistent with the model is rejected; the noise which is consistent with the model cannot be removed.

For linear, least square estimation, the error in the estimate is orthogonal to the estimators. The orthogonality of the estimate and the estimators is called the orthogonality principle. Orthogonality means that the estimate removes all of the information from the data. Because of the orthogonality principle, estimation is analogous to projection of one vector, the data, onto another vector, the estimators.

Two estimation problems were solved in Chapter 12, estimation of the data and estimation of the unknown. Estimation of the unknown required knowledge about the statistics of the unknown. It is easier to estimate the data, than to estimate the unknown. Both of these methods are common in radiologic reconstruction problems. Estimation of the data is applied to stochastic processes in Chapter 25 (Normal Equations). Estimation of the unknown is applied to stochastic processes in Chapter 26 (Wiener Filtering).

VIII. SUMMARY

Part I of this book has been concerned with explaining how to model systems, particularly systems which are used to collect data. We have described several different models, since each model sheds additional light on the basic idea of a system. The most important models for the remainder of the book will be the convolution model and the linear systems model.

Part II will describe transform methods which will be used to transform the description of a system into a format which is more natural to the system. The most useful concept for understanding Part II is the description of a signal in terms of an eigenfunction basis.

II. Transformations

Chapter 14

INTRODUCTION TO THE FOURIER TRANSFORM

Part II of this book will deal with transformations of a signal from one representation to a new representation. The most important of these transformations is the Fourier transform. It transforms a signal from a representation as a function of time into a representation as a function of frequency, or equivalently from a representation as a function of space into a representation as a function of spatial frequency. The Fourier transform is important both because it will provide the reader with a deeper understanding of signals and systems, and because it will provide an important mathematical method for solving problems.

Fourier transform techniques are used throughout Radiology. Fourier transform reconstruction is the primary method used in nuclear magnetic resonance imaging. The convolution back projection method used most commonly in computed tomography is analogous to Fourier reconstruction, and it is best understood in terms of the Fourier transform. Fourier transform methods are used for image processing in many fields of Radiology. Many of the properties of both nuclear magnetic resonance and ultrasound imaging can be best understood from the frequency domain description of their signals.

The signals which are the basis of the frequency representation are imaginary exponentials. In Chapter 5 we showed that the exponentials, including imaginary exponentials, are the eigenfunctions of linear, time invariant systems. In Chapter 4, we showed that representation of a signal in terms of the eigenfunctions of a system makes description of the operation of the system particularly simple. This is one of the major reasons why the Fourier transform is so useful for describing a radiological system.

In this chapter and the next, we shall introduce the Fourier transformation. Chapter 16 will describe the properties of the Fourier transformation. The main purpose of other chapters in this part is to help to understand the Fourier transform.

Chapter 17 introduces the polynomial transformation. This transformation is not useful for Radiologic problems; however, it does provide a better understanding of a property which is very important in the rest of the book — the transformations of convolution into multiplication. Chapter 18 examines the difference between digital, discrete, and continuous signals, and describes the transform which is appropriate for each type of signal. Chapter 19 describes rotation of a vector space from a description in terms of one set of basis vectors into a second set of basis vectors. Rotation is analogous to transformation, and this analogy will provide a geometrical interpretation for transformation. Chapter 20 describes some other relatives of the Fourier transform.

This chapter will start with an introduction to the frequency domain. The inverse Fourier transform will be introduced as a method of representing a signal in terms of frequencies. The forward Fourier transform will be introduced as a correlation — a method of determining how much a given signal is like a sinusoidal signal. This chapter will be descriptive; the next will present the same material from a mathematical perspective.

I. HEARING AND SIGHT

The idea of sinusoidal functions and of frequencies may still seem a bit foreign to the reader; however, humans have a natural understanding of frequencies. When we hear music, the parameters of which we are aware are the frequencies in the sound. If we were to look at an oscilloscope tracing of the input to a speaker, the tracing would be totally uninterpretable. However, our ears easily interpret the frequencies in the music. The oscilloscope tracing is the time domain representation of the music; our conscious sensation is the frequency domain representation of the same music.

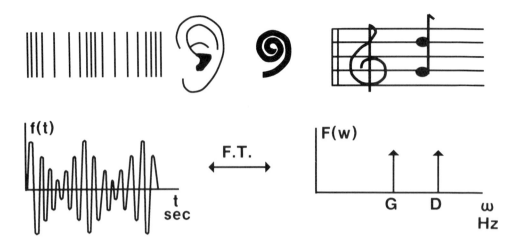

FIGURE 14.1. Hearing as a frequency domain operation: a sound wave consists of regions of compression and rarefaction. Because of the shape of the cochlea, the hair cells along the cochlea are stimulated maximally by compressions and rarefactions at a particular frequency. The effect of the cochlea is to change the time domain sound signal to a frequency domain signal. This figure shows a sound wave with two frequencies corresponding to G and D. The upper portion of this figure shows a representation of the compression and the rarefaction on the left and a musical representation of notes G and D. The lower portion of the figure shows a graphical representation of the signal and its Fourier transform. The frequency domain representation of the two notes, G and D, is more natural to the human.

The cochlea in the ear performs a Fourier transform. The endolymph in the cochlea carries the time domain representation of the sound, the sound wave. Because of the shape of the cochlea, the hair cells at any one point along the cochlea are activated most intensely by a single pitch or frequency. The information provided to the brain by the hair cells is a frequency description of the sound, not a time domain description. The data provided by the human auditory system to the brain is a frequency domain representation of the sound.

Figure 14.1 shows the analogy between hearing and the Fourier transform. On the left side of the figure is a representation of the sound wave. The sound wave enters the ear and the cochlea transforms the signal into a frequency description. The sound consists of two notes, G and D. The brain perceives the Fourier transform of the sound — the two notes — indicated diagrammatically as notes on a scale. On the bottom of the figure is the mathematical representation of this process. The sound wave is represented as a function of time. The Fourier transform has two delta functions, one at the frequency corresponding to G and the other at the frequency corresponding to D.

By contrast sight is a space domain representation. We see in terms of spatial position. The description of images in terms of spatial frequencies is not natural to the human. We have some understanding of the spatial frequencies differences between fine and coarse textures; but for images which do not have a texture, there is no natural understanding of spatial frequency. We have a natural sensory context for understanding images in terms of spatial positions, but we do not have a natural sensory context for understanding images in the spatial frequency domain. By contrast, we do have a natural sensory context for understanding sound in terms of frequencies, but we do not have a natural sensory context for understanding sounds in the time domain.

Figure 14.2 shows the Fourier transform of an image. It is a rather unusual image since it only contains a single sinusoid. The Fourier transform of the image is very simple; it consists of two delta functions at plus and minus the spatial frequency of the sinusoid.

We can try to combine our sensory understanding of the space domain from vision and the frequency domain from hearing. Sight can help us understand the time domain repre-

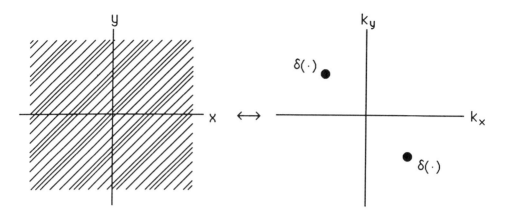

FIGURE 14.2. Spatial sinusoid: the left side of this figure is an artistic representation of a spatial sinusoid. The area where the lines are closer together indicates regions where the function is larger and the area where they are farther apart indicates regions where the function is smaller. The right side of the figure shows the Fourier transform of this sinusoid. It consists of two delta functions at the frequency of the spatial sinusoid.

sentation of sound, and hearing can help us understand the frequency domain representation of images. The cochlea gives us a physiological model of the Fourier transform operation.

II. SPECTROSCOPY

A. OPTICAL SPECTROSCOPY

Another example where the reader may already have an intuitive understanding of the frequency domain is in spectroscopy. The basic idea in spectroscopy is the representation of a signal in terms of its frequency components. For example, when a beam of white light passes through a prism, it is split up into the colors of the spectrum. The difference between the various spectral colors is the frequency of the electromagnetic radiation. The colors are a frequency representation of the light. The time domain representation is the variations in the electric or magnetic fields in the beam of light as a function of time. The colors in the spectrum are a representation of the Fourier transform of a light beam.

White light contains all of the spectral colors. Therefore, all colors are seen in its spectrum. The purple light is composed of red and blue light. If instead of white light, purple light is passed through the prism, then the colors present in the spectrum are red and blue. The prism performs a Fourier transform operation. The Fourier transform of the light shows which frequencies are contained in a beam of light.

Figure 14.3 shows a diagram of purple light being split into red and green light by the action of a prism. Below the purple light beam is a time domain description of the electric field of the light beam. The Fourier transform of the electric field intensity consists of two components, one representing the red light and one representing the green light. The spectrum shows the intensities in the light beam as a function of frequency.

B. NUCLEAR MAGNETIC RESONANCE SPECTROSCOPY

In nuclear magnetic resonance, the chemical properties of a sample are determined from spectroscopy. In the first type of nuclear magnetic resonance spectroscopy, called **continuous wave (CW) nuclear magnetic resonance**, the strength of interaction of the sample with a radio frequency signal was measured directly as a function of frequency. The frequency of the exciting signal was varied slowly and the intensity of the output was recorded as a function of frequency. The chemical environment of a nucleus influences the frequency at which it will interact with a radio frequency signal. Thus, the nuclei in a particular chemical environment will produce a signal at particular frequency.

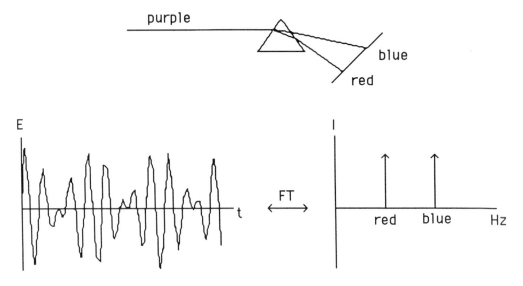

FIGURE 14.3.   Optical spectroscopy: optical spectroscopy can be performed with a prism. The top part of this figure shows a purple light beam split by a prism into two components, red and blue. The bottom of the figure shows a time domain representation of the signal on the left and a frequency domain representation, the spectrum, on the right. The time domain representation is very complicated, the spectrum is much simpler.

Now, most nuclear magnetic resonance spectroscopy is performed with the pulsed technique. After a radio frequency pulse, the sample produces magnetic field, which is picked up by a coil surrounding the sample. The time domain representation of the signal, called the **free induction decay,** is the electric signal induced by the magnetic field in the coil. A Fourier transform of the free induction decay is used to produce the nuclear magnetic resonance spectrum.

In the case of continuous wave nuclear magnetic resonance, the spectrum is sampled, while in the case of pulsed nuclear magnetic resonance, the free induction decay is sampled. The spectrum is obtained from the free induction decay by performing a Fourier transform operation on the time domain signal.

The continuous wave nuclear magnetic resonance spectroscopy experiment was shown in Figure 5.3. That diagram demonstrates that sinusoids are the eigenfunctions of nuclear magnetic resonance. The pulsed nuclear magnetic resonance spectroscopy experiment was shown in Figure 5.4. The advantage of the pulsed experiment is shown in Figure 14.4. The Fourier transform of the free induction decay provides information about all of the frequencies in the spectrum simultaneously. The continuous wave experiment provides information about one frequency at a time.

The other types of spectroscopy all involve representation of the signal in terms of its frequency components. A spectrum is a frequency domain representation of a signal. Sometimes, the instrument produces the frequency signal directly, similar to the auditory system. At other times the spectroscopic signal is obtained as a Fourier transform of the time domain signal, similar to the visual system.

III. FREQUENCY DOMAIN REPRESENTATION OF A SIGNAL

Now that we have some understanding of the difference between the time and frequency domain, let us develop a mathematical representation of a signal in terms of a frequency domain description. Below we shall call this description the inverse Fourier transform.

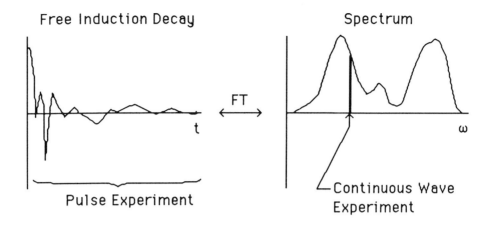

FIGURE 14.4. Pulse and continuous wave nuclear magnetic resonance spectroscopy: the left side of this figure shows the free induction decay which is obtained during a pulsed nuclear magnetic resonance experiment. The right side of this figure shows the spectrum which is the Fourier transform of the free induction decay. During a continuous wave nuclear magnetic resonance experiment, a single value of the spectrum is obtained at each point in time. The frequency of the input is changed to obtain values for the entire spectrum.

In Equation 6.28, the imaginary exponential was written:

$$e^{i\omega t} = \cos(\omega t) + i \cdot \sin(\omega t) \tag{14.1}$$

The real part of the $e^{i\omega t}$ is a cosine function, and the imaginary part is a sine function. The sine and cosine functions can be written in terms of the imaginary exponentials (Equations 6.47 and 6.48):

$$\cos(\omega t) = (1/2) \cdot (e^{i\omega t} + e^{-i\omega t}) \tag{14.2}$$

$$\sin(\omega t) = (1/2i) \cdot (e^{i\omega t} - e^{-i\omega t}) \tag{14.3}$$

Since we can define imaginary exponentials in terms of sines and cosines, and sines and cosines in terms of imaginary exponentials, it is possible to use either representation. For most of the mathematics we shall use the imaginary exponentials since they are easier to work with. For descriptions and figures we shall use sine or cosine functions since they are more easily drawn.

In Part I, we frequently found it useful to represent a signal as a linear combination of a set of basis functions. If we take the imaginary exponentials as the set of basis functions, then all linear combinations of these basis functions can be written in the form:

$$f(t) = (1/2\pi) \cdot \int_{-\infty}^{+\infty} F(\omega) \cdot e^{i\omega t} \, d\omega \tag{14.4}$$

where the factor, $1/2\pi$, is introduced to be compatible with the definition of the inverse Fourier transform below. This equation defines the signal, $f(t)$, as a scaled sum of imaginary exponentials. The $F(\omega)$ are the scale factors.

Figure 14.5 shows a very simple example of defining a signal in terms of a sum of scaled cosine functions. In this case the factors, $F(\omega)$, are nonzero for only a few values of ω.

Rather than thinking of the $F(\omega)$ as a set of scale factors for the respective sinusoidal

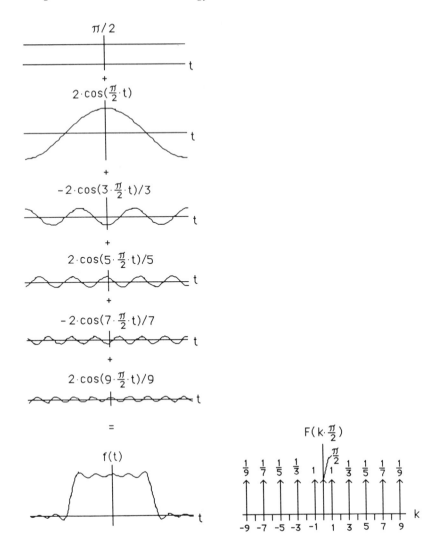

FIGURE 14.5.   Representation of a signal as the sum of sinusoidal components: the left side of this figure shows the time domain representation of a signal as the sum of a small number of sinusoids. The signal, f(t), is approximately equal to the rectangle function. Although the rectangle function is not at all sinusoidal, it can be reasonably well approximated with a small number of sinusoidal components. The right side shows the Fourier transform of the signal.

functions, we can think of $F(\omega)$ as a function of the frequency variable ω. This function is the frequency domain representation of f(t). If we are given the frequency domain representation, $F(\omega)$, then Equation 14.5 provides a formula for determining the time domain representation, f(t).

Recall in Chapter 3 that we wrote f(t) in terms of a set of shifted delta functions (Equation 3.3):

$$f(t) = \int_{-\infty}^{+\infty} f(\tau) \cdot \delta(t - \tau) \, d\tau \tag{14.5}$$

This equation expresses the idea that f(t) can be considered to be a scaled set of delta functions. $f(\tau)$ are the set of factors which scale the delta functions $\delta(t - \tau)$. As such, the time domain description of the signal is a representation in terms of a set of shifted delta functions.

In some sense, Equation 14.5 is a silly way of expressing something which we already understand. However, the analogy between Equations 14.4 and 14.5 should help the reader to understand that the frequency domain representation of the signal is not so different than the time domain representation. The major difference between these two representations is the underlying set of basis functions which is being used — imaginary exponentials or shifted delta functions.

There is an analogy between representing a signal in terms of a set of sinusoidal functions and representing a vector in terms of a set of basis vectors. The factors, $F(\omega)$, which give the weightings for each of the basis functions, $e^{i\omega t}$, are analogous to the components of a vector which give the weightings for each of the basis vectors. The difference between the space domain description of a signal and the frequency domain description of that same signal is analogous to the difference between the description of a single vector in terms of two different sets of basis vectors. There is an analogy between the Fourier transform and a rotation of coordinate axes. This analogy will be described further in Chapter 19.

IV. THE FOURIER TRANSFORM

Let us jump to the conclusion, the mathematical representation of the Fourier transform pair:

$$f(t) = 1/2\pi \int_{-\infty}^{+\infty} F(\omega) \cdot e^{i\omega t} \, d\omega \tag{14.6}$$

$$F(\omega) = \int_{-\infty}^{+\infty} F(t) \cdot e^{-i\omega t} \, dt \tag{14.7}$$

$f(t)$ is a time domain signal; it is a function of the time variable, t. $F(\omega)$ is a frequency domain signal; it is a function of the angular frequency variable, ω. In the next chapter we shall prove that this pair of equations provides a mechanism for transforming from one representation to the other. In general, we shall use capital letters for frequency domain signals and small letters for time domain signals. When the independent variable is position, t and ω are replaced by x and k_x.

A. THE TWO DOMAINS

The first equation is identical to Equation 14.4. It defines a signal, $f(t)$, as a linear combination of imaginary exponentials. This equation is called the **inverse Fourier transform.** Because the signal, $f(t)$, is synthesized from the imaginary exponentials, this equation is sometimes referred to as **Fourier synthesis.** The second equation is used to calculate the value of the scale factor, $F(\omega)$. This equation is called the **Fourier transform.** Because this equation can be used to determine the scale factors, it is sometimes referred to as **Fourier analysis.**

The two signals, $f(t)$ and $F(\omega)$, are two representations of the same signal. They differ only in that one is expressed in terms of the time domain and one is expressed in the frequency domain. One has basis functions which are shifted delta functions and the other has basis functions which are sinusoids. Since we shall frequently encounter a pair of signals which are related by the Fourier transform relationships, it is convenient to have a notation that indicates this relation. We shall use a two headed arrow:

$$f(t) \leftrightarrow F(\omega) \tag{14.8}$$

There are two ways of viewing the basis functions, $e^{i\omega t}$. One way is to consider them to be a function of t:

$$f(t) = e^{i\omega t} \tag{14.9}$$

From this point of view, ω is a parameter which determines the angular frequency. The other point of view is that $e^{i\omega t}$ is a function of ω:

$$F(\omega) = e^{i\omega t} \tag{14.10}$$

From this point of view the roles of t and ω are reversed. There is a duality between the two variables, which we shall explore more fully in the Chapter 15.

B. CALCULATION OF THE FOURIER TRANSFORM

There are several mathematical techniques for calculating the Fourier transform. If a signal can be written in the form of one of the equations in the Fourier transform pair, then the Fourier transform can be identified by inspection. We already know how to represent the cosine and sine function in terms of complex exponentials, Equations 14.2 and 14.3. We can rewrite Equation 14.2 into the form of an inverse Fourier transform:

$$\cos(\omega_0 t) = (1/2\pi) \int_{-\infty}^{+\infty} \pi \cdot \delta(\omega - \omega_0) \cdot e^{i\omega t}\, d\omega$$

$$+ (1/2\pi) \int_{-\infty}^{+\infty} \pi \cdot \delta(\omega + \omega_0) \cdot e^{i\omega t}\, d\omega \tag{14.11}$$

From this somewhat awkward equation we can see that:

$$\cos(\omega_0 t) \leftrightarrow \pi \cdot [\delta(\omega - \omega_0) + \delta(\omega + \omega_0)] \tag{14.12}$$

Similarly,

$$\sin(\omega_0 t) \leftrightarrow (\pi/i) \cdot [\delta(\omega - \omega_0) - \delta(\omega + \omega_0)] \tag{14.13}$$

The Fourier transform of $\cos(\omega_0 t)$ and $\sin(\omega_0 t)$ are nonzero for only two frequencies, ω_0 and $-\omega_0$. Figure 14.6 shows these Fourier transform pairs graphically.

Figure 14.7 shows another interesting Fourier transform pair. The Fourier transform of the Gaussian function also has the shape of a Gaussian function.

$$[1/\sqrt{(2\pi) \cdot \sigma}] \cdot e^{-x^2/2\sigma^2} \leftrightarrow e^{-\sigma^2\omega^2/2} \tag{14.14}$$

Among the many interesting properties of the Gaussian function, it has the same form in both the time and frequency domain. The width of the Gaussian in the time domain is related to the square root of the denominator of the exponent, σ. The width of the Gaussian function in the frequency domain is related to $1/\sigma$. Therefore, the width of the Gaussian in the frequency domain is inversely related to the width of the Gaussian in the time domain. We shall come back to the inverse relation between the widths of the signals in the two domains later.

V. FOURIER TRANSFORM AS A CORRELATION

We have argued that expressing f(t) in the form given by Equation 14.6 is a reasonable thing to do. However we have not yet explained by Equation 14.7 provides the correct scale

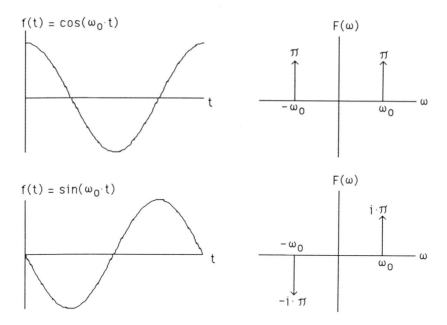

FIGURE 14.6. Time and frequency representations of the cosine and sine functions: the left side of this figure shows the time domain representation of the cosine and the sine functions. The right side shows the frequency domain representations of the same functions.

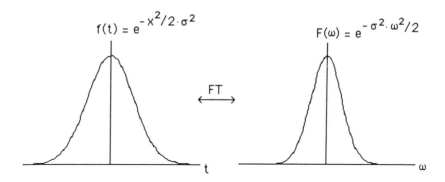

FIGURE 14.7. The Gaussian functions: the left side of this figure shows the time domain representation of the Gaussian functions. The right side of the figure shows the frequency domain representation of the same function. The frequency domain representation is also a Gaussian function. The width of the time domain representation is related to σ, and the width of the frequency domain representation is related to $1/\sigma$.

factors $F(\omega)$. The mathematical answer to this question will be provided in the next chapter. But let us first try to get a more intuitive understanding of why it works.

We have run into the idea of correlation at several points in the book, correlation of vectors (Equation 8.50), correlation of signals (Equation 13.17), correlation of random variables (Equation 10.31), and correlation of stochastic processes (Equation 11.6). In each case the correlation operation determines how similar two entities are. It determines the mutual power or energy in the two entities. Equation 14.7 is analogous to these correlation operations. It gives the correlation of the signal, $f(t)$, with the basis function $e^{i\omega t}$ ($e^{-i\omega t}$ is the complex conjugate of $e^{i\omega t}$).

Thus, each of the factors, $F(\omega)$, is the correlation of the time domain signal with the corresponding basis function. The Fourier transform of f(t) tells how much f(t) is like each of the sinusoidal functions $e^{i\omega t}$.

An analogy to linear algebra may also be useful. A signal, f(t), can be considered analogous to a vector, **f**, in an infinite-dimensional vector space. Correlation of **f** with a unit vector gives the projection of **f** along that vector. Thus, the Fourier transform is analogous to projection of a vector along the imaginary exponential. Representation of **f** as **F** amounts to a change of basis. But more of this in Chapter 19.

VI. RESPONSE OF A SYSTEM TO AN IMAGINARY EXPONENTIAL

One of the major reasons that we are interested in the Fourier transform is that it simplifies the description of the effects of a linear, time invariant systems. Recall from Chapter 4 that the effect of a linear, time invariant system, h(t), on the input signal, f(t), can be written with the convolution integral, Equation 3.10:

$$g(t) = \int_{-\infty}^{+\infty} f(t - \tau) \cdot h(\tau) \, d\tau \qquad (14.15)$$

Let us consider an input signal, f(t), which is the imaginary exponential function, $e^{i\omega t}$. Then,

$$f(t - \tau) = e^{i\omega(t - \tau)} = e^{i\omega t} \cdot e^{-i\omega \tau} \qquad (14.16)$$

Substituting into the convolution integral we obtain:

$$g(t) = \int_{-\infty}^{+\infty} e^{i\omega t} \cdot e^{-i\omega \tau} \cdot h(\tau) \, d\tau \qquad (14.17)$$

The factor, $e^{i\omega t}$, is not a function of τ; therefore, we can move it outside of the integral:

$$g(t) = \left\{ \int_{-\infty}^{+\infty} h(\tau) \cdot e^{-i\omega \tau} \, d\tau \right\} \cdot e^{i\omega t} \qquad (14.18)$$

The factor inside the brackets is the Fourier transform of h(t) (Equation 14.7). Therefore,

$$g(t) = H(\omega) \cdot e^{i\omega t} = H(\omega) \cdot f(t) \qquad (14.19)$$

Equation 14.19 is truly remarkable. The output of a linear, time invariant system to an imaginary exponential, $e^{i\omega t}$, is the same imaginary exponential times a scaling factor. We have already seen this property before, namely — the imaginary exponentials are the eigenfunctions of linear, time invariant systems. However, we have now identified the eigenvalues associated with these eigenfunctions; the eigenvalues are the values of the Fourier transform of the system function at the corresponding angular frequency, ω.

The Fourier transform of the system function, H(ω), gives the eigenvalues of the system. If we have a description of a signal in terms of the imaginary exponentials, then H(ω) provides a simple method for calculating the output of the system.

Figure 14.8 shows this fact diagrammatically. The system is represented by the Fourier transform of its impulse response, H(ω). We shall represent linear, time invariant systems by either their impulse response or the Fourier transform of their impulse response depending upon what feature of the system is being emphasized. The response of this system to an imaginary exponential is just H(ω) times the imaginary exponential.

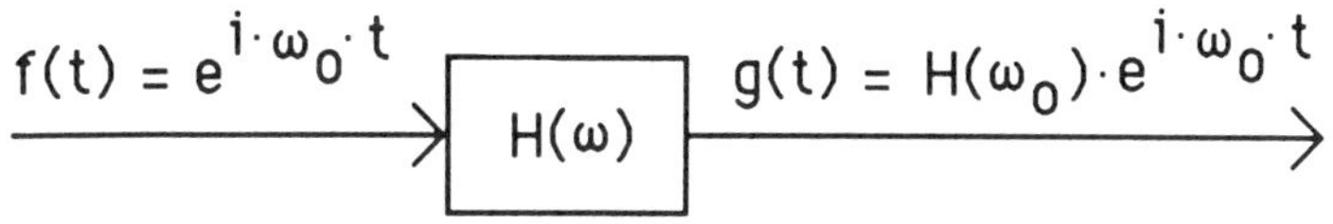

$$f(t) = e^{i \cdot \omega_0 \cdot t} \longrightarrow \boxed{H(\omega)} \longrightarrow g(t) = H(\omega_0) \cdot e^{i \cdot \omega_0 \cdot t} \longrightarrow$$

FIGURE 14.8.   Response of a system to an imaginary exponential: the output of a system in response to an input which is an imaginary exponential, $e^{i\omega_0 t}$, is equal to the same imaginary exponential scaled by the corresponding value of the frequency domain representation of the system function, $H(\omega_0)$. In this figure the system is represented by the frequency domain representation of the system function, $H(\omega)$.

A. MODULATION TRANSFER FUNCTION

The **line spread function** is the response of an imaging system to an object which is a very thin line. In the idealized case of a delta function input, the line spread function is the system function, $h(x)$. The Fourier transform of the line spread function, $H(k_x)$, is called the **modulation transfer function** (MTF). The MTF tells how a system will affect an input which is a sinusoidal function. The variation or modulation of the input at the spatial frequency k_x will be multiplied by the factor, $H(k_x)$.

One method of measuring the resolution of a system is to take closely spaced bars and determine if they can be resolved. An ideal phantom would have a sinusoidally varying density; however, for practical reasons it is easier just to use rectangular bars. The spatial frequency of the bars is often given in terms of line pairs per centimeter, where a pair of lines is one bar and one space. Since each pair of lines is equal to one cycle, line pairs per centimeter is equivalent to cycles per centimeter.

In order to determine the resolution of a system a different phantom must be imaged for each frequency. Instead a single image of a line source can be imaged. The whole modulation transfer function can be calculated with the Fourier transform. Using a single line source to measure the whole modulation transfer function is similar to using a single pulsed NMR experiment to measure the whole NMR spectrum.

Figure 14.9 shows two different line spread functions and their corresponding modulation transfer functions. The system with the wider line spread function will blur the input image more heavily and hence the resolution will be less. The modulation transfer function for the wider line spread function is smaller for the higher spatial frequencies. Thus, it will not transfer the modulation due to high frequency variation. The line spread function and the modulation transfer function provide similar information about the system.

VII. REAL AND IMAGINARY PARTS OF THE FOURIER TRANSFORM

The example of Fourier transforms which we have described so far are rather simple. Except for the sine function, they have had real Fourier transforms. However, in general, the Fourier transform of a function will be complex; it will have both real and imaginary parts. In Chapter 16, we shall learn that signals with complex symmetry will have real Fourier transforms; but, more of that later.

An example of a signal which has both real and imaginary parts to its Fourier transform is the exponential which starts at zero (see Equation 2.45):

$$f(t) = u(t) \cdot e^{-\lambda t} \tag{14.20}$$

where $u(t)$ is the step function which is zero for t less than zero and one for t greater than zero. Figure 14.10 shows this signal. This signal is used frequently in radiology. It describes the decrease in an X-ray beam as a function of thickness. It describes the radioactive decay

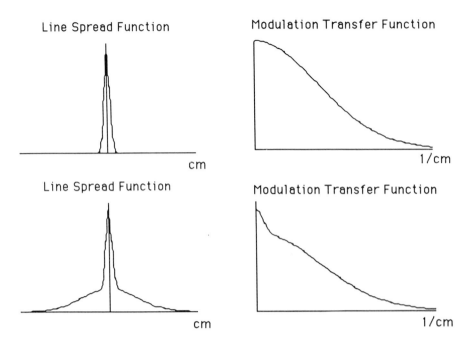

FIGURE 14.9.   Line spread functions and modulation transfer functions: this figure shows two line spread functions and the corresponding modulation transfer functions. The bottom line spread function is typical of that seen with a gamma camera when there is septal penetration.

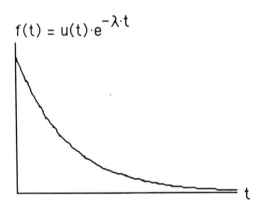

FIGURE 14.10.   Exponential signal: this graph shows an exponential signal which starts at the origin. The decay constant is λ. This signal is found in many applications in radiology.

of an isotope. It describes the decay of magnetization in nuclear magnetic resonance. Because this signal finds so many applications in radiology, we shall describe its Fourier transform in some detail.

We can use Equation 14.7 to calculate the Fourier transform. The effect of the step function, $u(t)$, is equivalent to changing the limits of integration:

$$F(\omega) = \int_{0}^{+\infty} e^{-\lambda t} \cdot e^{-i\omega t} \, dt \qquad (14.21)$$

We can solve this equation by integration:

$$F(\omega) = -1/(\lambda + i \cdot \omega) \cdot e^{-(\lambda + i\omega)t}\big|_0^\infty$$

$$= -[0 - 1/(\lambda + i \cdot \omega)] = 1/(\lambda + i \cdot \omega) \quad (14.22)$$

In the two headed arrow notation, we can write:

$$u(t) \cdot e^{-\lambda t} \leftrightarrow 1/(\lambda + i \cdot \omega) \quad (14.23)$$

The Fourier transform of this function has both real and imaginary parts. At ω equal to zero the value of the transform is purely real:

$$F(0) = 1/\lambda \quad (14.24)$$

When ω is much larger than λ the value of the transform is purely imaginary:

$$F(\omega) = -i/\omega, \qquad \omega \gg \lambda \quad (14.25)$$

In between these two extremes, the value of the transform is complex.

One method of obtaining a feel for the value of the transform is to separate Equation 14.22 into its real and imaginary parts. We shall use a trick from Chapter 6, multiplying both the numerator and denominator by the complex conjugate of the denominator:

$$F(\omega) = 1/(\lambda + i \cdot \omega) \cdot (\lambda - i \cdot \omega)/(\lambda - i \cdot \omega)$$

$$= \lambda/(\lambda^2 + \omega^2) - i \cdot \omega/(\lambda^2 + \omega^2) \quad (14.26)$$

Thus the real part of the transform is:

$$\text{Re}\{F(\omega)\} = \lambda/(\lambda^2 + \omega^2) \quad (14.27)$$

The imaginary part of the transform is:

$$\text{Im}\{F(\omega)\} = -\omega/(\lambda^2 + \omega^2) \quad (14.28)$$

The real and the imaginary parts of the transform are shown in Figure 14.11. As we have already shown, at zero the real part of the function is $1/\lambda$ and the imaginary part is zero. For large ω, the real part becomes small faster than the imaginary part so that it dominates the value. For each angular frequency, ω, there is single complex value, $F(\omega)$; however, it is easier to graph the real and imaginary values of this complex valued functions separately.

In nuclear magnetic resonance, the real part of the signal is called the **absorptive signal** and the imaginary part of the signal is called the **dispersive signal**. In Chapter 16 these signals will be described further in the section on quadrature signals.

VIII. MAGNITUDE AND PHASE OF THE FOURIER TRANSFORM

An alternate way of expressing a complex number is in terms of the magnitude and phase (see Chapter 6). We calculate the magnitude and the phase of Equation 14.22:

$$|F(\omega)|^2 = F(\omega) \cdot F^*(\omega) \quad (14.29)$$

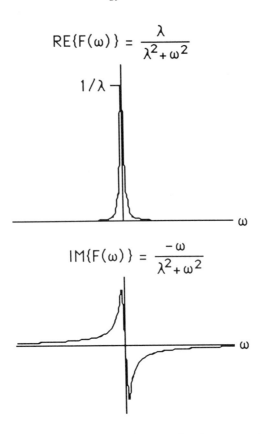

$$RE\{F(\omega)\} = \frac{\lambda}{\lambda^2 + \omega^2}$$

$$IM\{F(\omega)\} = \frac{-\omega}{\lambda^2 + \omega^2}$$

FIGURE 14.11. Real and imaginary parts of the frequency domain representation of an exponential signal: the top graph shows the real part and the bottom graph shows the imaginary part of the Fourier transform of the signal shown in Figure 14.10.

For $f(t)$ equal to $u(t) \cdot e^{-\lambda t}$:

$$|F(\omega)| = [1/(\lambda + i \cdot \omega) \cdot 1/(\lambda - i \cdot \omega)]^{1/2}$$

$$= [1/(\lambda^2 + \omega^2)]^{1/2} \tag{14.30}$$

The phase is equal to the inverse tangent of the real part divided by the imaginary parts of Equation 14.22:

$$\theta = \tan^{-1}(-\lambda/\omega) \tag{14.31}$$

At ω equal to zero, the magnitude, $1/\lambda$, is equal to the real part since the imaginary part is zero. The phase is zero since the value is a positive real number. For large values of ω, the magnitude, $1/\omega$, is equal to the imaginary part since the real part is nearly zero. The phase is $\pi/2$ since the value is a positive imaginary number.

Figure 14.12 shows the magnitude and the phase as a function of ω. Figure 14.13 shows the path of $F(\omega)$ in the complex plane. As ω increases, the value goes from $1/\lambda$ on the real axis up in a spiral toward the imaginary axis. It approaches zero along the imaginary axis. It is useful to compare Figures 14.11, 14.12, and 14.13. They are all representation of the same function from different perspectives. Understanding how they relate should provide insight about complex valued functions.

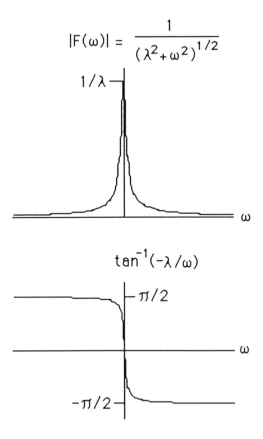

FIGURE 14.12.   Magnitude and phase of the frequency domain representation of an exponential signal: the top graph shows the magnitude and the bottom graph shows the phase of the Fourier transform of the signal shown in Figure 14.10. This figure and Figure 14.11 are two methods of representing the same signal.

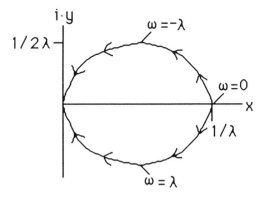

FIGURE 14.13.   Path on the complex plane of the frequency domain representation of an exponential signal: this figure shows the path that the value of the Fourier transform of the signal shown in Figure 14.10 follows in the complex plane. Figures 14.10 to 14.13 all show different representations of the same complex signal. It may be useful to compare these figures with Figures 6.5 and 6.6 which also show different representations of a single signal.

IX. TWO-DIMENSIONAL FOURIER TRANSFORM

In this book we are most concerned with two-dimensional images. In that case we must use a two-dimensional Fourier transform. The two-dimensional Fourier transform is quite similar to the one-dimensional transform, and most of the complexity associated with going from one to two dimensional is notational In fact, some authors simply state that the variable, t, stands for x,y and that ω stands for k_x, k_y.

The two-dimensional Fourier transform pair is:

$$f(x,y) = (1/2\pi)^2 \int_{-\infty}^{+\infty} \int_{-\infty}^{+\infty} F(k_x,k_y) \cdot e^{i(xk_x + yk_y)} \, dk_x dk_y \qquad (14.32)$$

$$F(k_x,k_y) = \int_{-\infty}^{+\infty} \int_{-\infty}^{+\infty} f(x,y) \cdot e^{-i(xk_x + yk_y)} \, dx dy \qquad (14.33)$$

x and y represent the two space variables. k_x and k_y represent two spatial frequency variables. If the units of x and y were centimeters, then the units of k_x and k_y would be 1/centimeters. Spatial frequency is the rate of change as a function of distance.

Many two-dimensional Fourier transforms are analogous to one-dimensional transforms. For example, the transform of a two dimensional Gaussian function is a two-dimensional Gaussian function. Knowledge of one-dimensional Fourier transforms usually lets one predict the form of a two-dimensional transform.

An exception to these rules is a two-dimensional Fourier transform pair which will be important in the discussion of computed tomography. In the space domain this function decreases in proportion to the inverse of the distance from the origin:

$$f(r,\theta) = 1/r \qquad (14.34)$$

where we have used polar notation. This function is most easily written in polar coordinate since it is circularly symmetric. Its Fourier transform is:

$$F(k,\phi) = 1/k \qquad (14.35)$$

where we have used k and ϕ as the polar coordinates in the spatial frequency domain. The transform of the signal, 1/r, has exactly the same form as the signal itself. There is no analog of this relationship in one dimension.

There are some special issues which arise for two dimensional Fourier transforms, but in general, they are remarkably similar to one-dimensional transforms. For that reason almost all of the development of Fourier transforms in this part of the book will be in terms of one-dimensional transform, while almost all of the applications in Part IV will be in terms of two-dimensional transforms.

X. SUMMARY

This chapter has attempted to introduce the Fourier transformation. The Fourier transform changes a signal from a time or space domain description into a frequency or spatial frequency domain description. The frequency domain description may at first seem obscure to the reader; however, we have shown that in some cases, such as hearing, there is a natural understanding of frequencies. Scientists are used to working with spectra in many fields, particularly nuclear magnetic resonance. Spectra are simply Fourier transforms of a time domain signal. Thus, the reader should now appreciate that the Fourier transform is not some obscure mathematics, but rather, it can be recognized as common to his experience.

One method of understanding the pair of Fourier transform operations is to understand that the time and frequency domain descriptions are merely two different representations of a single signal. The Fourier transform pair converts between these descriptions. Another method of understanding the Fourier transform pair is in terms of other mathematical operations. A signal can be represented in terms of a set of sinusoidal basis functions. This representation leads naturally to the inverse Fourier transform. The forward Fourier transform is analogous to a correlation operation. The frequency domain coefficients tell how much a signal is ''like'' the corresponding imaginary exponential.

Another method of motivating the Fourier transformation operation is to consider the effect of a linear, time invariant system on an imaginary exponential. The imaginary exponentials are eigenfunctions of linear, time invariant systems. The eigenvalues for these eigenvectors are the corresponding values of the Fourier transform of the system function. The reader may now appreciate why so much emphasis was placed on linear, time invariant systems, and on eigenvectors and eigenvalues in Part I.

The description of a signal in the time domain is analogous to defining a vector in terms of a set of basis vectors which are delta functions. The description of a signal in terms of its Fourier transform is analogous to defining a vector in terms of a new set of basis functions which are the imaginary exponentials. In Chapter 19 we shall see that the Fourier transform operation is analogous to a rotation from one set of basis vectors to a new set of the basis vectors.

This chapter has attempted to introduce the idea of representing a signal in the frequency domain and the notion that the Fourier transformation can be used to transform between time and frequency domain descriptions. The goal of the rest of this section of the book is to provide a further understanding and familiarity with the Fourier transform operation.

XI. FURTHER READING

There are several related Fourier transformation operations depending upon whether the time or frequency domain signals are continuous, discrete, or digital. These various Fourier transformations will be described in Chapter 18. In addition the Laplace transform and the z transform are also closely related operations. We have chosen to begin this part of the book using the transform from continuous time signals to continuous frequency signals. This transformation is the one which we shall use most frequently in Parts III and IV, and it is conceptually the simplest. The first chapter of the reasonably advanced book by Bracewell[1] takes this same approach. A brief introduction using this approach is also found in Appendix B of the book by Barrett and Swindell.[2]

The difficulty with this approach is that some of the mathematics (as described in the next chapter) is difficult. A more typical approach is first to introduce the transformation from a continuous time signal to a discrete frequency signal, called the Fourier series. Then to introduce the Fourier transformation as a limit in the case where the frequency signals are closely spaced. For example, the excellent book by Oppenheim and Willsky[3] takes this approach in Chapter 4. Chapter 1 of the radiologically oriented book by Kak and Slaney[4] also takes this approach.

Many of the more recent engineering books begin with discrete time signals. They often emphasize the z transform. For example, the reader is referred to the books by Oppenheim and Schafer,[5] Rabiner and Gold,[6] Gabel and Roberts,[7] and Siebert.[8] The Fourier transform uses mathematics, physics, chemistry, engineering, etc. Each field adds its own flavor to the Fourier transform operation. One field, which like radiology is primarily interested in images, is the field of optics. For example, Chapter 7 of the book by Gaskill[9] introduces the two-dimensional Fourier transform. The excellent, if terse, book by Goodman[10] also discusses the Fourier transform in the context of optics.

We have glossed over the special issues related to the two-dimensional Fourier transform since from a conceptual point of view these issues can often be ignored. There are, however, several interesting implementation issues. The book by Dudgeon and Mersereau[11] describes these issues more accurately.

REFERENCES

1. **Bracewell, R. N.,** *The Fourier Transform and Its Applications,* McGraw-Hill, New York, 1965.
2. **Barrett, H. H. and Swindell, W.,** *Radiological Imaging: The Theory of Image Formation, Detection, and Processing,* Academic Press, New York, 1981.
3. **Oppenheim, A. V. and Willsky, A. S.,** *Signals and Systems,* Prentice-Hall, Englewood Cliffs, NJ, 1983.
4. **Kak, A. C. and Slaney, M.,** *Principles of Computerized Tomographic Imaging,* IEEE Press, New York, 1988.
5. **Oppenheim, A. V. and Schafer, R. W.,** *Digital Signal Processing,* Prentice-Hall, Englewood Cliffs, NJ, 1975.
6. **Rabiner, L. R. and Gold, B.,** *Theory and Application of Digital Signal Processing,* Prentice-Hall, Englewood Cliffs, NJ, 1975.
7. **Gabel, R. A. and Roberts, R. A.,** *Signals and Linear Systems,* John Wiley & Sons, New York, 1973.
8. **Siebert, W. Mc. C.,** *Circuits, Signals, and Systems,* MIT Press, Cambridge, 1986.
9. **Gaskill, J. D.,** *Linear Systems, Fourier Transforms, and Optics,* John Wiley & Sons, New York, 1978.
10. **Goodman, J. W.,** *Introduction to Fourier Optics,* McGraw-Hill, New York, 1968.
11. **Dudgeon, D. E. and Mersereau, R. M.,** *Multidimensional Digital Signal Processing,* Prentice-Hall, Englewood Cliffs, NJ, 1984.

Chapter 15

FOURIER TRANSFORM

The last chapter introduced the Fourier transform and the inverse Fourier transform, and tried to explain why these operations were reasonable. This chapter will extend the description of the Fourier transform and it will prove mathematically the relationship between Fourier transform and inverse Fourier transform. In order to proceed with the proof, it is necessary to show that the imaginary exponentials are orthogonal to each other. In developing this important property we shall encounter some properties which will be important when we discuss the discrete Fourier transform.

This chapter has more of a mathematical flavor than many in the book. The mathematically sophisticated reader may find this material provides a more concrete explanation of the Fourier transform. The mathematically phobic reader may find these explanations more opaque and may wish to skim this chapter. The mathematically phobic reader should just accept the results of this chapter without being too concerned about how they are derived.

I. LINEARITY

The Fourier transform is a linear operation. In other words, the Fourier transform of a linear combination of signals is equal to the same linear combination of their Fourier transforms. In the last chapter we implicitly assumed this property. In this section we shall show this property mathematically.

The Fourier transform of $a \cdot f(t) + b \cdot g(t)$ is:

$$\int_{-\infty}^{+\infty} [a \cdot f(t) + b \cdot g(t)] \cdot e^{-i\omega t} \, dt \tag{15.1}$$

Because of the linearity of the integration operation, this integral can be written as:

$$= a \cdot \int_{-\infty}^{+\infty} f(t) \cdot e^{-i\omega t} \, dt + b \cdot \int_{-\infty}^{+\infty} g(t) \cdot e^{-i\omega t} \, dt \tag{15.2}$$

$$= a \cdot F(\omega) + b \cdot G(\omega) \tag{15.3}$$

where the capital letter frequency signals are the Fourier transforms of the corresponding small letter time signals. Using our double headed arrow notation:

$$a \cdot f(t) + b \cdot g(t) \leftrightarrow a \cdot F(\omega) + b \cdot G(\omega) \tag{15.4}$$

Similarly, the Fourier transform of any linear combination of signals can be shown to be the same linear combination of the transforms of the signals.

Linearity of the Fourier transform is very important. It means that it is possible to divide a signal up into parts and consider how each of the parts is transformed separately. If the Fourier transforms of a set of signals are known, then the Fourier transform of any linear combination of signals can be derived immediately. Even if a signal is not an exact linear combination of a set of known signals, it can often be approximated from a set of signals for which the Fourier transforms are known.

II. DUALITY

We have a natural understanding of the time domain, and therefore it seems that the time domain description of a signal, f(t), is the primary description and that the frequency domain description, F(ω), is subordinate. However, these two domains are really coequals. They both provide the same information. Similarly, we tend to think of the Fourier transform and the inverse Fourier transform as differnet operations. In the last chapter, we used different explanations of these two operations. However, in this section we shall show that they are exactly analogous. They differ only in our intuitions about the time and frequency description of signals. The analogy between the two domains and the two transforms is called **duality**.

We can show the mathematical relationship between the transforms by multiplying the inverse Fourier transform, Equation 14.6, by 2π and substituting −t′ for t:

$$2\pi \cdot f(-t') = \int_{-\infty}^{+\infty} F(\omega) \cdot e^{-i\omega t} \, d\omega \tag{15.5}$$

This equation is identical to the Fourier transform equation, Equation 14.7, except for the change of variables. Therefore, the Fourier transform of F(t) is $2\pi \cdot f(-t)$. We can express these relations symbolically:

$$f(t) \leftrightarrow F(\omega) \tag{15.6}$$

$$F(t) \leftrightarrow 2\pi \cdot f(-\omega) \tag{15.7}$$

In words, the Fourier transform of the Fourier transform of f(t) is equal to $2\pi \cdot f(-t)$. Two applications of the Fourier transform scale a signal by 2π and reflect it about the origin.

It is easy to get confused about when the sign changes and where the 2π goes, but the important point is the fact that the forward and inverse transforms result in signals of the same form. We shall see that all of the properties of the Fourier transform are also true for the inverse Fourier transform.

The equations defining the Fourier transform, Equations 14.6 and 14.7, show the duality between the time and frequency domains. The roles of f(t) and F(ω) are very similar. There are, however, two differences between the equations — the factor 1/2π and the sign of the exponent.

The factor 1/2π arises from the difference between frequency, ν, and angular frequency, ω. Recall that these variables are related by the Equation 6.56:

$$\omega = 2\pi \cdot \nu \tag{15.8}$$

Thus:

$$d\omega = 2\pi \cdot d\nu \tag{15.9}$$

Substituting into Equations 14.7 and 14.8, the Fourier transform pair could be defined:

$$F(\nu) = \int_{-\infty}^{+\infty} f(t) \cdot e^{-i2\pi\nu t} \, dt \tag{15.10}$$

$$f(t) = \int_{-\infty}^{+\infty} F(\nu) \cdot e^{i2\pi\nu t} \, d\nu \tag{15.11}$$

In this form the symmetry of the forward and inverse Fourier transforms is even more apparent. Using the frequency formulation, we can write the duality property:

$$f(t) \leftrightarrow F(\nu) \tag{15.12}$$

$$F(t) \leftrightarrow f(-\nu) \tag{15.13}$$

The disadvantage of using frequency as opposed to angular frequency is that all the exponents have the factor 2π. Another approach for emphasizing duality while using the angular frequency notation is to define the frequency domain values with a factor of $1\sqrt{(2\pi)}$. Then the factor in the inverse transform is also $1\sqrt{(2\pi)}$. In this book, we have chosen the angular frequency notation with $1/2\pi$ in the inverse transform. It is the more common notation in electrical engineering and in physics, and it is slightly more common in Radiology.

Understanding the reason for the difference between the signs in the exponents of the forward and inverse transform operations requires a deeper understanding of the Fourier transform. Basically, "the line of points in the complex plane along which the inverse Fourier transform is defined is rotated by $\pi/2$ compared to the line of points along which the Fourier transform is defined". But what this sentence means will not become apparent until Chapter 20, where we describe the Laplace transform. At this point, let us just note that if the forward transform is applied twice to $f(t)$, the result is $2\pi \cdot f(-t)$. If it is applied four times, we get back to a scaled version of the original signal, $4\pi^2 \cdot f(t)$.

In Radiology, duality is most clearly expressed in nuclear magnetic resonance imaging. In nuclear magnetic resonance, the time domain signal is called the free induction decay. Its Fourier transform, the spectrum, is the frequency domain representation of the signal (see Figure 14.4). The amplitude of the nuclear magnetic resonance spectrum is proportional to the number of nuclei at a particular magnetic field intensity. The number of nuclei at a particular magnetic field is related to position due to the gradient field (as explained more fully in Chapter 30). Thus, the spatial representation of the imaging data is equal to the nuclear magnetic resonance spectrum.

The Fourier transform of nuclear magnetic resonance image data gives the spatial frequencies of the object. Except for a sign here and a 2π there, the spatial frequency representation of the image is equivalent to the free induction decay. Thus the time domain is analogous to the spaital frequency domain, and the frequency domain is analogous to the spatial domain.

These relationships are shown in Figure 15.1. On the right side of Figure 15.1 the spectrum, $F(\omega)$, is related to the position data, $f(x)$, by the gradient field, G_x. The inverse Fourier transform of the spectrum is the free induction decay, $f(t)$. The Fourier transform of the image is the spatial frequency signal, $F(k_x)$. The spectrum, $F(\omega)$, and the image, $f(x)$, are signals of the same form, and the free induction decay, $f(t)$, and the spatial frequency data, $F(k_x)$, are signals of the same form.

There are two ways of viewing the data — in terms of the measured time domain signal or in terms of the object being imaged. In each case physical intuition clearly tells us which is the primary domain. However, the primary time domain free induction decay is related to the spatial frequency domain of the image, and the primary spatial domain image is related to the frequency domain spectrum. The mathematical property of duality helps to explain this apparent paradox. The two forms of the signal are coequals. Neither is the primary representation. Rather it depends upon the point of view with which the data are viewed. We shall return to this example in Chapter 30.

III. ORTHOGONALITY OF THE IMAGINARY EXPONENTIALS

One of the very important properties of a set of basis functions is orthogonality. In this section we shall show that the imaginary exponentials all are orthogonal to each other.

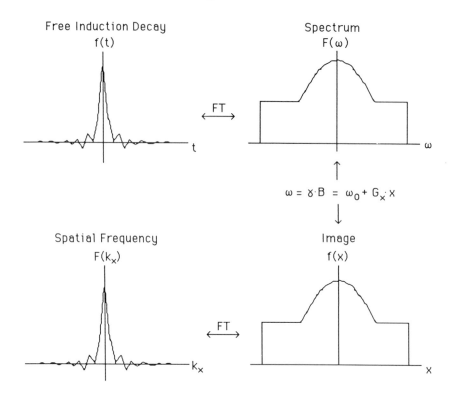

FIGURE 15.1. Duality in nuclear magnetic resonance imaging: the top left graph shows the free induction decay, f(t), which is measured in a nuclear magnetic resonanc experiment. The Fourier transform of the free induction decay is shown on the top right. This frequency domain signal is the spectrum, F(ω). The spectrum is related to the local magnetic field, B, by the Larmor equation; and the local magnetic field is related to the x position by the applied field gradient, G_x. Thus, the spectrum is related directly to the image, f(x). The Fourier transform of the image, $F(k_x)$, is therefore directly related to the free induction decay. The image domain is more natural to the radiologist than the spatial frequency domain, and the time domain is more natural than the frequency domain. But, the signals in these domains are a Fourier transform pair. These signals show the duality between domains.

Unfortunately, in order to show these properties we shall have to go through some complicated mathematical tricks. For the less mathematically oriented reader, the indented sections can be skipped without loss of continuity.

We shall start with consideration of a signal on a finite interval of length, T, extending from $-T/2$ to $T/2$ (Figure 15.2). We shall be inserted in the integral of $e^{i\omega t}$ over this interval. When ω is not equal to zero the integral is:

$$\int_{-T/2}^{+T/2} e^{i\omega t} \, dt = e^{i\omega t}/i\omega \Big|_{-T/2}^{+T/2}$$

$$= (e^{i\omega T/2} - e^{-i\omega T/2})/i\omega$$

$$= (2/\omega) \cdot \sin(\omega T/2) \qquad (15.14)$$

When ω is zero, then $e^{i\omega t}$ is equal to one, and the integral is equal to:

$$\int_{-T/2}^{+T/2} 1 \, dt = T \qquad (15.15)$$

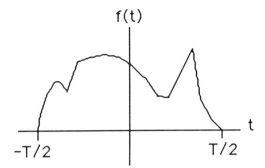

FIGURE 15.2. Limited extent signal: this figure shows a limited extent signal. It is defined only in the range $-T/2$ to $T/2$.

We can summarize these two results:

$$\int_{-T/2}^{+T/2} e^{i\omega t} \, dt = \begin{cases} T, & \omega = 0 \\ (2/\omega) \cdot \sin(\omega T/2), & \omega \neq 0 \end{cases} \tag{15.16}$$

Below, we shall be interested in the values for which the integral is equal to zero. The integral in Equation 15.16 is zero only when the argument of the sine function is equal to a multiple of π:

$$\omega T/2 = n \cdot \pi, \quad n \neq 0 \tag{15.17}$$

where n is an integer. In terms of the variable ω:

$$\omega = n \cdot 2\pi/T, \quad n \neq 0 \tag{15.18}$$

In Chapter 8 we defined two functions as orthogonal, when the integral of the first function times the complex conjugate of the second function was equal to zero, Equation 8.67. In that equation, the integral was from $-\infty$ to $+\infty$. Orthogonality over a finite interval is defined analogously:

$$\int_{-T/2}^{+T/2} f(t) \cdot g^*(t) \, dt = 0 \tag{15.19}$$

The correlation of $e^{i\omega_1 t}$ and $e^{i\omega_2 t}$ is given by:

$$\int_{-T/2}^{+T/2} e^{i\omega_1 t} \cdot e^{i\omega_2 t} \, dt = \int_{-T/2}^{+T/2} e^{i(\omega_1 - \omega_2)t} \, dt \tag{15.20}$$

(The complex conjugate of $e^{i\omega_1 t}$ is $e^{-i\omega_2 t}$.) Comparing Equations 15.19 and 15.20, $e^{i\omega_1 t}$ is orthogonal to $e^{i\omega_2 t}$ — their correlation is zero — when:

$$\omega_1 - \omega_2 = n \cdot 2\pi/T, \quad n \neq 0 \tag{15.21}$$

We have derived an important result — two imaginary exponentials are orthogonal on the interval $-T/2$ to $T/2$ when the difference in their angular frequency is $n \cdot 2\pi/T$, where

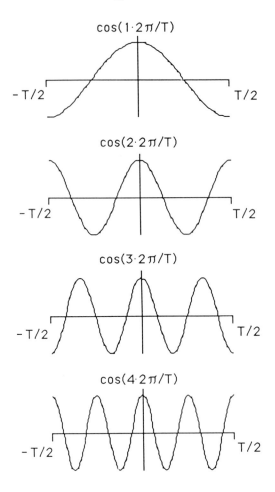

FIGURE 15.3. Orthogonal cosine functions: this figure shows four of the cosine functions, $\cos(n \cdot 2\pi \cdot t/T)$, which are orthogonal to each other on the interval $-T/2$ to $T/2$.

n is an integer. Thus, the countably infinite set of sinusoidal functions, $e^{int2\pi/T}$, is orthogonal on the interval $-T/2$ to $T/2$. Figure 15.3 shows the real parts, $\cos(nt2\pi/T)$, of four of these functions.

There is another important aspect to this result. The difference between the angular frequency of the successive orthogonal sinusoids is inversely related to the length of the interval:

$$\Delta\omega = 2\pi/T \tag{15.22}$$

In terms of frequency:

$$\Delta\nu = 1/T \tag{15.23}$$

As the interval increases in length, the frequency of the orthogonal imaginary exponentials comes closer together. We shall see this same behavior frequently with transforms. As the axis expands in one domain, the axis in the other domain contracts. But more of this later.

Now let us consider what happens as the length of the interval increases to infinity.

$$\lim_{T\to\infty} \Delta\omega = \lim_{T\to\infty} 2\pi/T = 0 \tag{15.24}$$

In other words, all of **the imaginary exponentials are orthogonal to each other on the interval $-\infty$ to $+\infty$.** This is the result that we sought to show.

Recall in Chapter 9 that we noted how useful it is to have a description of a vector in terms of a set of orthogonal basis vectors. The components of the vector in terms of the basis vectors can be determined from the projection of the vector onto the basis vector. Similarly, we shall see that it is useful to have a signal expressed in terms of a set of orthogonal basis functions. Since the imaginary exponentials are an orthogonal basis set, the inverse Fourier transform, Equation 14.6, gives an expansion of the signal, f(t), in terms of an orthogonal set of functions, which are the eigenfunctions of linear, time invariant systems!

IV. THE INTEGRAL OF AN IMAGINARY EXPONENTIAL

In order to prove that the Fourier transform pair is correct, we shall need to know the value of the integral of an imaginary exponential. The mathematics in this section is not strictly correct, but it provides us with some useful results. For anyone who is upset with the sloppy mathematics, the method of generalized functions puts these results on a more sound mathematical footing. We have opted for ease of exposition over mathematical rigor.

We are interested in finding the integral of the imaginary exponential, $e^{i\omega t}$, over the interval $-\infty$ to $+\infty$.

$$\int_{-\infty}^{+\infty} e^{i\omega t}\, dt \tag{15.25}$$

When ω is zero, $e^{i\omega t}$ is equal to one, and the integral is equal to ∞. When ω is not equal to zero, the value of the integral is more difficult to determine. What we shall do is to start with Equation 15.16 and then allow the interval to expand to $-\infty$ to $+\infty$.

The trick that we shall use is to consider only the angular frequencies for which 15.18 is equal to zero:

$$\omega = n \cdot 2\pi/T, \quad n \neq 0 \tag{15.26}$$

As we let T go to infinity, the integral of the imaginary exponential at these angular frequencies remains equal to zero. Above we have shown that for an infinite interval, all of the frequencies (except zero) are represented. Therefore:

$$\int_{-\infty}^{+\infty} e^{i\omega t}\, dt = \begin{cases} \infty, & \omega = 0 \\ 0 & \omega \neq 0 \end{cases} \tag{15.27}$$

(Although not of practical importance, mathematically it is worthy of note that the reason the integral is zero is due to the way we choose to let the limit go to infinity.)

The result, Equation 15.27, may remind the reader of the definition of the delta function, $\delta(\omega)$ in Chapter 2. However, the delta function also has the property that its integral is equal to one. In order to integrate Equation 15.27 with respect to ω, we shall go back to the definition of integration, Equation 2.18:

$$\int_{-\infty}^{+\infty} \left\{ \int_{-\infty}^{+\infty} e^{i\omega t}\, dt \right\} d\omega = \lim_{\Delta\omega \to 0} \sum_{\omega} \left\{ \int_{-T/2}^{+T/2} e^{i\omega t}\, dt \right\} \cdot \Delta\omega \tag{15.28}$$

Again, we shall only consider angular frequencies for which the integral inside the braces in Equation 15.28 is zero. Above we found that these angular frequencies are separated by an amount:

$$\Delta\omega = 2\pi/T \tag{15.29}$$

Or alternately the length of the interval is inversely related to the separation between the angular frequencies:

$$T = 2\pi/\Delta\omega \tag{15.30}$$

The integral given by Equation 15.28 can be rewritten using the relationship given in Equation 15.30:

$$\int_{-\pi/\Delta\omega}^{+\pi/\Delta\omega} e^{i\omega t}\, dt = \begin{cases} 2\pi/\Delta\omega, & \omega = 0 \\ \\ 0, & \omega \neq 0 \end{cases} \tag{15.31}$$

The only nonzero term in the summation in Equation 15.28 is when ω is equal to zero. Therefore,

$$\int_{-\infty}^{+\infty}\int_{-\infty}^{+\infty} e^{i\omega t}\, dt d\omega = \lim_{\Delta\omega\to 0} \{2\pi/\Delta\omega\} \cdot \Delta\omega = 2\pi \tag{15.32}$$

For the delta function, $\delta(\omega)$, the integral with respect to ω is one. For the imaginary exponential, the integral is 2π.

Thus we have established the important relationship:

$$\int_{-\infty}^{+\infty} e^{i\omega t}\, dt = 2\pi \cdot \delta(\omega) \tag{15.33}$$

Using exactly the same argument with the roles of ω and t exchanged we could also derive:

$$\int_{-\infty}^{+\infty} e^{i\omega t}\, d\omega = 2\pi \cdot \delta(t) \tag{15.34}$$

These two integrals can be viewed as Fourier transforms. The first integral gives the Fourier transform, $F(\omega)$, of the signal:

$$f(t) = 1 \tag{15.35}$$

We can identify the Fourier transform by inspection:

$$1 \leftrightarrow 2\pi \cdot \delta(\omega) \tag{15.36}$$

The second integral gives the inverse Fourier transform of:

$$F(\omega) = 1 \tag{15.37}$$

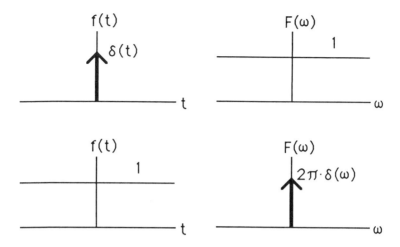

FIGURE 15.4. Fourier transform of the delta function: the Fourier transform of the delta function, $\delta(t)$, is the constant, one. The inverse Fourier transform of the delta function, $2\pi \cdot \delta(\omega)$, is the constant, one.

Therefore:

$$\delta(t) \leftrightarrow 1 \tag{15.38}$$

These two Fourier transform pairs are shown in Figure 15.4.

Equation 15.38 states that the delta function is composed of all frequencies, and that all frequencies have the same weighting factors, namely one. This explains why the delta function is so valuable. Below we shall see that this relation is a key to the fact that the output in response to a delta function input is the system function.

V. "PROOF" OF THE FOURIER TRANSFORM RELATIONSHIPS

We shall now show mathematically that the inverse Fourier transform reproduces the original signal. Substituting the Fourier transform relation, Equation 14.7, into the inverse Fourier transform, Equation 14.6:

$$f(t) = 1/2\pi \int_{-\infty}^{+\infty} \int_{-\infty}^{+\infty} f(t') \cdot e^{-i\omega t'} \, dt' \cdot e^{i\omega t} \, d\omega \tag{15.39}$$

We have used the variable, t', in the Fourier transformation in order not to confuse it with t in the inverse transformation. Changing the order of integration we get:

$$f(t) = 1/2\pi \int_{-\infty}^{+\infty} \int_{-\infty}^{+\infty} e^{i\omega(t-t')} \, d\omega \cdot f(t') \, dt' \tag{15.40}$$

The inner integral in Equation 15.40 is in the same general form as Equation 15.20. It is the correlation of two imaginary exponentials, $e^{i\omega t}$ and $e^{i\omega t'}$. Since these signals are orthogonal, the integral is equal to $2\pi \cdot \delta(t - t')$. Therefore Equation 15.40 reduces to:

$$f(t) = 1/2\pi \int_{-\infty}^{+\infty} 2\pi \cdot \delta(t - t') \cdot f(t') \, dt' = f(t) \tag{15.41}$$

Thus the inverse Fourier transformation of a Fourier transform is the original function. The key feature which simplified this operation is the fact that the imaginary exponentials are orthogonal.

We can do an analogous mathematical problem from a different point of view. We can consider that f(t) is defined in terms of a set of basis functions, $e^{i\omega't}$, by the inverse Fourier transform relationship:

$$f(t) = 1/2\pi \int_{-\infty}^{+\infty} F(\omega') \cdot e^{i\omega't} \, d\omega' \qquad (15.42)$$

The effect of the Fourier transform is that it picks out the single component, $e^{i\omega t}$. Due to the orthogonality of the basis functions, all the other functions are zero.

$$F(\omega) = \int_{-\infty}^{+\infty} \delta(\omega - \omega') \cdot F(\omega') \, d\omega' \qquad (15.43)$$

If the basis functions were not orthogonal, then these simple relationships would not exist.

VI. COMPLETENESS

One question which we have not addressed is what types of functions can be represented as the sum of complex exponentials, or equivalently, for which functions does the Fourier transform exist. Mathematical texts discuss at great length the requirements that a Fourier transform of a function exists. However, we can summarize these interesting mathematical questions very succinctly. **All signals which represent real physical entities have Fourier transforms**.

In Chapter 5 we showed that the eigenfunctions of linear, time invariant systems are the exponentials, including imaginary exponentials. The Fourier transform provides a method of representing all physical signals as linear combinations of the eigenfunctions of linear, time invariant systems!

It may at first seem surprising that all reasonable signals can be expressed in terms of sinusoidal functions. The sinusoidal functions are periodic, while most of the signals we are interested in are not periodic. It turns out that periodicity is a very important feature of the discrete Fourier series described in Chapter 18. In that chapter, we shall learn that periodicity in one domain is related to discrete sampling in the other domain. In that chapter, the apparent paradox of using periodic basis functions to represent nonperiodic signals will be resolved. But more of this later.

One way of understanding how any reasonable signal can be constructed using the inverse Fourier transform is to consider the delta function. Its Fourier transform is (Equation 15.38):

$$\delta(t) \leftrightarrow 1 \qquad (15.44)$$

In other words the Fourier transform of the delta function is equal to one for all angular frequencies. This transform is equivalent to having cosines of all angular frequencies which are weighed by one. Figure 15.5 shows the a number of cosines functions. At the point t equal to zero, they all add. At other points they tend to cancel each other. As the number of cosine frequencies increases, this cancellation becomes better and better.

Now let us calculate the Fourier transform of a shifted delta function.

$$F(\omega) = \int_{-\infty}^{+\infty} \delta(t - \tau) \cdot e^{-i\omega t} \, dt = e^{-i\omega\tau} \qquad (15.45)$$

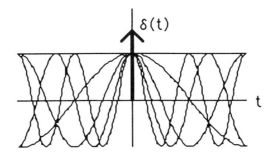

FIGURE 15.5. Synthesis of the delta function: a few of the sinusoidal components which make up the delta function are shown in this figure. At t equal to zero, all of the sinusoids add. At other points in time, the sinusoids cancel each other.

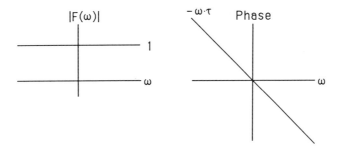

FIGURE 15.6. Fourier transform of $\delta(t - \tau)$: the left side of this figure shows the graph of the magnitude of the Fourier transform of $\delta(t - \tau)$. The right side shows the phase of the Fourier transform of $\delta(t - \tau)$.

Thus,

$$\delta(t - \tau) \leftrightarrow e^{-i\omega\tau} \tag{15.46}$$

The magnitude of the Fourier transform is equal to one for all angular frequencies, and the phase is equal to $-\omega \cdot \tau$. The phase increases in direct proportion to the angular frequency, ω. For this reason, $e^{-i\omega\tau}$ is referred to as a linear phase shift. Figure 15.6 shows the magnitude and the phase of $F(\omega)$. The dual relationship is:

$$e^{i\omega t}/2\pi \leftrightarrow \delta(\omega - \omega_0) \tag{15.47}$$

Equation 15.46 is equivalent to having an infinite set of cosine functions where each function is shifted in phase by $-\omega \cdot \tau$. Figure 15.7 shows a number of cosine functions where the phase of the functions is given by $-\omega \cdot \tau$. Notice that the cosine functions are all equal to one at time τ. At other times they tend to cancer each other out.

Since we can represent $\delta(t - \tau)$ as a Fourier transform, and since we can represent any time function as the sum of delta function (Equation 3.3), we can represent any signal as an inverse Fourier transform. This argument is not mathematically rigorous, but at least it gives some idea of the reason why all physically realizable functions can be represented using the Fourier transform.

VII. SUMMARY

The first two sections of this chapter showed two important properties of the Fourier transform pair, linearity and duality. In the remaining portion of this chapter we have

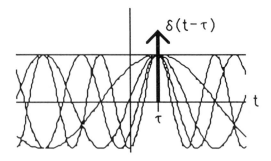

FIGURE 15.7. Synthesis of a shifted delta function: this figure shows a few of the sinusoidal components of a shifted delta function. The sinusoids which make up a shifted delta function all add at t equal to τ. At other points in time, the sinusoids cancel each other. A comparison with Figure 15.5 shows that the sinusoids are all shifted by the same amount, τ. The phase shift required to shift the sinusoids by an amount, τ, increases linearly with frequency.

"proved" that the inverse Fourier transform of a Fourier transform returns the original function. In order to prove this relation we showed that the imaginary exponentials have the important property of orthogonality. We have also discovered that the Fourier transform of a delta function is equal to one.

We have presented some rather tricky mathematics. Although this material is very important for mathematicians, from a radiological point of view, this material is much less important than trying to understand what the mathematics means. If the reader understands that the imaginary exponentials are orthogonal and that signals can be expressed as a linear combination of the imaginary exponentials, then he understands the meat of this chapter.

VIII. FURTHER READING

The references at the end of the last chapter also cover the material in this chapter. The importance of orthogonality of the basis functions of the Fourier transform is illuminated in Chapter 4 of the book by Strang,[1] in Chapter 5 of the book by Hildebrand,[2] and in Section 5-2 of the book of Papoulis.[3]

This book has been free and easy with its discussion of delta functions. The correct mathematical method of dealing with functions with singularities is to introduce the concept of generalized functions. The book by Bracewell[4] describes generalized functions in a readable fashion.

REFERENCES

1. **Strang, G.,** *Introduction to Applied Mathematics,* Wellesley-Cambridge Press, Wellesley, MA, 1986.
2. **Hildebrand, F. B.,** *Advanced Calculus for Applications,* Prentice-Hall, Englewood Cliffs, NJ, 1962.
3. **Papoulis, A.,** *Signal Analysis,* McGraw-Hill, New York, 1977.
4. **Bracewell, R. N.,** *The Fourier Transform and Its Applications,* McGraw-Hill, New York, 1978.

Chapter 16

PROPERTIES OF THE FOURIER TRANSFORM

The last two chapters introduced the Fourier transform and showed a few examples of Fourier transform pairs. This chapter will present several of the properties of the Fourier transform and show more examples. One of the reasons that we are interested in these properties is that they can be used to derive new Fourier transform pairs from ones that are already known. Although the properties of the Fourier transform are useful in calculations, the main reason for presenting them is to provide the reader with a better understanding of transformation operations.

The single most important property of the Fourier transform is the mapping of the complex operation of convolution into the simple operation of multiplication. We shall introduce that property in this chapter and further expand on it in the next chapter.

I. MAPPING OF CONVOLUTION TO MULTIPLICATION

The Fourier transform maps convolution in one domain to multiplication in the other domain. This relation provides an efficient method for performing convolution numerically on a computer. Although numerical efficiency is of great practical importance to radiology, our main interest in this property is that it will be very important in understanding image reconstruction from projections in Chapter 31.

In order to derive this property mathematically let us start with the convolution integral, Equation 3.4:

$$g(t) = \int_{-\infty}^{+\infty} f(\tau) \cdot h(t - \tau) \, d\tau \qquad (16.1)$$

Taking the Fourier transform of both sides of this equation:

$$G(\omega) = \int_{-\infty}^{+\infty} \int_{-\infty}^{+\infty} f(\tau) \cdot h(t - \tau) \, d\tau \cdot e^{-i\omega t} \, dt \qquad (16.2)$$

After changing the order of integration we can change the variable of integration:

$$t' = t - \tau \qquad (16.3)$$

Because of the change in the order of integration, τ is a constant within the inner integral; therefore:

$$dt' = dt \qquad (16.4)$$

We can rewrite Equation 16.2:

$$G(\omega) = \int_{-\infty}^{+\infty} \int_{-\infty}^{+\infty} f(\tau) \cdot h(t') \cdot e^{-i\omega(t' + \tau)} \, dt' d\tau \qquad (16.5)$$

Due to the properties of power functions (Table 2.3), the factors in t' and τ can be separated:

$$= \int_{-\infty}^{+\infty} f(\tau) \cdot e^{-i\omega\tau} \, d\tau \cdot \int_{-\infty}^{+\infty} h(t') \cdot e^{-i\omega t'} \, dt' \qquad (16.6)$$

Therefore,

$$G(\omega) = F(\omega) \cdot H(\omega) \tag{16.7}$$

We can summarize this result using the double headed arrow notation:

$$f(t) * h(t) \leftrightarrow F(\omega) \cdot H(\omega) \tag{16.8}$$

Using exactly the same mathematical manipulation the dual relationship can be derived:

$$f(t) \cdot h(t) \leftrightarrow (1/2\pi) \cdot F(\omega) * H(\omega) \tag{16.9}$$

We have formally shown that convolution in one domain maps into multiplication in the other domain. But let us derive this same property from a more intuitive point of view. We have stressed that the imaginary exponentials are the eigenfunctions of linear, time invariant systems. In Chapter 14 we showed that $H(\omega)$ is the eigenvalue associated with the imaginary exponential of angular frequency ω:

$$H\{e^{i\omega t}\} = H(\omega) \cdot e^{i\omega t} \tag{16.10}$$

where we have used the notation $H\{\cdot\}$ for the system (see Chapter 4).

The inverse Fourier transform provides a method of writing a signal in terms of a linear combination of imaginary exponentials.

$$f(t) = \int_{-\infty}^{+\infty} F(\omega) \cdot e^{-i\omega t} \, d\omega \tag{16.11}$$

Becuase the system is linear, the output is the same linear combination of imaginary exponentials scaled by the corresponding $H(\omega)$.

$$g(t) = \int_{-\infty}^{+\infty} F(\omega) \cdot [H(\omega) \cdot e^{-i\omega t}] \, d\omega \tag{16.12}$$

Figure 16.1 shows this relationship diagrammatically. Because of linearity, each component of the input signal can be considered separately. The output is the sum of the outputs from each portion of the input. $F(\omega)$ is a scale factor; $H(\omega)$ is an eigenvalue.

Equation 16.12 is in the form of an inverse Fourier transform. Therefore, the transform of the output can be identified by inspection:

$$G(\omega) = F(\omega) \cdot H(\omega) \tag{16.13}$$

This same equation was derived more analytically in Equation 16.7. This somewhat more intuitive argument is really equivalent to the mathematical argument above. The simplicity of this equation is related to the fact that the Fourier transform of the input signal represents the signal in terms of the eigenfunctions of linear, time invariant systems. Since the eigenfunctions of a system are characteristic of the system, they simplify the description of the operation of the system.

Figure 16.2 shows the mapping of convolution to multiplication diagrammatically. The upper panel shows the time domain signals. They are combined by convolution. The lower panel shows the frequency domain signals, they are combined by multiplication. In both cases we use a box to indicate the system.

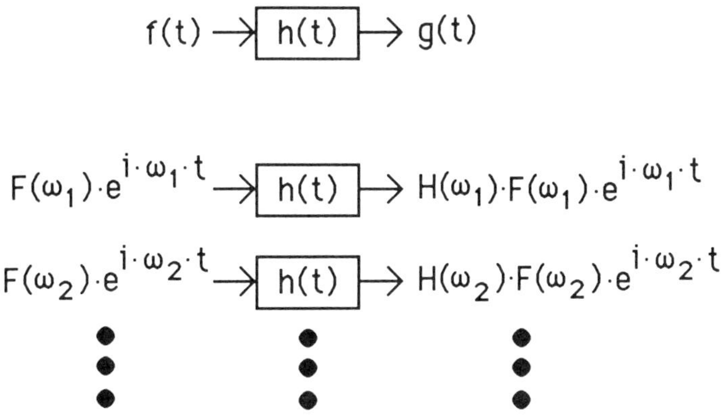

$$f(t) \rightarrow \boxed{h(t)} \rightarrow g(t)$$

$$F(\omega_1) \cdot e^{i \cdot \omega_1 \cdot t} \rightarrow \boxed{h(t)} \rightarrow H(\omega_1) \cdot F(\omega_1) \cdot e^{i \cdot \omega_1 \cdot t}$$

$$F(\omega_2) \cdot e^{i \cdot \omega_2 \cdot t} \rightarrow \boxed{h(t)} \rightarrow H(\omega_2) \cdot F(\omega_2) \cdot e^{i \cdot \omega_2 \cdot t}$$

$$\bullet \qquad\qquad \bullet \qquad\qquad \bullet$$
$$\bullet \qquad\qquad \bullet \qquad\qquad \bullet$$
$$\bullet \qquad\qquad \bullet \qquad\qquad \bullet$$

FIGURE 16.1.   Fourier transform of the system function as eigenvalues: in the time domain, the input, $f(t)$, to the system, $h(t)$, produces an output, $g(t)$. The Fourier transform of the input at angular frequency, ω_1 is $F(\omega_1)$. It is equal to the amount of the sinusoidal component, $e^{i\omega_1 t}$, in the input. Since $e^{i\omega_1 t}$ is an eigenfunction of the system, the output of the system in response to $F(\omega_1) \cdot e^{i\omega_1 t}$ is $H(\omega_1) \cdot F(\omega_1) \cdot e^{i\omega_1 t}$, where $H(\omega_1)$ is the Fourier transform of the system function.

$$f(t) \rightarrow \boxed{h(t)} \rightarrow g(t) = \int_{-\infty}^{+\infty} f(\tau) \cdot h(t-\tau) \, d\tau$$

$$F(\omega) \rightarrow \boxed{H(\omega)} \rightarrow G(\omega) = F(\omega) \cdot H(\omega)$$

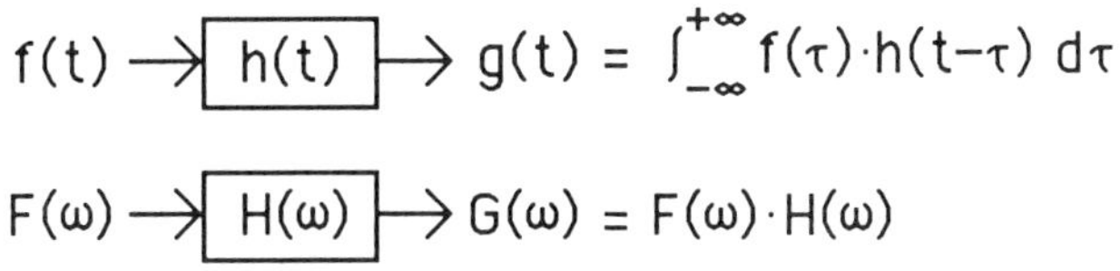

FIGURE 16.2.   Convolution $\leftrightarrow$ Multiplication: in the time domain, the output, $g(t)$, is equal to the convolution of the input, $f(t)$, and the system function, $h(t)$. In the frequency domain, the output, $G(\omega)$, is equal to the product of the input, $F(\omega)$, and the system function, $H(\omega)$.

A. RESPONSE OF A SYSTEM TO A DELTA FUNCTION INPUT

A delta function is composed of equal contributions of all angular frequencies (Equation 15.38):

$$\delta(t) \leftrightarrow 1 \tag{16.14}$$

Figure 15.5 shows that the sinusoids all add at t equal to zero; at other times they cancel each other. If the input to a system, $f(t)$, is a delta function, then the Fourier transform, $F(\omega)$, is equal to one for all angular frequencies. The output in the frequency domain is given by Equation 16.13:

$$G(\omega) = 1 \cdot H(\omega) \tag{16.15}$$

The output is equal to the system function. We already know that this result is true by definition, but this is another way to understand it.

Equations 16.14 and 16.15 help to explain why a delta function is such an important input. It contains equal amounts of all the imaginary exponential signals. Since it is composed of all the imaginary exponentials, the output will provide information about how the system interacts with all of the imaginary exponentials. Thus, the system function, the output in response to a delta function input, can be used to characterize a system.

B. AUDIO COMPONENT SYSTEM

Mapping of convolution in one domain into multiplication in the other domain may seem

Current from Amplifier   Speaker   Sound Wave

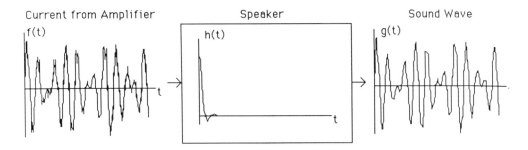

FIGURE 16.3.   Effect of a speaker in the time domain: the effect of a speaker in the time domain can be modeled as the convolution of the input, f(t), with the system function, h(t), of the speaker. The output, g(t), is a slightly smoother version of the input. The input to the speaker is the current from the amplifier. The output is the sound produced by the speaker.

Current from Amplifier   Speaker   Sound

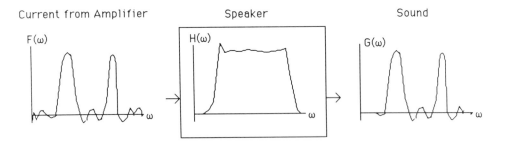

FIGURE 16.4.   Effect of a speaker in the frequency domain: the effect of a speaker in the frequency domain can be modeled as the product of the input, F(ω), and the system function, H(ω), of the speaker. The system function of a speaker tends to be flat in the middle range of frequencies. It attenuates the low and high frequencies. The output, G(ω), is similar to the input in the middle range of frequencies, but is near zero for the high and low frequencies.

strange to the reader; however, audio equipment provides an example which is very familiar to almost everyone. The output of a speaker in response to a current from an audio amplifier is a sound wave. In the time domain, the sound wave is the convolution of the input signal with the impulse response of the speaker, Figure 16.3. Although this model represents the physical signals accurately, it is totally unintelligible to the human.

However, the frequency domain representation of this system is much more natural. We can plot the input and the output of the speaker as a function of tone, i.e., as a frequency signal. The effects of the speaker on the signal are obvious (Figure 16.4). The input frequencies are multiplied by the system function to produce the output. When speakers are evaluated in *Consumer Reports,* the system functions of the speakers in the frequency domain are shown. Anyone familiar with audio equipment has a natural understanding that the frequency response of a speaker can be determined by the multiplication of the input music by the corresponding frequency response.

With audio equipment, we have a very natural understanding of how the complex time domain operation of the speaker on a signal is transformed into a simple description in the frequency domain. The frequency response of the speaker is the frequency domain representation of the system function.

C. SEQUENCE OF SYSTEMS

Let us suppose that we are passing a signal through a sequence of two of systems, $h_1(t)$ and $h_2(t)$. The output is given by:

$$g(t) = f(t) * h_1(t) * h_2(t) \tag{16.16}$$

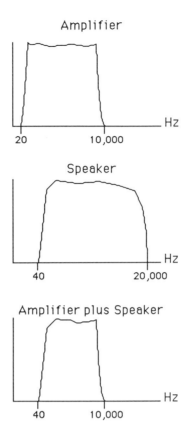

FIGURE 16.5. Sequence of systems: the effect of a sequence of systems in the frequency domain is the product of their system functions. In this example, the amplifier has a flat response in the range 20 to 10,000 Hz, and the speaker has a flat response in the range 40 to 20,000 Hz. The overall system including both the amplifier and the speaker has a flat response in the range 40 to 10,000 Hz.

Calculation of the output in the time domain is very complicated. It would require a double integration. In the frequency domain, the calculation becomes very simple. We can consider the systems in order. The output of the first system, $F(\omega) \cdot H_1(\omega)$, is the input to the second system. The effect of the second system on this signal is simply to multiply by $H_2(\omega)$. Thus the output of the two systems is:

$$G(\omega) = F(\omega) \cdot H_1(\omega) \cdot H_2(\omega) \tag{16.17}$$

In the frequency domain, the affect of two systems in sequence is simply the product of their effects. Similarly, the affect of any number of systems in sequence is simply the product of the frequency responses. One can easily get an idea of the effect of a complex system in the frequency domain when the time domain effects of the system are totally opaque.

Again, this property is well known to the audio buff. In order to determine the combined effects of an amplifier and a speaker, the frequency responses of the amplifier and the speaker are multiplied together. If an amplifier has a reasonably flat response from 20 to 10,000 Hz, and a speaker has a reasonable flat response from 40 to 20,000 Hz, then an audio buff who knows nothing about Fourier transforms can tell you that the combination will have a good response from 40 to 10,000 Hz (Figure 16.5). Of course any audio buff will also know that usually, the speakers limit the performance of the overall system.

The response of a sequence of systems is very important to understanding complex

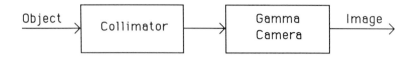

FIGURE 16.6.   Nuclear medical image formation: image formation in nuclear medicine can be modeled as a sequence of two systems, where one system represents the response of the collimator and the other system represents the intrinsic response of the gamma camera.

radiological systems. In fact the reader may already have some insight into this property from his radiological experience. We can consider a collimator and a gamma camera to be a sequence of image processing systems (see Figure 16.6). The resolution of a gamma camera is often given both as intrinsic resolution (without collimator) and extrinsic resolution (with collimator). The extrinsic resolution is the resolution of the combination of systems.

In Chapter 14, we showed that resolution can be given either in terms of the line spread function, LSF, or the modulation transfer function, MTF (Figure 14.9). In terms of the line spread function:

$$\mathrm{LSF_{intrinsic}} = \mathrm{LSF_{camera}} \qquad (16.18)$$

$$\mathrm{LSF_{extrinsic}} = \mathrm{LSF_{camera}} * \mathrm{LSF_{collimator}} \qquad (16.19)$$

In terms of the modulation transfer function:

$$\mathrm{MTF_{intrinsic}} = \mathrm{MTF_{camera}} \qquad (16.20)$$

$$\mathrm{MTF_{extrinsic}} = \mathrm{MTF_{camera}} \cdot \mathrm{MTF_{collimator}} \qquad (16.21)$$

If the intrinsic MTF of the camera and the MTF of the collimator are known, then the extrinsic MTF can be calculated with a simple multiplication.

D. MAPPING OF DECONVOLUTION TO DIVISION

Let us consider two signals which are combined by convolution:

$$g(t) = f(t) * h(t) \qquad (16.22)$$

The process of determining $f(t)$ given $g(t)$ and $h(t)$ is called deconvolution. Because of the symmetry of the convolution operation, this problem is equivalent to determining $h(t)$ given $g(t)$ and $f(t)$. Deconvolution is a very difficult problem. It involves the solution of an integral equation. However, in the transform domain, this problem is trivial:

$$G(\omega) = F(\omega) \cdot H(\omega) \qquad (16.23)$$

$$F(\omega) = G(\omega)/H(\omega) \qquad (16.24)$$

It is a simple division.

In the last section, we showed how to calculate the extrinsic resolution of a gamma camera from the intrinsic resolution and the resolution of the collimator. This calculation is not typically the problem of interest. More commonly we have measured the intrinsic and extrinsic resolutions, and we wish to calculate the resolution of the collimator. Solution of this problem in terms of the line spread functions is very difficult, a deconvolution. In terms of the modulation transfer function, this deconvolution is very simple:

$$\text{MTF}_{\text{collimator}} = \text{MTF}_{\text{extrinsic}}/\text{MTF}_{\text{intrinsic}} \qquad (16.25)$$

The Fourier transform maps deconvolution in one domain into division in the other domain.

Mapping of convolution into multiplication provides great numerical efficiency. The opposite relation, mapping of deconvolution into division, transforms a nearly impossible operation into a simple operation. In Part IV we shall learn more about deconvolution and the special considerations which come into play for systems with noise.

II. SHIFT/MODULATION

In this section we shall show that the shift of a signal in one domain results in the multiplication of its transform by an imaginary exponential. A shift of a signal in the time domain changes the phases of the frequency domain signal. The dual relation, a shift of the frequency domain signal, results in the multiplication of the time domain signal by an imaginary exponential. Although this is the same operation, we often think of it from two different points of view. The multiplication by an imaginary exponential in the frequency domain is viewed as a phase shift, while multiplication by an imaginary exponential in the time domain is viewed as **modulation** of a carrier signal by the original signal. Below we shall describe these points of view more fully.

Let us consider what happens when a signal, f(t), is shifted by an amount τ. The Fourier transform of the shifted signal is:

$$\int_{-\infty}^{+\infty} f(t - \tau) \cdot e^{-i\omega t} \, dt \qquad (16.26)$$

If we substitute for the variable of integration:

$$t' = t - \tau \qquad (16.27)$$

the transform is then:

$$= \int_{-\infty}^{+\infty} f(t') \cdot e^{-i\omega(t' + \tau)} \, dt' \qquad (16.28)$$

Since τ is a constant, the factor, $e^{-i\omega\tau}$, can be moved outside the integral:

$$= e^{-i\omega\tau} \cdot \int_{-\infty}^{+\infty} f(t') \cdot e^{-i\omega t'} \, dt' \qquad (16.29)$$

The remaining integral is the Fourier transform of f(t). Thus the transform of f(t − τ) is:

$$= e^{-i\omega\tau} \cdot F(\omega) \qquad (16.30)$$

A shift of a signal in one domain leads to the multiplication of the transform by an imaginary exponential:

$$f(t - \tau) \leftrightarrow e^{-i\omega\tau} \cdot F(\omega) \qquad (16.31)$$

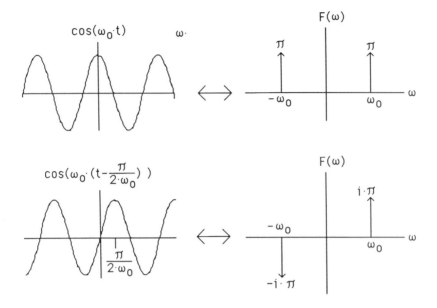

FIGURE 16.7.   Linear phase shift: In the time domain, shift of the cosine function by $\pi/(2 \cdot \omega_0)$ gives the sine function. In the frequency domain this corresponds to a phase shift of $e^{i\omega\pi/2\pi_0}$. At ω equal to ω_0, this phase shift is i. At ω equal to $-\omega_0$, this phase shift is $-i$. Multiplying the Fourier transform cosine function by these phase shifts gives the Fourier transform of the sine function.

The imaginary exponential has a magnitude of one; therefore, this factor changes the phase of the transform, but not the magnitude. Since the phase change is proportional to the angular frequency, it is called a **linear phase shift**. We can state Equation 16.31 in words — **a shift of f(t) in time leads to a linear phase shift of F(ω)**.

We can use this property of the Fourier transform to derive the transform of a sine function from the transform of a cosine function. The cosine and its transform were given by Equation 14.12:

$$\cos(\omega_0 t) \leftrightarrow \pi \cdot [\delta(\omega - \omega_0) + \delta(\omega + \omega_0)] \tag{16.32}$$

A shift of this cosine by $\pi/2\omega_0$, gives the sine function:

$$\cos(\omega_0(t - \pi/2\omega_0)) = \cos(\omega_0 t - \pi/2) = \sin(\omega_0 t) \tag{16.33}$$

In the transform domain, this shift results in multiplication by $e^{-i\omega\pi/2\omega_0}$. For ω equal to $-\omega_0$, the phase shift is $e^{-i\pi/2}$, which is equal to $-i$ (or 1/i). For ω equal to ω_0, the phase shift is i (or $-1/i$). Thus,

$$\sin(\omega_0 t) \leftrightarrow \pi/i \cdot [\delta(\omega - \omega_0) - \delta(\omega + \omega_0)] \tag{16.34}$$

Figure 16.7 shows this relationship diagrammatically.

Any sinusoidal function can be represented as a sum of a cosine and a sine function (see Equation 6.63). The factors in Equation 6.63 are equal to the real and imaginary parts of the phase shift, $e^{i\omega\pi/2\omega_0}$. As the cosine function shifts in the time domain, the delta functions rotate from the real to imaginary axis in the frequency domain (see Figure 16.8). Also notice that the amount of shift required to change a cosine function into a sine function is inversely related to the angular frequency, $\pi/2\omega_0$. The higher the angular frequency, the shorter the period.

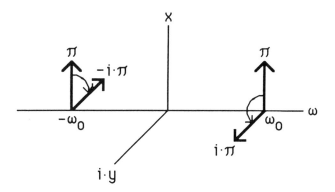

FIGURE 16.8. Frequency domain effect of a shift in the time domain: the frequency domain representation of a cosine function is two delta functions. As the cosine function is shifted, the effect of the linear phase shift in the frequency domain is to rotate the delta functions toward the imaginary plane.

The linear phase shift property has been used in nuclear magnetic resonance blood flow imaging. By intentionally moving the free induction decay with respect to the origin, a linear phase shift is introduced into the Fourier transform. The Fourier transform of the free induction decay, which is the spectrum of the nuclear magnetic resonance signal, corresponds to the spatial domain of the image (see Figure 15.1). A shift in the origin of the free induction decay results in multiplication of the image by an imaginary exponential. If the real part of the image is displayed, then this sinusoidally varying phase produces stripes in the image. Changes in the position of these stripes can be used to help determine the rate of blood flow.

A. MODULATION OF A CARRIER

A frequent problem in electrical engineering is the modulation of a carrier signal, often a sinusoidal signal, by a second signal. For example, a radio station is assigned a specific range of frequencies by the FCC. It transmits a sinusoidally varying electromagnetic wave at the center of that range. The voice or music to be broadcast is used to modulate that sinusoidal signal. AM radio stations modulate the amplitude of the carrier signal. FM radio stations modulate the frequency of the carrier signal.

AM modulation is similar to the problem just considered. AM modulation is performed by multiplying a carrier signal, $e^{i\omega_0 t}$, and the voice signal, $f(t)$. The same mathematical operations which were used to derive Equation 16.31 can be used to show that:

$$(e^{i\omega_0 t}/2\pi) \cdot f(t) \leftrightarrow F(\omega - \omega_0) \qquad (16.35)$$

Figure 16.9 shows the frequency domain representation of the signal before and after it has been multiplied by the carrier $e^{i\omega_0 t}/2\pi$. Multiplication by the carrier signal moves the frequency domain signal by an amount, ω_0. The carrier signal is modulated by the signal, $f(t)$. The voice signal can be moved to the set of frequencies assigned by the FCC simply by multiplying by an appropriate imaginary exponential.

Nuclear magnetic resonance can also be modeled using the ideas of a carrier signal. In nuclear magnetic resonance we are interested in the small variations in the output signal caused by the sample. The resonant frequency of a nucleus is in the radio frequency range while these small variations are in an audio frequency range. If we model the audio frequency signal as $f(t)$, then the radio frequency signal, $g(t)$, is given by:

$$g(t) = f(t) \cdot e^{i\omega_0 t}/2\pi \qquad (16.36)$$

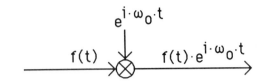

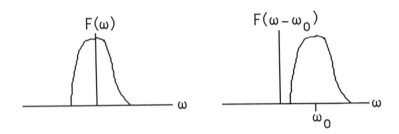

FIGURE 16.9.   Modulation: multiplication of a signal by a sinusoid, $e^{i\omega_0 t}$, in the time domain is equivalent to shifting the frequency domain function by ω_0.

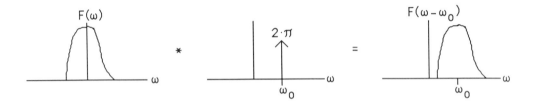

FIGURE 16.10.   Modulation as a convolution in the frequency domain: multiplication of a signal by $e^{i\omega_0 t}$ in the time domain is equivalent to convolution of the signal by a delta function at ω_0 in the frequency domain.

where ω_0 is the resonant angular frequency. Using this model, $e^{i\omega_0 t}/2\pi$ is a carrier signal which is modulated by $f(t)$.

The mapping of multiplication in the time domain into convolution in the frequency domain can be used to help understand modulation. In the time domain the signal, $f(t)$, is multiplied by $e^{i\omega_0 t}/2\pi$. The Fourier transform of $e^{i\omega_0 t}/2\pi$ is a delta function at angular frequency ω_0 (see Equation 15.47). Therefore, Equation 16.36 corresponds to:

$$G(\omega) = F(\omega) * \delta(\omega - \omega_0) \qquad (16.37)$$

In the frequency domain, the audio frequency signal convolved with a delta function at the resonant frequency.

Convolution with a delta function merely shifts the signal. Figure 16.10 shows how the audio frequency signal is shifted to a higher frequency by convolution with the delta function. In order to recover the audio frequency signal from the NMR signal, the first stage in processing is to democulate the signal. Demodulation is performed by multiplying the NMR signal by an imaginary exponential at the negative frequency:

$$g(t) \cdot (2\pi \cdot e^{-i\omega_0 t}) = f(t) \cdot (e^{i\omega_0 t}/2\pi) \cdot (2\pi \cdot e^{-i\omega_0 t})$$

$$= f(t) \qquad (16.38)$$

In nuclear magnetic resonance, the use of two coils at right angles to each other is referred to as quadrature detection. The two coils can be modeled as the real and imaginary parts of a complex signal. Quadrature nuclear magnetic resonance detection is most accurately modeled with imaginary exponential signals. Using an imaginary exponential carrier signal simplifies the modulation problem. Our description of AM radio modulation is not entirely accurate. Radio signals are more accurately modeled as real signals. When we are limited to real signals, modulation is slightly more complex. We shall come back to modulation of real carrier signals in Chapter 23.

III. CHANGE IN SCALE

When a signal becomes narrower, its transform becomes wider, and when a signal becomes wider, its transform becomes narrower. We have already been something of this behavior in the last chapter when we discussed the orthogonal, imaginary exponentials on a finite interval. This property will be very important in understanding the discrete Fourier transform in Chapter 18.

Mathematically, a signal, f(t), can be widened or narrowed by substituting, $a \cdot t$, for the independent variable t. $f(a \cdot t)$ will be narrower than $f(t)$ if a is greater than one. The Fourier transform of $f(a \cdot t)$ is

$$\int_{-\infty}^{+\infty} f(a \cdot t) \cdot e^{-i\omega t} \, dt \qquad (16.39)$$

In order to relate this Fourier transform to $F(\omega)$, we can change the variable of integration:

$$t' = a \cdot t \qquad (16.40)$$

The Fourier transform of $f(a \cdot t)$ is then:

$$\int_{-\infty}^{+\infty} f(t') \cdot e^{-i\omega t'/a} \, dt'/|a| \qquad (16.41)$$

The absolute value, $|a|$, arises because the limits switch depending upon the sign of a. By moving the terms around we can write this equation in terms of a Fourier transform:

$$1/|a| \cdot \int_{-\infty}^{+\infty} f(t') \cdot e^{-i(\omega/a)t'} \, dt' = 1/|a| \cdot F(\omega/a) \qquad (16.42)$$

We have shown the relationship:

$$f(a \cdot t) \leftrightarrow 1/|a| \cdot F(\omega/a) \qquad (16.43)$$

With the same mathematical argument, we could show:

$$1/|a| \cdot f(t/a) \leftrightarrow F(a \cdot \omega) \qquad (16.44)$$

These relationships are shown graphically in Figure 16.11. When the signal shrinks in the time domain, its transform expands.

A good radiological example of this property is the relation between the relaxation time, T_2^*, and the line width in the nuclear magnetic resonance spectrum. The audio frequency portion of the free induction decay from a sample with a single nuclear species can be modeled as an exponential. The frequency domain representation, the spectrum, is given by Equation 14.23. There is a single peak at the resonance frequency whose width is related

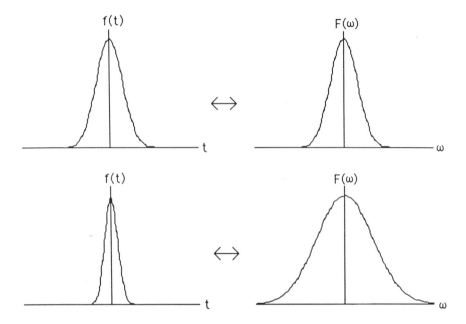

FIGURE 16.11. Scaling: the Fourier transform of a Gaussian function is also a Gaussian function. Scaling the independent variable changes the width of a signal. As the time domain signal becomes smaller, the frequency domain signal becomes larger.

to the relaxation time. Sharp line widths are associated with long relaxation times and narrow line widths are associated with short relaxation times:

$$\Delta\omega = 1/T_2^* \tag{16.45}$$

IV. MAPPING OF DIFFERENTIAL EQUATIONS TO POLYNOMIAL EQUATIONS

Another property of the Fourier transform is that it can be used to map differential equations to polynomial equations. This property is included primarily for readers who have some previous knowledge of differential equations. The mathematically phobic reader can skip to the next section.

$df(t)/dt$ can be expressed in terms of the inverse Fourier transform by:

$$\frac{d}{dt} (1/2\pi) \cdot \int_{-\infty}^{+\infty} F(\omega) \cdot e^{i\omega t} \, d\omega$$

$$= (1/2\pi) \cdot \int_{-\infty}^{+\infty} i\omega \cdot F(\omega) \cdot e^{i\omega t} \, d\omega \tag{16.46}$$

Therefore:

$$df(t)/dt \leftrightarrow i\omega \cdot F(\omega) \tag{16.47}$$

The dual relationship is:

$$-it \cdot f(t) \leftrightarrow dF(\omega)/d\omega \tag{16.48}$$

The derivative operation in one domain leads to multiplication by i times the variable in the other domain. The second derivative is given by:

$$d^2f(t)/dt^2 \leftrightarrow -\omega^2 \cdot F(\omega) \tag{16.49}$$

And so forth for higher derivatives.

This property is very important for solution of differential equations. A differential equation in one domain can be transformed into a polynomial equation in the other domain. For example, Equation 7.2 gives a general formula for the set of linear differential equation with constant coefficients. Using Equation 16.47, this equation can be expressed in the frequency domain as a polynomial equation. The system function, $H(\omega)$, represented by this equation, is equal to the ratio $G(\omega)/F(\omega)$. Using the frequency domain representation of Equation 7.2, this ratio can be expressed as a ratio of polynomials in the angular frequency variable, ω.

For a system which is initially at rest, the system function of any linear differential equation with constant coefficients can be expressed in the frequency domain as the ratio of two polynomials. The use of transform operations to assist in the solution of differential equations will not be covered in this book; however, this brief description should indicate to the reader that this property of the transform operation is very useful when working with differential equations.

V. FOURIER TRANSFORM OF EVEN AND ODD SIGNALS

It is often useful to divide a signal into two functions — one that is symmetric about zero and one that is asymmetric about zero. These functions are called the even and odd parts of the function. We shall use the notation $f_e(t)$ for the even part of $f(t)$, and $f_o(t)$ for the odd part of $f(t)$. Our goal will be to show that the Fourier transform of the even part of a real function is real and that the Fourier transform of the odd part of a real function is imaginary.

There are several symmetry relations between the even and odd parts of a signal and its transform. These relations can get confusing. One of the advantages of the complex notation is that it simplifies these relations. The complex Fourier transform pair is easily remembered, and these other relations can be easily derived from it.

We can define the even and odd parts of $f(t)$ as follows:

$$f_e(t) = [f(t) + f^*(-t)]/2 \tag{16.50}$$

$$f_o(t) = [f(t) - f^*(-t)]/2 \tag{16.51}$$

By substitution, the reader can check that:

$$f(t) = f_e(t) + f_o(t) \tag{16.52}$$

and the following summetry properties:

$$f_e(t) = f_e^*(-t) \tag{16.53}$$

$$f_o(t) = -f_o^*(-t) \tag{16.54}$$

We have defined the symmetry property using the complex conjugate operator, *, to allow for the case where $f(t)$ is complex.

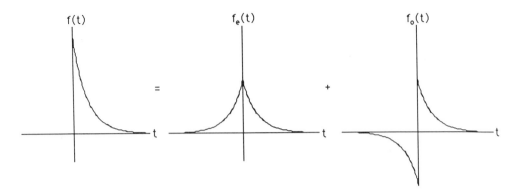

FIGURE 16.12.   Even and odd parts of a function: the exponential function on the left can be divided into its even and odd parts shown on the right.

Figure 16.12 shows a signal, f(t), which is an exponential function, $u(t) \cdot e^{-\lambda t}$, and the corresponding even and odd parts of the signal. Although the signal is zero for t less than zero, both the even and odd parts of the signal are nonzero for t less than zero. (Since the even and odd parts are opposite for t less than zero, the sum is zero.) Although one would not naturally think of f(t) in terms of even and odd signals, it can easily be divided into even and odd parts, and this separation provides some insights.

Since the Fourier transform is a linear operation (Equation 15.4), Equation 16.52 can be written in the frequency domain as:

$$F(\omega) = F_e(\omega) + F_o(\omega) \tag{16.55}$$

where $F_e(\omega)$ and $F_o(\omega)$ are the Fourier transforms of $f_e(t)$ and $f_o(t)$, respectively. ($F_e(\omega)$ and $F_o(\omega)$ are not necessarily even and odd.) We are now interested in finding the Fourier transform of the even and the odd parts separately. The Fourier transform of the even signal can be divided into two parts:

$$F_e(\omega) = \int_{-\infty}^{0} f_e(t) \cdot e^{-i\omega t}\, dt + \int_{0}^{+\infty} f_e(t) \cdot e^{-i\omega t}\, dt \tag{16.56}$$

In the first integral we can substitute for the variable of integration (see Equation 2.25):

$$t' = -t \tag{16.57}$$

Then, Equation 16.56 is equal to:

$$= \int_{0}^{+\infty} f_e(-t') \cdot e^{i\omega t'}\, dt' + \int_{0}^{+\infty} f_e(t) \cdot e^{-i\omega t}\, dt \tag{16.58}$$

Since $f_e(t)$ is equal to $f_e(-t)$, these integrals can be combined:

$$F_e(\omega) = \int_{0}^{+\infty} f_e(t) \cdot [e^{i\omega t} + e^{-i\omega t}]\, dt \tag{16.59}$$

But the factor inside the brackets is just twice the cosine function; therefore:

$$F_e(\omega) = \int_0^{+\infty} 2 \cdot f_e(t) \cdot \cos(\omega t) \, dt \tag{16.60}$$

Exactly the same argument applies to f_o except that $f_o(-t)$ is equal to $-f_o(t)$. Thus:

$$F_o(\omega) = \int_0^{+\infty} f_o(t) \cdot [e^{i\omega t} - e^{-i\omega t}] \, dt \tag{16.61}$$

and the function in brackets is 2i times the sine function.

$$F_o(\omega) = i \cdot \int_0^{+\infty} 2 \cdot f_e(t) \cdot \sin(\omega t) \, dt \tag{16.62}$$

Equations 16.60 and 16.62 lead to a number of interesting conclusions. The Fourier transform of a function can be determined entirely in terms of the sine and cosine functions. Some authors define **sine and cosine transforms,** and these equations show how they relate to the complex Fourier transform as we have defined it. The cosine Fourier transform can be used for the even part of a function. The sine Fourier transform can be used for the odd part of a function. Symbolically, we can write:

$$\text{even} \leftrightarrow \text{cosine transform} \tag{16.63}$$

$$\text{odd} \leftrightarrow \text{sine transform} \tag{16.64}$$

From Equation 16.60, we see that if $f_e(t)$ is real, then the Fourier transform is real. Thus, we have proved that the Fourier transform of an even real function is real. Similarly, from Equation 16.62 we see that the Fourier transform of an odd real function is pure imaginary. Symbolically, these conditions can be written:

$$\text{even \& real} \rightarrow \text{real} \tag{16.65}$$

$$\text{odd \& real} \rightarrow \text{imaginary} \tag{16.66}$$

Since these are sufficient, but not necessary conditions, we have used a one-headed arrow.
We can derive another relation which will be of use later in the book. The Fourier transform of $f^*(-t)$ is given by:

$$\int_{-\infty}^{+\infty} f^*(-t) \cdot e^{i\omega t} \, dt = \left[\int_{-\infty}^{+\infty} f(-t) \cdot e^{-i\omega t} \, dt \right]^* \tag{16.67}$$

where $e^{-i\omega t}$ is the complex conjugate of $e^{i\omega t}$.
We can substitute for the variable of integration:

$$t' = -t \tag{16.68}$$

Then, Equation 16.67 is equal to:

$$= \left[\int_{+\infty}^{-\infty} f(t') \cdot e^{i\omega t'} \, d(-t') \right]^* \tag{16.69}$$

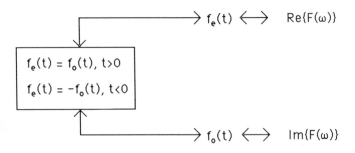

FIGURE 16.13.   Quadrature signals: the even and the odd parts of a causal signal are related by the equations shown in the box. The Fourier transform of the even part of a real, causal function is real and the Fourier transform of the odd part of a real, causal function is imaginary. The real and imaginary parts of the Fourier transform of a real, causal function are quadrature signals. They have the same information. Using the relations shown in this diagram, the real and imaginary parts of the Fourier transform can be derived from each other.

Switching the limits of integration:

$$= \left[\int_{-\infty}^{+\infty} f(t') \cdot e^{i\omega t'} \, dt' \right]^{*} \tag{16.70}$$

The integral in Equation 16.70 is the complex conjugate of the Fourier transform of f(t); therefore:

$$f^{*}(-t) \leftrightarrow F^{*}(\omega) \tag{16.71}$$

This is an interesting result. The complex conjugate of a time-reversed signal has a Fourier transform which is the complex conjugate of the Fourier transform of the signal. One might suspect that the frequency variable would also be reversed, but it is not. The symmetry properties of the two domains are not always obvious, but they can be easily derived.

A. QUADRATURE SIGNALS
We are often interested in real signals which are zero for t less than zero. For example, if a system does not have any output until there is an input, then the system function is zero for t less than zero. Such systems are called **causal**. The even part of a causal signal must be equal to the negative of the odd part of the signal for t less than zero:

$$f_e(t) = -f_o(t), \quad t < 0 \tag{16.72}$$

Because of Equation 16.53 and 16.54, these signals must be equal for t greater than zero:

$$f_e(t) = f_o(t), \quad t > 0 \tag{16.73}$$

These relations are shown in the box in Figure 16.13. An example of a causal signal was shown in Figure 16.12.
Causal signals can be determined entirely from either their even or odd parts.

$$f(t) = \begin{cases} 0, & t < 0 \\ 2 \cdot f(t) \quad \text{or} \quad 2 \cdot f_o(t), & t > 0 \end{cases} \tag{16.74}$$

The Fourier transform of the even part of a real signal is real, and the transform of the odd part of a real signal is imaginary. Therefore, the real and the imaginary parts of the Fourier transform of a real, causal signal are related since they can be calculated from even and odd parts of the signal. These somewhat confusing relationships are also shown in Figure 16.13.

The real and imaginary parts of the Fourier transform of a real, causal signal are called **quadrature signals**. Given either of the two quadrature signals, the other signal can be calculated. For example, given the real part of the Fourier transform, the even part of the causal signal can be calculated using the inverse Fourier transform; then, the odd part of the signal can be calculated using Equation 16.72 and 16.73; then, the imaginary part of the Fourier transform can be calculated from the odd part of the signal. Transformation between the real and imaginary parts of a quadrature signal is called the **Hilbert transform.**

The details of the Hilbert transform will not be of importance to us, but what is important is that quadrature signals are closely related. They carry the same information. We can determine a real, causal signal from either the real or imaginary parts of its Fourier transform, and we can determine the real part of the Fourier transform from the imaginary part and *vice versa*.

The free induction decay of a nuclear magnetic resonance experiment can be modeled as a real, causal signal. If time zero is set to the beginning of the experiment, then there is no signal prior to time zero. The signal intensity measured in a single coil is real by definition. Since the free induction decay is modeled as a real, causal signal, the real and imaginary parts of the nuclear magnetic resonance spectrum are quadrature signals.

The real part of the nuclear magnetic resonance spectrum is called the **absorptive signal**, and the imaginary part of the spectrum is called the **dispersive signal** (see Figure 14.11). Depending upon how the data are collected, it is possible to obtain either the absorptive signal, or the dispersive signal, or a combination of these signals. Either of these signals provide equivalent information about the nuclear magnetic resonance spectrum. A first step in processing is often to calculate the absorptive signal from experimental signal.

The word quadrature is often used somewhat loosely. Above we used the term quadrature detection to refer to nuclear magnetic resonance signal collection using two orthogonal coils. The orthogonal coils sample the real and imaginary parts of the free induction decay. This use of the word, quadrature, can be explained by duality. If the reference frequency is picked so that it is below all of the peaks in the spectrum, then we can model the spectrum using a frequency domain signal which is zero for ω less than zero. The spectrum is real by definition. Therefore, the spectrum can be modeled as a real, "causal" frequency domain signal. ("Causal" in the frequency domain.) Therefore the real and imaginary parts of the time domain signal must be quadrature signals.

In the first case, the free induction decay was modeled as a real, causal signal. Then the real part of the spectrum, the absorptive signal and the imaginary part of the spectrum, the dispersive signal are quadrature signals. In the second case, the spectrum was modeled as a real, "causal" signal. Then the real and imaginary parts of the free induction decay are quadrature signals. These relations again show the importance of understanding the duality between the time and frequency domains.

Causality is a frequent property of electrical signals so that it is often heavily stressed in electrical engineering texts. Causality is usually not an important feature of image processing applications. We have mentioned causality because it helps to explain nuclear magnetic resonance data collection; however, since our major goal is image processing, we shall not emphasize causality.

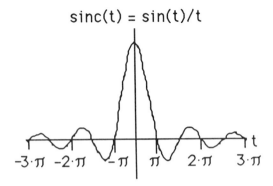

FIGURE 16.14.   Sinc function: this figure shows the function, sinc(t), which is defined to be sin(t)/t.

VI. THE SINC FUNCTION

In signal processing applications a function which appears frequently is sin(t)/t. For that reason it is given a special name, sinc (pronounced "sink"):

$$\text{sinc}(t) = \sin(t)/t \tag{16.75}$$

The sinc function is shown in Figure 16.14. For larger values of t, the function is a sine wave where the amplitude of the fluctuation decreases as t increases. For small values of t we can predict the behavior of this function t from the power series expansion of sin(t), (Table 2.5):

$$\text{sinc}(t) = (t - t^3/3! + t^5/5! - \ldots)/t$$
$$\approx 1 - t^2/3! \tag{16.76}$$

At t equal to zero, the value will be one. For small t, the value will be less than one.

The reason that this signal appears so frequently is that it is the Fourier transform of a common signal, the rectangle. Let us consider a signal, $F(\omega)$, which is one over the interval $-\Omega/2$ to $\Omega/2$, and zero elsewhere. The inverse Fourier transform of this function is given by:

$$\int_{-\Omega/2}^{+\Omega/2} 1 \cdot e^{i\omega t} \, d\omega = (1/it) \cdot (e^{i\Omega t/2} - e^{-i\Omega t/2})$$
$$= (1/t) \cdot 2 \cdot \sin(\Omega t/2) = \Omega \cdot \text{sinc}(\Omega t/2) \tag{16.77}$$

Therefore we can write:

$$\Omega \cdot \text{sinc}(\Omega t/2) \leftrightarrow u(\Omega/2 - \omega) \cdot u(\omega - \Omega/2) \tag{16.78}$$

where we have written the rectangle as the product of two step functions. Using the same argument we can show:

$$u(T/2 - t) \cdot u(t - T/2) \leftrightarrow 2\pi \cdot T \cdot \text{sinc}(\omega T/2) \tag{16.79}$$

Figure 16.15 shows two different rectangles and the corresponding sinc functions. As was seen above for the scaling property, the wider rectangle results in a narrower sinc

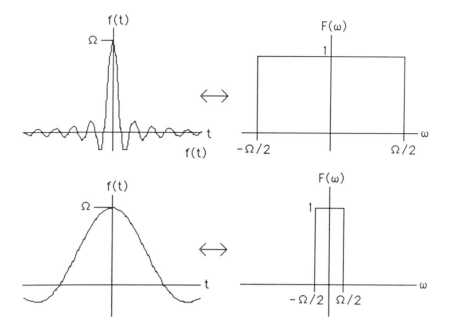

FIGURE 16.15. Sinc function ↔ Rectangle function: the sinc function and the rectangle functions form a Fourier transform pair. As the sinc function becomes wider, the rectangle function becomes narrower.

function. This example of a Fourier transform pair shows another general rule — sharp edges in one domain, like the edges of the rectangle, lead to wiggles in the other domain.

VII. VALUE AT THE ORIGIN AND THE INTEGRAL IN THE OTHER DOMAIN

The value of the signal at the origin in the time domain is related to the integral of the signal in the frequency domain. Substituting t equal to zero in the inverse Fourier transform relation, Equation 14.6, gives:

$$f(0) \; = \; (1/2\pi) \cdot \int_{-\infty}^{+\infty} F(\omega) \cdot e^0 \; d\omega \qquad (16.80)$$

Since e^0 is equal to 1:

$$f(0) \; = \; (1/2\pi) \cdot \int_{-\infty}^{+\infty} F(\omega) \; d\omega \qquad (16.81)$$

The value of the time domain signal at the origin, $f(0)$, is equal to the integral of the frequency domain signal divided by 2π.

Similarly, substituting ω equal to zero in the Fourier transform relation, Equation 14.7, gives:

$$F(0) \; = \; \int_{-\infty}^{+\infty} f(t) dt \qquad (16.82)$$

The value of the frequency domain signal at the origin, $F(0)$, is equal to the integral of the time domain signal. The zero frequency component is the constant part of the signal. Equation 16.82 states that the constant part of the signal is equal to the integral of the signal.

VIII. CONSERVATION OF ENERGY

In this section we shall develop **Parseval's relation**. Parseval's relation states that the correlation of two signals is proportional to the correlation of their Fourier transforms. We shall use this relationship to show that the energy in a signal is proportional to the energy in its transform. In other words there is a conservation of energy in transforming from one domain to the other domain.

The correlation of two signals is given by:

$$\int_{-\infty}^{+\infty} f(t) \cdot g^*(t) \, dt \tag{16.83}$$

We can substitute the inverse Fourier transform of $g^*(t)$:

$$= \int_{-\infty}^{+\infty} f(t) \cdot (1/2\pi) \cdot \int_{-\infty}^{+\infty} G^*(\omega) \cdot e^{-i\omega t} \, d\omega dt \tag{16.84}$$

where the minus sign in the exponent is due to the complex conjugation. Changing the order of integration and moving terms about:

$$= (1/2\pi) \cdot \int_{-\infty}^{+\infty} G^*(\omega) \cdot \int_{-\infty}^{+\infty} f(t) \cdot e^{-i\omega t} \, dt d\omega \tag{16.85}$$

The inner integral is the Fourier transform of $f(t)$; therefore:

$$= (1/2\pi) \cdot \int_{-\infty}^{+\infty} G^*(\omega) \cdot F(\omega) \, d\omega \tag{16.86}$$

In summary:

$$\int_{-\infty}^{+\infty} f(t) \cdot g^*(t) \, dt = (1/2\pi) \cdot \int_{-\infty}^{+\infty} F(\omega) \cdot G^*(\omega) \, d\omega \tag{16.87}$$

This relationship is called **Parseval's theorem**. The correlation of two signals is equal to $1/2\pi$ times the correlation of their Fourier transforms. The factor, $1/2\pi$, is due to the use of the angular frequency, ω. If the transforms are defined in terms of frequency, ν, then the correlation of the signals is equal to the correlation of their transforms.

In the case of an autocorrelation:

$$\int_{-\infty}^{+\infty} |f(t)|^2 \, dt = (1/2\pi) \cdot \int_{-\infty}^{+\infty} |F(\omega)|^2 \, d\omega \tag{16.88}$$

In other words, the energy in a signal is equal to $1/2\pi$ times the energy in its Fourier transform. There is a conservation of energy across the Fourier transform operation. In nuclear magnetic resonance where $f(t)$ can be used to represent the magnetic field, conservation of energy has a real physics meaning. In image processing, energy does not have any physical meaning; however, with these relationships we can use the concepts of correlation and energy across the two domains.

IX. UNCERTAINTY PRINCIPLE

The **uncertainty principle** states that a signal and its transform cannot both be narrower than a certain combined limit. The uncertainty principle is related to the scaling property. When a signal shrinks, its transform expands. The uncertainty principle appears in several fields. In electrical engineering, the duration of an electrical pulse is inversely related to the minimum frequency band width in the pulse. Therefore the **duration band width** product must be greater than a certain minimum. In physics, the **Heisenberg uncertainty principle** states that the accuracy of the measurement of the position of a particle is inversely related to the accuracy of the momentum of a particle. In ultrasound, the width of the beam and the size of the transducer are inversely related.

A full mathematical derivation of the uncertainty principle is beyond the scope of this book and the interested reader is referred to Chapter 16 of the book by Siebert,[1] and Chapter 8 of the book by Bracewell.[2] We shall, however, describe the form of the uncertainty principle. It is defined in terms of the variance of the power of a signal and its transform.

One measure of the width of a signal which is often used in Radiology is the full width at half maximum, FWHM. However, this measure only makes sense with reasonably well behaved unimodal signals. Therefore, we need a more robust measure. In Chapter 10, we found that the variance was a very robust statistic related to the width of the probability density function. Thus, one notion is that the width should be related to the variance.

A second notion which has been emphasized a number of times is the importance of the square of the signal, the signal power. We have just shown that the integral of the power, the energy in a signal, is equal to the energy in its Fourier transform.

In order to combine the idea of power and of variance, let us define a probability density function related to the power in a signal:

$$p(t) = |f(t)|^2/E_t \qquad (16.89)$$

where E_t is the energy in the signal:

$$E_t = \int_{-\infty}^{+\infty} |f(t)|^2 \, dt \qquad (16.90)$$

Division of the power by E_t normalizes $p(t)$ so that the total area under the curve is equal to one. Similarly, we can define:

$$p(\omega) = |F(\omega)|^2/E_\omega \qquad (16.91)$$

where

$$E_\omega = \int_{-\infty}^{+\infty} |F(\omega)|^2 \, d\omega \qquad (16.92)$$

· We can define the width of the signal to be equal to twice the standard deviation of these two probability density functions:

$$\Delta t = 2 \cdot \sigma_t \qquad (16.93)$$

$$\Delta\omega = 2 \cdot \sigma_\omega \qquad (16.94)$$

The standard deviation is defined in terms of the half width of the signal. We have chosen to define the width of the signal in terms of a full width, although there is no uniformity among authors on use of the half width or the full width. The 2s in Equations 16.93 and 16.94 are due to the use of half width in the definition of the standard deviation versus full width in the definition of the signal width. The uncertainty principle can be stated mathematically:

$$\Delta t \cdot \Delta \omega \geq 2 \qquad (16.95)$$

(In physics, Planck's constant, h, enters into the uncertainty principle because the Fourier transform relating position and momentum uses basis functions which are imaginary exponentials with h in the exponent.)

The product of the time and angular frequency widths of a signal is the smallest, equal to two, when the signal is a Gaussian function. For other signals the product of the time and angular frequency widths is greater than two. Figure 16.11 shows a Gaussian function and its Fourier transform, another Gaussian function. The width in the frequency domain is inversely related to the width of the time domain signal:

$$\Delta \omega = 2/\Delta t \qquad (16.96)$$

A good radiological example of this property occurs in nuclear magnetic resonance imaging. The radio frequency pulses used to affect the magnetization in the patient can be either high power, short duration pulses or low power, long duration pulses. The former are called hard pulses and the latter are called soft pulses. The short duration, hard pulses must contain a broad band of frequencies, while the long duration, soft pulses may contain only a narrow band of frequencies. The product of the duration and the band width of the frequencies cannot be arbitrarily small. If the duration is short, then the band width must be large.

The band width of the frequencies in the radio frequency pulses determines the thickness of the slice (see Chapter 30). Therefore, hard pulses, which have a large band width, must be nonselective (excite the entire object); whereas, soft pulse may be selective (excite a thin slice). The uncertainty property of the Fourier transform helps to explain this feature of nuclear magnetic resonance imaging.

Another place where the uncertainty principle is important in radiology is in computed tomography. A frequent problem is to measure the CT number in a small region of interest. The spatial frequencies sampled by a region of interest are determined by the Fourier transform of the region. We shall learn in Chapter 32 that the signal to noise ratio in computed tomography is best for the low spatial frequencies. To minimize the noise in a region of interest, it is best to use a region which has a narrow Fourier transform; however, to localize the measurement, it is best to use a small region of interest.

We wish to simultaneously minimize the width of the region of interest and the width of the Fourier transform of the region. But this is not possible because of the uncertainty principle. The best reduction in noise for a given width region of interest is provided by a circularly symmetric region of interest with a Gaussian profile.

The uncertainty principle is also important in Doppler ultrasound. In ultrasound, axial position is determined by the time between initial pulse and the returning echo. The position is related to time by the velocity of the sound in tissue. To obtain the best axial resolution, the pulse should be as short as possible. The doppler principle measures the speed of a reflector by the change in frequency of the reflected wave compared to the transmitted wave. To measure the speed most accurately, the band of frequencies in the transmitted wave should be as narrow as possible.

As in the other examples, there are simultaneous constraints in two domains — the transmitted pulse should be as short as possible, and the transmitted pulse should have as narrow a band width as possible. Because of the uncertainty principle, there is a trade off between the accuracy with which position of a reflector and its speed can be measured.

X. HEURISTICS

A heuristic is a rule of thumb. In this section we shall boldly extrapolate from the few properties we have derived and the few examples we have presented to a set of general rules about Fourier transform pairs. Recall from Chapter 15 that the Fourier transform is a linear operation. Therefore, we can divide a signal into a sum of components and consider each of them separately. Using linearity and these heuristics, we can predict the general form of the Fourier transform of a large number of signals.

If a signal is wide in one domain, then it is narrow in the other domain. We have seen various aspects of this rule. When the axis shrinks in one domain, it expands in the other (Equations 16.43 and 16.44, Figures 16.11 and 16.15). The uncertainty principle tells us that there is a minimum for the product of the widths in the two domains — a signal cannot simultaneously be of short duration and narrow band width.

Signals which are multiplied in one domain are convolved in the other domain (Equations 16.8 and 16.9, Figures 16.3, 16.4, and 16.5). This property is also important in understanding modulation (Figure 16.9). We shall revisit this important property in the next chapter.

If a signal has sharp edges in one domain, then it has ripples in the other domain. The ripples are often referred to as ringing. The prototypical example of this behavior is the rectangle in one domain and the sinc function in the other domain (Figure 16.15). In reconstruction problems, a sharp spatial frequency cut off is like the rectangle function. If too sharp a frequency cut off is used, then there is often ringing in the image. In computed tomography, this effect is particularly noticeable at bone tissue interfaces.

Smoothness in one domain results in a transform which is concentrated in the other domain. If the signal is real, then the transform is concentrated near the origin. Most often we think of this property in terms of smoothness in the time domain translating into low frequencies in the frequency domain. However, if a signal is smooth in the frequency domain, it will be narrow in the time domain.

Sinusoidal components in one domain lead to delta functions in the other domain (Equation 14.12). If the component is not a perfect sinusoidal, then in the other domain the delta function becomes a finite peak with some width.

Since a shift in one domain translates to a linear phase shift in the other domain, we know that the magnitude of the Fourier transform of a signal will not be affected by a shift of the signal. However, the signal will be multiplied by an imaginary exponential, changing the phase.

These heuristics can be used together. Suppose that in the frequency domain a signal resembles a Gaussian out to some cut-off frequency. Past that frequency, the signal is zero. This signal can be modeled as a Gaussian multiplied by a rectangle. In the time domain, the signal will be equal to the Gaussian which can be determined from Equation 14.14 convolved with a sinc function which can be determined from Equation 16.78.

Suppose instead that the time domain signal has two components. One component is slowly varying in time. The other component consists of oscillations predominately of near a single frequency. Then in the frequency domain, the signal is the sum of two components. One component is a peak concentrated at the origin. The other component is a peak near the frequency. Similarly, the general form of many transform pairs can be derived from the few examples which have been given, using these heuristics.

XI. SUMMARY

The purpose of this chapter was to present a number of properties of the Fourier transform. These properties help explain how the Fourier transform works and how features of a signal in one domain relate to the feature of the signal in the other domain. The most important property for the rest of the book is the mapping of convolution into multiplication. But understanding the other properties will also be useful. Hopefully this chapter has provided the reader with a better understanding of the Fourier transform.

XII. FURTHER READING

Almost all books which describe the Fourier transformation describe the properties of the Fourier transform. For example, a good description can be found in Chapter 4 of the book by Oppenheim and Willsky.[3] Chapter 7 of that book includes an extensive discussion of the modulation property. The properties of the Fourier transform are also well described in Chapter 6 of the book by Bracewell,[2] and Chapter 3 of the book by Papoulis.[4] The Hilbert transform is described in Chapter 12 of Bracewell's book, and Chapter 7 of Papoulis's book.

The line spread function, the modulation transfer function and their application in Radiology are described in the book by Barrett and Swindell.[5]

We have defined even functions in terms of conjugate symmetry (Equation 16.50 and 16.51). This follows the usage in Chapter 1 of the book by Oppenheim and Schafer.[6] Chapter 2 of Bracewell's book[2] has an excellent description of these properties, but defining even functions only in terms of symmetry, not conjugate symmetry.

REFERENCES

1. **Siebert, W. Mc. C.**, *Circuits, Signals, and Systems,* The MIT Press, Cambridge, MA, 1986.
2. **Bracewell, R. N.**, *The Fourier Transform and its Applications,* McGraw-Hill, New York, 1978.
3. **Oppenheim, A. V. and Willsky, A. S.**, *Signals and Systems,* Prentice-Hall, Englewood Cliffs, NJ, 1983.
4. **Papoulis, A.**, *Signal Analysis,* McGraw-Hill, New York, 1977.
5. **Barrett, H. H. and Swindell, W.**, *Radiological Imaging: The Theory of Image Formation, Detection, and Processing,* Academic Press, New York, 1981.
6. **Oppenheim, A. V. and Schafer, R. W.**, *Digital Signal Processing,* Prentice-Hall, Englewood Cliffs, NJ, 1975.

Chapter 17

POLYNOMIAL TRANSFORM

In this chapter we shall develop a method of describing a signal in terms of a polynomial. We shall find that the coefficients of terms in the polynomial are analogous to the frequency domain description of the signal. We can think of the coefficients as a signal just as we think of the values of the Fourier transform as a signal.

The polynomial transform will not be important to us from a practical point of view. However, the idea of a polynomial transform may help the reader understand the other transform operations. The analogy between the coefficient domain and the frequency domain may provide insight into defining a signal in terms of a set of basis functions. Like the Fourier transform, the polynomial transform maps the operation of convolution into multiplication. Furthermore, the polynomial transform will provide a bridge between the continuous transform operations and the discrete transform described in the next chapter.

I. SIGNALS OF LIMITED COMPLEXITY

In this chapter and the next we shall be interested in signals of limited complexity; signals that can be described by a finite set of parameters. For example, a signal which is constant can be described by a single parameter, the value of the constant. A signal which is a line can be described by two values, a signal which is a parabola can be described by three values, and so forth.

Our concepts of a constant, a line, and a parabola are very closely tied to the polynomial representation described in the next section. However, for this section let us try to think of these as concepts, not as their polynomial representations. Perhaps one method of separating the concept of a signal from the polynomial representation is to think of them graphically. Figure 17.1 shows a constant signal, a line, and a parabola. We have a graphical concept of these signals and of the fact that they are quite limited in form.

The next chapter will describe the discrete Fourier transform. The discrete Fourier transform also deals with signals of limited complexity, but in that case the signals are composed of a small number of sinusoidal functions. It is possible to consider a number of other models, where the underlying signals are in a variety of forms. The basic idea is that these signals are described by a small number of parameters. The actual shape of the signals is less important.

II. POLYNOMIAL REPRESENTATION OF A SIGNAL

Signals can be represented in terms of polynomials. In fact, our first exposure to modeling of signals is as polynomials in introductory algebra. In general, a polynomial is written:

$$f(t) = a_0 + a_1 \cdot t + a_2 \cdot t^2 \ldots \tag{17.1}$$

For a constant signal, all of the coefficients, a_k, are zero except for a_0. For a line, only a_0 and a_1 are nonzero. For a parabola, only a_0, a_1, and a_2 are nonzero. As more terms are added, the signal becomes more complex.

Representation of a signal as polynomial is very similar to representation of a signal as an inverse Fourier transform, Equation 14.6. The difference is that instead of using the imaginary exponentials as the basis functions, the basis functions are the powers of t. Figure 17.2 shows the first three basis functions, $a_0 \cdot t^0$, $a_1 \cdot t^1$, and $a_2 \cdot t^2$. Equation 17.1 states that the polynomial model of the signal is a linear combination of these basis functions.

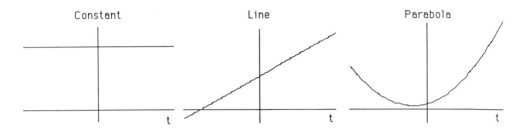

FIGURE 17.1.   Graphical representation of signals: three different signals are shown in graphical form. On the left is a constant; in the center is a line; and on the right is a parabola.

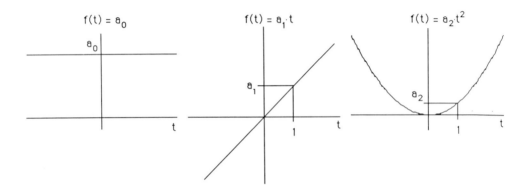

FIGURE 17.2.   Polynomial basis functions: the first three polynomial basis functions are shown in this figure.

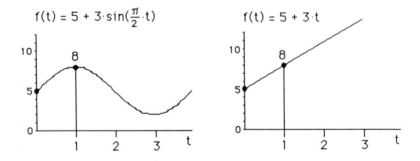

FIGURE 17.3.   Two functions with equal sample values at zero and one: although the graphical and algebraic representations of the two functions shown in this figure are very different, their values at t equal to zero and one are the same. The graph on the left is defined in terms of two components of an inverse sine transform, and the graph on the right is defined in terms of two polynomial components.

Figure 17.3 shows two signals. One signal is defined in terms of two components, ω equal 0 and $\pi/2$, of an inverse sine transform:

$$f(t) = 5 + 3 \cdot \sin((\pi/2) \cdot t) \qquad (17.2)$$

The other signal is made from two polynomial components, k equal 0 and 1:

$$f(t) = 5 + 3 \cdot t \qquad (17.3)$$

The signals are of quite different form due to the set of basis functions which have been used to model the signals. However, the basic idea of the model and the complexity of the models have obvious analogies. Both signals are equal to five at t equal to 0 and eight at t equal to one.

The set of functions which are powers of t share some features in common with the set of functions which are the imaginary exponentials. The powers of t are independent. It is not possible to express one power of t in terms of any combination of the other powers of t. The independence of a set of basis functions is analogous to the independence of a set of vectors (see Chapter 9).

However, unlike the imaginary exponentials, the set of functions which are the powers of t are not orthogonal.

$$\int_{-\infty}^{+\infty} t^{k_1} \cdot t^{k_2} \, dt \neq 0 \tag{17.4}$$

This difference between the powers of t and the imaginary exponentials is very important. It is one of the major reasons why the imaginary exponentials are a much more useful set of signals for describing systems that are the powers of t.

It is worth noting in passing that the powers of t do a bad thing at infinity; they become infinite. Therefore, they are not useful for describing signals over all time. Polynomials are used to represent signals over a limited interval. The Taylor series expansion is the most common polynomial representation of signals. It describes a signal in an interval around a point in terms of a power series. (Recall from Chapter 2, that the coefficients of the Taylor series are the derivatives of the function at that point.)

We can think of the coefficients of a polynomial as a discrete signal. We can emphasize this point of view by rewriting Equation 17.1 as follows:

$$f(t) = \sum_k a[k] \cdot t^k \tag{17.5}$$

where a[0] is equal to the coefficient a_0, a[1] is equal to the coefficient a_1, etc. We shall say that the signal a[k] is defined in the **coefficient domain**.

Equation 17.5 shows the relationship between the inverse Fourier transformation and the polynomial representation of a signal. Both are linear combinations of a set of basis functions with weighting factors $F(\omega)$ and a[k], respectively. The inverse Fourier transform is an integral relation whereas the polynomial representation is a summation. In Chapter 18, we shall introduce the discrete Fourier transform. It is also defined as a summation and it is even more analogous to the polynomial representation. From what has already been said, the reader could predict that an important property of the discrete Fourier transform is that it is used for signals which can be described by a limited set of parameters. But more of this later.

III. SAMPLE REPRESENTATION OF A SIGNAL

Another method of representing a signal is to give the values a particular set of times. For convenience of notation we shall consider the set of times 0, 1, 2, ... If we have a signal which is a constant, then a single sample, e.g., f(0), will suffice to describe the signal. Since a line is defined by two points, two samples will suffice, e.g., f(0) and f(1). For a parabola, three samples will suffice, e.g., f(0), f(1), and f(2).

If we have signals which are limited in form we need only a limited number of samples to exactly define the signals. There is an obvious analogy between the limited set of coefficients, a[k], and the limited set of values f(0), f(1) . . . . To further emphasize this

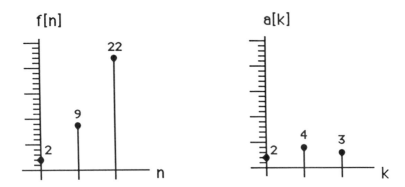

FIGURE 17.4.   Value and coefficient domain representations of a signal: on the left is a three point signal corresponding to the values of the polynomial given by Equation 17.6. On the right is a signal corresponding to the coefficients of the same equation. Equation 17.10 shows these two signals as a transform pair.

similarity, let us define a discrete signal, f[n], which is the value of the function f(t) at the times, 0, 1, ... Then we can represent the signal f(t) by a limited set of values f[n].

We have described three ways of representing a signal — as a concept, f(t), as a polynomial, a[k], and as samples, f[n]. The polynomial, a[k], and the samples, f[n], are well defined mathematically. The concept of a limited complexity signal underlies these models of the signal, but it may be a little difficult to separate the concept from the mathematical representations. The graph of a signal is the closest instantiation of what we are calling the concept of a signal.

For a signal of a certain complexity, a given number of parameters are needed to define it. For example, a constant can be defined by one coefficient, or by one sample. A line can be defined by two coefficients or by two samples. A parabola can be defined by three coefficients or by three samples. There is an exact relationship between the complexity of the signal and the number of coefficients or the number of samples which are needed to represent the signal. We shall see this same relationship with the discrete Fourier transform in the next chapter.

IV. EVALUATION

The method of transforming from the coefficient representation to the sample representation is very simple. It is called **evaluation**. For example, let us suppose that we have the polynomial:

$$f(t) = 2 + 4 \cdot t + 3 \cdot t^2 \qquad (17.6)$$

We can easily evaluate this signal at 0, 1, and 2:

$$f[0] = 2 \qquad (17.7)$$

$$f[1] = 2 + 4 + 3 = 9 \qquad (17.8)$$

$$f[2] = 2 + 4 \cdot 2 + 3 \cdot 4 = 22 \qquad (17.9)$$

In Figure 17.4 we have shown the coefficients and the values as signals. The coefficients and the values are defined for 0, 1, and 2. The evaluation operation transforms from the

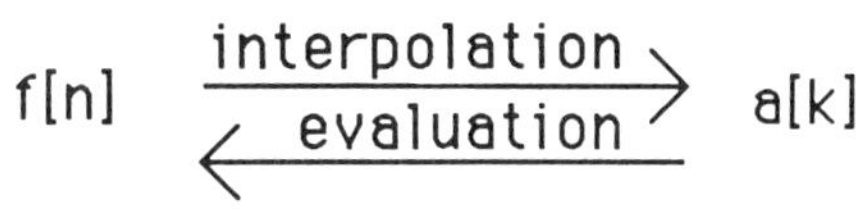

$$f[n] \quad \xrightarrow{\text{interpolation}} \quad a[k]$$
$$\xleftarrow{\text{evaluation}}$$

FIGURE 17.5. Transformations between value and coefficient domains: the transformation from the coefficients of a polynomial to the values of the polynomial is a process called evaluation. The transformation from a set of values to coefficients of a polynomial is a process called interpolation.

coefficient domain to the value domain. If we borrow the two headed arrow notation from the Fourier transform we can write this relation as:

$$2 \quad 9 \quad 22 \leftrightarrow 2 \quad 4 \quad 3 \qquad (17.10)$$

On the left side of the double arrow are the values f[n] for n equal to 0, 1, and 2. On the right side are the values of a[k] for k equal to 0, 1, and 2.

The evaluation operation is analogous to the inverse Fourier transform. The weighting factors are multiplied by the basis functions and the results are summed.

V. INTERPOLATION

The opposite operation is the transformation from samples to coefficients. We shall call this operation **interpolation**. The reader may be familiar with the use of the word interpolation to mean the operation of filling values in between known values in a curve. In order to perform this operation, the known sample values must be fit to some function, often a very simple polynomial, such as a line. Then the new values can be obtained by evaluation of the coefficients. We prefer to refer to the fitting operation as interpolation and then call the evaluation operation resampling. These definitions are consistent with the engineering literature.

Interpolation of a constant function is particularly simple:

$$a[0] = f[0] \qquad (17.11)$$

Similarly, it is easy to interpolate a line:

$$a[0] = f[0] \qquad (17.12)$$

$$a[1] = (f[1] - f[0])/(1 - 0) = f[1] - f[0] \qquad (17.13)$$

The general interpolation formula is somewhat complicated. Since we are not interested in the mechanics of interpolation, we shall just state that it is possible to interpolate any set of points to a polynomial.

What we are more interested in is the analogy between interpolation and the Fourier transform operation. Interpolation transforms from the sample domain to the coefficient domain just as the Fourier transform transforms from the time to the frequency domain. (One reason that the formula for interpolation is more complicated is that the basis functions are not orthogonal.) Figure 17.5 shows these relations diagrammatically.

$$f_1[n] \cdot f_2[n] \longleftrightarrow a_1[k] * a_2[k]$$

FIGURE 17.6.   Multiplication ↔ Convolution: multiplication of the values of two polynomials is equivalent to the convolution of the respective coefficients.

VI. POLYNOMIAL MULTIPLICATION

The method for multiplying two polynomials is to multiply each element of the first polynomial times all of the elements of the second polynomial. The following is the example of polynomial multiplication:

$$3t^2 - 4t + 1$$
$$2t^2 + 3t + 5$$
$$\overline{}$$
$$5 \cdot (3t^2 - 4t + 1)$$
$$3t \cdot (3t^2 - 4t + 1)$$
$$2t^2 \cdot (3t^2 - 4t + 1)$$
$$\overline{}$$

$$6t^4 + t^3 + 5t^2 - 17t + 5 \qquad (17.14)$$

Notice what happens to the coefficients when two polynomials are multiplied. The coefficients of the first polynomial are shifted over the appropriate number of spaces, then scaled by the coefficients of the second polynomial, and then the results are added. This process — shifting, scaling, and adding — should be familiar to the reader. (If not, review Chapter 3!) It is convolution. Polynomial multiplication is performed by convolution of the coefficients.

We can write polynomial multiplication symbolically as:

$$\sum_l a_1[k - 1] \cdot a_2[l] \cdot t^k \qquad (17.15)$$

where $a_1[k]$ are the coefficients of the first polynomial and $a_2[k]$ are the coefficients of the second polynomial. In the polynomial multiplication, the powers of t help to keep the places, but they are not really important to the multiplication process. We can rewrite Equation 17.15 without the powers of t:

$$\sum_l a_1[k - 1] \cdot a_2[l] \qquad (17.16)$$

In this form the relationship between polynomial multiplication and convolution of the coefficients is even more obvious.

The operation of polynomial multiplication is very complicated in the coefficient domain; it requires convolution. However, in the value domain it is very simple. In order to multiply two signals all one does is to multiply the values:

$$f_1[n] \cdot f_2[n] \qquad (17.17)$$

Thus, convolution in the coefficient domain is equivalent to multiplication in the value domain. This relationship is shown diagrammatically in Figure 17.6.

VII. MAPPING OF CONVOLUTION TO MULTIPLICATION

In this section we shall determine what property of the basis functions allows convolution in one domain to map to multiplication in the other domain. Some of the mathematics to determine this property is a little complex and not necessary for the rest of the book. The less mathematically inclined reader may wish to skip to the last paragraph of this section. The material toward the end of the indented section is most interesting in understanding the relation between the Fourier transform and other transform operation. The interested reader may wish to return to this section after having read Chapter 20.

Suppose that f(t) is convolved with h(t) to give g(t):

$$g(t) = \int_{-\infty}^{+\infty} f(\tau) \cdot h(t - \tau) \, d\tau \tag{17.18}$$

Further suppose that there is a linear transformation which uses the basis functions, $\phi(t,s)$. The linear transformation can be written:

$$G(s) = \int_{-\infty}^{+\infty} g(t) \cdot \phi(t,s) \, dt \tag{17.19}$$

It might be worth commenting just a bit about the form of the transformation in Equation 17.19. It is very general. The basis functions, $\phi(t,s)$, could be any function of the two variables, t and s. The integral is a linear combination of these functions with a weighting determined by g(t). Equation 17.19 can be used to represent any linear transformation.

The transform of the convolution is obtained by substituting Equation 17.18 into Equation 17.19:

$$G(s) = \int_{-\infty}^{+\infty} \left[\int_{-\infty}^{+\infty} f(\tau) \cdot h(t - \tau) \, d\tau \right] \cdot \phi(t,s) \, dt \tag{17.20}$$

Rearranging the terms and the order of integration:

$$G(s) = \int_{-\infty}^{+\infty} f(\tau) \cdot \left[\int_{-\infty}^{+\infty} h(t - \tau) \cdot \phi(t,s) \, dt \right] d\tau \tag{17.21}$$

We can substitute the variable of integration in the inner integral:

$$t' = t - \tau \tag{17.22}$$

Then:

$$G(s) = \int_{-\infty}^{+\infty} f(\tau) \cdot \left[\int_{-\infty}^{+\infty} h(t') \cdot \phi(t' + \tau, s) \, dt' \right] d\tau \tag{17.23}$$

It is possible to simplify Equation 17.23 if and only if the basis function, $\phi(t' + \tau,s)$ can be expressed as:

$$\phi(t' + \tau, s) = \phi(t',s) \cdot \phi(\tau,s) \tag{17.24}$$

Under this condition the terms of Equation 17.23 can be rearranged:

$$G(s) = \int_{-\infty}^{+\infty} f(\tau) \cdot \phi(\tau,s) \, d\tau \cdot \int_{-\infty}^{+\infty} h(t') \cdot \phi(t',s) \, dt'$$

$$= F(s) \cdot H(s) \tag{17.25}$$

Therefore, if the basis functions have the property given by Equation 17.24, convolution in the time domain is mapped into multiplication in the transform domain.

Now let us see what Equation 17.24 implies. An exponential function has this property:

$$e^{t+\tau} = e^t \cdot e^\tau \tag{17.26}$$

But does this property imply that $\phi(t,s)$ is an exponential?. The derivative of Equation 17.24 with respect to τ is:

$$d\phi(t + \tau, s)/d\tau = \phi(t,s) \cdot d\phi(\tau,s)/d\tau \tag{17.27}$$

For τ equal to zero:

$$d\phi(t + \tau, s)/d\tau|_{\tau=0} = \phi(t,s) \cdot d\phi(\tau,s)/d\tau|_{\tau=0} \tag{17.28}$$

The derivative of $\phi(t + \tau,s)$ with respect to τ evaluated at zero is equal to the derivative of $\phi(t,s)$ with respect to t. We can prove this from the definition of the derivative.

$$d\phi(t + \tau, s)/d\tau|_{\tau=0} = \lim_{\Delta\tau \to 0}[\phi(t + \Delta\tau, s) - \phi(t,s)]/\Delta\tau \tag{17.29}$$

$$d\phi(t,s)/dt = \lim_{\Delta t \to 0}[\phi(t + \Delta t, s) - \phi(t,s)]/\Delta t \tag{17.30}$$

Except for the change in variable, these two equations are identical. Therefore, Equation 17.28 can be rewritten:

$$d\phi(t,s)/dt = \phi(t,s) \cdot d\phi(\tau,s)/d\tau|_{\tau=0} \tag{17.31}$$

The last factor in Equation 17.31 is just a constant, the slope at zero. We shall call this constant, $-a$. Thus,

$$d\phi(t,s)/dt = -a \cdot \phi(t,s) \tag{17.32}$$

This equation is the equation for an exponential (see Equation 7.3); therefore,

$$\phi(t,s) = e^{-at} \tag{17.33}$$

The derivation used to get Equation 17.32 was based on mapping convolution in the time domain into multiplication in the transform domain. Since the roles of t and s are symmetric, this derivation could be repeated in order to obtain a relation where convolution in the transform domain maps into multiplication in the time domain. This derivation would lead to a basis function of the form:

$$\phi(t,s) = e^{-bs} \tag{17.34}$$

where b is another arbitrary constant.

By setting a equal to s and b equal to t, Equations 17.32 and 17.33 can be simultaneously satisfied:

$$\phi(t,s) = e^{-st} \tag{17.35}$$

Basis functions of the form given in Equation 17.33 will map convolution to multiplication from time to transform domains and from transform to time domains. The various types of transform operations can be derived by expressing the variables, s and t, in terms of other variables.

For the Fourier transform, Equation 17.35 is:

$$\phi(t, i \cdot \omega) = e^{-i\omega t} \tag{17.36}$$

The Laplace transform, which will be described in Chapter 20, uses a complex exponent, s, which is equal to $\sigma + i \cdot \omega$:

$$\phi(t,s) = e^{-st} = e^{-(\sigma + i\omega)t} \tag{17.37}$$

We can substitute the natural logarithm of t, ln(t), for t, and k for s in Equation 17.35 in order to get the polynomial transform:

$$\phi(\ln(t),k) = e^{k\ln(t)} = t^k \tag{17.38}$$

The z transform which is described in Chapter 20 comes from a similar type of substitution:

$$\phi(n,\ln(z)) = e^{\ln(z)n} = z^n \tag{17.39}$$

Convolution in the domain with the logarithm substitution is defined somewhat differently. It is called circular convolution. But these details are not of importance to us here. What is important is that for all of these transformation operations, multiplication in one domain maps to convolution in the other domain.

In summary, convolution maps to multiplication if and only if the basis functions are exponentials. They can be real as in the case of the polynomials, imaginary as in the case of the Fourier transform, or complex as in the case of the Laplace transform. In any case, the key relationship is that given by Equation 17.35.

VIII. SUMMARY

Representation of signals as polynomials is used widely in mathematics and in many applications. However, these basis functions have the disadvantage that they are not orthogonal. When working with linear, time invariant systems, orthogonality is a very useful property. Thus, we shall find that the Fourier representation will be more useful for most radiologic applications than the polynomial representation.

Although polynomials will not be of practical importance to us, they help to explain the most important property of the transform operations — mapping of convolution in one domain into multiplication in the other domain. This property at first seems somewhat mystical. However, we have shown that this property is already well known in terms of polynomial multiplication. Any transformation operation which has exponential basis functions maps convolution to multiplication.

The idea of a limited complexity signal, a signal which can be specified in terms of a limited set of parameters, is quite familiar from polynomials. In the next chapter, we shall introduce the discrete Fourier transform. The discrete Fourier transform uses a limited number of imaginary exponential to represent a signal. Although the signals are quite different in form, this method is exactly analogous to the polynomial representation. They can be tied together by the sample domain. If we have a fixed number of samples, then they can be represented by either a polynomial or a discrete Fourier transform. All three representations will give the same values at the sample points. At other points the representations may give very different values.

The goal of this chapter has been to provide some insight into the mapping of convolution to multiplication and to introduce the idea of a limited complexity signal. The other material in this chapter is only important for illuminating these two points.

IX. FURTHER READING

The analogy between the polynomial transform and the Fourier transform is not generally discussed in books about Fourier transforms. Chapter 3 of the book by Bracewell[1] describes the similarity of convolution and polynomial multiplication. The interested reader is directed to the book by Aho, Hopcroft, and Ullman[2] for the details. The reader who is interested in interpolating procedures is referred to the books by Press et al.[3] and by Aho et al.[2] Chapter 20 has references for the Laplace transform and the z transform.

REFERENCES

1. **Bracewell, R. N.,** *The Fourier Transform and its Applications,* McGraw-Hill, New York, 1965.
2. **Aho, A. V., Hopcroft, J. E., and Ullman, J. D.,** *The Design and Analysis of Computer Algorithms,* Addison-Wesley, Reading, PA, 1976.
3. **Press, W. H., Flannery, B. P., Teukolsky, S. A., and Vetterling, W. T.,** *Numerical Recipes: The Art of Scientific Computing,* Cambridge University Press, Cambridge, MA, 1986.

Chapter 18

DISCRETE FOURIER TRANSFORM

This chapter will describe the Fourier transform operation for discrete signals, the **discrete Fourier transform**. The discrete Fourier transform is analogous to the continuous Fourier transform, and the two operations share most of the same properties. Although most of the applications in this book use the continuous Fourier transform, the discrete Fourier transform is very important from a practical sense. Almost all applications of Fourier transform techniques use the discrete Fourier transform implemented on a digital computer.

However, the primary reason for describing the discrete Fourier transform in this book is to explain the process of sampling. Most measurements involve sampling of a continuous signal to produce a digital signal. If not properly performed, the process of sampling can produce some confusing artifacts. These artifacts are most obvious in nuclear magnetic resonance imaging, where parts of the body sometimes appear in the wrong place. Chapter 23, which describes sampling, will rely heavily on the concepts develop in this chapter.

In Chapter 15, the "proof" that the inverse Fourier transform of a Fourier transform returns the original signal was very complicated and not mathematically rigorous. We shall find that this proof is more easily understood for the discrete Fourier transform. A few readers may find that this proof helps to explain how the Fourier transform works.

The major goal of the last three chapters in this part of the book is to provide an understanding of the Fourier transform operation. Except for Chapter 23, this material is not integral to understanding the rest of the book. Some readers may wish to skip these chapters. Other readers may wish to skim these chapters skipping over most of the mathematical detail. The readers who find this material interesting should refer to the more complete descriptions of this material in the references mentioned at the end of the chapters.

I. CONTINUOUS, DISCRETE, DIGITAL

In Chapter 2, the difference between continuous, discrete, and digital signals was described. Recall that continuous signals are defined for all values of both the dependent and the independent variable. We have chosen to indicate continuous signals with parentheses around the independent variable, e.g., f(t). The continuous Fourier transform described in the first three chapters of this part of the book is used with these signals.

Discrete signals are defined for only a discrete set of values of the independent variable. Square brackets around the independent variable are used to indicate a discrete signal, f[n]. Like continuous signals, the values of the discrete signals are continuous; the dependent variable can assume a continuous set of values. Thus, the values which can be assumed by n are integers, while the values which can be assumed by f[n] are all the real numbers. The discrete Fourier transform described in this chapter is used with these signals.

In practical applications, discrete signals are often used to represent continuous signals. In Chapter 23 (Sampling) we shall discuss in more detail the conditions under which discrete signals can be used to approximate continuous signals.

In this book we shall always refer to the Fourier transform for discrete signals as "the discrete Fourier transform". Sometimes we shall refer to the Fourier transform for continuous signals as simply "the Fourier transform". When we wish to emphasize that we are referring to continuous signals, we shall call it "the continuous Fourier transform".

Some transformation operations use both continuous and discrete signals. For example, the Fourier series transforms between continuous signals in the time domain and discrete signals in the frequency domain. The Fourier series is mentioned briefly in Chapter 20.

Digital signals take on discrete values for both the dependent and the independent variables. The transforms which are used with digital signals are called **number theoretic transforms**. These transformations are beyond the scope of this book.

Digital signals can be exactly represented in a digital computer, while discrete and continuous signals can only be approximated in a computer. However, since operations with digital signals are more complex, they are rarely used. Since the computer approximation of discrete signals is very good, the signals in computers are often thought of as discrete signals. In this book, we shall not be concerned with the relatively minor problem caused by the digitization of the dependent variable.

II. PERIODIC SIGNALS

Below we shall define the discrete Fourier transform in terms of periodic signals. We shall find that periodicity is a very important property. In this section we shall describe some of the properties of periodic signals.

A periodic signal is one that repeats at regular intervals. For example, a sine wave repeats with an interval of 2π. The value of sine wave at some point, t, is the same as the value at $t + 2\pi$:

$$\sin(t) = \sin(t + 2\pi) \tag{18.1}$$

More generally, the value of a sine wave is the same at any multiple of 2π:

$$\sin(t) = \sin(t + m \cdot 2\pi) \tag{18.2}$$

where m is an integer.

Any signal which repeats itself with an interval, T, is said to be periodic with period, T. This property can be written mathematically:

$$f(t) = f(t + m \cdot T) \tag{18.3}$$

with m an integer. The same property for discrete signals is written:

$$f[n] = f[n + N] \tag{18.4}$$

where the period of this signal is said to be N.

A. REPRESENTATION OF A LIMITED EXTENT SIGNAL BY A PERIODIC SIGNAL

A **limited extent signal** is a signal which is nonzero over a finite region. For example, a discrete signal, f[n], might be nonzero only over the interval 0 to $N - 1$. Alternately, we could define a limited extent signal as a signal which is defined for only a finite interval, 0 to $N - 1$. Almost all of the signals in radiology are limited extent signals. For example, the attenuation coefficients in a CT scan are nonzero only within the cross section of the body. Elsewhere, the values are zero. In fact, almost all images are finite in extent. Mathematicians say that the area where a function is nonzero is the **support** of the function. Limited extent signals have a finite support.

The discrete Fourier transform can be defined in terms of limited extent signals; however, this definition results in several confusing properties. Instead we shall define the discrete Fourier transform in terms of periodic signals. The analogies between the properties of the discrete Fourier transform and the continuous Fourier transform are much more obvious in this format.

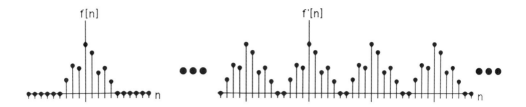

FIGURE 18.1. Periodic representation of a limited extent signal: on the left is a limited extent signal, f[n]. It is nonzero for only a small number of points. On the right is a periodic signal, f'[n], which is equal to f[n] in the region where f[n] is nonzero. The period of f'[n] must be greater than the region of nonzero values in f[n].

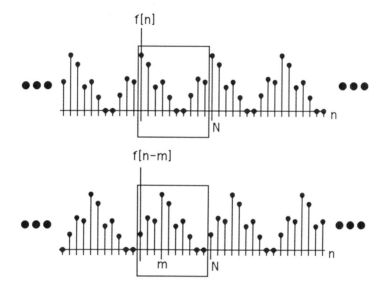

FIGURE 18.2. Circular shifting: on the top panel is a periodic signal, f[n]. On the bottom panel is the same signal shifted to the right by m positions, f[n − m]. The N points in the range 0 to N − 1 are shown in a box. If we consider only these points, then shifting produces an interesting effect. It is as if the values shifted out at the right wrap around to the left. This type of shifting is called circular shifting.

However, since the signals which are of most interest to us are limited extent signals, we need to represent a limited extent signal as a periodic signal. The obvious method is to replicate the finite signal at an interval which is equal to or larger than the area where the signal is nonzero. Figure 18.1 shows a limited extent signal, f[n], and a periodic signal, f'[n], which has been used to represent it. Notice that the period of f'[n] is larger than the extent of f[n]. We shall have more to say about what period should be used in Chapter 23.

B. SHIFTING

Shifting a periodic signal is mathematically the same as shifting an aperiodic signal. f[n − m] is shifted to the right by m units as compared to f[n]. Figure 18.2 shows a periodic signal f[n] and the shifted signal f[n − m].

When a periodic signal with period, N, is used to represent a limited extent signal which is defined for the values 0 to N − 1, some unusual artifacts arise from shifting. In Figure 18.2 the values from 0 to N − 1 are shown in a box. Shifting the periodic signal is different than shifting the limited extent signal. It is as if the values from the right side of the limited extent signal circle around to the left side of the signal. Representation of a limited extent signal by a periodic signal results in a new type of shifting operation, circular shifting.

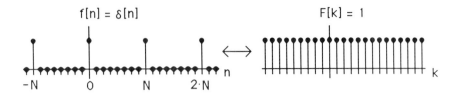

FIGURE 18.3.   Periodic delta function: this graph shows the periodic representation of a delta function. The signal is equal to one at n equal to m · N. The discrete Fourier transform of this signal is the constant, one.

Circular shifting of a limited extent signal is equivalent to shifting of a periodic signal. When we use a periodic signal to represent a limited extent signal, the relationship between shifting the periodic signal and circular shifting of the limited extent signal is very important. This relationship is how certain body parts appear on the opposite side of a nuclear magnetic resonance image.

III. DISCRETE FOURIER TRANSFORM

Let us start with the conclusion, the discrete Fourier transform relationships:

$$f[n] = (1/N) \cdot \sum_{k=0}^{N-1} F[k] \cdot e^{i2\pi kn/N} \tag{18.5}$$

$$F[k] = \sum_{n=0}^{N-1} f[n] \cdot e^{-i2\pi kn/N} \tag{18.6}$$

There are obvious analogies between these equations and the continuous Fourier transform pair, Equations 14.6 and 14.7. The integral signs have been replaced by the summation and there is an extra $2\pi/N$ in the exponent, but basically the two sets of equations are very similar. Since f[n] is analogous to the signal f(t), we shall refer to f[n] as the time domain signal. Since F[k] is analogous to $F(\omega)$, we shall refer to F[k] as the frequency domain signal.

A. EXAMPLES OF DISCRETE FOURIER TRANSFORM PAIRS

The delta function, $\delta[n]$, is equal to one for n = 0 and zero for all other values of n. The periodic representation of the delta function is a signal, f[n], which is equal to one for n equal to any multiple of N, and zero for all other values of n. Figure 18.3 shows this signal. The discrete Fourier transform is easily calculated from Equation 18.6. The only nonzero value in the summation is for n = 0. Thus,

$$F[k] = 1 \cdot e^{-i2\pi k0/N} = 1 \cdot 1 = 1 \tag{18.7}$$

The frequency domain signal, F[k], is also shown in Figure 18.3. This discrete Fourier transform is analogous to the continuous Fourier transform of $\delta(t)$, Equation 15.38.

Figure 18.4 shows a signal, F[k] which is one for k = 3 and k = N − 3, and zero for other values of k. Again we have shown this signal as a periodic signal. Below we shall learn that the discrete Fourier transform can be calculated over any N point interval. Over the interval −(N/2 − 1) to N/2 − 1, F[k] is analogous to the continuous Fourier transform of a cosine function. In fact, f[n], also shown in Figure 18.4, is a cosine function.

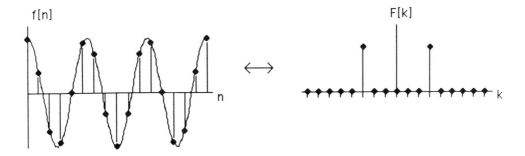

FIGURE 18.4. Discrete cosine function: this figure shows N + 1 points of a discrete cosine signal, $2 \cdot \cos(2\pi \cdot 3 \cdot n/N)$. A continuous cosine of the same frequency is shown on the same graph for comparison. The Fourier transform has two nonzero point at k equal to 3 and -3.

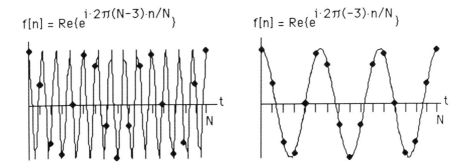

FIGURE 18.5. Discrete representation of negative frequencies: on the left is the real part of the sinusoidal signal, $e^{i2\pi(N-3)n/N}$. On the right is the real part of the sinusoidal signal $e^{i2\pi(-3)n/N}$. Also shown are the equivalent continuous sinusoids. These sinusoids correspond to angular frequencies, k, equal to $N-3$ and -3, respectively. Although the continuous sinusoids are quite different, at the sample points these two discrete sinusoids are the same. For a frequency domain signal defined in the interval, 0 to $N-1$, the frequencies in the range, $N/2$ to $N-1$, are equivalent to the negative frequencies, $-N/2$ to -1.

From this example, we see that the frequencies below N are like negative frequencies. Figure 18.5 shows the two sinusoids $e^{i2\pi(N-3)n/N}$ and $e^{i2\pi(-3)n/N}$. Notice that these two sinusoids have the same values at the integer values of n. Thus the frequencies greater than $N/2$ are "like" negative frequencies.

B. BASIS FUNCTIONS

The inverse discrete Fourier transform, Equation 18.5, expresses the signal, f[n], in terms of a weighted sum of functions, $e^{i2\pi kn/N}$. These functions are the basis functions for the discrete Fourier transform. They are analogous to the basis functions, $e^{i\omega t}$, for the continuous Fourier transform. We can consider these functions either in the time, n, or frequency, k, domains. The signal

$$f[n] = e^{i2\pi kn/N} \tag{18.8}$$

has an angular frequency of $2\pi \cdot k/N$, and a period of N/k. The signal

$$F[k] = e^{i2\pi kn/N} \tag{18.9}$$

has an angular frequency of $2\pi \cdot n/N$, and a period of N/n.

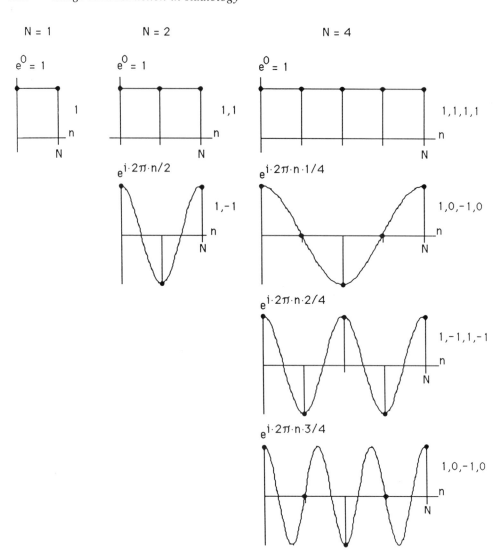

FIGURE 18.6. Basis functions for N equal to 1, 2, and 4: this figure shows N + 1 points of the real parts of the basis functions for N equal to 1, 2, and 4. Also shown are the corresponding continuous sinusoids. For N equal to 1, there is a single basis function with one point equal to 1. For N equal to 2, there are two basis functions with two points each, (1, 1) and (1, −1). For N equal to 4, there are four basis functions with four points each, (1, 1, 1, 1); (1, 0, −1, 0); (1, −1, 1, −1); and (1, 0, −1, 0). The second (k = 1) and fourth (k = N − 1) functions have the same real parts, but different imaginary parts.

Figure 18.6 shows the single basis function for N = 1, the two basis functions for N = 2, and the four basis functions for N = 4. The basis functions for the discrete Fourier transform are defined only for integer values of n; however, Figure 18.6 also shows the equivalent continuous sinusoidal signals. Sometimes it is helpful to think of the discrete signals as samples of a sinusoidal function. Notice that integral multiples of the sinusoidal functions just fit in the period N.

C. PERIODICITY OF THE DISCRETE FOURIER TRANSFORM

We can show that any signal, f[n], defined by the inverse discrete Fourier transform, Equation 18.5, is periodic with period, N.

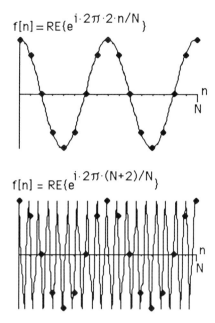

$$f[n] = RE\{e^{i \cdot 2\pi \cdot 2 \cdot n/N}\}$$

$$f[n] = RE\{e^{i \cdot 2\pi \cdot (N+2)/N}\}$$

FIGURE 18.7. Equivalence of frequencies separated by N: on the top is the real part of the sinusoid, $e^{i2\pi 2n/N}$, on the bottom is the real part of the sinusoid, $e^{i2\pi(N+2)n/N}$. Also shown are the corresponding continuous sinusoids. The frequencies of the two signals, 2 and $N + 2$, are separated by N. Although the continuous versions of the two signals are quite different, the signals have the same value at the discrete sample points.

$$f[n + N] = (1/N) \cdot \sum_{k=0}^{N-1} F[k] \cdot e^{i2\pi k(n + N)/N}$$

$$= (1/N) \cdot \sum_{k=0}^{N-1} F[k] \cdot e^{i2\pi kn/N} \cdot e^{i2\pi kN/N} \qquad (18.10)$$

The exponent of the last factor is equal to $i \cdot 2\pi \cdot k$, a multiple of $i \cdot 2\pi$; therefore, the last factor is equal to one. What we are left with is the inverse Fourier transform of f[n]. Thus,

$$f[n + N] = f[n] \qquad (18.11)$$

All signals, f[n], defined by the inverse Fourier transform, Equation 18.5, are periodic with period equal to N. For exactly the same reason, all signals, F[k], defined by the Fourier transform, Equation 18.6, are periodic with period N. Thus both the time and frequency domain signals defined by the discrete Fourier transform are periodic with period equal to N.

D. DEFINITION OF THE DISCRETE FOURIER TRANSFORM ON ANY N POINT INTERVAL

We can show that the discrete Fourier transform can be defined over any N point interval. The key feature is the periodicity of the basis functions. Above we found that $e^{i2\pi kn/N}$ can be thought of as a time signal with period N/k. Since k is an integer, this period is an integral function of N, i.e., k periods of $e^{i2\pi kn/N}$ are equal to N. Therefore, all of the basis functions are periodic with period, N.

Figure 18.7 shows the two signals $e^{i2\pi kn/N}$ and $e^{i2\pi(k + N)n/N}$. Although the continuous versions of these signals are very different, the values at integer values of n are exactly equal. This figure is similar to Figure 18.5 except that in this case the frequencies of both of the signals are positive. In both cases, the frequencies are separated by N.

In the definition of the inverse Fourier transform, Equation 18.5, there are two factors in the summation, F[k] and $e^{i2\pi kn/N}$. Since F[k] is equal to F[k + m · N], and since $e^{i2\pi kn/N}$ is equal to $e^{i2\pi(k+mN)n/N}$, any multiple of N can be added to any of the values of k without affecting the terms in the summation:

$$F[k + m \cdot N] \cdot e^{i2\pi(k+mN)n/N} = F[k] \cdot e^{i2\pi kn/N} \qquad (18.12)$$

Above we have defined the inverse discrete Fourier transform for k running from 0 to N − 1. However, because of Equation 18.12 we can define it using any sequence of N values. For example, we could let k run from −N/2 to (N/2) − 1, or from −N + 1 to 0, or any set of N distinct values of $e^{i2\pi kn/N}$.

The key feature in all of this is that everything is periodic with period N. Both the signal, f[n], and its transform, F[k], are periodic with period N. All of the basis functions are periodic over the period N. And now we have even shown that the range of values over which the Fourier transform can be defined is periodic, over the period N.

IV. SUM OF BASIS FUNCTIONS

An important property for development of the continuous Fourier transform was that the integral of the basis functions, $e^{i\omega t}$ was zero except for ω equal to zero:

$$\int_{-\infty}^{+\infty} e^{i\omega t} \, d\omega = \delta(t) \qquad (18.13)$$

We shall show that there is an analogous property which is important for the discrete Fourier transform.

When working with discrete signals, summations replace integrations. There is a whole style to working with summations. The engineer who works with discrete signals frequently becomes facile with summation operations. If the reader finds the following manipulations a bit difficult to follow, it is probably not worthwhile spending too much time working through the derivations, since we shall not make much use of summation operations. Instead, skip past the indented section.

Consider the following product:

$$(1 - x) \cdot \sum_{n=0}^{N-1} x^n = \sum_{n=0}^{N-1} (x^n - x^{n+1}) \qquad (18.14)$$

We can expand the right hand side of the equation as:

$$= (1 - x) + (x - x^2) + (x^2 - x^3) + \ldots + (x^{N-1} - x^N) \qquad (18.15)$$

Notice that for each term, except for the first and last terms, the left-hand member of each term cancels the right-hand member of the previous term. Thus we are left with:

$$= 1 - x^N \qquad (18.16)$$

Dividing both sides of Equation 18.14 by $(1 - x)$ gives the important relationship:

$$\sum_{n=0}^{N-1} x^n = (1 - x^N)/(1 - x) \tag{18.17}$$

(An alternate method of deriving this result is by polynomial division on the right hand side of Equation 18.14.)

Now let us consider the sum:

$$\sum_{k=0}^{N-1} e^{i2\pi kn/N} \tag{18.18}$$

Notice that the summation is over the variable, k. When n is equal to any multiple of N, the exponent is a multiple of 2π so that the value of the imaginary exponential is one, and Equation 18.18 reduces to:

$$\sum_{k=0}^{N-1} 1 = N \tag{18.19}$$

When n is not equal to a multiple of N, we can expand Equation 18.18 using Equation 18.17:

$$\sum_{k=0}^{N-1} e^{i2\pi kn/N} = (1 - e^{i2\pi Nn/N})/(1 - e^{i2\pi n/N})$$

$$= (1 - e^{i2\pi n})/(1 - e^{i2\pi n/N}) \tag{18.20}$$

Since $2\pi \cdot n$ is an integral multiple of 2π, $e^{i2\pi n}$ is equal to one, and $1 - e^{i2\pi n}$ is equal to zero. Since n is not a multiple of N, $e^{i2\pi n/N}$ is not equal to one, and the denominator is nonzero. Thus, the quotient is zero.

We can summarize these two results:

$$\sum_{k=0}^{N-1} e^{i2\pi kn/N} = \begin{cases} N, & n = m \cdot N \\ 0, & n \neq m \cdot N \end{cases} \tag{18.21}$$

where m is an integer. This result is similar to Equation 18.13. The sum is N for n equal to zero and zero for n equal to one to $N - 1$.

V. PROOF OF THE DISCRETE FOURIER TRANSFORM RELATION

We can show show that the inverse discrete Fourier transform of a discrete Fourier transform returns the original signal. Substituting Equation 18.6 into Equation 18.5 yields:

$$f[n] = (1/N) \cdot \sum_{k=0}^{N-1} \left[\sum_{n'=0}^{N-1} f[n'] \cdot e^{-i2\pi kn'/N} \right] \cdot e^{i2\pi kn/N} \tag{18.22}$$

We have used n′ for the inner summation so that it is not confused with the n in f[n]. Rearranging the order of summation and combining the exponentials gives:

$$f[n] = (1/N) \cdot \sum_{n'=0}^{N-1} f[n'] \cdot \sum_{k=0}^{N-1} e^{i2\pi k(n-n')/N} \qquad (18.23)$$

The last sum in Equation 18.23 is of the form given by Equation 18.21. We have shown that it is zero when n − n′ is not an integral multiple of N, and it is equal to N when n − n′ is a multiple of N. The only n′ in the range 0 to N − 1 for which the second sum is nonzero is for n′ equal to n. Therefore,

$$f[n] = (1/N) \cdot f[n] \cdot N = f[n] \qquad (18.24)$$

And we have proven that the inverse transform of a Fourier transform of f[n] is equal to f[n].

The mathematics of this proof is a little tricky with regard to keeping the summations and the variables straight, but it is not conceptually as complicated as the proof of the continuous Fourier transform. This proof is also mathematically correct while our proof of the continuous Fourier transform was only approximately correct. For very large N, we can approximate the continuous Fourier transform with the discrete Fourier transform (see Chapter 20). Thus, an alternate method of proving that the continuous Fourier transform pair is correct is to consider it as the limit of the discrete Fourier transform as N goes to infinity.

VI. ANALOGY BETWEEN VECTORS AND THE DISCRETE SIGNALS

Chapter 8, which described vectors, brought out the analogy between discrete signals and vectors. A limited extent signal, f[n], with N nonzero values, can be exactly represented by a vector, **f**, with N components. A limited extent frequency domain signal, F[k], can be exactly represented by a vector, **F**. Similarly, periodic signals can be represented by the same vectors.

There is a small notational problem. Recall that we used only small letters for vectors. Since we use capital letters for frequency domain signals such as F[k], it is natural to define the analogous vector using a capital letter, **F**. In this special case, where we have a vector representing a frequency domain signal, we shall break our rule and use a capital letter.

Each component of the frequency domain signal, given by the discrete Fourier transform operation (Equation 18.6) is a linear combination of the components of the time domain signal. Thus, the frequency domain signal is a linear transformation of the time domain signal. Recall that in Chapter 9, we found that all linear transformations could be represented by matrix operations.

Let us define a matrix, W, which performs the discrete Fourier transform operation. Then in vector notation the discrete Fourier transform can be written:

$$\mathbf{F} = (1/\sqrt{N}) \cdot \mathbf{W} \cdot \mathbf{f} \qquad (18.25)$$

The components of the matrix, W, can be determined from Equation 18.6:

$$w_{kn} = (1/\sqrt{N}) \cdot e^{-i2\pi(k-1)(n-1)/N} \qquad (18.26)$$

where we have used n and k instead of the more usual indices i and j. The " -1 "'s are included since the matrix indices start at one not zero. The constant, $1/\sqrt{N}$, makes the energy in $\mathbf{w}_k$ equal to one. The inverse discrete Fourier transform is written:

$$\mathbf{f} = \sqrt{N} \cdot W^{-1} \cdot \mathbf{F} \tag{18.27}$$

where:

$$w_{nk}^{-1} = (1/\sqrt{N}) \cdot e^{i2\pi(k-1)(n-1)/N} \tag{18.28}$$

In the next chapter we shall come back to the linear algebra formulation of the discrete Fourier transform pair. We shall find that the discrete Fourier transform is analogous to a rotation of the basis vectors which are used to define the vector space. But more of that later.

VII. FAST FOURIER TRANSFORM

One of the major reasons that the Fourier transform operation is of importance in Radiology today is the discovery of the fast Fourier transform algorithm. The fast Fourier transform algorithm has transformed a vast amount of image processing from being impractical to being very practical.

In Chapter 13 we emphasized the complexity of the various system models described in Part I. The complexity of the models is closely related to the efficiency with which the output of a system can be calculated. A branch of engineering called complexity theory attempts to measure the difficulty of implementing various algorithms. The most important factor in determining how difficult an algorithm is to perform is how the number of operations required varies with the size of the input, N.

The most obvious way to calculate the output signal, F[k], is to apply Equation 18.6 for each of the N points in the output. Each application of Equation 18.6 requires that we calculate $f[n] \cdot e^{i2\pi kn/N}$ for the N different values of n. Thus we need to do N operations to calculate each of the N values of F[k]. The total complexity of the algorithm is on the order of N^2 operations.

If we consider the vector formulation of the discrete Fourier transform operation (Equation 18.25) we come to the same conclusion. Multiplication of an N by N matrix times an N-dimensional vector requires N multiplication for each component of the output. The total complexity is on the order of N^2 operations. However, we can get a clue that there might be a better algorithm by considering the elements of the matrix, W:

$$w_{nk} = (1/\sqrt{N}) \cdot e^{-i2\pi(k-1)(n-1)/N} \tag{18.29}$$

The N^2 elements, w_{nk}, have only N different values, $e^{i2\pi 0/N}$ to $e^{i2\pi(N-1)/N}$. Thus, the matrix W is much more simple than the usual N by N matrix. The fast Fourier transform algorithm makes use of this simplicity.

The key feature of the fast Fourier transform algorithm is that it divides the problem of calculating a discrete Fourier transform for a signal of length, N, into the problem of calculating two discrete Fourier transforms of length, N/2. Computer science algorithms that use this strategy are called divide and conquer. In order to use this algorithm, it is convenient if N is a power of two. This is one of many reasons why most digital radiological images are powers of two.

Let us start with the discrete Fourier transform:

$$F[k] = \sum_{n=0}^{N-1} f[n] \cdot e^{i2\pi kn/N} \tag{18.30}$$

The trick is to divide this sum up into the terms for which n is even and odd. If we define a new variable n' which varies from 0 to $(N/2) - 1$, then the even terms are given by $2n'$ and the odd terms are given by $2n' + 1$. We can rewrite Equation 18.30:

$$F[k] = \sum_{n'=0}^{n-1} f[2n'] \cdot e^{i2\pi k 2n'/N} + \sum_{n'=0}^{(N/2)-1} f[2n' + 1] \cdot e^{i2\pi k(2n' + 1)/N} \tag{18.31}$$

We can rearrange the factors in Equation 18.31:

$$F[k] = \sum_{n'=0}^{(N/2)-1} f[2n'] \cdot e^{i2\pi kn'/N/2} + e^{i2\pi k/N} \cdot \sum_{n'=0}^{(N/2)-1} f[2n' + 1] \cdot e^{i2\pi kn'/N/2} \tag{18.32}$$

The first term in Equation 18.32 is an N/2 point discrete Fourier transform, and the second term is an N/2 point discrete Fourier transform multiplied by the factor, $e^{i2\pi k/N}$. The factor, $e^{i2\pi k/N}$, is constant for a single value of k. Separating the discrete Fourier transform into even and odd terms has allowed us to divide an N point transform into two N/2 point transforms. The fast Fourier transform algorithm applies this trick recursively until there are N one-point transforms. If N is equal to 2^m, then this trick must be applied m times.

Now let us calculate how difficult it is to apply this algorithm. At each stage in the algorithm it is necessary to combine the results of the next stage for all N different values of k, using Equation 18.32. However, the total number of stages needed is only m, where m is equal to $\log_2(N)$. The total complexity of the algorithm goes as $N \cdot \log_2(N)$. $N \cdot \log_2(N)$ is only slightly larger than N, and a great deal smaller than N^2. Thus the fast Fourier transform algorithm is much faster than the straight forward method of calculating the Fourier transform.

Calculation of the convolution sum requires N operations for each of the N points in the output. Convolution is an N^2 algorithm. However, we said that it could be accomplished by performing a fast Fourier transform, a multiplication, and an inverse fast Fourier transform. The multiplication step can be done in an amount of time equal to N, and the Fourier transforms can be done in an amount of time proportional to $N \cdot \log_2(N)$. The total time will be dominated by the slower $N \cdot \log_2(N)$ process. Thus, the fast Fourier transform algorithm also transforms convolution from an N^2 to an $N \cdot \log_2(N)$ algorithm.

VIII. SUMMARY

This chapter has introduced the discrete Fourier transform. In explaining Radiologic applications we rely heavily on the continuous Fourier transform. However, there are three major reasons for introducing the discrete Fourier transform. First, there are several important effects that sampling has on Radiologic images. The description of sampling in Chapter 23 relies heavily on the ideas developed in this chapter. Second, the relations between continuity and periodicity for the different Fourier transforms (described in Chapter 20) helps to explain how the time and frequency domains are related. Third, the analogy between the discrete Fourier transform and multiplication of a matrix and a vector provides some insight about the Fourier transform. Developing this insight is the major goal of the next chapter.

In addition the discrete Fourier transform allowed us to prove that the inverse Fourier transform of a Fourier transform returns the original signal. This proof was much more simple than the proof for the continuous Fourier transform, and it is mathematically more rigorous. From a practical sense, the discrete Fourier transform is very important. Almost all actual computer implementation of a Fourier transform operation is in terms of the discrete Fourier transform, using the fast Fourier transform algorithm.

IX. FURTHER READING

Our description of the discrete Fourier transform is designed primarily to provide insights about the operation of the continuous Fourier transform. Several authors give the discrete Fourier transform a much more central position in their expositions. For example, this approach is taken in the books by Oppenheim and Schafer[1] and by Dudgeon and Mersereau.[2] Since the discrete Fourier transform is very important for actual implementation of image processing methods, this approach is more appropriate for an engineer. Since we are more interested in general concepts than in practical implementation, we have made the continuous Fourier transform central to our exposition.

The discrete Fourier transform is described in several texts, for example see Chapter 5 of the book by Oppenheim and Willsky.[3] The fast Fourier transform algorithm is described in Chapter 6 of the book by Oppenheim and Schafer,[1] and Chapter 5 of the book by Strang.[4] The analogy between the discrete Fourier transform and multiplication of a matrix times a vector is described in Chapter 4 of the book by Strang.[4]

In this chapter we have used periodic signals to represent limited extent signals. There are some mathematical considerations about the use of periodic signals which we have totally ignored. For example, periodic signals are nonintegrable and have infinite energy. These problems are really of no concern to us; however, the reader who is interested in the mathematical details is referred to Chapter 5 of the book by Hildebrand.[5]

The continuous Fourier transform is used for continuous signals; the discrete Fourier transform is used for discrete signals; and the number theoretic transform is used for digital signals. Number theoretic transforms are not discussed in this book; however, the reader who is interested in mathematics may find the book by McClellan and Rader[6] very interesting.

We have generally assumed that the digital representation of discrete numbers by a computer is sufficiently accurate. In general this is a safe assumption, but on occasion the limited precision of the computer representation can cause problems. The effects of approximating the continuous values of a discrete signal are described in Chapter 9 of the book by Oppenheim and Schafer.[1]

REFERENCES

1. **Oppenheim, A. V. and Schafer, R. W.,** *Digital Signal Processing,* Prentice-Hall, Englewood Cliffs, NJ, 1975.
2. **Dudgeon, D. E. and Mersereau, R. M.,** *Multidimensional Digital Signal Processing,* Prentice-Hall, Englewood Cliffs, NJ, 1984.
3. **Oppenheim, A. V. and Willsky, A. S.,** *Signals and Systems,* Prentice-Hall, Englewood Cliffs, NJ, 1983.
4. **Strang, G.,** *Introduction to Applied Mathematics,* Wellesley-Cambridge Press, Wellesley, MA, 1986.
5. **Hildebrand, F. B.,** *Advanced Calculus for Applications,* Prentice-Hall, Englewood Cliffs, NJ, 1962.
6. **McClellan, J. H. and Rader, C. M.,** *Number Theory in Digital Signal Processing,* Prentice-Hall, Englewood Cliffs, NJ, 1979.

Chapter 19

VECTOR SPACE ROTATION

In this chapter we shall return to the description of systems using the linear algebra model. Our primary goal will be to describe the process of transforming from one set of basis vectors to a new set of basis vectors. We shall loosely refer to this transformation operation as rotation. The rotation of a vector space is analogous to the other transformation operations which are described in this section, and it will provide a geometrical insight into these operations. Prior to reading this chapter it may be useful for the reader to briefly review Chapters 8 and 9.

If we have a vector which is defined in terms of one coordinate system, it is often necessary to be able to define the vector in another coordinate system. For example, if we know the position of a mass lesion on a computed tomography image, it is necessary to translate that description into physical coordinates before a needle biopsy can be performed. Changing from one coordinate system to another coordinate system may require a translation of the origin of the coordinate system, or a rotation of the coordinate system, or both operations. Only the rotation operation will be described in this chapter.

I. EXAMPLE OF A ROTATION OPERATION

Let us start by considering a 2 by 2 matrix, S, defined as follows:

$$S = \begin{pmatrix} \cos\theta & -\sin\theta \\ \sin\theta & \cos\theta \end{pmatrix} \qquad (19.1)$$

The columns of S are the two vectors, s_1 and s_2. The x component of s_1 is $\cos\theta$ and the y component of s_1 is $\sin\theta$. The x component of s_2 is $-\sin\theta$ and the y component of s_2 is $\cos\theta$. Figure 19.1 shows these two vectors. We can define a new coordinate system x', y' where the x' axis lies along the direction of s_1, and the y' axis lies along the direction of s_2. From Figure 19.1 we see that the x', y' coordinate system is rotated by an angle, θ, with respect to the x,y coordinate system.

The vectors s_1 and s_2 have some special properties. Both vectors have a length of 1:

$$s_1^T \cdot s_1 = \cos\theta \cdot \cos\theta + \sin\theta \cdot \sin\theta = \cos^2\theta + \sin^2\theta = 1 \qquad (19.2)$$

$$s_2^T \cdot s_2 = -\sin\theta \cdot (-\sin\theta) + \cos\theta \cdot \cos\theta = \sin^2\theta + \cos^2\theta = 1 \qquad (19.3)$$

and they are orthogonal to each other:

$$s_1^T \cdot s_2 = -\cos\theta \cdot \sin\theta + \sin\theta \cdot \cos\theta = 0 \qquad (19.4)$$

Thus, the columns of S are orthonormal (orthogonal vectors of length 1). These two vectors are very similar to the vectors, d_1 and d_2, defined in Chapter 9.

Recall that the set of basis vectors, d_1, d_2, d_3 . . . , were defined to be orthonormal vectors with a single nonzero value (Equation 9.6).

$$d_1 = (1 \quad 0 \quad 0 \quad ...)^T \qquad (19.5)$$

$$d_2 = (0 \quad 1 \quad 0 \quad ...)^T \qquad (19.6)$$

$$d_3 = (0 \quad 0 \quad 1 \quad ...)^T \qquad (19.7)$$

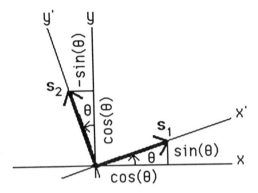

FIGURE 19.1.   Orthonormal basis vectors: this figure shows the two vectors, s_1 and s_2, which are the columns of matrix, S, given by Equation 19.1.

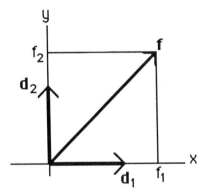

FIGURE 19.2.   Components of a vector: the components of a vector, f, in the vector space defined by the canonical vectors, d_1 and d_2, are f_1 and f_2. The canonical basis vectors are typically associated with the x,y coordinate system.

In the case of a two-dimensional vector space, these vectors point along the direction of the x and y axes. This set of basis vectors is particularly easy to work with, since the projection of a vector along one of the basis vectors is equal to the corresponding component of the vector e.g., the projection of $(3\ 5)^T$ along d_2 is 5.

Now suppose that we have some vector f which is defined in the x,y coordinate system (see Figure 19.2). f_1 is the x coordinate of the vector and f_2 is the y coordinate of the system. Now let us consider the vector, f', which is the product of S^T and f

$$f' = S^T \cdot f \qquad (19.8)$$

the components of f' are

$$f'_1 = \quad \cos\theta \cdot f_1 + \sin\theta \cdot f_2 \qquad (19.9)$$

$$f'_2 = -\sin\theta \cdot f_1 + \cos\theta \cdot f_2 \qquad (19.10)$$

Figure 19.3 shows that f'_1 is equal to the projection of f along the x' coordinate system, and Figure 19.4 shows that f'_2 is the projection of f along the y' coordinate. Therefore, f and f' can be considered to be different representations of the same vector, where f is defined in the x,y coordinate system, and f' is defined in the x',y' coordinate systems (see Figure

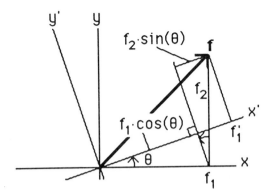

FIGURE 19.3. Calculation of f'_1: the two components of f'_1 given by Equation 19.9 are shown in this diagram. The first portion is $f_1 \cdot \cos(\theta)$, and the second portion is $f_2 \cdot \sin(\theta)$. From the geometrical relations, it can be seen that f'_1 is the projection of f on the x' coordinate axis.

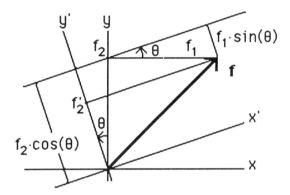

FIGURE 19.4. Calculation of f'_2: the two components of f'_2 given by Equation 19.10 are shown in this diagram. The first portion is $f_2 \cdot \cos(\theta)$, and the second portion is $-f_1 \cdot \sin(\theta)$. The second portion is subtracted from the first. From the geometrical relations, it can be seen that f'_2 is the projection of f on the y' coordinate axis.

19.5). f_1 is the distance along the x axis, $\mathbf{d}_1$, to a perpendicular from the vector. f_2 is the distance along the y axis, $\mathbf{d}_2$, to a perpendicular from the vector. f'_1 is the distance along the x' axis, $\mathbf{s}_1$, to a perpendicular from the vector. f'_2 is the distance along the y' axis, $\mathbf{s}_2$, to a perpendicular from the vector.

The transformation of $\mathbf{f}$ to $\mathbf{f}'$ is equivalent to a rotation of the underlying coordinate system by an angle θ. Recall that a vector space can be defined in terms of a set of basis vectors. The transformation of $\mathbf{f}$ by the matrix S^T can be viewed as a rotation of the basis vectors which define the vector space from $\mathbf{d}_1$ and $\mathbf{d}_2$ to $\mathbf{s}_1$ and $\mathbf{s}_2$.

Any vector in the original coordinate system, including the basis vectors, can be transformed to the new system. For example,

$$s_1 = S^T \cdot d_1 \qquad (19.11)$$

$$s_2 = S^T \cdot d_2 \qquad (19.12)$$

An alternate point of view is that the matrix S^T rotates f by an angle $-\theta$ in the opposite direction. Figure 19.6 shows these two methods of viewing the same operation. The top row shows the rotation of the coordinate system by an angle θ and the bottom row shows

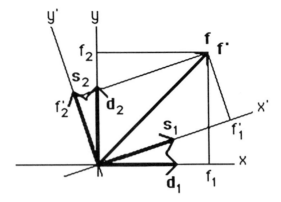

FIGURE 19.5.   Rotation of the basis vectors: the transformation of **f** to **f′** by the matrix given by Equation 19.1 can be viewed as a rotation of the basis vectors. From this point of view, **f** and **f′** are the same vector. What has changed is the basis vectors. The canonical basis vectors, d_1 and d_2, are rotated to the vectors, s_1 and s_2, given by the columns of the matrix, S.

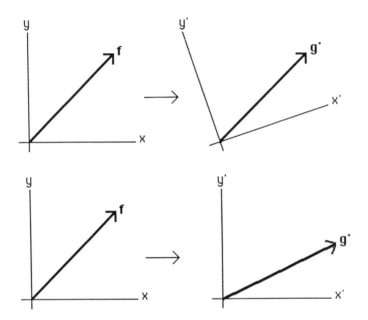

FIGURE 19.6.   Two conceptualizations of rotation: rotation by the matrix, S, can be viewed as a rotation of the coordinate axes by angle, θ, or the same operation can be viewed as rotation of the vector by angle, $-\theta$. These points of view are mathematically equivalent; they relate to how the vector space is viewed with respect to the rest of the world.

the rotation of the vector by an angle $-\theta$. The relation between **f′** and the coordinate system is the same with these two points of view; the difference is how they relate to the rest of the world. The relation to the rest of the world is important for us conceptually, but it does not matter to the mathematics.

With multi-dimensional vectors there is no geometrical interpretation for multiplication by a matrix with orthonormal rows. However, we shall refer to this operation as a rotation of the coordinate system.

II. ROTATION OF A VECTOR SPACE

In the description of vector space rotation, we shall use the description of a matrix as a set of vectors which was introduced in Chapter 9. Recall that a matrix, H, can be viewed as a set of column receptors $\mathbf{h}_j$ (Equation 9.17):

$$H = (\mathbf{h}_j) = (\mathbf{h}_1 \quad \mathbf{h}_2 \quad \mathbf{h}_3) = \begin{pmatrix} | & | & | \\ h_{i1} & h_{i2} & h_{i3} \\ | & | & | \end{pmatrix} \tag{19.13}$$

Alternately, we can think of a matrix as a collection of row vectors $\mathbf{h}_i^T$ (Equation 9.18):

$$H = (\mathbf{h}_i^T) = \begin{pmatrix} \mathbf{h}_1^T \\ \mathbf{h}_2^T \\ \mathbf{h}_3^T \end{pmatrix} = \begin{pmatrix} -h_{1j}- \\ -h_{2j}- \\ -h_{3j}- \end{pmatrix} \tag{19.14}$$

In order to rotate to a new set of basis vectors, we shall use a special matrix, S. We can write S as a set of column vectors:

$$S = (\mathbf{s}_j) = (\mathbf{s}_1 \quad \mathbf{s}_2 \quad \mathbf{s}_3 \quad ...) \tag{19.15}$$

As in the example above, the columns of S are defined to be orthonormal vectors; each column of S is length one, and the product of any two different columns of S is zero. The orthonormal vectors, $\mathbf{d}_j$, are one possible choice for the column vectors, $\mathbf{s}_j$; however, there are infinitely many other possible sets of orthonormal vectors.

In order to understand the mathematics of the rotation operation, we shall have to take an excursion into the properties of a matrix, S, with orthonormal columns. The product of the transpose of S times S is:

$$S^T \cdot S = (\mathbf{s}_i^T \cdot \mathbf{s}_j) \tag{19.16}$$

where we have written the elements of the product matrix in terms of the products of the columns of S. By definition, the vectors are orthonormal; thus

$$\mathbf{s}_i^T \cdot \mathbf{s}_j = \begin{cases} 1 & \text{for } i = j \\ 0 & \text{for } i \neq j \end{cases} \tag{19.17}$$

Therefore

$$S \cdot S^T = \begin{pmatrix} 1 & 0 & 0 & ... \\ 0 & 1 & 0 & ... \\ 0 & 0 & 1 & ... \\ & ... & & \end{pmatrix} \tag{19.18}$$

Because the columns of S are orthonormal, the product of the transpose of S and S is equal to the identity matrix:

$$S^T \cdot S = I \qquad (19.19)$$

However, this relationship is just the definition of the inverse matrix, Equation 8.31. Therefore, a matrix with orthonormal rows has the very special property that its transverse is its inverse:

$$S^T = S^{-1} \qquad (19.20)$$

An example of a matrix, S, which has orthonormal columns is the identity matrix, I, with columns equal to d_i. The transpose of I is I, and the inverse of I is also I.

In order to understand how to use this matrix, we shall need to do one bit of tricky mathematics. The transpose of a matrix with orthonormal columns is a matrix with orthonormal rows:

$$S^T = (s_i^T) \qquad (19.21)$$

The product of S^T and a vector, f, is a new vector, f'.

$$f' = S^T \cdot f = \left(\sum_j s_{ij} \cdot f_j \right) = \sum_j s_i \cdot f_j \qquad (19.22)$$

In the last equality we have made a considerable change in notation. The parenthesis on the left indicates that we are showing one element of the vector, f', namely, f'_i. On the right-hand side of the equality we have switched to a vector notation where s_i are the rows of S^T.

What this fancy notational footwork accomplishes is that we can see how the columns of S contribute to the vector, f'. For each component of f, the result has a term which is a scaled vector s_i. f' is a linear combination of vectors which are the columns of S

$$f' = f_1 \cdot s_1 + f_2 \cdot s_2 + f_3 \cdot s_3 + \ldots \qquad (19.23)$$

We used this same method of decomposition in Chapter 9 when examining the vector spaces associated with a matrix.

This point of view is very interesting. If we consider the orthonormal columns of S as a set of basis vectors, then the components of f' are the coordinates of the same vector as f in terms of this new basis. In other words, if f is a vector in terms of the canonical basis set, d_i, then f' represents the same vector in terms of the basis set consisting of s_i.

Figure 19.5 shows these relationships graphically in terms of a two-dimensional coordinate system. The vector, f, is defined in terms of the canonical basis set d_i, using the unprimed coordinates. We can consider that the vectors, s_i, are the basis for another coordinate system, axes x', y'. Since f can be written in terms of s_i, using the scalar factors, f'_i, f' is the same vector as f, but expressed in terms of the new coordinate system.

Since the transpose of S is equal to the inverse of S we can solve Equation 19.8 for f

$$S \cdot S^T \cdot f = S \cdot f' \qquad (19.24)$$

$$S \cdot S^{-1} \cdot f = S \cdot f' \qquad (19.25)$$

$$f = S \cdot f' \qquad (19.26)$$

This equation says that in order to transform a vector which is written in terms of the set of basis vectors, s_i, into a vector which is written in terms of a canonical basis, d_i, the vector should be multiplied by the matrix, S.

We have found a method for transforming a vector, f, from one coordinate system into another coordinate system. If the new coordinate system is given by the orthonormal vectors s_j, then a vector f', equal to $S^T \cdot f$, is the same vector as f, but f' is expressed in terms of the new coordinates. To return to the original coordinate system we multiply f' by S; $S \cdot f'$ is equal to f. The simplicity of this transformation between coordinate systems is due to the fact that the basis vectors are orthonormal. If the basis vectors are not orthonormal, then the transformation is considerably more complicated, and not necessarily invertible.

III. THE DISCRETE FOURIER TRANSFORM AS A ROTATION

It is possible to consider the discrete Fourier transform as a matrix operation (see Chapter 18). The space domain signal, f[n], is equivalent to a vector, f. We run into a notational difficulty when we try to write the equivalent of the frequency domain signal, F[k]. We have used capital letters to indicate frequency domain signals in our linear systems description. Capital letters are reserved for matrices in our linear algebra description. For this section we shall break our rule and define the vector, F, as the equivalent of F[k].

We can define a matrix, W, with components given by Equation 18.26:

$$w_{kn} = (1/\sqrt{N}) \cdot e^{-i2\pi(n-1)(k-1)/N} \tag{19.27}$$

The "-1"s in the exponent are due to the fact that we have defined discrete signals for 0 to $N - 1$ and vector components from 1 to N. The discrete Fourier transform, Equation 18.25, is given by:

$$F = (1/\sqrt{N}) \cdot W \cdot f \tag{19.28}$$

The rows of W are discrete sinusoids in the variable, n, of different frequencies, $k - 1$. They are equivalent to the discrete signals:

$$w_k[n] = (1/\sqrt{N}) \cdot e^{-i2\pi n(k-1)/N} \tag{19.29}$$

where the frequency is $(k - 1)/N$. In Chapter 18 it was shown that these signals are orthogonal to each other. Furthermore, the product of any of these signals with itself is equal to one (see Equation 18.23). The rows of W are an orthonormal set of vectors, analogous to S^T. Thus, the discrete Fourier transform operation, Equation 19.28, is analogous to the rotation operation, Equation 19.8. (The factor, $1/\sqrt{N}$, simply performs a scaling operation.)

Figure 19.7 shows a very simple signal, f[n], with only two components. Its transform, F[k], is also shown. On the bottom of the figure is a vector, f, with components equal to the values of the signal, f[n], in the d_1, d_2 coordinate system. The sinusoidal basis set for the frequency domain representation can be determined from Equation 19.27:

$$w_1^T = (1/\sqrt{2} \quad 1/\sqrt{2}) \tag{19.30}$$

$$w_2^T = (1/\sqrt{2} \quad -1/\sqrt{2}) \tag{19.31}$$

The vector, F, defined in the w_1, w_2 coordinate system is the same vector as f defined in the d_1, d_2 coordinate system.

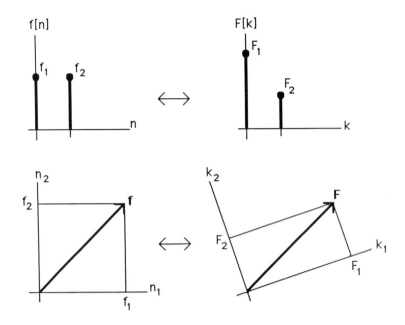

FIGURE 19.7.   Analogy between the Fourier transform and rotation: the top
panel shows a two point signal, and the two points in its discrete Fourier transform.
The bottom panel shows two vectors, **f** and **F**, which have components equal to
the points in the two signals. The vectors, **f** and **F**, are the same vector; the axes
are different. The Fourier transform operation is analogous to the rotation of the
basis vectors.

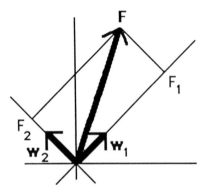

FIGURE 19.8.   Vector representing a frequency domain signal: the two vectors, w_1 and w_2, define the
first and second components of the frequency domain signal. The projection of **F** on the w_1 axis gives
the first component, F_1. The projection of **F** on the w_2 axis gives the second component, F_2.

The discrete Fourier transformation can be written in terms of the rows of **W**:

$$\mathbf{F} = (1/\sqrt{N}) \cdot (\mathbf{w}_k^T) \cdot \mathbf{f} = (1/\sqrt{N}) \cdot (\mathbf{w}_k^T \cdot \mathbf{f}) \qquad (19.32)$$

This form of the equation emphasizes that the components, F_k, of the frequency domain
vector are equal to the product of the rows of **W** and the time domain vector, **f**. Recall that
multiplication of a vector by a unit vector (a vector of length 1) is equivalent to calculating
the projection of that vector along the direction of the unit vector. Thus the discrete Fourier
transform operation calculates the projection of **f** along the new basis vectors, $\mathbf{w}_k^T$. Figure
19.8 shows the components, F_k, as the projections of **f** along the sinusoidal vectors, $\mathbf{w}_k^T$.

Vector multiplication is like correlation. Another way of viewing the discrete Fourier transform (Equation 19.28), is as a correlation between the vector, $\mathbf{f}$, and the sinusoidal vectors $\mathbf{w}_k^T$. The components, $\mathbf{F}_k$, tell how much $\mathbf{f}$ is like the basis vector, $\mathbf{w}_k^T$. This same point of view was used with the continuous Fourier transform in Chapter 14.

The discrete Fourier transform operation can be viewed as a rotation of the basis vector set from the canonical basis set, $\mathbf{d}_n$, to a basis set, $\mathbf{w}_k$, which consists of sinusoidal waves. The space domain vector, $\mathbf{f}$, and the frequency domain vector, $\mathbf{F}$, are the same vector defined in terms of two different sets of basis vectors. From this point of view, the space and frequency domain signals are used to define a single point in an N-dimensional space. The difference between the two signals is how we define the set of basis vectors.

This point of view brings out the equivalence of the space and frequency domain descriptions of a signal. Both descriptions refer to the same point in a multidimensional vector space. The difference between the descriptions is simply a matter of which basis we use to describe the vector space. The space domain signal is the most natural description for viewing the signal. The frequency domain description is most natural for linear time invariant systems. In order to understand why this is true, we must see how matrices transform to a new vector space (*vide infra*).

The inverse discrete Fourier transform can be defined as

$$\mathbf{f} = \sqrt{N} \cdot W^{-1} \cdot \mathbf{F} \tag{19.33}$$

where

$$w_{nk}^{-1} = (1/\sqrt{N}) \cdot e^{i2\pi(k-1)(n-1)/N} \tag{19.34}$$

In the following section we show that W^{-1}, as defined by this equation, is the inverse of W. This section can be skipped without loss of continuity.

The rows of W^{-1} are orthogonal to the columns of W:

$$\mathbf{w}_n^{-1} \cdot \mathbf{w}_{n'} = \sum_{n=1}^{N} (1/N) \cdot e^{i2\pi(k-1)(n-1)/N} \cdot e^{-i2\pi(k-1)(n'-1)/N}$$

$$= (1/N) \cdot \sum_{n=1}^{N} e^{i2\pi(k-1)(n-n')/N} \tag{19.35}$$

where we have used n for the index of the row of W^{-1} and the index, n', for W. The last sum is equal to N for n equal to n' and 0 otherwise (see Equation 18.23). Thus,

$$\mathbf{w}_n^{-1} \cdot \mathbf{w}_{n'} = \begin{cases} 1, & n = n' \\ 0, & n \neq n' \end{cases} \tag{19.36}$$

Therefore, $W^{-1} \cdot W$ is equal to I, and W^{-1} is in fact the inverse of W.

IV. MATRIX ROTATION

The effect of a rotation on a matrix is somewhat more complicated than the effect on a vector. However, understanding this change will provide new insight into a matrix as a system.

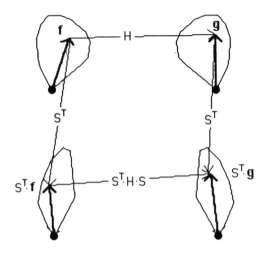

FIGURE 19.9.   Vector spaces associated with a system: the blobs in this figure represent the vector spaces associated with the operation of a system as represented with both the canonical basis vectors and the basis vectors rotated with S. The blob in the upper left is the vector space of the input vector, **f**. The blob on the right represents the vector space of the output vector, **g**. This vector space is the column space of H. The blob on the lower left is the vector space associated with $S^T \cdot$ **f**. The blob on the right is the vector space associated with $S^T \cdot$ **g**. The operation of $S^T \cdot H \cdot S$ on $S^T \cdot$ **f** to produce $S^T \cdot$ **g** is equivalent to the operation of H on **f** to produce **g**.

Let us start with the equation representing the operation of a system, H, on a signal **f** (Equation 9.1):

$$\mathbf{g} = H \cdot \mathbf{f} \tag{19.37}$$

If **f** and **g** are expressed in terms of one set of basis functions, then $S^T \cdot$ **f** and $S^T \cdot$ **g** are the same vectors in terms of a set of basis functions, s_j. Let us try to express Equation 19.37 in terms of $S^T \cdot$ **f** and $S^T \cdot$ **g**. Multiplying both sides of the equation by $S^T \cdot$ **g** gives:

$$S^T \cdot \mathbf{g} = S^T \cdot H \cdot \mathbf{f} \tag{19.38}$$

From Equation 19.19 we know that $S \cdot S^T$ is equal to I, the identity matrix; therefore we can expand Equation 19.38 as

$$S^T \cdot \mathbf{g} = S^T \cdot H \cdot S \cdot S^T \cdot \mathbf{f} \tag{19.39}$$

Let us rewrite Equation 19.39 to emphasize the various factors

$$(S^T \cdot \mathbf{g}) = (S^T \cdot H \cdot S) \cdot (S^T \cdot \mathbf{f}) \tag{19.40}$$

$S^T \cdot$ **g** is the output signal, **g**, written in terms of a new set of basis vectors, s_i. $S^T \cdot$ **f** is the input signal, **f**, written in terms of the new set of basis vectors. The remaining factor, $S^T \cdot H \cdot S$, must therefore represent the system in terms of the new set of basis functions. Figure 19.9 shows these relationships artistically.

In order to rotate a matrix to a new coordinate system we need to multiply it on both sides by the rotation matrix. On the left side we use S^T and on the right side we use S. Recall from Chapter 9 that the right most matrix in a product determined the row space and the left most matrix in a product determined the column space. One reason we need to multiply the matrix, H, on both sides is that we need to modify both the row space, associated with the input, and the column space, associated with the output, into the new coordinate system.

V. ROTATION TO AN EIGENVECTORS BASIS

Throughout the book there is a considerable emphasis on eigenvector representation of signals since the operation of systems on eigenvectors is particularly simple. In this section we shall see how it is possible to rotate the basis vectors to a representation in terms of eigenvectors. However, we first must explore the properties of diagonal matrices.

A diagonal matrix, D, is a matrix with all zero entries except for the diagonal. We can write:

$$d_{ij} = \begin{cases} d_i, & i = j \\ 0, & i \neq j \end{cases} \tag{19.41}$$

where we have written the element d_{ii} as d_i to emphasize that the diagonal elements can be seen as a one-dimensional set of numbers.

$$D = \begin{pmatrix} d_1 & 0 & 0 & \dots \\ 0 & d_2 & 0 & \dots \\ 0 & 0 & d_3 & \dots \\ & \dots & & \end{pmatrix} \tag{19.42}$$

Thus, the form of diagonal matrix is particularly simple. (In this section, we shall use d_i to indicate an element of the diagonal matrix, D. Hopefully, the reader will not confuse d_i with the canonical basis vectors, $\mathbf{d}_i$.)

Multiplication of a diagonal matrix times another matrix can be written:

$$D \cdot H = \left(\sum_k d_{ik} \cdot h_{kj} \right) \tag{19.43}$$

However, the only nonzero element in the sum is when k is equal to i. Therefore, we can write the product as:

$$D \cdot H = (d_i \cdot h_{ij}) = (d_i \cdot \mathbf{h_i^T}) \tag{19.44}$$

where the last equality uses the vector notation for a matrix. Equation 19.44 states that the product of a diagonal matrix and a second matrix is equal to the second matrix with each of the rows multiplied by the corresponding diagonal element, d_i.

Similarly, multiplication on the right by a diagonal matrix leads to a simple result.

$$H \cdot D = (h_{ij} \cdot d_j) = (d_j \cdot \mathbf{h_j}) \tag{19.45}$$

The product of a matrix and a diagonal matrix is equal to the columns of the matrix multiplied by the corresponding diagonal elements of the diagonal matrix.

The product of two diagonal matrices, D and D′, is also very simple:

$$D \cdot D' = \left(\sum_k d_{ik} \cdot d'_{kj} \right) \tag{19.46}$$

The only nonzero element, d_{ik}, is when i equals k:

$$D \cdot D' = (d_i \cdot d'_{ij}) \tag{19.47}$$

and the only nonzero element, d'_{ij}, is when i equals j:

$$D \cdot D' = \begin{cases} d_i \cdot d'_i, & i = j \\ 0, & i \neq j \end{cases} \tag{19.48}$$

Thus, the product of two diagonal matrices is just a diagonal matrix with the elements equal to a simple product of the corresponding diagonal elements.

We can now return to the problem of rotating a system, H, into an eigenvector basis. If we have an n by n matrix, H, which has N linearly independent eigenvectors, s_j, then we can rotate H into a description in terms of its eigenvectors $S^T \cdot H \cdot S$. Let us start with the product of H and S:

$$H \cdot S = (H \cdot s_j) \tag{19.49}$$

where we have expressed the product in terms of the columns of S. By definition the columns of S are the eigenvectors of H; therefore:

$$H \cdot S = (\lambda_j \cdot s_j) \tag{19.50}$$

The product takes a very simple form — the columns of S are simply multiplied by the corresponding eigenvectors.

We can define a diagonal matrix, Λ, where the elements on the diagonal are equal to the eigenvalues, λ_j.

$$\Lambda = \begin{pmatrix} \lambda_1 & 0 & 0 & \dots \\ 0 & \lambda_2 & 0 & \dots \\ 0 & 0 & \lambda_3 & \dots \\ \dots & \dots & \dots & \dots \end{pmatrix} \tag{19.51}$$

Because of the multiplicative property of diagonal matrices (Equation 19.45) we can write 19.50 as:

$$H \cdot S = S \cdot \Lambda \tag{19.52}$$

Multiplying both sides of Equation 19.52 by S^{-1} gives:

$$S^{-1} \cdot H \cdot S = S^{-1} \cdot S \cdot \Lambda = \Lambda \tag{19.53}$$

If the eigenvectors are also orthonormal, then S^{-1} is equal to S^T, so we can write:

$$S^T \cdot H \cdot S = \Lambda \tag{19.54}$$

Rotation of H into a basis, which is made up of its eigenvectors, transforms H into a very simple form — a diagonal matrix where the elements on the diagonal are equal to the corresponding eigenvalues.

Multiplication of a vector by a diagonal matrix is very simple. Each component of the vector is multiplied by the corresponding eigenvalue. This operation is equivalent in complexity to the multiplication of two vectors. Thus, transforming to an eigenvector set of basis vectors changes the complexity of calculating the effect of a system from a matrix multiplication to a simple vector multiplication.

In the derivation of Equation 19.54 we have assumed that the matrix, H, is a square matrix with a complete set of orthonormal eigenvectors. These assumptions put considerable limitations on the systems, H, which can be described by this simple form. These assumptions are, however, not quite as severe as it might at first seem. Derivation of the eigenvectors of a matrix is beyond the scope of this book; however, we shall state some facts about the eigenvectors of a matrix.[1] Nonsingular matrices often have linearly independent eigenvectors. If there is a set of linearly independent eigenvectors, then they can be scaled so that they are of length one. Thus, an orthonormal eigenvector set can be constructed.

In particular, we know that the eigenvectors of linear, time invariant systems are complex exponentials. If properly scaled, these eigenfunctions are a complete orthonormal set. Thus, all linear, time invariant systems can be transformed to a set of basis vectors, where the systems are diagonal matrices!

Since there are many systems which are linear and not time invariant and which have a complete set of orthonormal eigenvectors, it may seem that we have discovered a powerful method for solving problems. Unfortunately, almost all radiological systems which are linear and not time invariant are too complex to be modeled by such systems. Thus, our use of Equation 19.54 is to obtain a better understanding of transform operations rather than as a practical method to solve radiological problems.

VI. EXAMPLE OF THE ROTATION OF A SYSTEM TO AN EIGENVECTOR BASIS

Let us return to an example in Chapter 9. We defined a system with a diagonal matrix (Equation 9.30) which operated on a two-dimensional vector space.

$$H = \begin{pmatrix} 2 & 0 \\ 0 & 1 \end{pmatrix} \tag{19.55}$$

H expands a vector in the x direction by 2, and does not change the vector in the y direction. We found that the eigenvectors of this system were $\mathbf{d}_1$ and $\mathbf{d}_2$. The effect is to stretch the vector space in the x direction.

A second system was defined by Equation 9.34:

$$H = \begin{pmatrix} 1.8 & .4 \\ .4 & 1.2 \end{pmatrix} \tag{19.56}$$

This system performs the same operation; however, this time the expansion was along the direction of the vector $(1\ 2)^T$. We noted that these two systems were similar except that the second system was rotated with respect to the first system. However, the rotation made calculation of the effects of this second system more complex. The operation of this system was shown graphically in Figure 9.18.

In Chapter 9, we found that the eigenvectors of the matrix described in Equation 19.56 are in the directions of the two vectors, $(2\ 1)^T$ and $(-1\ 2)^T$. The length of both of these vectors is $\sqrt{5}$. Thus, a set of orthonormal eigenvectors for the matrix given by Equation

19.56 is $(1/\sqrt{5}) \cdot (2 \; 1)^{\mathrm{T}}$ and $(1/\sqrt{5}) \cdot (-1 \; 2)^{\mathrm{T}}$. Let us rotate this system with a matrix, S, given by:

$$S = 1/\sqrt{5} \cdot \begin{pmatrix} 2 & -1 \\ 1 & 2 \end{pmatrix} \tag{19.57}$$

If we multiply Equation 19.56 on the left by S^{T} and on the right by S we get:

$$1/5 \cdot \begin{pmatrix} 2 & 1 \\ -1 & 2 \end{pmatrix} \cdot \begin{pmatrix} 1.8 & .4 \\ .4 & 1.2 \end{pmatrix} \cdot \begin{pmatrix} 2 & -1 \\ 1 & 2 \end{pmatrix} = \begin{pmatrix} 2 & 0 \\ 0 & 1 \end{pmatrix} \tag{19.58}$$

The matrix in Equation 19.56 is transformed into a simple diagonal matrix, the matrix given in Equation 19.55.

Rotation of the basis vectors so that they lie along the eigenvectors of the system has made the system very simple, a diagonal matrix. Recall that we noted that the eigenvectors are natural to the matrix. The effect of a system on an eigenvector is only to change the magnitude, not the direction of the vector. Thus, when we rotate the basis vectors to lie along the eigenvectors, we get a particularly simple result. The system multiplies each of the components by the eigenvalue for that basis vector.

VII. ANALOGY BETWEEN MATRIX ROTATIONS AND LINEAR SYSTEMS

Above, the similarity between the discrete Fourier transform operation and a rotation has been noted. The discrete Fourier transform rotates from a description in terms of the canonical set of basis vectors to a description in terms of sinusoidal basis vectors. We have frequently noted that the sinusoids are the eigenfunctions of linear, time invariant systems. Thus, the discrete Fourier transform the systems to an eigenvector basis.

The Fourier transform matrix, W, has orthogonal columns — the sinusoids. These orthonormal columns are the eigenvectors for linear, time invariant systems. Thus rotation of a matrix, H, to a basis set of eigenvectors will produce a simple, diagonal matrix, Λ. By rotating the axes to this eigenvector set, the operation of the matrix is made very simple — each component of the input is simply multiplied by the corresponding eigenvalue. Description in terms of the eigenvectors has rotated the signals into a description in terms of the characteristic directions of a system. Like our example the axes lie along the directions of operation of the system.

In the time domain, the operation of a linear, time invariant system is described by convolution. Transforming to the frequency domain simplifies the operation to multiplication. Similarly, transformation to eigenvector basis, changes the complicated matrix multiplication operation into a simple operation, multiplication by a diagonal matrix.

The imaginary exponentials are eigenfunctions for all linear, time invariant systems. Therefore, the same transformation, the Fourier transform, can be used to express this whole set of systems in terms of an eigenfunction basis. Instead of finding the eigenfunctions for each system separately, we automatically know the eigenfunctions of a very large class of systems.

If we have two sequential linear, time invariant systems defined in terms of the imaginary exponentials, then they are both diagonal matrices. Instead of performing matrix multiplication, their product can be calculated by simply multiplying their eigenvalues (Equation 19.48). We have already met this property of Fourier transforms several times in this part of the book. It is the key property of the eigenfunction description of a system.

Description of the system which stretched vectors along $(2 \; 1)^{\mathrm{T}}$ was not natural in the canonical basis set, $\mathbf{d}_1, \mathbf{d}_2$. The components of the input vectors warped in peculiar ways.

By rotating to an eigenvector basis, the operation became very natural. The eigenvectors lie along the direction of the stretching. The description of linear, time invariant systems in terms of the sinusoids is natural to the system in the same way that description of the stretching operation is natural when the basis lies along the direction of stretch.

VIII. SUMMARY

The goal of this chapter is to provide some geometrical insight into transformation operations. They are similar to the rotation of the set vectors which define the basis of the system. The time and the frequency domain signal are two representations of the same signal. One is in terms of the delta functions and one is in terms of the imaginary exponentials. Both representations can be viewed as representing a single point in an N-dimensional space. The transform operation amounts to changing the basis vectors which are used to define this point.

For linear systems a particularly valuable transformation is to a description in terms of the eigenfunctions of the system. If the system is described in terms of the operation of a matrix on a vector, then the analogous operation is the rotation of the basis vectors to an eigenvector basis. Rotation to an eigenvector basis transforms the matrix to a diagonal matrix. For all linear, time invariant systems, this transformation can be performed by rotation with a matrix with columns which are the imaginary exponentials. This operation is exactly analogous to the discrete Fourier transform operation.

The system which performs the stretching operation is a good example for understanding eigenvectors. The stretching occurs along the eigenvectors. When the system is defined in terms of a basis which is not in the direction of the eigenvectors, then the stretching appears to be a complicated operation, affecting many or all of the components of the vector. When the system is defined along the stretching direction(s), then the system becomes much simpler, affecting only one component. The discrete Fourier transform transforms the description of linear, time invariant systems into the directions of their characteristic effects.

IX. FURTHER READING

Rotation of a basis set of vectors is described in Chapter 5 of the book by Strang.[1] Chapter 4 of the more advanced book by the same author[2] describes the discrete Fourier transform in terms of matrix operations.

REFERENCES

1. **Strang, G.,** *Linear Algebra and Its Applications,* Academic Press, New York, 1980.
2. **Strang, G.,** *Introduction to Applied Mathematics,* Wellesley-Cambridge Press, Wellesley, MA, 1986.

Chapter 20

OTHER TRANSFORMS

This chapter will briefly introduce a number of other transform operations — the multi-dimensional Fourier transform, the Fourier series, the z transform, the Laplace transform, the Hankel transforms, and the Radon transform. These transforms are not used in this book; however, they are briefly introduced to help explain aspects of the Fourier transform. The task in this chapter will be to understand how the various transforms relate to each other, rather than to learn about these transforms for their own sake.

Two portions of this chapter will be used later in the book. In the section on the multi-dimensional Fourier transform, we shall find that rotation of the coordinate system in one domain results in a similar rotation in the other domain. This property is very useful for understanding reconstruction in computed tomography. The section on the relationship between the discrete and continuous Fourier transform is important for understanding the process of sampling in Chapter 23.

This chapter is more mathematical than most of the rest of the book. It is particularly useful for the reader who has some previous familiarity with other transform operations and wishes to understand how the Fourier transform relates to other transform operations. This chapter can be skipped on first reading.

I. MULTI-DIMENSIONAL FOURIER TRANSFORMS

In Chapter 14, we introduced the one- and two-dimensional Fourier transforms (Equations 14.6, 14.7, 14.32, and 14.33). In this section we shall extend this description to allow any number of dimensions. Multi-dimensional signals occur naturally in radiological applications. Up to three spatial dimensions and a time dimension are used in many fields. In addition, velocity and chemical shift dimensions can occur in nuclear magnetic resonance imaging.

We shall use the vectors, $\mathbf{x}$ and $\mathbf{k}$, to represent the independent variables in the space and frequency domains, respectively. The components of the variables are:

$$\mathbf{x} = (x_1 \quad x_2 \quad x_3 \quad ...)^T \tag{20.1}$$

$$\mathbf{k} = (k_1 \quad k_2 \quad k_3 \quad ...)^T \tag{20.2}$$

Both vectors have N components. For N equal to 1, we have the usual one-dimensional Fourier transform where x_1 and k_1 are either t and ω or x and k_x. For N equal to 2, we have the two-dimensional Fourier transform where x_1 and x_2 represent x and y, and k_1 and k_2 represent k_x and k_y.

Previously we have used vectors with the Fourier transform to represent the dependent variable, e.g., we used $\mathbf{f}$ to represent f(t). In this section we are using vectors for the independent variables. The space domain signal is f($\mathbf{x}$) and the frequency domain variable is F($\mathbf{k}$). An N-dimensional vector as an independent variable is equivalent to N independent variables, $f(x_1,x_2,x_3, \ldots)$ and $F(k_1,k_2,k_3, \ldots)$.

Using these vectors, we can write the multi-dimensional Fourier transform quite simply:

$$f(\mathbf{x}) = [1/(2\pi)^N] \int_{-\infty}^{+\infty} F(\mathbf{k}) \cdot e^{i\mathbf{x}^T \cdot \mathbf{k}} \, d\mathbf{k} \tag{20.3}$$

$$F(\mathbf{k}) = \int_{-\infty}^{+\infty} f(\mathbf{x}) \cdot e^{-i\mathbf{x}^T \cdot \mathbf{k}} \, d\mathbf{x} \tag{20.4}$$

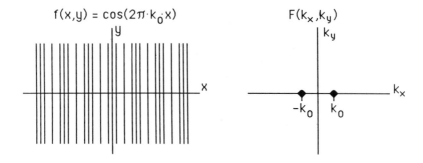

FIGURE 20.1. Two-dimensional Fourier transform: on the left is a diagrammatic representation of a two-dimensional cosine wave which varies along the x direction with a spatial frequency given by k_0. The areas where the lines are closely spaced indicate places where the signal has a large magnitude. On the right is a diagrammatic representation of the two-dimensional Fourier transform of the signal on the cosine wave. The Fourier transform consists of two delta functions on the k_x axis at position k_0 and $-k_0$.

The basis functions can be expanded in terms of their components:

$$e^{i\mathbf{x}^T \cdot \mathbf{k}} = e^{i(x_1 k_1 + x_2 k_2 + x_3 k_3 + \ldots)} \tag{20.5}$$

In this form, the basis functions can be more easily recognized as functions of a multi-dimensional space. Although we have written these equations with a single integral sign for simplicity, the integration is actually over N dimensions. Thus, these two equations are deceptively simple.

Except for the N on the 2π, Equations 20.3 and 20.4 look remarkably like the one-dimensional Fourier transform equations. In fact, this book largely ignores the difference between the one-dimensional Fourier transform and the multi-dimensional Fourier transform. The applications of the Fourier transform in Part IV deal largely with two- and three-dimensional signals, while the first three parts deal almost exclusively with one-dimensional signals. Although there is relatively little conceptual difference between the one- and multi-dimensional Fourier transform, the reader should keep in mind that Equation 20.3 and 20.4 are quite complex mathematical operations.

A. ROTATION OF A SIGNAL AND ITS TRANSFORM

Now let us consider what happens when we rotate a signal. Figure 20.1 shows a two-dimensional signal which is a cosine along the x direction:

$$f(x,y) = \cos(2\pi \cdot k_0 \cdot x) \tag{20.6}$$

Its Fourier transform is a pair of delta functions on the k_x axis at $2\pi \cdot k_0$. The signal rotated by an angle, θ, is shown in Figure 20.2. Its Fourier transform is a pair of delta functions on a line rotated by θ from the k_x axis. When a signal is rotated, its transform is rotated in the same way. Below we shall prove that this property is true in general.

In the last chapter we described rotation of a coordinate system. Rotation of a coordinate system is equivalent to rotating a signal in the opposite directions (see Figure 19.6). Consider a signal $g(\mathbf{x})$ which is a rotated version of $f(\mathbf{x})$:

$$g(\mathbf{x}) = f(S^T \cdot \mathbf{x}) \tag{20.7}$$

where S is defined to have orthonormal columns (see Equation 19.17).

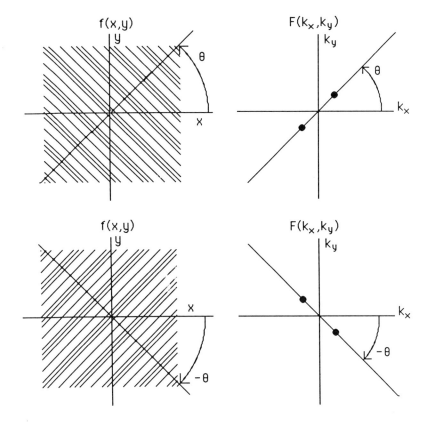

FIGURE 20.2. Rotation of a signal and its Fourier transform: on the left are two cosine waves which are similar to the cosine shown in Figure 20.1. On the top the cosine is rotated by an angle, θ, and on the bottom the cosine is rotated by an angle, −θ. The Fourier transforms of these two signals are similar to the Fourier transform of the signal shown in Figure 20.1. On the top, the Fourier transform has been rotated by an angle, θ, and on the bottom, the Fourier transform has been rotated by an angle, −θ.

Consider for example S given by Equation 19.1:

$$S = \begin{pmatrix} \cos\theta & -\sin\theta \\ \sin\theta & \cos\theta \end{pmatrix} \qquad (20.8)$$

Recall there are two ways of visualizing the effects of S — it rotates the x,y coordinate system by an angle θ to the x′,y′ coordinate system, or it rotates the signal, f(**x**), by an angle −θ to the signal g(**x**). Figure 20.3 shows an example of a signal on a two coordinate system and two signals on the same coordinate system.

Now let us try to calculate the Fourier transform of g(**x**):

$$G(\mathbf{k}) = \int_{-\infty}^{+\infty} f(S^T \cdot \mathbf{x}) \cdot e^{-i\mathbf{x}^T \cdot \mathbf{k}} \, d\mathbf{x} \qquad (20.9)$$

We can substitute for the variable of integration:

$$\mathbf{x}' = S^T \cdot \mathbf{x} \qquad (20.10)$$

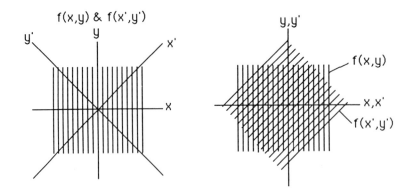

FIGURE 20.3.   Rotation of a signal: on the left is a diagram of a two-dimensional signal. There are two coordinate systems, x,y and x',y', which are rotated with respect to each other. On the right the coordinate systems are made to align with each other. The two representations of the signal are then rotated with respect to each other. This diagram shows two mathematically equivalent points of view of the rotation operation. Either the coordinate axes are rotated by a positive angle, or the signals are rotated by a negative angle.

Then the Fourier transform becomes:

$$G(\mathbf{k}) = \int_{-\infty}^{+\infty} f(\mathbf{x}') \cdot e^{-i(S \cdot \mathbf{x}')^T \cdot \mathbf{k}} \, d(S \cdot \mathbf{x}') \qquad (20.11)$$

In general this type of change of variable is very complicated. However, this change of variables is simplified by the fact that the limits of integration are all from $-\infty$ to $+\infty$, and S is defined to be an orthonormal transformation. Because of the orthonormality, the new differential can be written:

$$d(S \cdot \mathbf{x}') = d\mathbf{x}' \qquad (20.12)$$

The exponent on the basis functions can be transformed using Equation 8.43:

$$(S \cdot \mathbf{x}')^T \cdot \mathbf{k} = \mathbf{x}'^T \cdot (S^T \cdot \mathbf{k}) \qquad (20.13)$$

Using Equations 20.12 and 20.13, we can rewrite the Fourier transform:

$$G(\mathbf{k}) = \int_{-\infty}^{+\infty} f(\mathbf{x}') \cdot e^{-i\mathbf{x}'^T \cdot (S^T \cdot \mathbf{k})} \, d\mathbf{x}' \qquad (20.14)$$

However, this integral is the Fourier transform of $f(\mathbf{x})$ with respect to the frequency $S^T \cdot \mathbf{k}$, using $\mathbf{x}'$ as a dummy variable of integration. Therefore:

$$G(\mathbf{k}) = F(S^T \cdot \mathbf{k}) \qquad (20.15)$$

In summary, the Fourier transform of the rotated signal, $f(S^T \cdot \mathbf{x})$, is the rotated Fourier transform, $F(S^T \cdot \mathbf{k})$. When a signal is rotated, its transform is rotated in exactly the same fashion. Using our two headed notation, we can write:

$$f(S^T \cdot \mathbf{x}) \leftrightarrow F(S^T \cdot \mathbf{k}) \qquad (20.16)$$

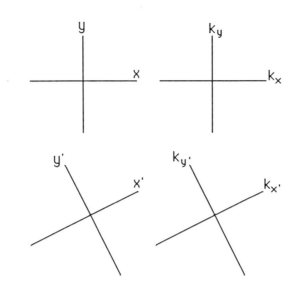

FIGURE 20.4. Rotation in the space and spatial frequency domains: the top panel shows the spatial and spatial frequency coordinate axes for a two-dimensional signal. The bottom panel shows that when the spatial coordinate axes are rotated, the spatial frequency coordinate axes are rotated by the same angle.

Figure 20.4 shows the relationship between the two pairs of coordinate systems, x,y and x′,y′, and k_x,k_y and k′$_x$,k′$_y$. This property will be important for understanding the reconstruction from projections.

II. CORRESPONDENCE BETWEEN THE CONTINUOUS AND THE DISCRETE FOURIER TRANSFORMS

In Chapter 23 (Sampling) we shall see how discrete signals can be obtained from continuous signals by sampling, and we shall see the effects that sampling in one domain has on the other domain. These effects will be very important for understanding some of the artifacts which are produced in nuclear magnetic resonance imaging. Chapter 23 will depend upon understanding how the discrete and continuous Fourier transforms are related. In this section we are interested in developing an understanding of the correspondence of the discrete and continuous Fourier transforms.

It is possible to consider discrete signals with more and more points. As the number of points increases, the discrete signal f[n] will approximate the continuous signal, f(t), or the discrete signal, F[k], will approximate the continuous signal, F(ω), or both. There are a number of ways to associate the discrete variables n and k with the continuous variables t and ω. The relation between the variables will determine which signals become continuous.

Table 20.1 shows the four combinations of discrete and continuous variables which can be used to define different types of Fourier transforms. The first transform is the discrete Fourier transform. The second transform is the **Fourier series**. The third transform is analogous to the second, but the roles of the time and frequency variables is switched. Since these two transforms are related by the duality property of the Fourier transform (see Chapter 15), we shall call this transform the dual of the Fourier series. In a slightly different form it is referred to as the **z transform**. The fourth transform is the continuous Fourier transform.

TABLE 20.1
Relation Between Continuous and Discrete Transforms

	Variable	Period	Step	Signal
Discrete Fourier Transform: Discrete Time Discrete Frequency				
Time	n	N	1	$f[n]$
Frequency	k	N	1	$F[k]$
Fourier Series: Continuous Time, Discrete Frequency				
Time	$t = n/N$	1	$1/N$	$f(t) = N \cdot f[N \cdot t]$
Frequency	k	N	1	$F[k]$
Dual of the Fourier Series: Discrete Time, Continuous Frequency				
Time	n	N	1	$f[n]$
Frequency	$\omega = 2\pi \cdot k/N$	2π	$2\pi/N$	$F(\omega) = F[N \cdot \omega/2\pi]$
Fourier Transform: Continuous Time, Continuous Frequency				
Time	$t = n/\sqrt{N}$	$\sqrt{N}$	$1/\sqrt{N}$	$f[n] = \sqrt{N} \cdot f(\sqrt{N} \cdot t)$
Frequency	$\omega = 2\pi \cdot k/\sqrt{N}$	$2\pi \cdot \sqrt{N}$	$2\pi/\sqrt{N}$	$F(\omega) = F[\sqrt{N} \cdot \omega/2\pi]$

A. DISCRETE FOURIER TRANSFORM: DISCRETE TIME, DISCRETE FREQUENCY

Because $f[n]$ and $F[k]$ are periodic signals, the discrete Fourier transform can be defined over any interval (see Equations 18.10 and 18.12). In this section it will be convenient to define it from $-N/2$ to $(N/2) - 1$. (We have assumed that N is even, but the following could be extended to the case where N is odd.) Using the interval $-N/2$ to $(N/2) - 1$, the discrete Fourier transform is written:

$$f[n] = (1/N) \cdot \sum_{k=-N/2}^{(N/2)-1} F[k] \cdot e^{i2\pi kn/N} \tag{20.17}$$

$$F[k] = \sum_{n=-N/2}^{(N/2)-1} f[n] \cdot e^{-i2\pi kn/N} \tag{20.18}$$

To understand the relationships between the various transforms it is useful to understand how the time and frequency domain signals are related. The time and frequency domain axes for the four transforms are shown in Figure 20.5. The two most important factors relating the signals are the period of the signals and the step between the points where the signals are defined. For the discrete Fourier transform both of the signals, $f[n]$ and $F[k]$, are periodic with period N. The size of the step between points on both axes is 1. The period and the step size are listed in Table 20.1.

B. FOURIER SERIES: CONTINUOUS TIME, DISCRETE FREQUENCY

The Fourier series relates a continuous time signal to a discrete frequency signal. The Fourier series can be obtained from the discrete Fourier transform by associating the discrete time variable, n, with the continuous time variable, t, as follows:

$$t = n/N \tag{20.19}$$

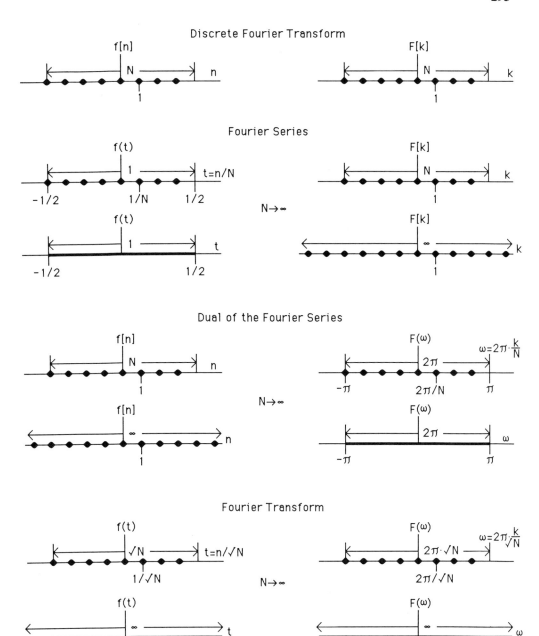

FIGURE 20.5. Relation between transform operations: this figure shows the relation between the discrete Fourier transform, the Fourier series, the dual of the Fourier series, and the Fourier transform. These relations are also summarized in Table 20.1. The time and frequency domains for the discrete Fourier transform are shown on the top panel. For the other transformation operations, two graphs of the time and frequency domain are shown. First, the relation to the discrete Fourier transform is shown, and then, the number of points, N, is set equal to infinity. If the period in one domain is a function of N, then the interval in the other domain is a function of N. As N goes to infinity, the signal becomes aperiodic in one domain and continuous in the other domain.

As n varies from $-N/2$ to $(N/2)-1$, t varies from $-1/2$ to $(1/2)-(1/N)$. Using the variable t, the basis functions can be rewritten:

$$e^{i2\pi kn/N} = e^{i2\pi kt} \tag{20.20}$$

Figure 20.5 shows the time and frequency domain axes. The time domain signal, f(t), is periodic with the period 1, and the frequency domain signal, F[k] is periodic with period N. The size of the step between points on the t axis is 1/N, and the size of the step between points on the k axis is 1. These relations are listed in Table 20.1.

As the number of points, N, increases, the period of the signal, f(t), remains 1. The step, 1/N, decreases. As N goes to infinity, f(t) becomes continuous over the interval −1/2 to 1/2 (Figure 20.5). As N increases, the period of F[k], which is equal to N, increase, and the step size, 1, does not change. As N goes to infinity, F[k] remains discrete, and the period becomes infinite, i.e., it becomes aperiodic. The continuity of the time variable, t, is associated with an infinite period for the frequency signal, F[k]. The finite period of the time signal is associated with a discrete frequency variable.

We have defined a relation between the discrete and the continuous time variable, but we have not yet defined the relation between the discrete and continuous signals. We shall select the following relation:

$$f(t) = N \cdot f[N \cdot t] \qquad (20.21)$$

where we have chosen to write the discrete variable, n, as $N \cdot t$ using Equation 20.19.

It is now possible to rewrite the discrete Fourier transform equations using t and k:

$$N \cdot f[N \cdot t] = \sum_{k=-N/2}^{(N/2)-1} F[k] \cdot e^{i2\pi kt} \qquad (20.22)$$

$$F[k] = \sum_{N \cdot t = -N/2}^{(N/2)-1} N \cdot f[N \cdot t] \cdot e^{-i2\pi kt} \cdot (1/N) \qquad (20.23)$$

where we have expressed the discrete variable, n, as $N \cdot t$. Notice that we have added two factors N and 1/N in the second equation. These two factors cancel each other.

Now consider what happens to these relations as N goes to infinity. The second equation will take on the form of an integral equation (see Equation 2.18). The factor 1/N in the second equation is equal to Δt, the spacing between points on the t axis. Thus as N goes to infinity:

$$f(t) = \sum_{k=-\infty}^{\infty} F[k] \cdot e^{i2\pi kt} \qquad (20.24)$$

$$F[k] = \int_{-\infty}^{+\infty} f(t) \cdot e^{-i2\pi kt} \, dt \qquad (20.25)$$

This pair of equations define the **Fourier series**. The Fourier series transforms between a continuous periodic time signal, f(t), and a discrete aperiodic frequency signal, F[k]. The Fourier series is particularly useful when the signal, f(t), can be modeled by a small number of sinusoidal components. In that case, F[k], is nonzero only for a small number of components, and it provides a simple representation for the signal.

C. DUAL OF THE FOURIER SERIES: DISCRETE TIME, CONTINUOUS FREQUENCY

The second method of associating the continuous and discrete variables is the dual relation of the Fourier series. It will lead to a relation between a continuous, periodic frequency domain signal and a discrete, aperiodic time domain signal. Below we shall see that with a modification of the frequency domain variable this transform is equivalent to a transform used extensively in electrical engineering known as the z transform.

Let us associate the continuous frequency variable, ω, with the discrete frequency variable, k, as follows:

$$\omega = 2\pi \cdot k/N \tag{20.26}$$

Figure 20.5 and Table 20.1 show these relations. As k runs from $-N/2$ to $(N/2) - 1$, ω runs from $-\pi$ to $\pi - \pi/N$. The period of $F(\omega)$ is 2π. The step on the ω axis is $2\pi/N$. Substituting into the basis functions gives:

$$e^{i2\pi kn/N} = e^{i\omega n} \tag{20.27}$$

As N goes to infinity, the period of f[n] becomes infinite, and the step remains 1. The period of $F(\omega)$ remains 2π, and the step goes to zero. f[n] becomes an infinite, discrete signal, and $F(\omega)$ becomes a periodic, continuous signal. We have selected the correspondence between k and ω (Equation 20.26), but we also need to choose the relation between $F(\omega)$ and F[k]. Let us choose:

$$F(\omega) = F[N \cdot \omega/2\pi] \tag{20.28}$$

We have chosen to write the discrete frequency variable, k, in terms of the continuous frequency variable, ω.

Now we can substitute into the discrete Fourier transform relation:

$$f[n] = (1/2\pi) \cdot \sum_{N\cdot\omega/2\pi = -N/2}^{(N/2)-1} F[N \cdot \omega/2\pi] \cdot e^{i\omega n} \cdot 2\pi/N \tag{20.29}$$

$$F[N \cdot \omega/2\pi] = \sum_{n = -N/2}^{(N/2)-1} f[n] \cdot e^{-i\omega n} \tag{20.30}$$

Again we have used $N \cdot \omega/2\pi$ for the frequency variable k.

The first equation of the pair, Equation 20.29, is in the form of an integral definition where $2\pi/N$ is equal to $\Delta\omega$. As N goes to infinity, this pair of equations becomes:

$$f[n] = (1/2\pi) \cdot \int_{-\infty}^{+\infty} F(\omega) \cdot e^{i\omega n} \, d\omega \tag{20.31}$$

$$F(\omega) = \sum_{n = -\infty}^{\infty} f[n] \cdot e^{-i\omega n} \tag{20.32}$$

These equations relate a discrete, aperiodic, time domain signal, f[n], to a continuous, periodic, frequency domain signal, $F(\omega)$.

This transform is rarely used in this form. Instead a new variable, z, is defined as:

$$z = e^{i\omega} \tag{20.33}$$

The basis functions are then equal to z^n. In this form, this transform is called the z transform. We shall briefly come back to the z transform below.

D. FOURIER TRANSFORM: CONTINUOUS TIME, CONTINUOUS FREQUENCY

The third method of relating the discrete and continuous variables is:

$$t = n/\sqrt{N} \tag{20.34}$$

$$\omega = 2\pi \cdot k/\sqrt{N} \tag{20.35}$$

This relationship is shown in Figure 20.5. The period of $f(t)$ is $\sqrt{N}$, and the period of $F(\omega)$ is $2\pi \cdot \sqrt{N}$. The step between points on the time axis is $\sqrt{N}$, and the step between points on the frequency axis is $2\pi/\sqrt{N}$(see Table 20.1). Substituting into the basis function gives:

$$e^{i2\pi kn/N} = e^{i\omega t} \tag{20.36}$$

As N goes to infinity, the period of $f(t)$ goes to infinity, and the step on the time axis goes to zero. The period of $F(\omega)$ also goes to infinity and the step on the frequency axis also goes to zero. Both $f(t)$ and $F(\omega)$ becomes continuous, aperiodic signals. The continuity of $f(t)$ is associated with the aperiodicity of $F(\omega)$ as in the case of the Fourier series, and the continuity of $F(\omega)$ is associated with the aperiodicity of $f(t)$ as in the last example.

As in the previous examples, in addition to defining the relation between the discrete and continuous variables, we need to define the relation between the discrete and continuous signals.

$$f(t) = \sqrt{N} \cdot f[\sqrt{N} \cdot t] \tag{20.37}$$

$$F(\omega) = F[\sqrt{N} \cdot \omega/2\pi] \tag{20.38}$$

Using t and ω, the discrete Fourier transform relations can be rewritten:

$$\sqrt{N} \cdot f[\sqrt{N} \cdot t] = (1/2\pi) \cdot \sum_{N\cdot\omega/2\pi = -N/2}^{(N/2)-1} F[\sqrt{N} \cdot \omega/2\pi] \cdot e^{i\omega t} \cdot 2\pi/\sqrt{N} \tag{20.39}$$

$$F[\sqrt{N} \cdot \omega/2\pi] = \sum_{N t = -N/2}^{(N/2)-1} \sqrt{N} \cdot f[\sqrt{N} \cdot t] \cdot e^{-i\omega t} \cdot 1/\sqrt{N} \tag{20.40}$$

As N goes to infinity, both of these equations take on the form of integrals. $2\pi/\sqrt{N}$ becomes $d\omega$, and $1/\sqrt{N}$ becomes dt. Thus:

$$f(t) = (1/2\pi) \cdot \int_{-\infty}^{+\infty} F(\omega) \cdot e^{i\omega t} \, d\omega \tag{20.41}$$

$$F(\omega) = \int_{-\infty}^{+\infty} f(t) \cdot e^{-i\omega t} \, dt \tag{20.42}$$

These equations are identical to the definition of the continuous Fourier transform (Equations 14.6 and 14.7).

The major reason for discussing the Fourier series and its dual operation is to understand how continuity and aperiodicity are related. Table 20.1 shows the steps and the periods for the four types of transforms. It is easy to get confused about where the "2π"'s go in these various transforms, but it is more important to understand that the step between points in one domain is inversely related to the period in the other domain. When the period is finite in one domain, then the step is finite in the other domain; when the period is infinite in one domain, then the step is zero in the other domain. Discrete signals have periodic transforms, and continuous signals have aperiodic transforms.

The basis functions for the discrete Fourier transform are periodic with period N/k. Since k is an integer, all of the basis functions are periodic with period N. Thus, the signals being represented by the periodic sinusoids are themselves periodic. When the frequency axis becomes continuous, the period on the time axis becomes aperiodic. The basis functions are no longer all multiples of the same period. For example, we can pick ω small enough so that the period of $e^{i\omega t}$ is arbitrarily long. This fact helps to explain why the periodic sinusoids can be used to represent an aperiodic signal.

III. LAPLACE TRANSFORM

Many times in this book we have emphasized the value of complex numbers in providing a more accurate description of a problem. Our description of the various transforms has relied heavily on the fact that the signals had complex values. However, so far the dependent variables, t and ω, have always been real. (The exceptionally astute reader may have noticed that the dependent variable, z, in the z transform is complex.) The major difference between the Fourier transform and the Laplace transform is that the frequency variable is complex.

Let us start with the conclusion, the Laplace transform pair:

$$f(t) \, = \, (1/2\pi i) \cdot \int_{\sigma - i\infty}^{\sigma + i\infty} F(s) \cdot e^{st} \, ds \tag{20.43}$$

$$F(s) \, = \, \int_{-\infty}^{+\infty} f(t) \cdot e^{-st} \, dt \tag{20.44}$$

This transform looks a great deal like the Fourier transform except that the basis function is e^{st} instead of $e^{i\omega t}$, and the inverse Laplace transform has some "i"'s in it.

For the inverse Laplace transform, the variable of integration, s, runs from $\sigma - i\infty$ to $\sigma + i\infty$. The real part of s is a constant equal to σ. The imaginary part of s varies from $-i\infty$ to $i\infty$. We can define the variable, s, in terms of its real and imaginary parts:

$$s \, = \, \sigma \, + \, i \cdot \omega \tag{20.45}$$

Due to the path of integration, σ, the real part of s does not vary, but ω varies from $-\infty$ to $+\infty$.

The basis functions, e^{st}, can be written in terms of the real and imaginary parts of the exponent:

$$e^{st} \, = \, e^{(\sigma + i\omega)t} \, = \, e^{\sigma t} \cdot e^{i\omega t} \tag{20.46}$$

The basis functions consist of an exponential factor, $e^{\sigma t}$, and a sinusoidal factor, $e^{i\omega t}$.

If σ is negative, then the basis functions decrease over time. If σ is positive, the basis functions increase over time. Figure 20.6 shows two basis functions, one with σ negative and one with σ positive. The function, $e^{\sigma t}$, forms an envelope for the sinusoidally varying factor, $e^{i\omega t}$.

Since σ is constant,

$$ds \, = \, i \cdot d\omega \tag{20.47}$$

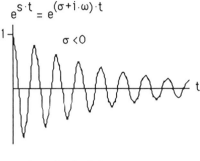

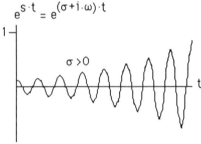

FIGURE 20.6.   Basis functions for the Laplace transform: this figure shows the real parts of two signals from two sets of the basis functions for the Laplace transform. σ is the real part of the frequency variable, s. For σ less than zero, the sinusoidal variations decrease with time. For σ greater than zero, the sinusoidal variations increase with time.

With some fancy footwork on the variable of integration and the limits of integration, we can rewrite the Laplace transform:

$$f(t) = (1/2\pi) \cdot \int_{-\infty}^{+\infty} F(\sigma + i \cdot \omega) \cdot e^{-\sigma t} \cdot e^{i\omega t} \, d\omega \tag{20.48}$$

$$F(\sigma + i \cdot \omega) = \int_{-\infty}^{+\infty} f(t) \cdot e^{-\sigma t} \cdot e^{-i\omega t} \, dt \tag{20.49}$$

Since the factor $e^{\sigma t}$ is a constant within the inverse Laplace transform, we can move it to the other side of the equation:

$$\{f(t) \cdot e^{-\sigma t}\} = (1/2\pi) \cdot \int_{-\infty}^{+\infty} F(\sigma + i \cdot \omega) \cdot e^{i\omega t} \, d\omega \tag{20.50}$$

$$F(\sigma + i \cdot \omega) = \int_{-\infty}^{+\infty} \{f(t) \cdot e^{-\sigma t}\} \cdot e^{-i\omega t} \, dt \tag{20.51}$$

In this form we can see the relationship between the Laplace transform and the Fourier transform. The Laplace transform of f(t) is equal to the Fourier transform of $f(t) \cdot e^{-\sigma t}$. In Chapter 22 we shall refer to multiplication in the time domain as a windowing operation. Using that terminology, the Laplace transform is equal to a Fourier transform of signal windowed by $e^{-\sigma t}$.

The Laplace transform of a signal depends both on the signal and the choice of the constant, σ. With σ equal to zero, the Laplace transform is equal to the Fourier transform. With other values of σ, the Laplace transform may have much different values than the

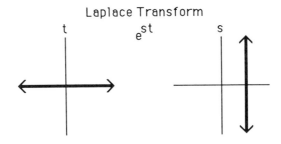

FIGURE 20.7. Path of integration for the Laplace transform: the basis functions for the Laplace transform are e^{st}. The path of integration of the inverse Laplace transform is a line parallel to the imaginary axis. The path of integration of the Laplace transform is the real axis. The paths of integration are rotated by $\pi/2$ with respect to each other.

Fourier transform. In applications, the Laplace transform and the Fourier transform are often used interchangeably. The Laplace transform is preferable to the Fourier transform when the set of basis functions, e^{st}, are more similar to the signals being modeled than the basis functions, $e^{i\omega t}$. In Chapter 29 we shall get some insight into when this might occur.

Our description of the Laplace transform has been very selective. We have ignored many very important aspects of the theory of Laplace transforms. One of these has to do with when a Laplace transform exists. Recall that we largely ignored the question of existence for Fourier transforms since all of the signals of interest in Radiology have Fourier transforms. One area where Laplace transforms are used extensively is for signals which do not have Fourier transforms. A central issue for Laplace transforms is the values of the constant, σ, for which the transform exists. These values are known as the **region of convergence**. We shall not discuss this important topic.

In mathematics and physics text, the limits of integration of the Laplace transform are defined from 0 to $+i\infty$, instead of from $-i\infty$ to $+i\infty$. In this form the Laplace transform is particularly useful for solving differential equations with initial conditions. This definition of the Laplace transform is sometimes called the unilateral Laplace transform, and our definition is called the bilateral Laplace transform. The bilateral Laplace transform is used more commonly in electrical engineering.

IV. PATH OF INTEGRATION IN THE COMPLEX PLANE

The Laplace transform is a bridge to considering all of the transform operations in terms of complex independent variables for both the time and frequency domains. We do not naturally think of the time or space variables as having complex values; however, the definitions of the various transform operations can be extended to allow the independent variables to be complex. Complex variables are defined on a plane (see Chapter 6). Thus, a new consideration which is introduced by allowing complex independent variables is the path of integration for the transform equations.

Figure 20.7 shows the path of integration for the time and frequency variables for the Laplace transform. The path of integration for the time variable is the real axis. The path of integration for the frequency variable is a line parallel to the imaginary axis. When σ is equal to zero, i.e., the Fourier transform, the path of integration is along the imaginary axis.

When we described the Fourier transform pair we noted that the forward transform had a negative exponent for the basis functions while the inverse transform had a positive exponent. By considering Figure 20.7 we see that the frequency domain signal is defined in terms of a path of integration which is rotated by $\pi/2$ as compared to the time domain.

Applying the forward transform twice results in a rotation by π, i.e., two applications of the Fourier transform produce f($-$t) (see Equation 15.7). Four applications of the forward transform rotates by 2π, returning the original signal. The change in sign of the basis functions rotates in the other direction.

The time domain signal, f(t), defined by the inverse Laplace transform (Equation 20.43) is defined for all points on the complex plane, not just the points on the real axis. Similarly, the frequency domain signal, F(s), defined by the Laplace transform (Equation 20.44), is defined for all frequencies, s, not just the points for which the real part of s is equal to σ. A function defined on the complex plane is analogous to a two-dimensional function defined in terms of real variables.

The astute reader may find it strange that it is possible to transform between signals defined on the whole complex plane using integration that includes only the values of the signals along a line in that plane. The explanation is found in the theory of analytic functions (see Chapter 6). If our derivation had been more rigorous, we would have stressed the fact that the Laplace transform is valid only for the set of signals which are analytic in a strip along the path of integration.

The theory of analytic functions on the complex plane is beyond the scope of this book. All we need to know is that requiring the signals to be analytic in a strip along the path of integration puts marked mathematical constraints on the set of functions which can be represented. This limited set of functions is completely defined by the values along the path of integration. From a practical point of view, all physical signals of interest in radiology are analytic, and therefore, this limited set of functions includes all of the functions of interest in this book. The theory of complex variables is very rich, and the reader who finds the material in this chapter interesting may wish to investigate this theory more deeply.

Let us consider which values of the independent variable are used in the other transforms. Figure 20.8 shows the points for which the discrete Fourier transform is defined. The time and frequency domain signals repeat every N points — the time domain is periodic along the real axis, and the frequency domain is periodic along the imaginary axis.

Figure 20.8 also shows the relation for the Fourier series. The Fourier series is periodic along the real axis in the time domain, and it is discrete along the imaginary axis in the frequency domain.

Figure 20.8 also shows the relation for the dual relation to the Fourier series. The dual of the Fourier series is periodic along the imaginary frequency axis, and it is discrete along the real time axis. Also shown is the relation for the z transform where z is given by Equation 20.33:

$$z = e^{i\omega} \tag{20.52}$$

Notice that the imaginary axis in Figure 20.8 maps to the unit circle in the z axis. The periodicity along the imaginary frequency axis corresponds to circular motion in the z plane.

In Chapter 17 we introduced the polynomial transform. The inverse polynomial transform, called evaluation, uses coefficient values, a[k], defined on a set of discrete points along the real frequency axis:

$$f(t) = \Sigma\ a[k] \cdot t^k \tag{20.53}$$

When the summation is from 0 to ∞, this equation is known as the Taylor series. When the summation is from $-\infty$ to $+\infty$, this equation is known as the Laurent series.

The forward polynomial transform, called interpolation, was only briefly discussed in Chapter 17. One possible way to define interpolation is in terms of the values of t defined around a circle in the complex plane. Using this type of interpolation, the polynomial

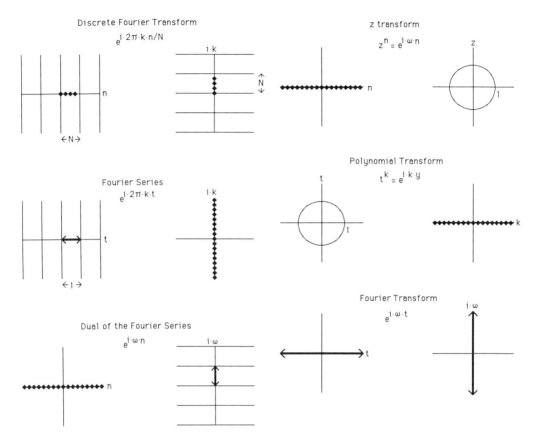

FIGURE 20.8. Path of summation or integration for several transforms: the basis functions and the points of definition for several transform operations are shown. Periodic signals are indicated by vertical or horizontal lines in the case of the discrete Fourier transform, the Fourier series, and the dual of the Fourier series. The periodicity of the z transform and the polynomial transform is related to the circular path of integration. The path of integration shown for the polynomial transform is not the usual method of interpolation, but it shows the analogy between the z transform and the polynomial transform.

transform is the dual of the z transform. Figure 20.8 shows the points for which such a transform is defined.

V. COMPLEXITY OF THE SIGNALS REPRESENTED BY VARIOUS TRANSFORMS

One way of categorizing the transforms is in terms of the complexity of the signals which can be represented. The complexity of the signals is related to the number of points at which values of the signals need to be defined in order to specify the signals. In general, to define a signal on the complex plane, the value of a signal needs to be given for every point in the complex plane.

The signals, used with the Laplace and Fourier transforms, are less complex. They can be completely defined by specifying the values of the signals at a continuous set of points along a line. For the Fourier series, the z transform, and the polynomial transform, the signals can be defined in one domain by a set of discrete points along an infinite length line and in the other domain by a set of continuous points along a finite length line. For the discrete Fourier transform, both time and frequency domain signals are completely defined by the values at N points.

Thus, the transform operations fall into three groups based on the complexity of the signals which can be represented. In general, the complexity of the signal in one domain must be equal to the complexity of the signal in the other domain in order to allow transformation back and forth between domains. A signal defined in terms of N values in one domain will also be defined in terms of N values in the other domain.

VI. HANKEL TRANSFORMS

The Bessel functions are used as the basis functions for the Hankel transforms. The different types of Bessel functions are used for the different Hankel transforms. The Hankel transform using the Bessel function of the first kind is particularly useful when there is radial symmetry in a two-dimensional problem. In that case the two-dimensional Fourier transform can be expressed in terms of a one-dimensional Hankel transform.

Hankel transforms are used frequently in solving optical problems where there is radial symmetry. Optical elements, such as lenses, are often constructed with radial symmetry. Bessel functions and Hankel transforms are beyond the scope of this book.

VII. RADON TRANSFORM

In 1917, Johann Radon, a German mathematician, described a method of transforming between a function and an infinite set of line integrals through the function. This transformation is known in radiology as the Radon transform. The infinite set of line integrals through the function is similar to the finite data set which is collected in computer tomography. The inverse Radon transform is similar to reconstruction of noiseless computed tomographic data (see Chapter 31).

The Radon transform provides sophisticated mathematical justification for computed tomographic reconstruction. However, it is not of much practical utility. Therefore, we have chosen not to include it in our discussion of reconstruction.

VIII. SUMMARY

This chapter began with the multi-dimensional Fourier transform. Most radiology problems deal with signals with more than one dimension. Thus, the multi-dimensional Fourier transform is of great practical importance. However, there is relatively little conceptual difference between the one-dimensional Fourier transform and the multi-dimensional Fourier transform. Therefore, we have given a brief description of the multi-dimensional Fourier transform. The one property of interest to us is that the rotation of a signal results in a similar rotation of its transform.

This chapter has shown how the discrete Fourier transform is related to the continuous Fourier transform. Periodicity in one domain is related to discrete values for the independent variable in the other domain. Aperiodicity is related to continuity of the independent variable. This relation will be important for understanding the effects of sampling.

The relationship between several transforms was described in this chapter. The purpose was to help the reader to better understand the Fourier transform. Use of complex independent variables should provide the reader with some idea of the more mathematical description of the transform operations. The idea that a transform is an alternate description of the same signal helps to explain why the signal and its transform must both have the same complexity.

IX. FURTHER READING

Multi-dimensional transform operations are described in several sources. For example, the multi-dimensional Fourier transform is described in Chapter 12 of the book by Bracewell.[1] The multi-dimensional discrete Fourier transform is described in Chapter 2 of the book by Dudgeon and Mersereau.[2]

The Laplace transform is described in several books; for example, see Chapter 11 of the book by Bracewell.[1] Descriptions of the differences between the unilateral and the bilateral Laplace transform can be found in that book and in the book by Siebert.[3] Descriptions of the z transform can be found in Chapter 10 of the book by Oppenheim and Willsky,[4] and in Chapter 2 of the book by Oppenheim and Schafer.[5]

The relationship between discrete and continuous signals is described in Chapter 1 of the book by Papoulis.[6] Chapter 3 of that book describes the relationships between the discrete Fourier transform, the Fourier series, and the continuous Fourier transform.

Description of the Taylor and the Laurent series for functions of a complex variable is described in Chapter 10 of the book by Hildebrand.[7]

Radon's original description of the transform between a function and line integrals through the function is in German.[8] The book by Barrett and Swindell[9] uses the Radon transform space much more extensively than this book, although not the Radon transform itself.

REFERENCES

1. **Bracewell, R. N.**, *The Fourier Transform and Its Applications*, McGraw-Hill, New York, 1965.
2. **Dudgeon, D. E. and Mersereau, R. M.**, *Multidimensional Digital Signal Processing*, Prentice-Hall, Englewood Cliffs, NJ, 1984.
3. **Siebert, W. Mc. C.**, *Circuits, Signals, and Systems*, MIT Press, Cambridge, MA, 1986.
4. **Oppenheim, A. V. and Willsky, A. S.**, *Signals and Systems*, Prentice-Hall, Englewood Cliffs, NJ, 1983.
5. **Oppenheim, A. V. and Schafer, R. W.**, *Digital Signal Processing*, Prentice-Hall, Englewood Cliffs, NJ, 1975.
6. **Papoulis, A.**, *Signal Analysis*, McGraw-Hill, New York, 1977.
7. **Hildebrand, F. B.**, *Advanced Calculus for Applications*, Prentice-Hall, Englewood Cliffs, NJ, 1962.
8. **Radon, J.**, Uber die bestimmung von funktionen durch ihre integralwerte langs gewisser mannigfaltigkeiten, *Ber. Verh. Saechs. Akad. Wiss. Leipzig*, 69, 262, 1917.
9. **Barrett, H. H. and Swindell, W.**, *Radiological Imaging: The Theory of Image Formation, Detection, and Processing*, Academic Press, New York, 1981.

Chapter 21

SUMMARY OF TRANSFORMATIONS

The goal of this part of the book is to introduce the Fourier transform. Several other transformation operations are described, but the major purpose of introducing these other transforms is to provide a better understanding of the Fourier transform. The Fourier transform allows signals to be described in terms of their frequency components. The Fourier transform is essential to understanding filtering and image reconstruction in Parts III and IV of this book. The Fourier transform is the major mathematical tool used in this book.

The Fourier transform changes signals to a form that simplifies the description of the operation of linear, time invariant systems. The basis functions for the Fourier transform are the imaginary exponentials. The imaginary exponentials are the eigenfunction of linear, time invariant systems. Throughout this book, the importance of the eigenfunctions of a system to understanding the operation of systems on signals is emphasized.

This chapter will review several of the most important properties of the Fourier transform, and several of the most common Fourier transform pairs. There are several themes which have recurred throughout this part of the book — description of signals in terms of basis functions; the similarity between correlation, projection, and the forward Fourier transform; the transformation operation as rotation; the value of eigenfunctions; mapping of convolution to multiplication; duality between the time and frequency domains; the relation between discrete and continuous signals; and the effects of a sequence of systems. We shall try to bring these ideas together in this chapter.

I. THE FREQUENCY DOMAIN

One of the most important concepts in this part of the book is the frequency domain representation of a signal. Chapter 14 gave several examples where the reader may already have some intuition about the frequency domain. The prime example of the natural understanding of signals in terms of the frequency domain is hearing. We listen to tones in a music; the tones are a frequency domain representation of the sound wave. In school we have learned that the sound wave consists of alternating regions of compression and rarefaction in air, but this description is not natural to us. Rather, it is the frequency domain representation which is natural to us.

Spectroscopy provides another example where the frequency domain description is more natural than the time domain description. Colors of the rainbow represent electromagnetic radiation of different frequencies. Separating a light beam into a spectrum is reasonably natural to us, since in general colors can be understood in terms of its spectral components. The many special properties of color vision make this analogy between perception and the frequency domain representation less exact than the sound analogy, but it is still useful.

Other forms of spectroscopy, particularly nuclear magnetic resonance spectroscopy, may also provide some readers with an appreciation of other frequency domain signals. The nuclear magnetic resonance spectrum is logically interpreted in terms of the magnetic environment of different nuclear species. The time domain signal, the free induction decay, provides no such easy interpretation.

The most important signals in this book are images. We naturally think of images in terms of their space domain representation. Hopefully, the analogies to these other types of signals will provide the reader with some understanding of images in terms of spatial frequencies. Just as these other signals can be understood using a frequency domain description, images can be understood using a spatial frequency domain description.

The Fourier transform and the inverse Fourier transform provide a method of changing back and forth between the space and the spatial frequency domain representations of a signal. The two representations provide the same information. This part of the book should have convinced the reader that these two descriptions of an image are equivalent.

II. PROPERTIES OF THE FOURIER TRANSFORM

Several properties of the Fourier transform were introduced in this part of the book. These properties are summarized in this section with a brief description of the importance of each property. These properties can often be used to guess the general shape of an unknown Fourier transform, by analogy to a known Fourier transform.

The **linearity** property was given by Equation 15.4:

$$a \cdot f(t) + b \cdot g(t) \leftrightarrow a \cdot F(\omega) + b \cdot G(\omega) \tag{21.1}$$

where we have used the two headed arrow notation to indicate the Fourier transform operation. Linearity means that different portions of a signal can be considered independently. The Fourier transform of a linear combination of signals can be calculated from the Fourier transform of each of the signals separately. This property is key to deriving new transform pairs from a small set of known transforms. It is often possible to describe a signal as being approximately equal to the sum of a set of signals whose Fourier transforms are known. The Fourier transform of the unknown signal is just the sum of the transforms of the component signals.

The **duality** property was given by Equations 15.6 and 15.7:

$$f(t) \leftrightarrow F(\omega) \tag{21.2}$$

$$F(t) \leftrightarrow 2\pi \cdot f(-\omega) \tag{21.3}$$

The duality property means that except for a minus sign here and a 2π there, the Fourier transform is equivalent to the inverse Fourier transform. Below we shall expand upon the equivalence of the time and frequency domain description of signals.

Mapping of convolution to multiplication was given by Equations 16.8 and 16.9:

$$f(t) * h(t) \leftrightarrow F(\omega) \cdot H(\omega) \tag{21.4}$$

$$f(t) \cdot h(t) \leftrightarrow (1/2\pi) \cdot F(\omega) * H(\omega) \tag{21.5}$$

This property is the major reason why the radiologist is interested in the Fourier transform. Below we shall expand upon this property.

Parseval's relationship was given by Equation 16.87:

$$\int_{-\infty}^{+\infty} f(t) \cdot g^*(t) \, dt = (1/2\pi) \cdot \int_{-\infty}^{+\infty} F(\omega) \cdot G^*(\omega) \, d\omega \tag{21.6}$$

Parseval's relation means that the correlation between two signals is equal to the correlation of their Fourier transforms (multiplied by $1/2\pi$). The relationship between signals is not changed by the Fourier transform. How well two signals are "lined up", the "angle" between two signals, is not changed by the Fourier transform.

The **energy relationship** was given by Equation 16.88:

$$\int_{-\infty}^{+\infty} |f(t)|^2 dt = (1/2\pi) \cdot \int_{-\infty}^{+\infty} |F(\omega)|^2 \, d\omega \tag{21.7}$$

The energy in a signal is conserved by the Fourier transform (save a factor of $1/2\pi$). The ideas of energy and length are very useful in understanding signal processing. The energy relation means that these concepts can be translated between the time and the frequency domains.

The uncertainty principle was given by Equation 16.95:

$$\Delta t \cdot \Delta\omega \geqslant 2 \tag{21.8}$$

The uncertainty principle means that a signal cannot be simultaneously narrow in both the time and the frequency domain. This principle has important implications for signal processing. We frequently wish to confine a signal in terms of both space and spatial frequency. The uncertainty principle puts a limit on this process. The signal which is maximally narrow in both domains is the Gaussian.

The relation between **even and odd** real signals and their transforms were given by Equations 16.65 and 16.66:

$$\text{even and real} \rightarrow \text{real} \tag{21.9}$$

$$\text{odd and real} \rightarrow \text{imaginary} \tag{21.10}$$

where even and odd are defined by Equations 16.50 and 16.51. The dual relation between **real and imaginary** signals and their transforms are given by:

$$\text{real} \leftrightarrow F(\omega) = F^*(-\omega) \tag{21.11}$$

$$\text{imaginary} \leftrightarrow F(\omega) = -F^*(-\omega) \tag{21.12}$$

These relations are of particular importance in understanding some of the properties of nuclear magnetic resonance data collection.

The **shift/modulation** relation was given by Equations 16.31 and 16.35:

$$f(t - \tau) \leftrightarrow e^{-i\omega\tau} \cdot F(\omega) \tag{21.13}$$

$$(1/2\pi) \cdot e^{i\omega_0 t} \cdot f(t) \leftrightarrow F(\omega - \omega_0) \tag{21.14}$$

The shift and modulation properties are important in nuclear magnetic resonance, but they are also important for understanding how various Fourier transforms are related.

A **change in scale** in one domain is related to the change in the other domain by Equations 16.43 and 16.44:

$$f(a \cdot t) \leftrightarrow 1/|a| \cdot F(\omega/a) \tag{21.15}$$

$$1/|a| \cdot f(t/a) \leftrightarrow F(a \cdot \omega) \tag{21.16}$$

When a signal shrinks in one domain, it expands in the other domain. This property is related to the uncertainty principle above.

Mapping of differential equations to polynomial equation results from the properties given by Equation 16.47 and 16.48:

$$df(t)/dt \leftrightarrow i\omega \cdot F(\omega) \tag{21.17}$$

$$-\text{it} \cdot \text{f(t)} \leftrightarrow \text{dF}(\omega)/\text{d}\omega \tag{21.18}$$

These properties are very important in understanding how Laplace transforms are used to solve differential equations. However, we do not make much use of this property in this book.

III. SELECTED FOURIER TRANSFORM PAIRS

We have shown examples of the Fourier transforms of only a few signals. However, using these few signals and the properties given above, it is possible to construct a large number of Fourier transform pairs. Even if the exact form of a signal cannot be constructed, it is often possible to get a rough idea of the shape of a Fourier transform using this method.

The Fourier transform of the delta function was given by Equations 15.38 and 15.36:

$$\delta(t) \leftrightarrow 1 \tag{21.19}$$

$$1 \leftrightarrow 2\pi \cdot \delta(\omega) \tag{21.20}$$

A delta function is composed of equal portions of all frequency components. This transform pair is shown in Figure 15.4.

The shifted delta function can be derived using the shift/modulation properties, Equations 21.13 and 21.14:

$$\delta(t - \tau) \leftrightarrow e^{-i\omega\tau} \tag{21.21}$$

$$e^{i\omega_0 t} \leftrightarrow \delta(\omega - \omega_0) \tag{21.22}$$

This transform pair is shown in Figure 16.7.

Using the definition of the cosine and sine in terms of imaginary exponentials (Equations 14.2 and 14.3), their Fourier transforms can be derived from the shifted delta functions:

$$\cos(\omega_0 t) \leftrightarrow \pi \cdot [\delta(\omega - \omega_0) + \delta(\omega + \omega_0)] \tag{21.23}$$

$$\sin(\omega_0 t) \leftrightarrow (\pi/i) \cdot [\delta(\omega - \omega_0) - \delta(\omega + \omega_0)] \tag{21.24}$$

This transform is shown in Figure 14.6.

The Gaussian function is special for a large number of reasons. One of those reasons is that the Fourier transform of a Gaussian is also a Gaussian function (Figure 14.7). This relation is given by Equation 14.14:

$$(1/\sqrt{(2\pi)}\sigma) \cdot e^{-1/2(t/\sigma)^2} \leftrightarrow e^{-1/2(\sigma\omega)^2} \tag{21.25}$$

In two dimensions, another interesting signal has the same form in the two domains, Equations 14.34 and 14.35:

$$1/r \leftrightarrow 1/k \tag{21.26}$$

The reciprocal will be important in understanding reconstruction from projections.

The exponentially decaying signal which starts at time zero is used throughout radiology — in radioactive decay, in the decay of the nuclear magnetic resonance signal, in X-ray and ultrasound attenuation, etc. The Fourier transform of this signal was given by Equation 14.23:

$$u(t) \cdot e^{-\lambda t} \leftrightarrow 1/(\lambda + i\omega) \tag{21.27}$$

This Fourier transform is diagrammed in several ways in Chapter 14 (see Figures 14.10 to 14.13). These different ways of plotting the same complex signal each highlight different aspects of the signal.

A very common signal is the rectangle (Figure 16.15). It will be used extensively in the next part of the book. Its transform was given by Equations 16.78 and 16.79:

$$\Omega \cdot \text{sinc}(\Omega t/2) \leftrightarrow u(\Omega/2 - \omega) \cdot u(\omega - \Omega/2) \tag{21.28}$$

$$u(T/2 - t) \cdot u(t - T/2) \leftrightarrow 2\pi \cdot T \cdot \text{sinc}(\omega T/2) \tag{21.29}$$

Chapter 16 gave some heuristics which help determine the Fourier transform of a signal. If a signal is wide in one domain, then it is narrow in the other domain. If a signal has sharp edges in one domain, then it has ripples in the other domain. Smoothness in one domain results in concentration about the origin in the other domain. Sinusoidal components in one domain result in delta functions in the other domain. Periodicity in one domain results in a discrete signal in the other domain. With these few transforms and rules of thumb, one can often make a good guess at the general shape of the Fourier transform of a signal.

IV. BASIS FUNCTIONS

A theme in both Parts I and II has been the representation of a signal as a linear combination of a set of basis functions. The time domain description represents a signal as a linear combination of delta functions, Equation 14.5:

$$f(t) = \int_{-\infty}^{+\infty} f(\tau) \cdot \delta(t - \tau) \, d\tau \tag{21.30}$$

The frequency domain description represents a signal as a linear combination of imaginary exponentials, Equation 14.6:

$$f(t) = 1/2\pi \int_{-\infty}^{+\infty} F(\omega) \cdot e^{i\omega t} \, d\omega \tag{21.31}$$

The coefficient domain description represents a signal as a linear combination of power functions, Equation 17.5:

$$f(t) = \Sigma \, a[k] \cdot t^k \tag{21.32}$$

Analogously, a vector can be represented as a linear combination of basis vectors. In terms of the canonical set of basis vectors, a vector can be written:

$$\mathbf{f} = \Sigma \, f_i \cdot \mathbf{d}_i \tag{21.33}$$

In terms of some other orthonormal set of basis vectors, the vector can be written:

$$\mathbf{f} = \Sigma \, (\mathbf{f} \cdot \mathbf{s}_i) \cdot \mathbf{s}_i \tag{21.34}$$

where the components of $\mathbf{f}$ along the vectors, $\mathbf{s}_i$, have been written as the projection, $(\mathbf{f} \cdot \mathbf{s}_i)$, of $\mathbf{f}$ along $\mathbf{s}_i$.

All of these representations are similar. They all represent a signal as a linear combination of basis functions or basis vectors. The type of signals that can be represented are defined by the basis functions or the basis vectors. The "space" of allowed signals is all possible combinations of these basis functions or vectors.

We normally think of the time domain description of a signal as the primary description. But, the frequency domain and coefficient domain descriptions are equivalent to the time domain; they are coequals. On an abstract level, we can think of a signal independent of its representation. The description of the signal depends upon the choice of the basis functions or the basis vectors. The form of the $f(\tau)$, $F(\omega)$, $a[n]$, f_i, or $(\mathbf{f} \cdot \mathbf{s}_i)$ is determined by the basis functions or vectors.

V. TRANSFORMATION, CORRELATION, AND PROJECTION

If the basis functions or basis vectors are orthogonal, then it is particularly easy to calculate the factors, $f(\tau)$, $F(\omega)$, f_i, or $(\mathbf{f} \cdot \mathbf{s}_i)$. These factors are the correlation of the signal with the basis functions or basis vectors. If the basis functions or basis vectors are orthonormal, then these factors are the projection of the signal along the basis functions or vectors. (The basis functions, t^n, are not orthogonal; thus, calculation of the interpolation of the factors, $a[k]$, is somewhat more complicated.)

Each of the following operations is a correlation.

$$f(\tau) = \int_{-\infty}^{+\infty} f(t) \cdot \delta(t - \tau) \, dt \tag{21.35}$$

$$F(\omega) = \int_{-\infty}^{+\infty} f(t) \cdot e^{-i\omega t} \, dt \tag{21.36}$$

$$f_i = \mathbf{f} \cdot \mathbf{d_i} \tag{21.37}$$

and:

$$(\mathbf{f} \cdot \mathbf{s}_i) = \mathbf{f} \cdot \mathbf{s}_i \tag{21.38}$$

Each of these operations determines the projection of the signal along the basis function or basis vector; each determines how much the signal is like the basis function or basis vector; and each determines how well the signal is correlated with the basis function or basis vector.

VI. TRANSFORMATIONS AND ROTATIONS

The reason for including both linear systems and linear algebra in this book is to bring out the analogies between signals and vectors. Vectors provide geometrical insight into operations on signals. Transformation of a signal from the time domain to the frequency domain is analogous to representing a vector in terms of a new set of basis vectors. We have loosely referred to changes in the set of basis vectors as rotating the basis vectors.

By rotating the basis vectors we change the description of a vector. The vector does not change, rather it is the basis vectors that change. Similarly, transformation from a description of a signal in the time domain to a description in the frequency domain does not change the signal — it changes the basis functions. Figure 19.5 shows the representation of a vector in terms of two different sets of basis vectors, where one set of basis vectors is rotated with respect to the other. This figure provides a geometric analogy to the Fourier transform operation.

If **f** is a vector defined in the canonical coordinate system, then $S^T \cdot f$ is the vector defined using the columns of S as the basis set. The vector, matrix representation of a system was rewritten in Equation 19.40:

$$(S^T \cdot g) = (S^T \cdot H \cdot S) \cdot (S^T \cdot f) \tag{21.39}$$

In this form, it can be seen that the representation of the system, H, in terms of the new basis vectors is $S^T \cdot H \cdot S$. These relationships are shown in Figure 19.9.

VII. EIGENFUNCTIONS

Throughout the book we emphasize the value of describing a signal in terms of the eigenfunctions or eigenvectors of a system. The eigenfunctions or eigenvectors of a system are signals which are not changed in shape or in direction as they go through a system. Mathematically, this property was given by Equation 5.1:

$$H\{f(t)\} = \lambda \cdot f(t) \tag{21.40}$$

These signals have a special relationship to the system. They can be used to characterize the operation of the system on the class of signals which are linear combinations of the eigenfunctions.

The transformation of a system to a description in terms of an eigenvector basis set, transforms the matrix representing the system into a diagonal matrix, Equation 19.54:

$$S^T \cdot H \cdot S = \Lambda \tag{21.41}$$

where Λ is a diagonal matrix with components equal to the eigenvalues of the matrix, H. The operation of a diagonal matrix on any input vector is particularly simple. This relation again emphasizes the value of the eigenvector description of systems.

The Fourier transform is a method of transforming a signal into a description in terms of the set of imaginary exponentials. The imaginary exponentials are eigenfunctions of all linear, time invariant systems. Thus, the frequency domain description of a signal is an eigenfunction description. The frequency domain is a more natural representation for understanding linear, time invariant systems. Transformation of a signal to a representation in terms of eigenfunctions is the whole point of Part II.

VIII. MAPPING OF CONVOLUTION TO MULTIPLICATION

The Fourier transform is the major tool which will be used in this book. The property of the Fourier transform which is most important for solving radiological problems is the mapping of the complex operation of convolution into the simple operation of multiplication. This property will be used in the next part of the book to understand how systems can be used to filter signals. In Part IV, this property will be essential to understanding reconstruction.

The reason for introducing the polynomial transformation in Chapter 17 was to provide an example of the mapping of convolution to multiplication using functions with which the radiologist is more familiar. In the case of polynomials, we saw that convolution in the coefficient domain mapped into multiplication in the time domain. In Chapter 17, we showed that this property is dependent upon use of basis functions which are exponentials.

This truly remarkable property is related to the fact that the exponentials are the eigenfunctions of linear, time invariant systems. The simplicity of the representation of a system in the frequency domain is due to the simplicity of the operation of a system on its eigen-functions (Equation 21.40).

IX. RELATION OF DISCRETE AND CONTINUOUS SIGNALS

Some of the relationships between discrete and continuous signals were discussed in relation to the discrete Fourier transform in Chapter 18. A discrete signal in one domain results in a periodic signal in the other domain. As the points in the discrete signal are closer together in one domain, the period in the other domain becomes longer. For a continuous signal in one domain, the signal in the other domain is aperiodic (an infinite period). These relations will be used in Chapter 23 to understand the process of sampling a continuous signal. The samples which produce a discrete signal in the time domain produce a periodic signal in the frequency domain.

The discrete Fourier transform of a signal which has N points in one period in one domain will also have N points in one period in the other domain. This relation is an example of a more general principle. The complexity of the signal in the time domain and the frequency domain is the same. If one can be described by N distinct points, then the other can also. Since it is possible to transform back and forth between representations, the representations must carry the same information.

The Laplace transform, described in Chapter 20, allowed us to consider signals with complex valued, independent variables. These signals were limited to the class of functions which are called analytic functions. Although an understanding of analytic functions is beyond the scope of this book, the property of most interest to us is that these signals can be defined in terms of the values of the signal along one line in the complex plane. Given the value along a single line, the value of the signal at any point in the whole plane can be calculated.

The time domain signal is defined in terms of the values along the real axis; the frequency domain signal is defined in terms of the values along the imaginary axis. Thus, the Laplace transform introduces a $\pi/2$ rotation. This rotation provides an explanation of the difference in the sign of the exponent of the forward and reverse Fourier transforms.

X. SEQUENCE OF SYSTEMS

In the time domain, a sequence of systems is very complicated — a series of convolutions. In the frequency domain the series is much simpler — a series of multiplications. One of the great advantages of the frequency domain description of complex systems is the ease of understanding a sequence of systems. Equations 16.16 and 16.17 provide the relation:

$$f(t) * h_1(t) * h_2(t) \leftrightarrow F(\omega) \cdot H_1(\omega) \cdot H_2(\omega) \qquad (21.42)$$

This property may already be known to the audiophile. The response of a sequence of audio systems is the product of the individual components. This relation is shown in Figure 16.5.

The modulation transfer function described in Chapter 16 is the spatial frequency domain description of an imaging system. The modulation transfer function of a sequence of systems is the product of the modulation transfer functions of the component systems. The line-spread function is the space domain representation of an imaging system. It provides the same information as the modulation transfer function, but the line spread function of a sequence of systems is the convolution of the line spread functions of the systems. One of the reasons that the modulation transfer function is used extensively in Radiology is the simplicity with which the effects of a sequence of imaging components can be understood.

XI. SUMMARY

The first chapter in this part of the book attempted to show that description of a signal in terms of its frequency components is natural to the radiologist in several application. The human naturally thinks of sound in terms of the frequency components of the signal. The cochlea of the ear performs a Fourier transform on the time domain signal represented by the sound wave and sends a frequency domain signal to the brain. Similarly, various types of spectroscopy are familiar to the radiologist, particularly now that nuclear magnetic spectroscopy is becoming important in radiology.

The Fourier transform is just a method of changing the representation of a signal from the time or space domain to the frequency or spatial frequency domain. The advantage of the frequency domain representation of a signal is that the basis functions of the frequency domain description are the eigenfunctions of all linear, time invariant systems. The transformation to an eigenfunction description simplifies the operation of systems on signals. This simplification is important for practical reasons; it leads to an efficient method of implementation using the fast Fourier transform algorithm. But more importantly for this book, this simplification will be essential in understanding image reconstruction in Part IV.

The goal of this part of the book is to provide the reader with an understanding of a major mathematical tool, the Fourier transform. It also should provide the reader with enough familiarity with how signals are transformed so that, in a general way, the relation between the representation of a signal in the two domains is understood.

III. Filtering

Chapter 22

INTRODUCTION TO FILTERING

Part III of this book describes an operation known as filtering. Filtering is often presented as an application of signal processing. It is a method which can be used to enhance certain aspects of actual radiological images. However, the major use of filtering in this book will not be as an application, but rather as a technique used in image reconstruction. Most radiologists have already heard of filtering with regard to reconstruction in computed tomography. The major method of reconstruction in computed tomography is usually called filtered back projection.

The first chapter of this part of the book will introduce the concept of filtering. Filtering is the modification of the amplitudes of the frequency components of a signal. Filtering is a signal processing operation which is defined in the frequency domain. We shall find that filtering is performed by passing an input signal through a system to produce an output signal — a process which has already been described many times in this book. There is very little new mathematical content in this chapter. Rather what is new is the point of view. Filtering is the operation of a system viewed from the frequency domain.

This chapter will also introduce an operation called windowing, defined in the time domain. The operation of filtering is analogous to the operation of windowing. Filtering and windowing are dual operations — filtering is a modification of the amplitudes of the frequency domain components of a signal; windowing is the modification of the time domain components of a signal.

The next chapter is primarily concerned with sampling signals. It is included in this part of the book because the operation of filtering is needed in order to understand sampling. Chapter 24 will explain the operation of a filter on stochastic signals. Chapter 25 will return to the vector and matrix description of signals and systems. It will introduce the normal equations of linear algebra. The normal equations provide a method for solving a set of simultaneous linear equations in the presence of noise. Chapter 26 will introduce the Wiener filter. The Wiener filter for linear, time invariant systems is analogous to the normal equation for linear systems. Finally, Chapter 27 will present a few applications of filtering for enhancement of images.

I. DEFINITION OF FILTERING

Filtering is the modification of the amplitude of the frequency components of a signal. If the initial signal is $F(\omega)$, then the modified signal, $G(\omega)$, can be defined by:

$$G(\omega) = F(\omega) \cdot H(\omega) \tag{22.1}$$

$H(\omega)$ is called the filter. The amplitudes of the frequency components of input signals are multiplied by the values of the filter to produce the output signal.

Often $H(\omega)$ is one for a certain range of values of ω and zero for all other values of ω. For example, Figure 22.1 shows the input signal, $F(\omega)$, the filter, $H(\omega)$, and the output signal $G(\omega)$. $G(\omega)$ is equal to $F(\omega)$ for the values of ω for which $H(\omega)$ is one. These frequency components are "passed through" the filter. $G(\omega)$ is equal to zero for the values of ω for which $H(\omega)$ is zero. These frequency components are "stopped" or "filtered out" by $H(\omega)$.

This type of filtering operation is performed by a radio receiver to select a particular station. Out of the whole range of electromagnetic waves, a radio receiver picks out a narrow band of frequencies transmitted by a radio station. It filters out all of the frequencies except for this narrow band of frequencies.

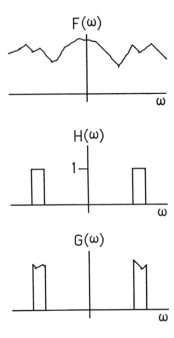

FIGURE 22.1.   Band pass filter: F(ω) is the frequency domain representation of an input signal. H(ω) is a filter which is equal to one for a band of frequencies and zero for all other frequencies. The output signal, G(ω), is equal to the input in the pass band, and it is zero in the stop band. The filter, H(ω), passes only a certain range of frequencies from the input to the output.

The common sense meaning of the word "filter" applies to this simple type of filtering operation. Certain frequencies are filtered out by the system. However, in linear system theory, the word filter is used for any type of signal, H(ω), not just signals which are either zero or one. For example, Figure 22.2 shows a filter which is equal to one for a middle range of frequencies, is greater than one for lower and higher frequencies, and is zero for very low and very high frequencies. The filtered signal, G(ω), has increased low and high frequency components as compared with the unfiltered signal, F(ω). The very low and very high frequency components of the unfiltered signal are not passed by the filter.

This type of filtering operation is performed by the base and treble adjustment of an audio amplifier. Turning up the treble adjustment on an audio amplifier increases the amplitude of the high frequency sound waves. Turning up the base adjustment on an audio amplifier increases the amplitude of the low frequency sound waves. Very high frequencies (above about 20 MHz) and very low frequencies (below about 20 Hz) are stopped by an audio amplifier. This type of modification of the amplitude of the frequencies of a signal is typical of filtering operations.

II. IMPLEMENTATION

The filtering operation described by Equation 22.1 can be implemented by a linear, time invariant system, h(t), which has a frequency response given by H(ω). In the time domain, the filtering operation is performed by the convolution operation:

$$g(t) = h(t) * f(t) \tag{22.2}$$

As has been pointed out several times, the convolution operation, given by Equation 22.2, is much more complicated than the multiplication operation, given by Equation 22.1. Thus,

319

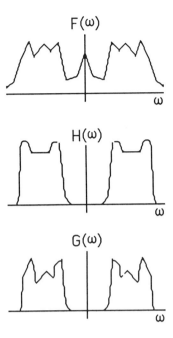

FIGURE 22.2. Treble and bass accentuation: F(ω) is the frequency domain representation of an input signal. H(ω) is a filter which passes the mid range of frequencies, accentuates the high and low frequencies, and stops the very high and very low frequencies. The output, G(ω), is similar to the input except that the low and high frequencies are accentuated and the very low and very high frequencies are zero. This type of filtering is similar to an audio amplifier with the treble and bass knobs turned up.

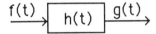

FIGURE 22.3. Filter model: the filter, h(t), is a linear, time invariant system with input, f(t), and output, g(t). This model is the same as the model in Figure 3.4.

filtering is a simple operation in the frequency domain, and a complicated operation in the time domain.

Filtering a signal is the same as passing a signal through a system (Figure 22.3). In the time domain, filtering is equivalent to convolving a signal with a system function, h(t). The term "filtering" is used when it is logical to specify the system in the frequency domain. The term "convolution" is used when it is logical to specify the system in the time domain.

In the case of an audio amplifier, we understand what it means to increase the treble or the base. Our natural description of the operation of the system is in terms of the frequency domain description of the signal. In these cases we say that the system is filtering the signal. We often have better intuition about image operations as space domain convolutions. However, below we shall see that it is also useful to understand these operations as spatial filtering operations.

All linear, time invariant systems are filters. They filter the input signal with the system function to produce the output signal. We use the term, filter, for some systems to indicate that it is natural to specify the system in terms of the frequency domain instead of the time domain. But it is possible to think of all linear, time invariant systems as filters.

III. SPATIAL FILTERING

The examples of filtering which are most natural to the nonengineer deal with sound, since humans have a natural understanding of sounds in terms of frequencies. However, filtering can also be applied to images. A frequent image-processing operation is to smooth an image. For example, if there is too much noise in the image, then smoothing the image can often improve its appearance.

The image in Figure 22.4A shows a nuclear magnetic resonance image which is very noisy. Figure 22.4B shows the same image after smoothing the image. The smoothing operation decreases the noise in the image. But, it also decreases the resolution of the image.

Smoothing can be performed by averaging adjacent pixels in the image. Typically, the averaging operation weighs the pixels by their proximity to the pixel being smoothed. Figure 22.5 shows an example of a set of weighting factors, $h(x,y)$, for a nine point smoothing operation. The center pixel is given the greatest weight and the surrounding pixels are given less weight.

The set of weights given in Figure 22.5 is shifted to the pixel of interest. The surrounding pixels are multiplied by the weighing factors. The new value at that position is the sum of the pixel values multiplied by the weights. We recognize this smoothing operation as a convolution — shift, scale, and add.

We can also view this operation from the frequency domain. The Fourier transform of the system function, $h(x,y)$, given by Figure 22.5 is shown for the x axis in Figure 22.6. Convolution of the image with $h(x,y)$ is equivalent to filtering the image with $H(k_x,k_y)$. $H(k_x,k_y)$ is about equal to one for low spatial frequencies and it is about equal to zero for high spatial frequencies. The smoothing operation can be described in the frequency domain as filtering out the high frequencies.

We can obtain a better understanding of the smoothing operation by considering it in terms of the two different domains. The smoothing operation reduces noise since it averages several pixels together. It decreases the resolution of the image since it filters out the high spatial frequencies which help to define the detail in the image.

Another common type of spatial filtering operation is edge enhancement. Figure 22.7A is a nuclear magnetic resonance image of the brain. Figure 22.7B is the same image with edge enhancement. Figure 22.8 shows the x axis of the space domain, $h(x,0)$, and spatial frequency domain, $H(k_x,0)$, representations of the edge enhancement system. In the space domain, the edge enhancement is accomplished by subtracting adjacent pixels from the center pixel.

Figure 22.9 shows the effect of an edge enhancement operation in the space domain for a pixel in a constant region, and for pixels on either side of an edge. In a region of constant value, the subtraction of the surrounding pixel values decreases the output value. Near an edge, the subtraction of pixels on the other side of the edge tends to increase the magnitude of the output value.

In the frequency domain, the effect is to amplify the higher frequencies, and decrease the lower frequencies. The higher frequencies are the most important for defining edges, so amplification of these frequencies tends to emphasize the edges. The lower frequencies are the most important for defining the constant regions, so decreasing their values tends to decrease the value of the pixels in constant regions.

In summary, if the space domain representation of the system has positive values in a central region, then the system averages surrounding pixels. As a general rule, this type of system tends to smooth the image, decreasing both noise and resolution. If the space domain representation of a system has positive values in the center and surrounding negative values, then it compares the center region to its surrounding. As a general rule, this type of system tends to enhance edges and increase noise. Many image enhancement operations are vari-

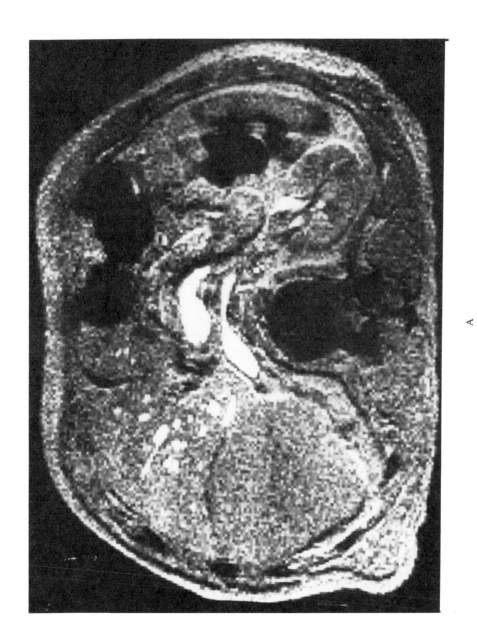

A

FIGURE 22.4. Smoothing: (A) A nuclear magnetic resonance image of a liver. (B) The same image after being smoothed. Smoothing reduces the noise in the image.

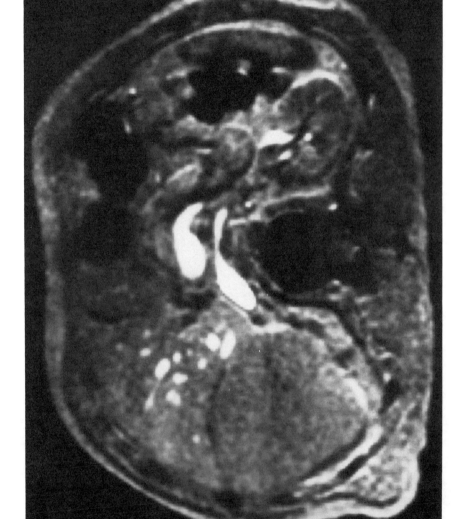

FIGURE 4B

h(x,y)

$\frac{1}{16}$	$\frac{1}{8}$	$\frac{1}{16}$
$\frac{1}{8}$	$\frac{1}{4}$	$\frac{1}{8}$
$\frac{1}{16}$	$\frac{1}{8}$	$\frac{1}{16}$

FIGURE 22.5. Smoothing operation: the nonzero elements in a simple nine-point smoothing operation are shown. Convolution by this smoothing kernel is particularly easy to implement on a digital computer since the elements are powers of two.

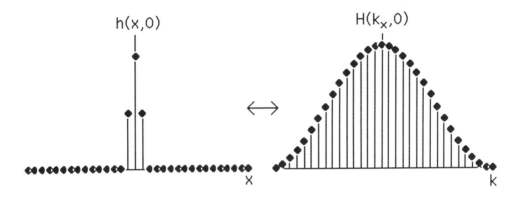

FIGURE 22.6. Smoothing in the space and spatial frequency domains: the x axis of the space domain representation of the smoothing operation shown in Figure 22.5 is shown on the left. On the right is the k_x axis of the frequency domain representation of this operation. The filter is in the general shape of a low pass filter; it has the highest value at zero and the value decreases for higher frequencies.

ations on these two general types of operations. We shall describe image enhancement more fully in Chapter 27.

IV. WINDOWING

We shall define the operation of windowing as the modification of the amplitudes of a time domain signal, f(t), by a window, h(t), to produce an output signal, g(t). Mathematically:

$$g(t) = f(t) \cdot h(t) \qquad (22.3)$$

This operation is the dual relation to the filtering operation, Equation 22.1. In the frequency domain this operation is a convolution:

$$G(\omega) = (1/2\pi) \cdot F(\omega) \cdot H(\omega) \qquad (22.4)$$

The most frequent radiological application of the windowing operation is the selection of a region of interest. Inside a region of interest the window value, h(x,y), is equal to one, and outside the region of interest the window value is equal to zero. A region of interest is used to determine the value of the image pixels which lie within a certain range of positions. This operation is analogous to the filtering operation which selects values which lie within a certain range of frequencies.

Regions of interest are often restricted to have values of only zero or one; a pixel is

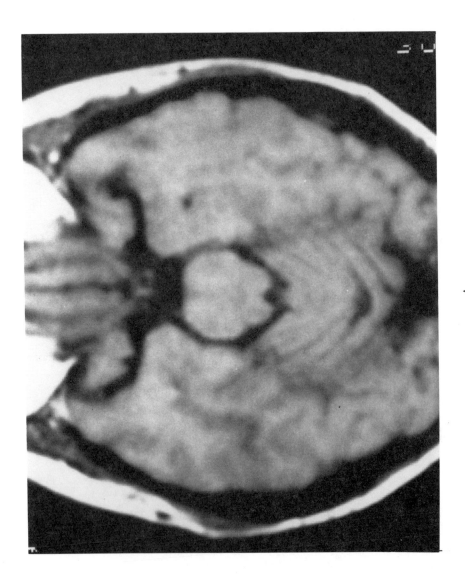

A

FIGURE 22.7. Edge enhancement: (A) A nuclear magnetic resonance image of a brain. (B) The same image after application of an edge enhancing filter. The edges in the image stand out, but also note that the noise is more apparent.

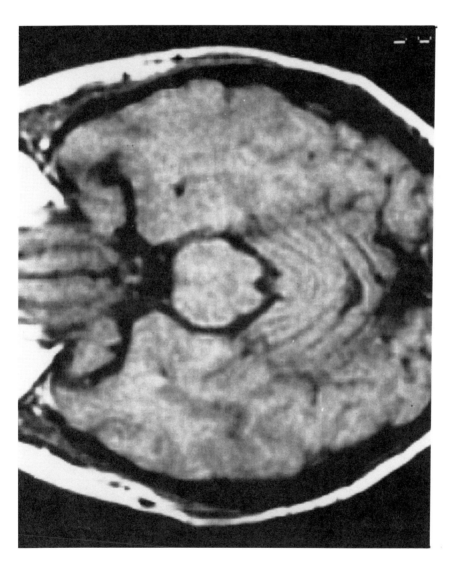

FIGURE 22.7B

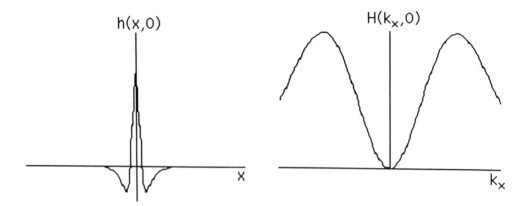

FIGURE 22.8.   High pass filter: on the left is the x axis of the space domain representation of a high pass filter. On the right is the frequency domain representation of the same filter. The filter attenuates the low frequencies, accentuates the high frequencies, and attenuates the very high frequencies. This type of filter will enhance the edge in a picture. Since the integral of h(x,0) is zero, regions of constant intensity will be set equal to zero.

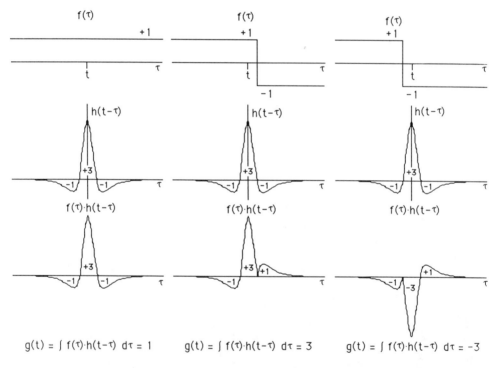

FIGURE 22.9.   Edge enhancing filter: this figure shows the effect of an edge enhancing filter. The top panel shows the values of an input image, $f(\tau)$. The middle panel show the edge enhancing filter, time reversed and shifted to position, t. The bottom panel show the product, $f(\tau) \cdot h(t - \tau)$. The output for position, t, is the integral of this product. On the left, the position is in a region of constant intensity; the integral is one. In the center, the position is on the positive side of an edge; the integral is three. On the right, the position is on the negative side of an edge; the integral is negative three. The values around an edge are amplified compared to values in a constant region.

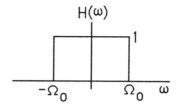

FIGURE 22.10. Ideal low pass filter: an ideal low pass filter has value of one in the pass zone and a value of zero for higher frequencies. Ω_0 is the cut-off frequency.

either outside or inside the region. We shall define windows in a more general fashion. A window may have any values for, h(t), just as filters may have any values for H(ω).

The very astute reader will have notice that Equations 22.3 and 22.4 are equivalent to Equation 16.9. In Chapter 16, we used this same operation to describe modulation. When a signal is multiplied by an imaginary exponential in the time domain, it is shifted in the frequency domain. The mathematics is the same, only the point of view is different.

V. IDEAL LOW PASS FILTER

An ideal low pass filter is shown in Figure 22.10. It is equal to one for frequencies below the cut-off frequency, Ω_0, and it is equal to zero for frequencies above the cut-off frequency. An ideal low pass filter is a rectangle function in the frequency domain.

We have encountered the rectangle function before; the time domain representation of the rectangle function is the sinc function (see Equation 16.78). (Recall that sinc(x) is equal to the sin(x)/x.) Multiplication of the frequency domain signal by an ideal low pass filter is equivalent to convolution of the time domain signal with a sinc function. The sinc function is a somewhat bizarre function. However, one of the reasons we have emphasized it is that ideal low pass filters are very common.

An ideal low pass filter is an example of a smoothing filter — it discards the higher spatial frequencies. However, the sinc function has ripples. (Recall from Chapter 16 that signals with sharp edges in one domain have ripples in the other domain.) Convolution with the sinc function will tend to produce ripples in the output. Thus, the ideal low pass filter is not typically used for smoothing. In general, filters with sharp edges are not used for smoothing since they cause ripples in the output.

The ideal low pass filter will be very important in the next chapter (Sampling). The sampling rate determines the highest frequency in the input signal which is faithfully reproduced in the output signal. In the next chapter we shall learn that the higher frequencies cause artifacts in the output signal by a process called aliasing. Prior to sampling a signal with an analog to digital converter, an ideal low pass filter is used to remove these artifacts.

A. MODULATION, DEMODULATION

The process of sending two or more signals over the same channel is called multiplexing. There are two typical methods of multiplexing. One, called time domain multiplexing, is often used in telephone transmission. The channel is switched very rapidly between different telephone calls. Each call is given multiple small time windows. The other method, called frequency domain multiplexing, is similar to time domain multiplexing; however, instead of using time windows, frequency filters are used. Frequency domain multiplexing is performed by modulating each signal with a different carrier before combining the signals. They are then demodulated at the other end of the channel.

Chapter 16 introduced modulation and demodulation. In that chapter modulation and

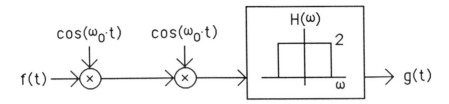

FIGURE 22.11.   Modulation, demodulation with real sinusoids: multiplication of a signal, f(t), by $\cos(\omega_0 \cdot t)$ modulates the signal to a carrier frequency, ω_0. Demodulation can be performed by multiplying the modulated signal by $\cos(\omega_0 \cdot t)$ and then by filtering with an ideal low pass filter with a gain of two.

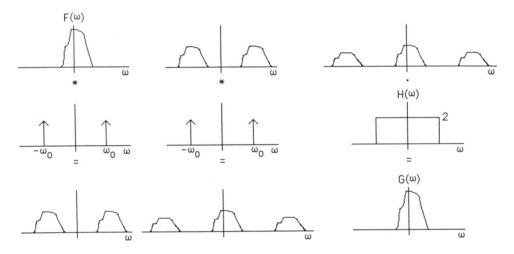

FIGURE 22.12.   Modulation, demodulation with real sinusoids: this diagram shows the effects of the algorithm shown in Figure 22.11. Multiplication of f(t) by $\cos(\omega_0 \cdot t)$ is equivalent to convolution of $F(\omega)$ with $1/2 \cdot \delta(\omega - \omega_0) + 1/2 \cdot \delta(\omega + \omega_0)$. This convolution results in two, half height copies of $F(\omega)$ located at ω_0 and $-\omega_0$. The modulated signal is again convolved with $1/2 \cdot \delta(\omega - \omega_0) + 1/2 \cdot \delta(\omega + \omega_0)$. This convolution results in a half height copy of $F(\omega)$ at the origin, and two quarter-height copies of $F(\omega)$ at $2 \cdot \omega_0$ and $-2 \cdot \omega_0$. Filtering of this signal with an ideal low pass filter, $H(\omega)$, with gain of two gives an output, $G(\omega)$, which is equal to $F(\omega)$ so long as the original signal was band limited to the range, $-\omega_0$ to ω_0.

demodulation were performed with an imaginary exponential, $e^{i\omega t}$. The advantage of using an imaginary exponential is that a single copy of the original signal is produced at the modulating frequency. Demodulation can then be performed with $e^{-i\omega t}$. However, it is unusual to be able to use this form of modulation, demodulation. Frequently, only the real component of the signal is available. In that case, modulation and demodulation must be performed with a real sinusoids.

Figure 22.11 shows the modulation, demodulation process diagrammatically. The modulation is performed by multiplication of the signal with a cosine function. The modulated signal can then be transmitted over a channel to the demodulator. The demodulator consists of two components. First the modulated signal is again multiplied by a cosine function, and then it is passed through an ideal low pass filter. This type of modulation, demodulation is used by AM radio stations.

Figure 22.12 shows the frequency domain representations of the signals associated with modulation and demodulation process diagrammed in Figure 22.11. The Fourier transform of the original signal is shown on the first line in the panel on the left. The frequency domain representation of the cosine function used for modulation is shown on the second line. The frequency domain representation of the modulated signal, the convolution of $F(\omega)$ with the transform of $\cos(\omega_0 \cdot t)$, is shown on the third line.

The transform of the product of the modulated signal with $\cos(\omega_0 \cdot t)$ is shown in the middle panel. In the time domain this signal is equal to:

$$
\begin{aligned}
f(t) \cdot {}^{1}/_{2} \cdot (e^{i\omega_0 t} &+ e^{-i\omega_0 t}) \cdot {}^{1}/_{2} \cdot (e^{i\omega_0 t} + e^{-i\omega_0 t}) \\
&= f(t) \cdot ({}^{1}/_{4} \cdot e^{i2\omega_0 t} + {}^{1}/_{2} + {}^{1}/_{4} \cdot e^{-i2\omega_0 t}) \\
&= {}^{1}/_{2}\, f(t) + {}^{1}/_{2}\, f(t) \cdot \cos(2\omega_0 t)
\end{aligned} \tag{22.5}
$$

This signal contains the original signal plus a signal modulated at twice the carrier angular frequency. These two components can be separated by passing the signal through an ideal low pass filter. The frequency domain representation of the demodulated signal, shown in the right panel of Figure 22.12, has the same form as the original signal. Demodulation is a common use of the ideal low pass filter.

VI. BAND PASS FILTER

A band pass filter is shown in Figure 22.1. A band pass filter is equal to one for a certain range of frequencies and equal to zero for the remaining frequencies. It passes a certain range of frequencies. A band pass filter is similar to an ideal low pass filter except that the range of frequencies which it passes does not include zero.

Multiplexing is a term that means that two signals are combined to be transmitted over a common medium. Frequency domain multiplexing means that each signal is allowed to use only a specific range of frequencies. For example, each program on a cable television system is transmitted with a certain range of frequencies. The television tuner, demultiplexes the cable television signal by extracting a single program. The television tuner is an example of a band pass filter.

In nuclear magnetic resonance, the signal is contained in a narrow band of frequencies around the resonant frequency. The first step in processing the signal is to select this narrow band of frequencies and reject all of the other radio frequencies.

When demultiplexing a signal, it is often desirable not only to select a range of frequencies, but also to demodulate the signal — shift the frequencies from some carrier frequency to zero frequency. Both the television tuner and the nuclear magnetic resonance detection circuit demodulate the signal. In this case, it is often easier to demodulate the signal first, and then pass the signal through an ideal low pass filter. These two filters are very closely related.

VII. APPROXIMATE LOW PASS FILTERS

Ideal low pass filters are impossible to implement in hardware. Because low pass filters are very commonly used, considerable effort has been extended on the design of approximate low pass filters. Different approximate low pass filters have different properties. For a particular application, one property may be very important and another less important. Thus, there are several types of low pass filters which are in common use. Understanding the properties of each will help explain the advantages and disadvantages for each application.

One property is how much the filter resembles an ideal low pass filter — how much the shape of the filter resembles a rectangle function. This property is often stated in terms of how the filter behaves in three zones — the pass band, the stop band, and the transition zone between the pass band and the stop band. A good approximation of an ideal low pass filter should be equal to one in the pass band, equal to zero in the stop band, and have a rapid transition between the pass band and the stop band. In electronics, this property is often the most important property. In image processing and image reconstruction the approximation to an ideal low pass filters is often less important than other properties.

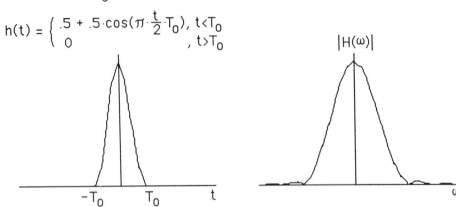

FIGURE 22.13.   Hanning window: on the left is the time domain and on the right is the frequency domain representations of the Hanning window. The Hanning window has a very simple time domain representation, and it is a reasonable low pass filter.

A property which often conflicts with close approximation of an ideal low pass filter is the extent of the time domain representation of the filter. Having a limited extent in the time domain is very important if the filter is to be implemented as a convolution in the time domain. If the impulse response of the filter is to be of short duration, then it is difficult to approximate a rectangularly shaped filter. Design of limited extent filters low pass filters is a major topic in electrical engineering.

One problem with an ideal low pass filter is that it has ripples in the time domain. The ripples may introduce very conspicuous artifacts in the output. Thus, a property that is important for some applications is that the time domain representation of the filter is smooth.

When the task is windowing as opposed to filtering, then the requirements are stated in terms of the alternate domain. Since windowing is the dual operation of filtering, the properties are the dual properties. At times even the distinction between windowing and filtering is blurred.

A. HANNING WINDOW

The Hanning window is a raised cosine function defined in the time domain. It is shown in Figure 22.13. Mathematically it is defined as:

$$h(t) = \begin{cases} .5 + .5 \cdot \cos(\pi \cdot t/2 \cdot T_0), & t < T_0 \\ 0, & \text{otherwise} \end{cases} \qquad (22.6)$$

The frequency response of the Hanning window is also shown in Figure 22.13. It is nearly equal to one for low frequencies; it is nearly zero for high frequencies; and the transition between the pass band and the stop band is reasonably rapid. The frequency response of the Hanning window is in the general form of a low pass filter.

In the time domain, the Hanning window is reasonably well confined. It is very smooth, and it does not have any ripples.

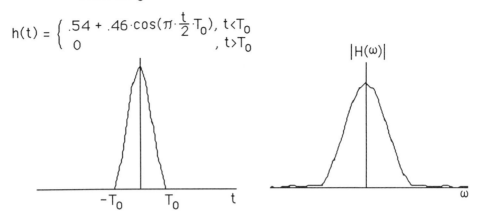

Hamming Window

$$h(t) = \begin{cases} .54 + .46 \cdot \cos(\pi \cdot \frac{t}{2} \cdot T_0), & t < T_0 \\ 0 & , t > T_0 \end{cases}$$

FIGURE 22.14.   Hamming window: on the left is the time domain and on the right is the frequency domain representation of the Hamming window. Like the Hanning window (Figure 22.13), the Hamming window has a very simple time domain representation, and it is a reasonable low pass filter. There is a small difference between these two filters in terms of their stop zone performance.

B. HAMMING WINDOW

The Hamming window is very similar to the Hanning window, but it is defined with slightly different constant factors. It is shown in Figure 22.14. Mathematically:

$$h(t) = \begin{cases} .54 + .46 \cdot \cos(\pi \cdot t/2 \cdot T_0), & t < T_0 \\ 0, & \text{otherwise} \end{cases} \tag{22.7}$$

The frequency response of the Hamming window is also a low pass filter. It is even closer than the frequency response of the Hanning window to an ideal low pass filter. Like the Hanning window, the Hamming window does not have any ripples; however, it is somewhat less confined in the space domain.

The Hanning and Hamming windows have been defined as time domain approximations to an ideal low pass filter. This definition is typical in electrical engineering. In image reconstruction, it is common to use Hanning and Hamming filters, where the filters are defined in the frequency domain. Hanning and Hamming filters are the duals of Hanning and Hamming windows. The time and frequency characteristics of the filter are merely interchanged.

There is some room for confusion — the Hanning and the Hamming windows are reasonably good approximations to an ideal low pass filter. Since the Hanning and the Hamming filters have large transition zones, they are not very good approximations of an ideal low pass filter. By duality, they are good approximations of an ideal time window.

C. BUTTERWORTH FILTER

The Butterworth filter is shown in Figure 22.15. Mathematically:

$$H(\omega) = 1/\sqrt{(1 + (\omega^2/\Omega_0^2)^n)} \tag{22.8}$$

where n is a parameter called the order of the Butterworth filter, and Ω_0 is a parameter which can be adjusted to change the frequency range. The Butterworth filters have the

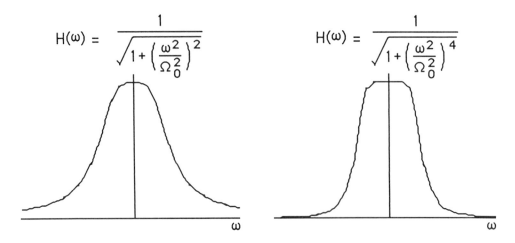

FIGURE 22.15.   Butterworth filters: this diagram shows two Butterworth filters with different exponents. The exponent determines the sharpness of the transition between the pass zone and the stop zone. The Butterworth filters have a simple mathematical expression in the frequency domain.

advantage that among the set of filters which are equally difficult to implement it is maximally flat at ω equal zero. That property is rarely very important in image processing; however, the Butterworth filter is still useful. It has a convenient shape; its position can be easily adjusted with Ω_0; and the transition between the pass band and the stop band can be easily adjusted with n. For large n, the Butterworth filter is a very good approximation to an ideal low pass filter.

D. GAUSSIAN FILTER

The Gaussian function can be used as a filter. The inverse Fourier transform of a Gaussian is also a Gaussian (see Equation 14.14). The main advantage of the Gaussian is that it has the lowest time, band width product of any function where the time, band width product is defined by Equation 16.95. (See the discussion of the uncertainty principle in Chapter 16.) Thus, the Gaussian is used when there are simultaneous constraints for both a narrow frequency and a narrow time domain response.

VIII. SUMMARY

Filtering and windowing are simple operations in the frequency and the time domain, respectively. They involve the multiplication of an input signal with a filter or a window signal. They are more complicated, a convolution, when viewed from the opposite domain. Filtering is really not a new operation; it is equivalent to passing an input signal through a system. The difference between a filter and another linear, time invariant system is the way the process is conceptualized.

Much of the description of filters has dealt with low pass filters. In fact, the vast majority of filtering is low pass filtering or some variation of low pass filtering. Another frequent operation in image processing is edge enhancement. Later in this part of the book we shall see that filtering can also be used to selectively reduce noise when the noise and the signal are different power spectral density functions.

IX. FURTHER READING

Filtering is described in all of the books which describe the Fourier transform. A good introduction can be found in Chapter 6 of the book by Oppenheim and Willsky.[1] A complete discussion of filtering is given in the book by Rabiner and Gold.[2] Filtering applied to images is described in the books by Gonzalez and Wintz,[3] and by Castleman.[4]

REFERENCES

1. **Oppenheim, A. V., and Willsky, A. S.,** *Signals and Systems,* Prentice-Hall, Englewood Cliffs, NJ, 1983.
2. **Rabiner, L. R. and Gold, B.,** *Theory and Application of Digital Signal Processing,* Prentice-Hall, Englewood Cliffs, NJ, 1975.
3. **Gonzalez, R. C. and Wintz, P.,** *Image Processing,* Addison-Wesley, London, 1977.
4. **Castleman, K. R.,** *Digital Image Processing,* Prentice-Hall, Englewood Cliffs, NJ, 1979.

Chapter 23

SAMPLING

Sampling is a frequent operation in radiological applications. Whenever a continuous signal is represented by a discrete signal, it must be sampled. All of the computerized imaging methods in radiology use digital samples of analog signals. Understanding the sampling process is important since sampling can introduce an important artifact called aliasing. Aliasing occurs when one frequency is misrepresented, or aliased, as another frequency. Aliasing is a particularly common cause of artifacts in nuclear magnetic resonance imaging.

This chapter will begin with a discussion of aliasing. In order to better understand the process of sampling, a new signal, the comb signal, will be introduced, and its Fourier transform will be derived. The comb function will allow us to understand sampling in terms of continuous signals. Much of this exposition will be reminiscent of Chapter 18 (Discrete Fourier Transform).

Sampling transforms a continuous signal into a discrete signal. Interpolation performs the opposite operation. It transforms a discrete signal into a continuous signal. In this chapter, it will be shown that under certain condition, interpolation performed with an ideal low pass filter will exactly reconstruct a sampled signal.

One of the most important results of this chapter is the sampling theorem. The sampling theorem states that a signal should be sampled at twice the highest frequency in the signal. Signals sampled according to the sampling theorem are exact representations of the original signal in the sense that the original signal can be reproduced using an ideal low pass filter.

I. ALIASING

Figure 23.1 shows two cosine waves and a number of sample points. Although the cosine waves are of much different frequencies, they both have exactly the same values at each of the sample points. There are an infinite number of sinusoidal functions which have exactly the same sample points given by:

$$f(t) = e^{i(\omega + k2\pi/T)t} \tag{23.1}$$

where k is an integer and T is the sampling interval. At sample points, $t = n \cdot T$:

$$f(n \cdot T) = e^{i\omega nT} \cdot e^{ikn2\pi} \tag{23.2}$$

Since k and n are integers, the second term is equal to one. Thus, sampling at interval, T, produces the same value for all of the angular frequencies, $\omega + k \cdot 2\pi/T$.

For a sinusoid signal at either angular frequency, ω, or angular frequency, $\omega + k \cdot 2\pi/T$, the sample values will be identical. It is impossible to distinguish which of these angular frequencies exists in the original signal from this set of samples. Given the set of sampled values, there is a basic ambiguity about the frequencies in the original signal. It is natural to think of the lowest frequency as the primary frequency; however, mathematically all frequencies are equally valid.

Multiple equivalent frequencies should be reminiscent of the discrete Fourier transform. We defined the discrete Fourier transform in terms of periodic signals in the time and frequency domain. We found that any range of N values in the frequency domain could be used to define the signal. Recall that the periodicity in one domain corresponded to discrete samples in the other domain.

$$\cos(\omega \cdot t) = \cos(\omega \cdot t + \frac{2\pi \cdot t}{T}), \quad t = n \cdot T$$

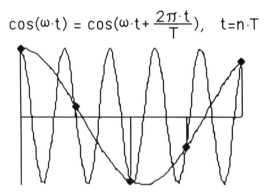

FIGURE 23.1.   Two different cosine functions with identical sample values: the two cosine function, $\cos(\omega \cdot t)$ and $\cos(\omega \cdot t + 2\pi \cdot t/T)$, have the same values at t equal to n $\cdot$ T. Notice the similarity between this figure and Figure 18.7.

When we sample a signal, all of the angular frequencies which are multiples of $2\pi/T$ will result in the same set of values. Thus, we cannot distinguish them. If we make the usual assumption that the signal contains only the lowest range of frequencies, then the higher frequencies will be incorrectly identified. Misinterpretation of a higher frequency due to sampling is called **aliasing**. The high frequency component is said to be aliased to a lower frequency.

A common example of aliasing occurs in old cowboy movies. As the wheels on a wagon speed up, the spokes in the wheels appear to change direction and rotate backwards. As the wheels go even faster, they again rotate forward, but at an inappropriately slow speed. As the wagon speeds up, the wheels may go through several cycles of backward and forward motion until they finally blur.

The frames of a motion picture are discrete samples in time. There may be 24 samples each second. When the motion picture is played back, we perceive the motion as continuous; we interpolate the images in time. When the wagon wheels are moving slowly, the spokes move only a short distance between each frame, and the motion is faithfully reproduced. As the wheels move more rapidly, the spokes may move so that they are nearly to the position of the next spoke in one frame time (see Figure 23.2).

The human observer's interpretation of this sequence of images is that the next spoke has moved backwards a small amount. The human interpretation uses the lowest frequency which is consistent with the data. Notice that the motion appears to change direction. As the wheels go even faster, a spoke may actually move more than one position between frames. When this happens, the wheels again go forward, but at a rate which is aliased to a much lower frequency.

An example of aliasing from Radiology is shown in Figure 23.3. This figure shows three images of a bar phantom collected using different size matrices. Figure 23.3A shows the "true" image, collected with a 512 by 512 matrix. The image in Figure 23.3B collected with a 128 by 128 matrix shows some change in the bars. Figure 23.3C, collected with a 64 by 64 matrix, shows the bars in a much different orientation. The actual orientation of the bars are not changed, rather the spatial frequencies are misrepresented due to aliasing. The net effect is that the direction of the bars is changed.

The effect of aliasing in this example may remind the reader of Moiré patterns. Moiré patterns occur when two regular patterns overlap. In this case, one pattern is the bar pattern, and the other pattern is the sampling pattern. The strange result shown in Figure 23.3 can be interpreted as a Moiré pattern. However, the view point in this chapter will be to interpret this phenomenon in the frequency domain. The under-sampling of the signal results in aliasing of the high spatial frequency to a lower spatial frequency.

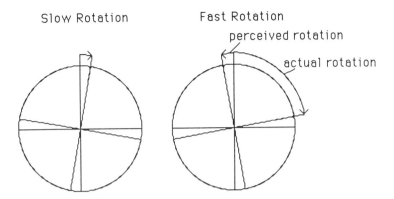

FIGURE 23.2. Wagon wheel aliasing: on the left is a diagram of two images of a wagon wheel which is rotating slowly. The spokes in the wagon wheel move only a short distance between the two images. The actual and perceived rotations are both in the clockwise direction. On the right is a diagram of two images of a wagon wheel which is rotating rapidly. A spoke moves almost to the position of the next spoke in the time between the two images. The actual rotation is in the clockwise direction; however, the perceived rotation is in the counter clockwise direction.

A common radiological example of aliasing occurs in nuclear magnetic resonance imaging. In Chapter 30 it will be shown that the positions in an image correspond to the nuclear magnetic resonance frequency spectrum. This relationship was shown diagrammatically in Figure 15.1. The Fourier transform of the image positions give the spatial frequencies in the image; and the inverse Fourier transform of the spectrum is the free induction decay. Since the image positions and the spectral frequencies are similar signals, their respective Fourier transforms, the spatial frequencies, and the free induction decay, are also similar signals.

During image collection the time domain signal, the free induction decay, is sampled by an analog to digital converter in the nuclear magnetic resonance scanner. Since the time signal is sampled, there can be ambiguity about the spectral frequencies and hence about the positions in the image. This ambiguity is expressed by wrap around of signals from one side of the image to another. Figure 23.4 shows an example of aliasing in nuclear magnetic resonance imaging. The physics of nuclear magnetic resonance image collection will be dealt with more fully in Chapter 30.

II. COMB SIGNAL

A comb signal is a sequence of equally spaced delta functions. Mathematically,

$$h(t) = \sum_{n=-\infty}^{\infty} \delta(t - nT) \tag{23.3}$$

The comb signal is shown in Figure 23.5. The comb signal will be useful for understanding sampling, since multiplication of a signal by a comb signal is analogous to sampling the signal. In this section we shall derive the Fourier transform of the comb signal.

Figure 23.6 shows various components of the comb signal, along with their Fourier transforms. The component at t equal to zero is a constant function in the frequency domain. The two adjacent components give a cosine function:

$$H(\omega) = e^{i\omega T} + e^{-i\omega T} = 2 \cdot \cos(\omega \cdot T) \tag{23.4}$$

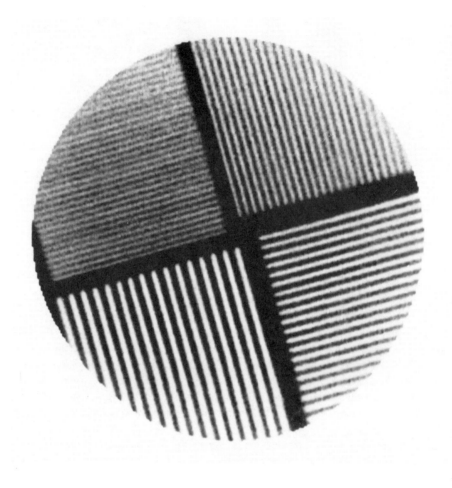

A

FIGURE 23.3.   Bar phantom aliasing: (A) a 512 by 512 gamma camera image of a bar phantom; (B) a 128 by 128 image of the same phantom; (C) a 64 by 64 image of the same phantom. Although the bars have not been physically moved, they appear to change direction due to aliasing.

The next two components give a cosine of twice the frequency:

$$H(\omega) = 2 \cdot \cos(2 \cdot \omega \cdot T) \qquad (23.5)$$

Subsequent pairs of delta functions give rise to cosines which are 3, 4, 5, etc. times the base "angular frequency", T. (Since these are cosine functions in the frequency domain, the "angular frequency" of the cosines is given in terms of the time domain.)

All of the cosine functions will line up at ω equal to $k \cdot 2\pi/T$, where k is an integer. In between, the different components will tend to cancel. This behavior may be reminiscent of the delta function described in Chapter 15. The delta function is made up of cosines which only line up at zero. The delta function is made up of equal contributions of every cosine function. The comb function does not have contributions from all of the cosine function, but rather it has contributions from a discrete set of evenly spaced cosine functions. The set of evenly spaced cosine functions line up at a set of evenly spaced frequencies.

The difference between the delta function and the comb function is analogous to the difference between the continuous and the discrete Fourier transform. A continuous signal

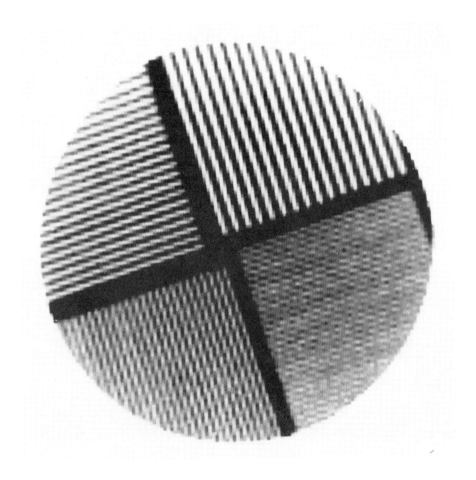

FIGURE 23.3B

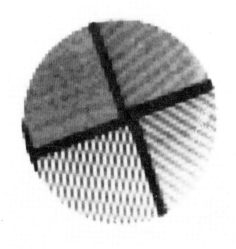

FIGURE 23.3C

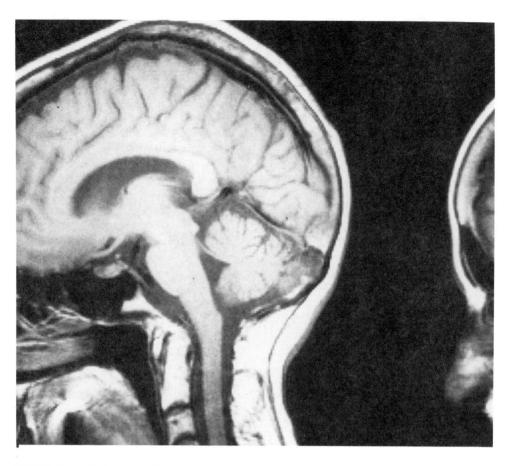

FIGURE 23.4.   Nuclear magnetic resonance position aliasing: in nuclear magnetic resonance, image positions correspond to precisional frequency. Aliasing of the frequency results in miss-positioning of the data. In this case, part of the image has "wrapped around" from the left to the right of the image.

Comb Signal

$$f(t) = \sum_{n=-\infty}^{\infty} \delta(t - n \cdot T)$$

t

FIGURE 23.5.   Comb signal: the comb signal is a sequence of equally spaced delta functions.

in one domain leads to an aperiodic signal in the other domain, while a discrete signal in one domain leads to a periodic signal in the other domain. The repetition of the comb signal in the frequency domain is related to the discrete set of values in the time domain.

Due to the similarity of the frequency domain representation of the comb function and the delta function, we can surmise that the Fourier transform of a comb function is also a

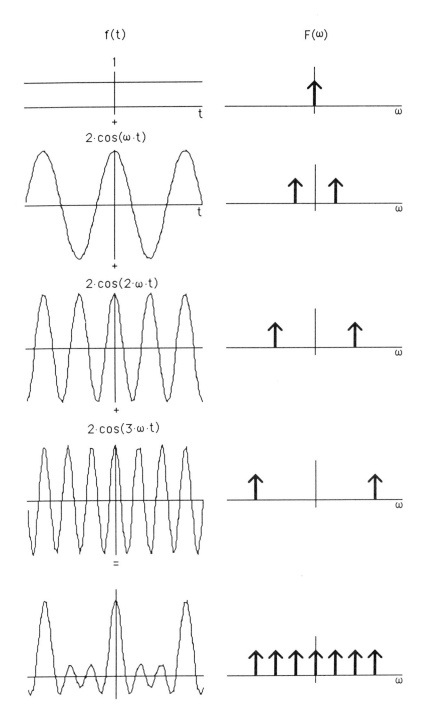

FIGURE 23.6. Approximation of a comb signal: a series of cosine functions, 2 · cos(n · ω · t) can be used to approximate the Comb signal. The cosine functions tend to reinforce each other at regular intervals. In between they tend to cancel. As more and more cosines are added, the sum of the cosine signals approaches a comb signal. The right side of the figure shows the Fourier transforms of the signals.

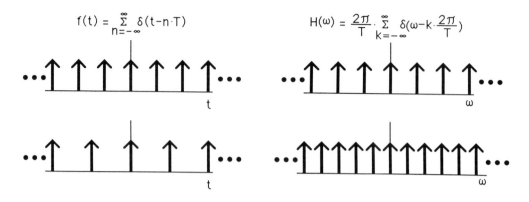

FIGURE 23.7. Comb signal: this figure shows two comb signals and their Fourier transform. As T increases, the delta functions in the time domain spread out and the delta functions in the frequency domain come closer together.

comb function. Figure 23.7 shows the comb function and its Fourier transform. The following section shows this result mathematically.

Because of linearity, the Fourier transform of each term in Equation 23.3 can be calculated separately. The delta function selects one time from the Fourier transform integral giving:

$$H(\omega) = \sum_{n=-\infty}^{\infty} e^{-i\omega nT} \tag{23.6}$$

For ω equal to $k \cdot 2\pi/T$, the exponent is equal to $-i \cdot k \cdot 2\pi \cdot n$. Since n and k are integers, the exponent is a power of 2π, and the exponential function is equal to one:

$$H(\omega) = \sum_{n=-\infty}^{\infty} 1 = \infty, \quad \omega = k \cdot 2\pi/T \tag{23.7}$$

For ω not equal to $k \cdot 2\pi/T$, the sum is a sum of exponentials similar to Equation 18.20. In Chapter 18, it was shown that these exponentials cancel each other. Therefore,

$$H(\omega) = \begin{cases} \infty, & \omega = k \cdot 2\pi/T \\ 0, & \omega \neq k \cdot 2\pi/T \end{cases} \tag{23.8}$$

The Fourier transform of the comb function in the time domain is a series of delta functions at ω equal to $k \cdot 2\pi/T$ — namely, it is a comb function in the frequency domain. In order to determine the magnitude of the delta functions, we can do some fancy foot work by integrating $H(\omega)$ over the interval from $-\pi/T$ to π/T. Within these limits there is a single delta function, so the value of the integral will give the size of the delta function. Choosing the interval $-\pi/T$ to π/T produces some very convenient cancellation of terms.

Using Equation 23.6 for $H(\omega)$:

$$\int_{-\pi/T}^{+\pi/T} H(\omega)\ d\omega = \int_{-\pi/T}^{+\pi/T} \sum_{n=-\infty}^{\infty} e^{i\omega nT}\ d\omega \qquad (23.9)$$

Because of linearity, we can switch the order of integration and summation:

$$\int_{-\pi/T}^{+\pi/T} H(\omega)\ d\omega = \sum_{n=-\infty}^{\infty} \int_{-\pi/T}^{+\pi/T} e^{i\omega nT}\ d\omega \qquad (23.10)$$

For n not equal to zero, the integral is equal to $(2/n \cdot T) \cdot \sin(n \cdot \pi)$. Since n is an integer, $\sin(n \cdot \pi)$ is zero, and the integral is zero. For n equal to zero, the exponential is equal to one, and the integral is equal to $2\pi/T$. Summarizing:

$$\int_{-\pi/T}^{+\pi/T} e^{i\omega nT}\ d\omega = \begin{cases} 2\pi/T, & n = 0 \\ \\ 0, & n \neq 0 \end{cases} \qquad (23.11)$$

Therefore, the only nonzero term in the summation in Equation 23.6 is for n equal to zero. Thus, the sum is equal to $2\pi/T$. The same argument applies to each of the delta functions in $H(\omega)$.

We can summarize the results of the tricky mathematics of the previous section with the Fourier transform pair:

$$h(t) = \sum_{n=-\infty}^{\infty} \delta(t - nT) \qquad (23.12)$$

$$H(\omega) = 2\pi/T \cdot \sum_{k=-\infty}^{\infty} \delta(\omega - k \cdot 2\pi/T) \qquad (23.13)$$

This Fourier transform pair was shown in Figure 23.7. The familiar inverse relation between the time and frequency axes is apparent. As T gets smaller, the delta functions in the time domain get closer together, and the delta functions in the frequency domain get farther apart, and *vice versa*.

III. SAMPLING USING THE COMB FUNCTION

We can model sampling a signal, $f(t)$, as multiplication of the signal by a comb function, $h(t)$. The sampled signal, $g(t)$, is given by:

$$g(t) = f(t) \cdot h(t) \qquad (23.14)$$

Multiplication in the time domain is equivalent to convolution in the frequency domain (Equation 16.9):

$$G(\omega) = (1/2\pi) \cdot F(\omega) * H(\omega) \qquad (23.15)$$

This model is shown graphically in Figure 23.8. Convolution by a comb function in the frequency domain will help to explain the sampling process.

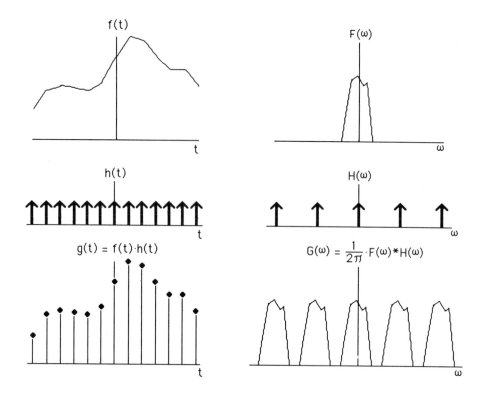

FIGURE 23.8. Sampling: the top panel shows a function, f(t), and its Fourier transform, F(ω). The middle panel shows the sampling signal, h(t), and its Fourier transform, H(ω). The bottom panel shows the sampled signal, g(t), and its Fourier transform, G(ω). In the time domain the sampling signal, h(t), is multiplied by f(t) to produce g(t). In the frequency domain the sampling signal is convolved with F(ω) to produce G(ω). G(ω) consists of an infinite series of replicates of F(ω).

Sampling involves transformation of a continuous signal into a discrete signal. However, it is difficult to relate the continuous and discrete signals since the basic representations are different. Using the comb function we can represent a discrete function by a continuous function which has nonzero values at only a discrete number of locations. It is then easier to see how the continuous and the "discrete" functions are related.

Convolution by the comb function in the frequency domain results in multiple replications of the transform of the signal. For example, consider F(ω) shown in Figure 23.8. Sampling, f(t), using an interval of T results in replication in the frequency domain at intervals of $2\pi/T$. The sampled signal is discrete in the time domain and periodic in the frequency domain. (It is reminiscent of the dual of the Fourier series.) Multiplication by the comb function, h(t), transforms the time domain signal into a "discrete" signal. Convolution by the comb function, H(ω), transforms the frequency domain signal into a periodic signal.

If the original signal, F(ω), extends only from $-\pi/T$ to π/T, then there is no problem. If, however, the signal extends past $-\pi/T$ or π/T, there will be a problem. Figure 23.9 shows an example of a signal with a single frequency which is slightly larger than $2\pi/T$. The transform of the sampled signal is a periodic signal with frequencies repeated at intervals of $2\pi/T$. One of the frequencies is near zero. If we interpret the sampled signal in the usual fashion, then the high frequency has been aliased to a frequency near zero. This aliasing is analogous to what happens with the wagon wheels.

Although the example in Figure 23.9 shows what happens when a single high frequency is aliased to a low frequency, more commonly the spectrum is more complex. In that case the copies of F(ω) may overlap. Figure 23.10 shows an example where there is overlap

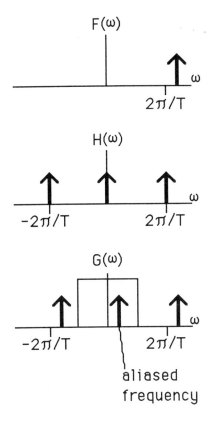

FIGURE 23.9. Aliasing: the signal, $F(\omega)$, contains a single frequency just above, $2\pi/T$. The sampling signal is shown on the second line. The sampled signal, $G(\omega)$, has frequencies repeated every $2\pi/T$ radians. Using the range $-\pi/T$ to π/T, the single frequency from $F(\omega)$ is aliased to a position near zero.

between the copies of $F(\omega)$. This overlapping leads to a more complicated form of aliasing. There is no way to recover the original signal from the sampled signal.

IV. INTERPOLATION

The term interpolation is often used to mean inserting additional points in between points in a discrete signal. This process can be broken down into two separate processes. The first process involves fitting two or more of the discrete points to a continuous model of the function, e.g., a spline function. The second part involves resampling this model at the intervening points. We shall restrict the meaning of the term **interpolation** to the first process — namely fitting discrete points to a continuous model. The term resampling will be used for the second process.

Often interpolation is performed in the time domain. A small set of points in some region is fit to a spline function. However, it is also possible to interpolate using the frequency domain representation of the signal. In that case, the signal is modeled by a limited range of sinusoidal components. Interpolation amounts to selecting a range of frequencies in the Fourier transform. The interpolated signal is continuous, but it is composed of a limited number of sinusoidal components.

Let us consider the discrete signal, $g(t)$, which is shown in Figure 23.8. This discrete signal is derived from sampling the continuous signal, $f(t)$. Suppose that we choose to use a model which includes the range of frequencies from $-\pi/T$ to π/T. Selecting the values

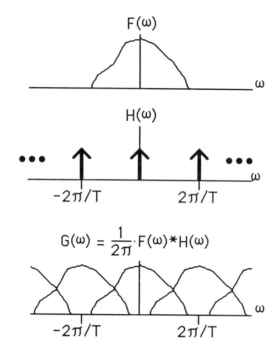

FIGURE 23.10.   Aliasing: the frequency domain representation of a signal, F(ω), is shown in the top panel. A sampling signal, H(ω), is shown in the second panel. The effect of the sampling is shown diagrammatically in the third panel. The different copies of F(ω) overlap in the sampled signal, G(ω). In this case it is not possible to recover the original signal from the sampled signal.

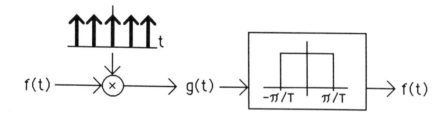

FIGURE 23.11.   Interpolation of a sampled signal: sampling of the signal, f(t), is represented by multiplication with a comb signal to produce the sampled signal, g(t). If the sampling rate meets the requirements of the sampling theorem, then interpolation of the sampled signal can be performed by an ideal low pass filter with cut-off frequency at the half the sampling rate.

of G(ω) in the range from $-\pi/T$ to π/T produces an interpolated signal which is equal to H(ω), the Fourier transform of the original signal. This result is truly remarkable. Interpolation of this sampled signal reproduces the original signal!

Selection of the frequencies $-\pi/T$ to π/T can be performed by an ideal low pass filter as discussed in the last chapter. This process is shown in Figure 23.11. The original signal, f(t), is multiplied by h(t) to produce the sampled signal g(t). The sampled signal is then passed through an ideal low pass filter with cut off π/T to produce the original signal, f(t). The sampled signal is an exact representation of the original signal in the sense that the original signal can be reproduced using the ideal low pass filter.

There is no way the signal, f(t), shown in Figure 23.10 can be reproduced from the samples, g(t). Application of an ideal low pass filter to g(t) will result in aliasing of all of the frequencies which are outside of the range $-\pi/T$ to π/T into that range. Thus, only certain sampled signals can be reproduced by ideal low pass filtering.

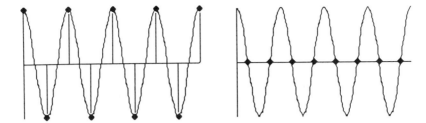

FIGURE 23.12.   Sampling at the Nyquist rate: if a sinusoidal signal is sampled at exactly the Nyquist rate, then the results depend upon the phase of the sinusoid and the sampling. On the left, sampling at the Nyquist rate accurately reflects the peaks and the valleys in the sinusoid. On the right, sampling at the Nyquist rate results in all zeros.

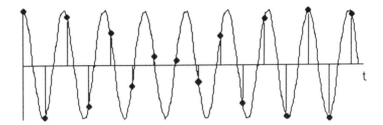

FIGURE 23.13.   Sampling above the Nyquist rate: if a sinusoid is sampled just above the Nyquist rate, then it is always possible to correctly identify the sinusoid from its samples. Some of the samples will reflect the peaks and the valleys accurately.

V. SAMPLING THEOREM

The sampling theorem defines the conditions under which a signal, f(t), can be exactly reproduced from a sampled signal, g(t), using an ideal low pass filter as shown in Figure 23.11. From the examples, we have seen that there is no problem with aliasing so long as F(ω) is nonzero only in the range $-\pi/T$ to π/T, where T is the sampling interval. The sampled signal, g(t), is an accurate representation of f(t) in the sense that f(t) can be created from g(t).

For a sampling interval of T, the angular frequency of the signal must be in the range $-\pi/T$ to π/T. The sampling interval, T, corresponds to an angular frequency of $2\pi/T$. Thus, a signal which has angular frequencies in the range $-\pi/T$ to π/T must be sampled at a rate greater than $2\pi/T$. The sampling frequency must be twice the highest frequency in the signal. This sampling frequency is known as the **Nyquist rate**.

This very important result is worth stating one more time. **A signal which has a limited frequency range can be exactly reproduced from its samples if the sampling frequency is greater than twice the highest frequency in the signal.**

There is a problem in sampling at exactly twice the highest frequency. Figure 23.12 shows two examples of sampling a cosine wave at exactly twice its frequency. In the first case the cosine wave will be faithfully reproduced; in the second case, it will not be accurately represented. In order to be sure that all of the frequencies are included, the sampling rate has to be just larger than the highest frequency. Figure 23.13 shows a case where the sampling rate is slightly higher than the cosine frequency. In this case the cosine can always be correctly identified with the discrete Fourier transform.

In order to understand the relationship between the Fourier transform of the original signal and the sampled signal, we have represented the sampled signal as a continuous signal which is nonzero at only a finite number of points. The sampled signal is actually equivalent to a discrete signal, g[n]. A discrete signal is considerably less complex than a continuous signal. Although the number of points at which a discrete signal is defined is infinite, the number of points that a continuous signal is defined is much larger. Mathematicians like to say that a discrete signal is defined for a countably infinite number of points whereas a continuous signal is defined for an uncountably infinite number of points.

It may seem strange that a continuous signal can be exactly represented by a discrete signal. But, the key factor is that not all continuous signals can be represented by samples. Only signals which have a finite range of nonzero frequencies can be represented by sampling. Sampling assumes that the signals can be modeled by a sum of sinusoidal components which are limited to a certain frequency range. Limitation of the extent of the frequency domain signal produces signals of complexity equivalent to discrete signals.

VI. PREVENTION OF ALIASING IN UNDER-SAMPLED SIGNALS

One method of preventing aliasing is to sample a signal at greater than twice the highest frequency in the signal. However, this may not always be possible, or desirable. For example, the signal of interest may be limited to a certain range of frequencies, but it may contain noise at a higher frequency. If the signal is under sampled, then the noise from the higher frequency will be aliased into the data. Once it is aliased into the data, it is no longer possible to remove it.

There is an easy solution to this problem. Prior to sampling, the analog signal should be filtered with an ideal low pass filter with a cut-off frequency equal to the sampling rate. This filtering will prevent aliasing of the higher frequency data by the sampling. Of course the higher frequency data are lost, but at least they are not misrepresented in the samples.

A radiological example where filtering before sampling is very important is in the receiver of a nuclear magnetic resonance imager. Given a certain gradient field strength and field of view, the frequencies which correspond to the object can be calculated. The signal of interest will be limited to this frequency range. Radio frequency noise occurs at all frequencies. If the receiver signal is not filtered prior to sampling, then noise from all of the frequencies received by the coil will be aliased into the image. By filtering the signal prior to sampling, only the noise which is in the same frequency range as the data will be included in the samples.

VII. IMPLEMENTATION OF SAMPLING

Throughout this chapter sampling has been defined in terms of the value of the signal during a single instant in time. This model of sampling is quite unrealistic. More often the average value of the signal during the sampling interval is sampled. For example, in computed tomography the X-ray attenuation is the average value over the region defined by the beam profile. Use of an average value is desirable. The average value is usually much more reliable than the value at a single instant in time.

To sample the average value, the continuous signal is convolved with a rectangle function with a width of T. Then, this signal is sampled with a comb function. The value at the sample point is equal to the average in the interval. The implementation of sampling is modeled as a filtering step followed by the ideal sampling used above.

This model of the sampling process shows that sampling the average value in the interval is equivalent to filtering the signal with a system with a time domain response which is a rectangle function. Figure 23.15 shows the time and frequency domain representations of this filter. In the frequency domain, this filter is a sinc function. In the range $-\pi/2$ to $\pi/2$, this function is reasonably flat; there is relatively little effect from the averaging process. At very high frequencies, there is considerable filtering. In the frequency range just above '

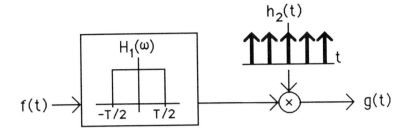

FIGURE 23.14. Filtering before sampling to avoid aliasing: if a signal, f(t), is filtered with an ideal low pass filter, $H_1(\omega)$, with a cut-off frequency equal to the Nyquist rate before it is sampled, then sampling with a comb signal, $h_2(t)$, will not result in aliasing of the high frequency components of f(t). Although, the high frequency components of f(t) will not be represented in the sampled signal, g(t), at least they will not be misrepresented.

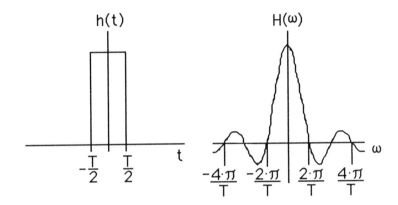

FIGURE 23.15. Average value sampling: the sample value will equal the average value in an interval if the signal is convolved with the rectangle function, h(t), prior to sampling. This convolution is equivalent to filtering the signal with the sinc function, $H(\omega)$. In the region $-\pi/T$ to π/T, this function is reasonably flat. Thus, in this region an average value sample is similar to a single-sample value. Frequencies out of this range will be aliased by sampling. Average value sampling reduces the effect of aliasing for very high frequencies, but it does poorly in the range just above the Nyquist rate.

the Nyquist frequency, this filter passes a considerable amount of the input signal. Thus, sampling the average signal intensity in the interval is not equivalent to low pass filtering.

In the last section we discussed the desirability of low pass filtering prior to sampling. In nuclear magnetic resonance imaging, it is reasonably simple to filter the electronic signals prior to sampling. In X-ray imaging it is less simple to smooth the input signal prior to sampling. However, Figure 23.14 suggests that if it is possible to design the shape of the sampling function, then the filtering step can be incorporated into the sampling process.

Sequential slices in computed tomography are defined by the X-ray beam profile. Design of the X-ray beam shape can be used to filter the attenuation signal in the axial direction prior to sampling. There are constraints in both the space and spatial frequency domains. In the space domain, the slice needs to be localized to a narrow slice; in the spatial frequency domain, the beam profile should perform a loss pass filtering operation. Because of the uncertainty principle (Equation 16.95) these goals cannot be simultaneously realized. However, proper selection of a beam profile (e.g., a Gaussian beam profile) will maximize the performance in the two domains.

VIII. SUMMARY

All of the digital imaging methods in radiology obtain their data from sampling of continuous signals. Therefore, it is important to understand the sampling process and the artifact which is produced by sampling. The artifact produced by sampling is called aliasing since higher frequency data are misrepresented or aliased as lower frequency data.

Aliasing in nuclear magnetic resonance takes a special form. Since the image domain signal corresponds to the frequency domain of the free induction decay which is sampled by the scanner, the image positions are aliased. Body parts wrap around from one side of the image to the opposite side. Although this is a dramatic artifact, it is easily recognized. The effects of aliasing in the other modalities may be less readily understood since they involve spatial frequency misrepresentations. In every day practice it is even more important to be aware of these problems in order to recognize these artifacts.

A very important result in this chapter is the sampling theorem. The sampling theorem states that the sampling frequency should be greater than twice the highest frequency in the data. If the sampling rate must be limited to less than this Nyquist rate, then the data should be filtered prior to sampling in order to prevent aliasing.

IX. FURTHER READING

All of the books which describe discrete Fourier transforms discuss the effects of sampling and the sampling theorem. The reader is referred in particular to Chapter 8 of the book by Oppenheim and Willsky,[1] and to Chapter 14 of the book by Siebert.[2] I have written an article with Drs. Kenyon and Troxel[3] on interpolating methods. Chapter 5 of the book by Kak and Slaney[4] describes aliasing in computed tomography. The references at the end of Chapter 30 describe aliasing in nuclear magnetic resonance imaging.

REFERENCES

1. **Oppenheim, A. V. and Willsky, A. S.,** *Signals and Systems,* Prentice-Hall, Englewood Cliffs, NJ, 1983.
2. **Siebert, W. Mc. C.,** *Circuits, Signals, and Systems,* McGraw-Hill, New York, 1986.
3. **Parker, J. A., Kenyon, R. V., and Troxel, D. E.,** Comparison of interpolation methods for image resampling, *IEEE Trans. Med. Imaging,* MI-2, 31, 1983.
4. **Kak, A. C. and Slaney, M.,** *Principles of Computerized Tomographic Imaging,* IEEE Press, New York, 1987.

Chapter 24

FILTERING STOCHASTIC PROCESSES

This chapter will combine the statistical model of signals introduced in Chapter 11 with the idea of filtering. The concept of noisy signals will be merged with the Fourier transform description of signals and systems. Understanding the effect of systems on noisy signals will explain how the signal to noise ratio is affected by systems. These concepts are important not only for understanding how to design filters to improve the signal to noise ratio (Chapter 26), but also to understand the noise texture in computed tomography (Chapter 32).

In order to understand the effect of a system on a stochastic process, the Fourier transform of the autocorrelation function will be introduced. The Fourier transform of the autocorelation function is called the power spectral density function. We have emphasized a number of times that the operation of linear, time invariant systems on deterministic signals is much simpler in the frequency domain (multiplication) than in the time domain (convolution). We shall similarly find that the effect of a linear, time invariant system on the statistical properties of a random signal is also most easily understood in the frequency domain using the power spectral density function.

The next chapter will be a slight diversion from linear systems theory. It will introduce the normal equations of linear algebra. The normal equations are a least-mean-square estimation method using the linear algebra model. Chapter 26 will return to the ideas of filtering statistical signals. It will introduce the Wiener filter. The Wiener filter is a least-mean-square estimation method using filtering methods. The normal equations provide a least-mean-square estimation method for linear systems, and the Wiener filter provides a least-mean-square estimation method for linear, time invariant systems.

I. STOCHASTIC PROCESSES

The concept of a random variable was introduced in Chapter 10. Recall that a random variable, f, represents an experiment which has outcomes, f_i, where f_i is the value of the outcome for the ith experiment. The outcomes of a set of experiments is not known until the experiments are performed; however, the statistics of the outcomes may be known. The ability to model this *a priori* statistical knowledge about the experiment is one of the major values of using the random variable model.

The most useful statistics are the mean, m, and the second moment, R. (In biomedical applications the variance, σ^2, is often used instead of the second moment.) The mean and the second moment are the first and second order statistics, respectively. Gaussian random variables are defined in terms of the first- and second-order statistics. Therefore, the first- and second-order statistics provide a complete description of experiments which are modeled by Gaussian statistics.

The concept of a stochastic process was introduced in Chapter 11. Recall that a stochastic process, $f(t)$, is a random signal, which has outcomes, $f_i(t)$, where $f_i(t)$ is the signal which is produced by the ith experiment. Like the case of the random variable, the outcome of an experiment is not known until the experiment is performed; however, the statistics of a set of outcomes may be known. Modeling of this *a prior* statistical knowledge is one of the major values of using the stochastic process model. Like the case of the random variable, the first and second order statistics are the most useful.

For example, in Chapter 11, liver spleen scintigraphy was modeled using stochastic processes (Equation 11.1):

$$p(x,y) = f(x,y) + n(x,y) \qquad (24.1)$$

The stochastic process which represents the liver spleen scan image, $p(x,y)$, is the sum of two processes, $f(x,y)$ and $n(x,y)$. The first process, $f(x,y)$, is called the signal. The outcomes of this process are noiseless, liver spleen scans. The statistics of this process are used to model the *a priori* information provided by knowing that the image is a liver spleen scan. The other process, $n(x,y)$, is called the noise. It is used to model the noise involved in the imaging process. This model of the medical imaging process will be used extensively in Part IV of this book.

The first-order statistics of a stochastic process is given by the mean (Equation 11.3)

$$m_f(t) = E\{f(t)\} \tag{24.2}$$

where $E\{\cdot\}$ is the expectation operator described in Chapter 10. The second-order statistics are given by the autocorrelation function (Equation 11.5)

$$R(t_1,t_2) = E\{f(t_1) \cdot f^*(t_2)\} \tag{24.3}$$

The autocorrelation function for t_1 equal to t_2 is equal to the second moment of $f(t_1)$:

$$R(t_1,t_1) = E\{|f(t_1)|^2\} \tag{24.4}$$

Recall that the second moment is also called the power. Although $R(t_1,t_2)$ is related to a statistical signal, $f(t)$, it is a deterministic function. Therefore, it can be operated on any deterministic signal.

A very important property for stochastic processes is stationarity. Recall from Chapter 11 that strict sense stationary means that all of the statistics of a process are invariant over time. Wide-sense stationary means that the first- and second-order statistics are invariant over time. (For Gaussian processes, wide sense stationarity implies strict sense stationarity.) For stationary processes the autocorrelation function can be defined in terms of a single variable, τ, equal to $t_1 - t_2$:

$$R(\tau) = E\{f(t) \cdot f^*(t - \tau)\} \tag{24.5}$$

For τ equal to zero the autocorrelation function is equal to the second moment, the power in the stochastic process:

$$R(0) = E\{|f(t)|^2\} \tag{24.6}$$

The power in the stochastic process is the average of the powers in the individual outcomes, $f_i(t)$. Because of stationarity, the power does not change with time, t. $R(\tau)$ is related to the square of $f(t)$; therefore, operations on $f(t)$ will result in "squared" operations on $R(\tau)$, where "squared" is used somewhat loosely in a mathematical sense.

II. POWER SPECTRAL DENSITY FUNCTION

The power spectral density function, $S(\omega)$, is defined as the Fourier transform of the autocorrelation function. Using the two headed arrow notation:

$$R(\tau) \leftrightarrow S(\omega) \tag{24.7}$$

This Fourier transform pair breaks our usual notational convention. Generally, the time domain signal is indicated by a small letter, and the frequency domain signal is indicated by the same letter capitalized. However, the literature is reasonably consistent in using $R(\cdot)$

for the autocorrelation function and S(·) for the power spectral density function, so we shall follow this convention.

Since R(τ) is a deterministic function, its Fourier transform, S(ω), is well defined. The relation between R(τ) and S(ω) should be easily understood; it is just the same as any Fourier transform pair. A more difficult problem is understanding the relation between S(ω) and f(t).

R(0) is equal to the power in the stochastic process, Equation 24.6. The value of R(0) is also equal to the integral of its Fourier transform, S(ω), (see Equation 16.81):

$$R(0) = (1/2\pi) \cdot \int_{-\infty}^{+\infty} S(\omega) \, d\omega \qquad (24.8)$$

Since R(0) is equal to the power in f(t), the integral of S(ω) with respect to the angular frequency variable, ω, is also equal to the power in f(t).

Since the integral of S(ω) is equal to the power in f(t), S(ω) is equal to the spectral density of the power — the power per radian. The unit of the integral of S(ω) is power; the unit of S(ω) is power per radian. Thus, S(ω) is related to the power per angular frequency unit. These angular frequency units are in terms of the time variable, τ. Below it will be shown that this frequency is also related to the frequencies in the stochastic process, f(t).

One of the main advantages of the power spectral density function is that the *a priori* information which we have about a stochastic process is often information about the power spectral density. For example, consider the case of liver spleen scintigraphy (Equation 24.1). Metastases from gastrointestinal malignancies tend to produce relatively large defects in a liver spleen scan. The power spectral density function of a stochastic process which represents liver spleen scans with gastrointestinal metastases will have most of its power at lower frequencies. By comparison, the noise which is dominated by counting statistics will tend to have most of its power at high frequencies. Thus, smoothing will improve the signal to noise ratio by preferentially, decreasing the high-frequency noise.

The meaning of the power spectral density function may still seem quite obscure. One of the best ways of understanding the power spectral density function is by considering the effect on the power spectral density function of band pass filtering a stochastic process. We shall see that a band pass filter which passes only a narrow range of frequencies in f(t) will pass that same band of frequencies in the power spectral density function. Thus, the power spectral density function gives the power in f(t) as a function of frequency. But before we can proceed with this explanation, we must first go through a considerable amount of mathematical detail.

III. DEFINITION OF FILTERING A STOCHASTIC PROCESS

We shall define the filtering of a stochastic process to be the operation of filtering each experimental value, $f_i(t)$, to produce an output, $g_i(t)$:

$$g_i(t) = f_i(t) * h(t) \qquad (24.9)$$

where h(t) is the filter. The filter is part of the experiment. It works on individual experimental outcomes; for each outcome this operation is deterministic. This is the same operation we have considered many times before. Although the effect of this operation on a single outcome, $f_i(t)$, is very familiar to us, we shall find that the effect of this operation on the statistics of the stochastic process, f(t), is more complicated.

The filtering operation is defined in terms of a single outcome, but we can also con-

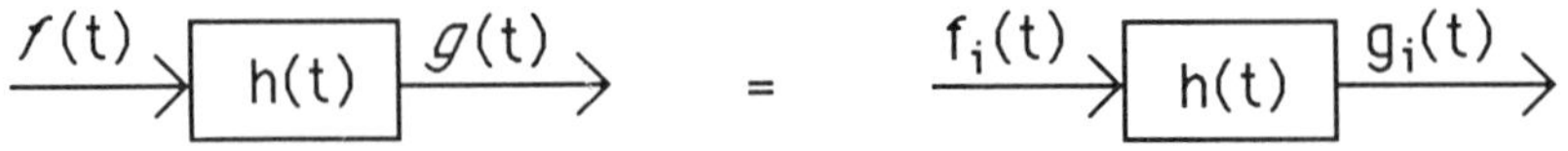

$$\xrightarrow{\;f(t)\;} \boxed{\;h(t)\;} \xrightarrow{\;g(t)\;} \quad = \quad \xrightarrow{\;f_i(t)\;} \boxed{\;h(t)\;} \xrightarrow{\;g_i(t)\;}$$

FIGURE 24.1.   Filtering a stochastic process: on the left is a diagrammatic representation of filtering a stochastic process. $f(t)$ is the input stochastic process; $g(t)$ is the output stochastic process; and $h(t)$ is a linear, time invariant system. On the right, $f_i(t)$ is an experimental outcome of the stochastic process, $f(t)$. $g_i(t)$ is the output a signal for this same experimental outcome. Filtering a stochastic process is defined to be equivalent to filtering each of the experimental outcomes.

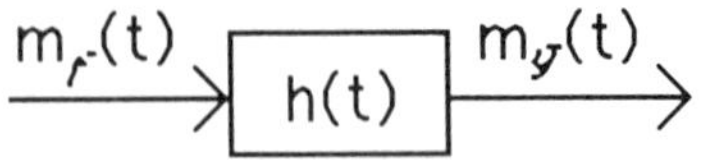

$$\xrightarrow{\;m_f(t)\;} \boxed{\;h(t)\;} \xrightarrow{\;m_g(t)\;}$$

FIGURE 24.2.   Effect of a system on the mean: the affect of a system on the mean of a stochastic process is the same as if the mean were passed through the system. $m_f(t)$ is the mean of the input stochastic process; $m_g(t)$ is the mean of the output stochastic process; and $h(t)$ is a linear, time invariant system.

ceptualize this operation in terms of stochastic processes. When we are trying to indicate the effect of a filter on a stochastic process, we shall write:

$$g(t) = f(t) * h(t) \tag{24.10}$$

However, this notation is meant to indicate the same operation as Equation 24.9. Figure 24.1 shows a diagrammatic representation of this. The stochastic process, $f(t)$, is filtered by a system, $h(t)$, to produce and output stochastic process, $g(t)$.

The *a priori* information about $f(t)$ provided by the statistical model is defined in terms of the relationships between different outcomes. The operation of a system on a stochastic process is defined in terms of a single outcome. In order to describe the statistics of the outcome process, the operation of a system on a single outcome must be combined with the description of the statistics of a stochastic process in terms of an ensemble of outcomes.

IV. MEAN OF AN OUTPUT PROCESS

The effect of a system on the mean of a stochastic process can be calculated from the definition of the mean and the definition of convolution. The mean of the output process, $g(t)$, is defined as (Equation 24.2):

$$m_g(t) = E\{g(t)\} \tag{24.11}$$

The output can be expressed as a convolution of the input with the system function:

$$m_g(t) = E\left\{ \int_{-\infty}^{+\infty} h(\tau) \cdot f(t - \tau)\, d\tau \right\} \tag{24.12}$$

The order of expectation and integration operations in Equation 24.12 can be interchanged. Since $h(\tau)$ is a deterministic factor, it can be moved outside of expectation. Therefore,

$$m_g(t) = \int_{-\infty}^{+\infty} h(\tau) \cdot m_f(t - \tau)\, d\tau \tag{24.13}$$

where $m_f(t - \tau)$ is the expected value of $f(t - \tau)$. Equation 24.13 is just a convolution of the mean of $f(t)$ with the system function:

$$m_g(t) = m_f(t) * h(t) \tag{24.14}$$

This relationship is shown diagrammatically in Figure 24.2. When a stochastic process is filtered with a linear, time invariant system, $h(t)$, the mean of the output process, $m_g(t)$, is equal to a filtered version of the mean of the input process, $m_f(t)$. The effect of a system on the first order statistics is particularly simple.

V. AUTOCORRELATION OF AN OUTPUT PROCESS

Calculation of the autocorrelation of the output process is more complicated than calculation of the mean. We can get some insight into the result by considering a heuristic argument. The autocorrelation is related to the "square" of the process. Therefore, the effect of a system on the autocorrelation should be a "squared" effect. The autocorrelation function is defined in the time domain. The effect of the system in the time domain is complicated; it is a convolution. Thus, the one might guess that the "squared" effect is a double convolution.

The actual calculation of the autocorrelation function of an output process is a little bit complicated. It is easiest to first calculate the cross-correlation function of the input and the output process, and then use this result to calculate the autocorrelation of the output process. The cross correlation of the input and the output process is:

$$R_{fg}(t_1,t_2) = E\{f(t_1) \cdot g^*(t_2)\} \tag{24.15}$$

The output process, $g(t_2)$, can be expanded as the convolution of the input with the system function:

$$R_{fg}(t_1,t_2) = E\left\{f(t_1) \cdot \int_{-\infty}^{+\infty} h^*(\tau) \cdot f^*(t_2 - \tau)\, d\tau\right\} \tag{24.16}$$

Since $f(t_1)$ is not a function of τ, it can be moved inside the integral. The order of the expectation and integration operations can be switched. Then, since $h^*(\tau)$ is deterministic, it can be moved outside the expectation operator:

$$R_{fg}(t_1,t_2) = \int_{-\infty}^{+\infty} h^*(\tau) \cdot E\{f(t_1) \cdot f^*(t_2 - \tau)\}\, d\tau \tag{24.17}$$

The expected value in Equation 24.17 is an autocorrelation of $f(t)$. Therefore,

$$R_{fg}(t_1,t_2) = \int_{-\infty}^{+\infty} h^*(\tau) \cdot R_{ff}(t_1, t_2 - \tau)\, d\tau \tag{24.18}$$

But this equation is simply a convolution:

$$R_{fg}(t_1,t_2) = R_{ff}(t_1,t_2) * h^*(t_2) \tag{24.19}$$

where the convolution is with respect to the second variable in the autocorrelation function.

Using this cross correlation, we are now ready to calculate the autocorrelation function.

$$R_{gg}(t_1,t_2) = E\left\{\int_{-\infty}^{+\infty} h(\tau) \cdot f(t_1 - \tau) \, d\tau \cdot g^*(t_2)\right\} \tag{24.20}$$

The order of the expectation and integration operations can be exchanged. Since $h(\tau)$ is deterministic, it can be moved outside the expectation operation. The expectation can then be recognized as a cross correlation:

$$R_{gg}(t_1,t_2) = \int_{-\infty}^{+\infty} h(\tau) \cdot R_{fg}(t_1 - \tau, t_2) \, d\tau \tag{24.21}$$

The integral in Equation 24.21 can be recognized as a convolution:

$$R_{gg}(t_1,t_2) = h(t_1) * R_{fg}(t_1,t_2) \tag{24.22}$$

We can use Equation 24.19 to substitute for the cross correlation, $R_{fg}(t_1, t_2)$:

$$R_{gg}(t_1,t_2) = h(t_1) * R_{ff}(t_1, t_2) * h^*(t_2) \tag{24.23}$$

where the first convolution is with respect to t_1 and the second convolution is with respect to t_2.

The autocorrelation of the output process is derived from the autocorrelation function of the input process by a double convolution. The first variable of the autocorrelation function is convolved with the system function and the second variable is convolved with the complex conjugate of the system function. As we had predicted from our heuristic argument, the system has a "square like" effect on the autocorrelation function. This time-domain description is very complicated and does not provide much insight into the operation of a system on a stochastic process. The frequency domain description will provide a better understanding of this filtering operation.

VI. POWER SPECTRAL DENSITY FUNCTION OF AN OUTPUT PROCESS

In the frequency domain, the affect of a system on an outcome of a stochastic process is described by a multiplication operation:

$$G_i(\omega) = H(\omega) \cdot F_i(\omega) \tag{24.24}$$

In terms of the stochastic process we shall write this operation:

$$G(\omega) = H(\omega) \cdot F(\omega) \tag{24.25}$$

The power spectral density function is the frequency domain representation of the autocorrelation function. It is a second order statistic like the variance. From Equation 10.12 it can be seen that when a random variable is multiplied by a constant, h, the variance is multiplied by $|h|^2$. Thus, we might expect that the effect on the power spectral density function will be related to $|H(\omega)|^2$.

Equation 24.23 is correct for both stationary and nonstationary processes. If the process is stationary, then Equation 24.23 can be rewritten:

$$R_g(t) = H(\tau) * R_f(\tau) * h^*(-\tau) \tag{24.26}$$

Using Equation 16.71, this equation can be written in the transform domain as:

$$S_g(\omega) = H(\omega) \cdot S_f(\omega) \cdot H^*(\omega) \tag{24.27}$$

However, $H(\omega)$ times $H^*(\omega)$ is just the squared magnitude of $H(\omega)$:

$$S_g(\omega) = |H(\omega)|^2 \cdot S_f(\omega) \tag{24.28}$$

The affect of filtering on the power spectral density function is multiplication of the power spectral density function by the square of the amplitude of the filter. Our heuristic argument about second-order statistics accurately predicted this result. Equation 24.28 is very important. It is the major link between our linear, time invariant model of systems and our statistical description of signals.

It is possible to be confused about why the autocorrelation function and the power spectral density are not simply filtered by the system like any other signal. The key point is that the autocorrelation function and the power spectral density function do not go through the system. A particular statistical outcome, $f_1(t)$, of the stochastic process goes through the system; it is filtered. The autocorrelation function and the power spectral density function are signals which describe the stochastic process, not signals which are filtered by the system. Since these signals do not directly pass through the system, there is no reason why they should be simply filtered by the system.

Figure 24.2 can also be confusing. The effect of the system on the mean of a stochastic process is the same as if the mean had passed through the system, but the mean does not pass through the system. Figure 24.2 is a model. Like the autocorrelation function and the power spectral density function, the mean is a description of a stochastic process. It just so happens that the affect of a system on the mean is the same as if the mean passed through the system.

VII. POWER SPECTRAL LOCALIZATION

We are now in a position to obtain a better understanding of the power spectral density function. Let us consider the effects of a band pass filter on a stochastic process. For each experiment, the band pass filter will remove all of the frequencies except those in the pass band. The output, $G_i(\omega)$, will be identical to the input, $F_i(\omega)$, in the pass band and zero elsewhere. If the band is small, then the output can be used to determine the spectral content of the input at some frequency, or at a number of different frequencies.

Let us try to understand the affect of an ideal band pass filter on the power spectral density function. The first graph in Figure 24.3 shows a power spectral density function for an input stochastic process. The second graph in the figure shows the squared magnitude of an ideal band pass filter:

$$|H(\omega)|^2 = \begin{cases} 1, & \text{within the band} \\ 0, & \text{outside the band} \end{cases} \tag{24.29}$$

The third line shows the power spectral density function of the output process.

The integral of the power spectral density function of the output process is equal to $R_g(0)$ (Equation 24.8), and $R_g(0)$ is the power in the output process (Equation 24.6). From Figure 24.3 we can see that this power is located in the power spectral density function at the narrow band of frequencies in the filter. The only portions of the input signal, $f_i(t)$,

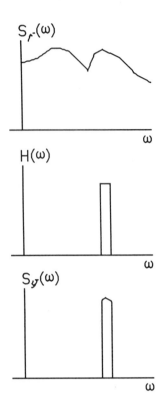

FIGURE 24.3.   Power localization in the frequency domain: the top panel shows the power spectral density function, $S_f(\omega)$ of an input stochastic process. The middle panel shows an ideal band pass filter, $H(\omega)$. The bottom panel shows the power spectral density function of the output process, $S_g(\omega)$. The only power in the output process is the power from the input process in the narrow band of the filter.

which are present in the output signal, $g_i(t)$, are the frequency components in the same band. Thus the average power in the signals, $f_i(t)$, at a given frequency is given by the power density function in the same range of frequencies. As the name implies, the power spectral density function gives the power in a stochastic process as a function of frequency.

Let us consider an example of a stochastic process. We can define a stationary, stochastic process to be imaginary exponentials of fixed frequency, ω_0, with a statistical phase, ϕ:

$$f_i(t) = e^{i(\omega_0 t + \phi_i)} \tag{24.30}$$

Each outcome process, $f_i(t)$, has the same, deterministic frequency, but the phase varies in a statistical fashion. The real part of a few outcomes of this process are shown in Figure 24.4. This stochastic process produces sinusoids which are shifted in some statistical manner. (We shall not be interested in the statistics of the phase, ϕ.)

The autocorrelation function is given by:

$$R(\tau) = E\{e^{i(\omega_0(t-\tau)+\phi_i)} \cdot e^{-i(\omega_0 t + \phi_1)}\}$$

$$= E\{e^{-i\omega_0\tau}\} \tag{24.31}$$

But the expression within the expectation operator is deterministic; therefore:

$$R(\tau) = e^{-i\omega_0\gamma} \tag{24.32}$$

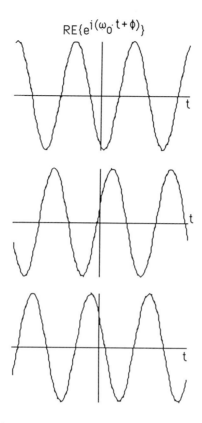

$$RE\{e^{i(\omega_0 t + \phi)}\}$$

FIGURE 24.4.   Outcomes of a process with random phase: this figure shows a few of the experimental outcomes of a process which is a sinusoid of fixed frequency, but a random phase.

The autocorrelation function does not depend upon the phase, ϕ. (The cross correlation will depend upon the statistics of ϕ.) The Fourier transform of $R(\tau)$, the power spectral density function, is given by:

$$S(\omega) = \delta(\omega - \omega_0) \tag{24.33}$$

The autocorrelation function and the power spectral density function are shown in Figure 24.5. Each outcome process has all of its power at the single angular frequency, ω_0. Therefore, the power spectral density function is nonzero only for angular frequency, ω_0. A band pass filter which includes frequency, ω_0, will have no effect on any of the outcomes shown in Figure 24.4. Similarly, it will not effect the power spectral density function shown in Figure 24.5. A filter which stops angular frequency, ω_0, will make each outcome zero and will make the power spectral density function zero.

This process is a special case. Each outcome has exactly the same frequency content. Thus, the effect of the filter on the power spectral density function is the same as the effect on every outcome of the stochastic process. In general, the outcomes need not have the same frequency content. In that case, the effect on the power spectral density is the average effect on the individual outcomes.

VIII. NOISE

Equation 24.1 presents a model of medical imaging with additive noise. An important feature of this model is the power spectral density functions of the signal and noise. If the

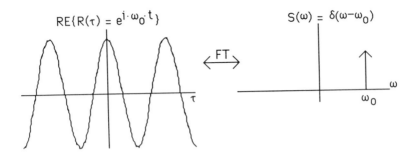

FIGURE 24.5.   Second order statistics of a random phase process: on the left is the autocorrelation function and on the right is the power spectral density function of the random phase process shown in Figure 24.4.

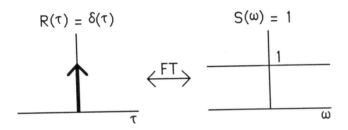

FIGURE 24.6.   White-noise process: on the left is the autocorrelation function and on the right is the power spectral density function of a white-noise process.

signal and the noise have different power spectral density functions, then it may be possible to selectively decrease the noise by filtering. There are some common models used to describe noise.

One stationary stochastic process commonly used to model noise has equal power at all frequencies. This noise model is similar to white light in that white light has equal power at all spectral frequencies. Therefore, this type of noise is called **white noise**. Figure 24.6 shows the power spectral density function and the autocorrelation function of a white-noise process. The power spectral density function is a constant:

$$S(\omega) = 1 \tag{24.34}$$

Therefore, the autocorrelation function is a delta function:

$$R(\tau) = \delta(\tau) \tag{24.35}$$

Since a white-noise process has energy at an infinite range of frequencies, the average power of a white-noise process, $R(0)$, is infinite — $R(\tau)$ is a delta function. Therefore, white noise cannot exist physically. However, frequently, the noise is constant over the range of interest in some application. The system may ignore any frequencies outside some range. In that case, the noise can be modeled as a white-noise process.

In some applications, the noise does not have the same power at all frequencies. This type of noise is sometimes called colored noise to contrast it with white noise. We can define a stochastic process with a nonconstant power spectral density function to model this type of noise. However, in practice it is often simpler to use a white-noise process which is filtered by a filter which is equal to the square root of the power spectral density function.

The colored noise is produced by passing a white-noise process through the appropriate filter.

Let us next consider the white noise process from the frequency domain. The Fourier transform of a stochastic process, $f(t)$, is also a stochastic process, $F(\omega)$:

$$F(\omega) = \int_{-\infty}^{+\infty} f(t) \cdot e^{i\omega t} \, dt \tag{24.36}$$

The process, $F(\omega)$, is a frequency domain representation of the process, $f(t)$. The autocorrelation function of this process is:

$$R_F(\omega_1, \omega_2) = E\{F(\omega_1) \cdot F^*(\omega_2)\} \tag{24.37}$$

Equation 24.36 can be substituted into Equation 24.37 for both $F(\omega_1)$ and $F(\omega_2)$; the integrals can be combined; and the order of the expectation and the integration can be changed:

$$R_F(\omega_1, \omega_2) = \int_{-\infty}^{+\infty} \int_{-\infty}^{+\infty} F\{f(t_1) \cdot f^*(t_2)\} \cdot e^{-i(\omega_1 t_1 - \omega_2 t_2)} \, dt_1 dt_2 \tag{24.38}$$

The expectation is equal to $R_f(t_1, t_2)$. Thus, the autocorrelation function of the Fourier transform is the Fourier transform of autocorrelation function. (Note, however, that Equation 24.38 is a two-dimensional Fourier transform; it is different from the power spectral density which is the Fourier transform with respect to the variable, τ, of a stationary process.)

Now let us consider the autocorrelation function of frequency domain representation of a white-noise process. The autocorrelation function, $R_f(t_1, t_2)$, of a white-noise process is a delta function, $\delta(t_2 - t_1)$. Substituting this value into Equation 24.38 gives:

$$R_F(\omega_1, \omega_2) = \int_{-\infty}^{+\infty} e^{-i(\omega_1 - \omega_2)t_2} \, dt_2 \tag{24.39}$$

where the delta function picks the single value t_1 equal to t_2 from the inner integral.

The integral in Equation 24.39 is of the form given by Equation 15.33. Therefore,

$$R_F(\omega_1, \omega_2) = 2\pi \cdot \delta(\omega_1 - \omega_2) \tag{24.40}$$

This equation says that $F(\omega)$ is a white-noise process in the frequency domain as well as the time domain.

The white-noise process is also a white-noise process in the frequency domains; the Fourier transform of white noise is white noise. It is possible to get confused about the stochastic processes, the statistics, and the Fourier transforms of each. $f(t)$ is a white-noise stochastic process. $F(\omega)$ is a stochastic process which is the Fourier transform of $f(t)$; it is the frequency domain representation of $f(t)$; it is also a white-noise process. $R_f(\tau)$ is the autocorrelation function of $f(t)$; it is deterministic; it is a delta function. $R_f(\omega_1, \omega_2)$ is the autocorrelation function of the frequency domain stochastic process, $F(\omega)$; it is deterministic; the previous section has shown that it is equal to 2π times a delta function. Since the autocorrelation functions are both delta functions, their Fourier transforms, the respective power density functions, are constants.

IX. SIGNAL TO NOISE RATIO

The signal to noise ratio is usually defined as the ratio of the average power in the signal to the average power in the noise. The signal to noise ratio is a very useful parameter since it describes the quality of the image independently of any scaling parameters. In nuclear magnetic resonance imaging, signal to noise ratio is commonly used by engineers to describe the free induction decay signal. It is also useful in describing the final image.

In terms of the stochastic process model, the average power is given by the autocorrelation function at zero (Equation 24.6). Thus, the signal to noise ratio can be written:

$$SNR = R_f(0)/R_n(0) \qquad (24.41)$$

where SNR is the signal to noise ratio. Using the power spectral density functions, it is possible to define the signal to noise ratio as a function of angular frequency:

$$SNR(\omega) = S_f(\omega)/S_n(\omega) \qquad (24.42)$$

In this case, the signal to noise ratio is the ratio of the power spectral densities.

In the case of liver spleen scans with gastrointestinal metastases described above, the signal to noise ratio will be high at lower spatial frequencies and low at higher spatial frequencies. As was discussed we can improve the overall signal to noise ratio by filtering out the high spatial frequencies where the signal to noise ratio is low.

There is often some confusion about the exact mathematical definition of the signal to noise ratio. For example, Equation 24.41 defines the signal to noise in terms of power while Equation 24.42 defines it in terms of power per radian. This difference is relatively small, and it is often obvious from the application what is meant.

A more important difference in definition occurs frequently. The signal to noise ratio is sometimes defined in terms of the absolute value of the signal and the noise instead of the power in the signal and noise. In this case the signal to noise ratio is related to the square root of the definition in Equation 24.41

Some of the confusion about the definition of the signal to noise ratio is ameliorated by the use of the decibel scale. Decibels are defined in terms of the logarithm of the signal to noise ratio; however, the definition varies depending upon whether the ratio is a ratio of the absolute signal intensities or a ratio of powers. For powers, decibels are defined:

$$10 \cdot \log_{10}(R_f(0)/R_n(0)) \qquad (24.43)$$

For signal intensities, decibels are defined:

$$20 \cdot \log_{10}(E\{|f(t)|\}/E\{|n(t)|\}) \qquad (24.44)$$

Therefore, the signal to noise ratio in terms of decibels is the same no matter how the original signal is defined. Table 24.1 gives some decibel values and the approximate signal to noise ratios for both power and amplitude.

X. SUMMARY

This chapter has brought together the linear system model of systems and the stochastic process model of signals. The stochastic process model allows us to describe noisy signals. The linear systems model describes the effects of a linear, time invariant system on a signal. This chapter has shown how the linear system model can be extended to include the operation of a system on a stochastic process.

TABLE 24.1
Approximate Decibel Values

Decibel	Power ratio	Amplitude ratio
1	1.26	1.12
3	2.0	1.41
6	4.0	2.0
10	10	3.2
13	20	4.5
16	40	6.3
20	100	10
23	200	14
26	400	20
30	1000	32
33	2000	45
36	4000	63
40	10,000	100
43	20,000	140
46	40,000	200
50	100,000	320
53	200,000	450
56	400,000	630
60	1,000,000	1000
63	2,000,000	1400
66	4,000,000	2000
70	10,000,000	3200
73	20,000,000	4500
76	40,000,000	6300
80	100,000,000	10,000
83	200,000,000	14,000
86	400,000,000	20,000
90	1,000,000,000	32,000
93	2,000,000,000	45,000
96	4,000,000,000	63,000
100	10,000,000,000	100,000
$n \cdot 10$	10^n	$10^{n/2}$

The power spectral density function, introduced in this chapter, is an important method for describing the statistics of stationary stochastic processes. The power spectral density function is the Fourier transform of the autocorrelation function with respect to the variable, τ. In radiology, the *a priori* information about a system is often known in terms of the power spectral density functions of the biological signal and the detector noise. Thus, this function is well suited to characterization of radiological imaging.

At several points in this book, we have emphasized the importance of the first- and second-order statistics of stochastic signals, the mean and the autocorrelation function. The affect of a linear, time invariant system on the mean of a stochastic process is given by Equation 24.14:

$$m_g(t) = m_f(t) * h(t) \tag{24.45}$$

where $m_g(t)$ is the mean of the output process, $m_f(t)$ is the mean of the input process, and $h(t)$ is the system. The result is the same as if the mean were filtered by the system.

For stationary processes, the affect of a linear, time invariant system on the second order statistics is best understood in the frequency domain. The power spectral density function of the output process is given by Equation 24.28:

$$S_g(\omega) = |H(\omega)|^2 \cdot S_f(\omega) \tag{24.46}$$

where $S_g(\omega)$ is the power spectral density function of the output process, $H(\omega)$ is the system function, and $S_f(\omega)$ is the power spectral density function of the input process. These two equations will be very important. They allow the statistics of an output process to be calculated from the statistics of the input process and the system function.

Equation 24.46 also provides insight about the meaning of the power spectral density function. If a process is filtered with a band pass filter, then only frequencies in the output process will be in the band which is passed by the filter. Similarly, the only power in the power spectral density function will be the power in the same band of frequencies. This shows that the power spectral density function does in fact represent the power in the signal as a function of frequency.

The next chapter will be a slight change of direction. It will deal with estimation using linear systems. In Chapter 26, we shall return to linear, time invariant systems. The power spectral density function will be important in deriving an optimal linear, time invariant, least-mean-square estimation of the unknown.

XI. FURTHER READING

The treatment of filtering of stochastic processes in this chapter is similar to the treatment in many linear systems texts. For example, see Chapter 19 of the book by Siebert.[1] A more advanced exposition can be found in Chapter 9 of the book by Papoulis.[2]

REFERENCES

1. **Siebert, W. Mc. C.,** *Circuits, Signals, and Systems,* McGraw-Hill, New York, 1986.
2. **Papoulis, A.,** *Signal Analysis,* McGraw-Hill, New York, 1977.

Chapter 25

NORMAL EQUATIONS

In this chapter we shall present the normal equations from linear algebra. The normal equations are the linear, least mean square solution to a set of inconsistent linear equations. The normal equations are not usually presented along with filtering. However, we wish to emphasize the similarity between the normal equations and Wiener filtering. Both can be used to provide a linear, least mean square estimate of a signal from a set of measurements.

There are two differences which we wish to emphasize between the normal equations and Wiener filtering. The first difference is that the normal equations deal with linear estimation whereas Wiener filtering deals with linear, time invariant estimation. Consequently, the normal equations come from linear algebra while Wiener filtering comes from linear system theory.

The second difference is that the normal equations produce an estimate which minimizes the error in terms of the measured signal while Wiener filtering produces an estimate which minimizes the error in terms of the unknown signal. Recall from Chapter 12 that the first approach leads to a simpler result while the second approach often produces the more desirable result. In this chapter we shall solve the former problem; in the next chapter we solve the latter problem.

Some of the concepts from this chapter will be used in Chapter 33 (Iterative Reconstruction: Single Photon Emission Computed Tomography); however, the major value of this chapter is in a fuller understanding of estimation. This chapter can be skipped without loss of continuity. It may be useful to review Chapter 9, Chapter 12, and Chapter 19 prior to reading this chapter.

I. PROJECTION OF A VECTOR ONTO A SUBSPACE

We shall start with a geometrical problem, estimation of a vector in terms of a set of vectors. This approach is exactly analogous to the approach taken in Chapter 12. Recall that first problem which we solved in that chapter was estimation of a vector in terms of a second vector. When we went to the real estimation problem, we found that most of the work had already been done. In this chapter, we shall estimate the vector in terms of a set of vectors instead of a single vector.

We wish to find the linear, least mean square error estimate of a vector, $\mathbf{p}$, in terms of a set of vectors, $\mathbf{a}_j$. Any linear estimate of $\mathbf{p}$ in terms of the vectors, $\mathbf{a}_j$, can be written as:

$$\hat{\mathbf{p}} = \sum_j \hat{f}_j \cdot \mathbf{a}_j \tag{25.1}$$

The estimation process involves determination of the factors, $\hat{f}_j$. This problem does not involve statistical quantities or noise, but we shall use the estimation terminology because of the similarity between this problem and the next problem.

The set of vectors, $\mathbf{a}_j$, forms a basis of a vector space. Since $\hat{\mathbf{p}}$ is a linear combination of $\mathbf{a}_j$, all of the estimates, $\hat{\mathbf{p}}$, must be in this vector space. We shall call this vector space the estimation space.

In Chapter 9 we found that a linear combination of vectors can be written as multiplication of a matrix times a vector (see Equation 9.19). If we find a matrix, A, where the columns of A are the vectors, $\mathbf{a}_j$, then Equation 25.1 can be written:

$$\hat{\mathbf{p}} = A \cdot \hat{\mathbf{f}} \tag{25.2}$$

$\hat{\mathbf{f}}$ is a vector made up of the factors $\hat{f}_j$.

$$\hat{\mathbf{p}} = A \cdot \hat{\mathbf{f}}$$

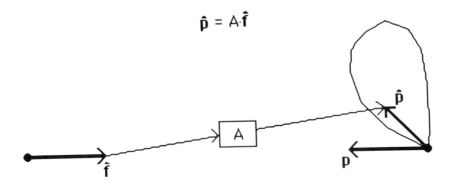

FIGURE 25.1.   Estimation of a vector by a set of vectors: this diagram shows the estimation of a vector, **p**, by a set of vectors, $\mathbf{a}_j$. The set of vectors are the columns of the matrix, A. The blob on the right represents the vector space defined by the set of vectors, $\mathbf{a}_j$, the column space of A. The estimate, $\hat{\mathbf{p}}$, of **p** must be in the column space of A. On the left is a vector, $\hat{\mathbf{f}}$, representing a set of estimation factors. The estimation factors times the columns of A, A $\cdot \hat{\mathbf{f}}$, give the estimate $\hat{\mathbf{p}}$.

$$\hat{\mathbf{p}} = A \cdot \hat{\mathbf{f}}$$

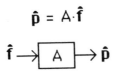

FIGURE 25.2.   System model: the linear combination of the columns of A shown in Figure 25.1 is equivalent to a linear system. The input is represented by the vector of factors, $\hat{\mathbf{f}}$, the system is represented by the matrix, A, and the output is represented by the estimate, $\hat{\mathbf{p}}$.

The multi-dimensional vector spaces considered in this chapter cannot be shown accurately in a two-dimensional diagram. As in Chapter 9, we shall diagram these vector spaces as blobs. The diagrams provide some geometric intuition about multi-dimensional vector spaces, but the reader is cautioned not to try to stretch the geometric relationships shown in these diagrams too far.

The estimation space defined by the columns of A is shown as a blob in Figure 25.1. The vector, **p**, will in general not lie in the estimation space. The estimation problem amounts to picking the vector, $\hat{\mathbf{p}}$, in the estimation space which is "closest" to **p**. The vector of estimation factors, $\hat{\mathbf{f}}$, is defined in its own vector space. This figure shows an alternate way of viewing this problem. The estimation factors, $\hat{\mathbf{f}}$, are transformed by a system represented by the matrix, A, into the estimate, $\hat{\mathbf{p}}$.

Equation 25.2 shows the equivalence of linear estimation and a linear system. The factors, $\hat{\mathbf{f}}$, are equivalent to an input signal; the matrix of estimators, A, is equivalent to a system; and the estimate, $\hat{\mathbf{p}}$, is equivalent to the output of the system in response to $\hat{\mathbf{f}}$. Figure 25.2 is a diagram showing the signal, $\hat{\mathbf{f}}$, going through the system, A, to produce the signal, $\hat{\mathbf{p}}$.

In Chapter 9, we discussed the various vector spaces associated with a matrix, A. Recall that the output vector must be in the column space of A. The column space of A is the estimation space, since the columns are the basis of the estimation space. Therefore, from the linear system point of view, we derive the same result as above — the estimate, $\hat{\mathbf{p}}$, which is the output of A must lie in the estimation space defined by the basis vectors, $\mathbf{a}_j$.

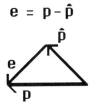

FIGURE 25.3.   Error vector: the error vector, **e**, is defined as $\mathbf{p} - \hat{\mathbf{p}}$.

The error vector is defined as the difference between the given vector and the estimate:

$$\mathbf{e} = \mathbf{p} - \hat{\mathbf{p}} = \ = \mathbf{p} - A \cdot \hat{\mathbf{f}} \tag{25.3}$$

The error, **e**, is shown in Figure 25.3, We wish to minimize the square of the error, $\mathbf{e}^T \cdot \mathbf{e}$, with respect to the choice of the parameters $\hat{f}_i$.

As in chapter 12, the minimization is performed by differentiating with respect to the factors, $\hat{f}_i$, and setting the results equal to zero:

$$\partial e^2 / \partial \hat{f}_i = 2 \cdot \partial \mathbf{e}^T / \partial \hat{f}_i \cdot \mathbf{e} = 0, \qquad \text{for all i} \tag{25.4}$$

The error, **e**, depends on two terms **p** and $\hat{\mathbf{p}}$. The given vector, **p**, is not a function of $\hat{f}_i$ since the $\hat{f}_i$ have to do only with the estimation process. $\hat{\mathbf{p}}$, is given by Equation 25.1. The only term in $\hat{\mathbf{p}}$ which is a function of f_i is the term where j is equal to i. Thus, there will be only one nonzero term in the differentiated sum.

$$\partial e^2 / \partial \hat{f}_i = 2 \cdot \mathbf{a}_i^T \cdot \mathbf{e} = 0, \qquad \text{for all i} \tag{25.5}$$

Recall from Chapter 12 that the orthogonality principle was important in all of the linear, mean square estimation problems. We have again found an example of the orthogonality principle:

$$\mathbf{a}_i^T \cdot \mathbf{e} = 0, \qquad \text{for all i} \tag{25.6}$$

The error is orthogonal to the vectors with which we are going to estimate, **p**. Equation 25.6 represents a set of equations, one equation for each value of i. We can write this set of equations in matrix notation as:

$$A^T \cdot \mathbf{e} = \mathbf{0} \tag{25.7}$$

where **0** is the zero vector.

Equation 25.7 states that the error is in the null space of A^T; therefore, the error is orthogonal to the column space of A (see the discussion of the vector spaces associated with a matrix in Chapter 9). In Chapter 12, we found that the error was orthogonal to the **vector** used to estimate **p**. Here we find that the error is orthogonal to the **vector space** used to estimate **p**.

Figure 25.4, shows the vector, **p**, and two vector spaces — the columns space of A and the null space of A^T. **p** can be represented as the sum of two vectors, $\hat{\mathbf{p}}$ in the column space of A and **e** in the null space of A^T (see Chapter 9). Geometrically, the orthogonality of **e** and A means that the estimate, $\hat{\mathbf{p}}$, is the projection of **p** onto the column space of A.

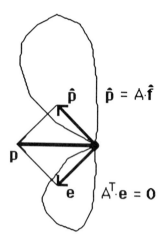

FIGURE 25.4. Orthogonality of the error and the estimation space: the upper blob represents the column space of A; and the lower blob represents the null space of A^T. The vector, **p**, is made up of two parts, the estimate, $\hat{\mathbf{p}}$, and the error, **e**. The model of the estimation process (Equation 25.2) requires the estimate to be in the column space of A. The orthogonality principle (Equation 25.7) requires the error, **e**, to be in the null space of A^T.

The system represented by A maps the vector, $\hat{\mathbf{f}}$, into the vector, $\hat{\mathbf{p}}$, in the column space of A; the factors, $\hat{\mathbf{f}}$, are mapped into an estimate, $\hat{\mathbf{p}}$, in the estimation space.

We can use the orthogonality principle, Equation 25.7, to derive the normal equations of linear algebra.

$$A^T \cdot \mathbf{e} = A^T \cdot (\mathbf{p} - A \cdot \hat{\mathbf{f}}) = A^T \cdot \mathbf{p} - A^T \cdot A \cdot \hat{\mathbf{f}} = \mathbf{0} \tag{25.8}$$

Therefore,

$$A^T \cdot A \cdot \hat{\mathbf{f}} = A^T \cdot \mathbf{p} \tag{25.9}$$

The set of equations represented by the matrix (Equation 25.9) are called the normal equations of linear algebra. They relate the estimation factors, $\hat{\mathbf{f}}$, the model, A, and the data, **p**.

If $(A^T \cdot A)^{-1}$ exists, then Equation 25.9 can be solved for $\hat{\mathbf{f}}$:

$$\hat{\mathbf{f}} = (A^T \cdot A)^{-1} \cdot A^T \cdot \mathbf{p} \tag{25.10}$$

A sufficient condition for the inverse $(A^T \cdot A)^{-1}$ to exist is that the columns, $\mathbf{a}_j$, of A are independent. (In terms of simultaneous linear equations, this requirement means that the equations are not under determined.) From a statistical point of view this means that the measurements are uncorrelated, a common situation. The estimate, $\hat{\mathbf{p}}$, is given by $A \cdot \hat{\mathbf{f}}$:

$$\hat{\mathbf{p}} = A \cdot (A^T \cdot A)^{-1} \cdot A^T \cdot \mathbf{p} \tag{25.11}$$

Comparing this result with equation 12.21, we see that this is the matrix analog of the simpler vector problem.

We can define a projection matrix, which projects a vector onto the column space of A:

$$A \cdot (A^T \cdot A)^{-1} \cdot A^T \tag{25.12}$$

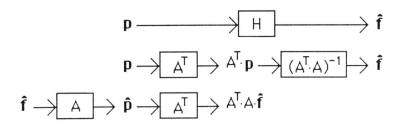

FIGURE 25.5. Model of the estimation process: the top line shows a model of the estimation process. The given vector, $\mathbf{p}$, is the input, the system is represented by the matrix, H, and the output is the estimation factors, $\hat{\mathbf{f}}$. The second line shows an alternate diagram using the relation given in Equation 25.14. The given vector, $\mathbf{p}$, goes through A^T to produce $A^T \cdot \mathbf{p}$. $A^T \cdot \mathbf{p}$ then goes through $(A^T \cdot A)^{-1}$ to produce the estimation factors, $\hat{\mathbf{f}}$. On the third line, the estimation factors, $\hat{\mathbf{f}}$, go through the matrix A to produce the estimate, $\hat{\mathbf{p}}$. The estimate can then go through A^T to yield $A^T \cdot A \cdot \hat{\mathbf{f}}$. The normal equations equate $A^T \cdot \mathbf{p}$ and $A^T \cdot A \cdot \hat{\mathbf{f}}$.

When A is square and the columns of A are independent, the projection matrix is very simple. When A is not square and when the columns of A are not independent, the projection matrix can be quite complicated. If one recognizes that this complicated matrix product merely serves to project a vector onto a subspace, then it does not seem so formidable.

Equation 25.10 can be viewed as representing a system which transforms the input signal, $\mathbf{p}$, into the output signal, $\hat{\mathbf{f}}$. We shall call this system, H. Mathematically,

$$\hat{\mathbf{f}} = H \cdot \mathbf{p} \qquad (25.13)$$

where the system is defined:

$$H = (A^T \cdot A)^{-1} \cdot A^T \qquad (25.14)$$

Figure 25.5 shows the operation of the system, H, diagrammatically. H transforms the vector, $\mathbf{p}$, into the estimation factors, $\hat{\mathbf{f}}$. On the second line, H is subdivided into two systems, A^T and $(A^T \cdot A)^{-1}$. The matrix, A^T, transforms the vector, $\mathbf{p}$, into the vector $A^T \cdot \mathbf{p}$. The third line shows the effect of A and A^T on $\hat{\mathbf{f}}$. A transforms the factors, $\hat{\mathbf{f}}$, into the estimate, $\hat{\mathbf{p}}$. $\hat{\mathbf{p}}$ times A^T results in the vector $A^T \cdot A \cdot \hat{\mathbf{f}}$. The normal equation of linear algebra (Equation 25.9) equate $A^T \cdot \mathbf{p}$ and $A^T \cdot A \cdot \hat{\mathbf{f}}$. This figure demonstrates one method of viewing these relationships.

Figure 25.6 shows the estimation problem from the point of view of the vector spaces associated with the matrix. A. The model says that estimation factors, $\hat{\mathbf{f}}$, are mapped into the estimate, $\hat{\mathbf{p}}$, by the system A (Equation 25.2). Therefore the vector, $\hat{\mathbf{p}}$, is in the column space of A. The given vector, $\mathbf{p}$, is mapped to the vector, $A^T \cdot \mathbf{p}$, by the system A^T. $A^T \cdot \mathbf{p}$ is in the row space of the matrix, A. Since the estimate, $\hat{\mathbf{p}}$, is the projection of $\mathbf{p}$ onto the column space of A (Equation 25.11), $\hat{\mathbf{p}}$, is mapped by A^T into the same vector, $A^T \cdot \mathbf{p}$.

The given vector is the sum of the estimate and the error:

$$\mathbf{p} = \hat{\mathbf{p}} + \mathbf{e} \qquad (25.15)$$

The estimate, $\hat{\mathbf{p}}$, is in the estimation space, which is the column space of A. The error, $\mathbf{e}$, is in the null space of A^T (Figure 25.6). The estimation process removes $\mathbf{e}$, which is the portion of $\mathbf{p}$ which is inconsistent with the model. The portion of $\mathbf{p}$ which is consistent with the model, $\hat{\mathbf{p}}$, is retained in the estimate.

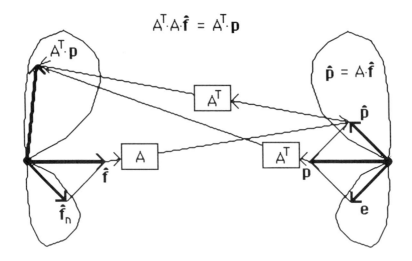

FIGURE 25.6. The estimation process and the vector spaces associated with A: the four blobs represent the vector spaces associated with the matrix, A. The upper left blob is the row space of A; the lower left blob is the null space of A; the upper right blob is the column space of A; and the lower right blob is the null space of A^T. Due to the model, the estimation factors, $\hat{f}$, are mapped by A to the estimate, $\hat{p}$, in the column space of A. Due to the normal equations, both the estimate, $\hat{p}$, and the given vector, p, are mapped by A^T to the same vector, $A^T \cdot p$ in the row space of A. The portion of $\hat{f}$ in the null space of A, $\hat{f}_n$, is mapped by A to the zero vector. $\hat{f}_n$ is the part of $\hat{f}$ which does not affect the estimate. The portion of p in the null space of A^T, e, is mapped by A^T to the zero vector. e is the part of p which is inconsistent with the model.

The vector of estimation factors, $\hat{f}$, can be divided into two parts, $A \cdot A^T \cdot \hat{f}$, in the row space of A, and $\hat{f}_n$ in the null space of A (Figure 25.6). The portion of $\hat{f}$ in the null space of A does not affect the estiamte, $\hat{p}$; therefore, this portion of the estimation factors is not determined by the normal equations. We can consider this portion of $\hat{f}$ from the terminology of simultaneous equations. If the system is under determined, then there is a family of solutions which satisfy the equations. Similarly, $\hat{f}$ can contain any component, $\hat{f}_n$, without affecting the estimate.

Figure 25.6 also shows the relationship defined by the normal equations of linear algebra. The normal equations say that mapping of $\hat{f}$ to the column space of A (by multiplication with A) and then to the row space of A (by multiplication with A^T) is equal to the mapping of the vector, p, to the row space of A (by multiplication with A^T); $A^T \cdot A \cdot \hat{f}$ is equal to $A^T \cdot p$. The mapping $A \cdot \hat{f}$ removes the part of $\hat{f}$ which does not affect the result; the mapping $A^T \cdot p$ removes the part of p which is inconsistent with the model.

Although we have not done a real estimation problem, we have accomplished a great deal in this section. Most of the mathematical framework has been developed. It may appear that we have made a reasonably simple problem more complicated than it really is; however, understanding this problem in excruciating detail will simplify our task later on.

Let us summarize the results of this section:

Given:	Vectors p and a_j	(25.16)
Estimate:	$\hat{p} = A \cdot \hat{f}$	(25.17)
Error:	$e = p - \hat{p}$	(25.18)

$$\text{Orthogonality:} \qquad A^T \cdot \mathbf{e} = \mathbf{0} \qquad\qquad (25.19)$$

$$\text{Solution:} \qquad \hat{\mathbf{f}} = (A^T \cdot A)^{-1} \cdot A^T \cdot \mathbf{p} \qquad\qquad (25.20)$$

The problem in this section has been to estimate a vector, $\mathbf{p}$, in terms of a set of vectors, $\mathbf{a}_j$. The estimate, $\hat{\mathbf{p}}$, must lie in the column space of A, a matrix made up of the vectors, $\mathbf{a}_j$. From the orthogonality principle, we see that the error will lie in the null space of A^T. The solution is defined in terms of the factors, $\hat{\mathbf{f}}$. The estimate, $\hat{\mathbf{p}}$, is the orthogonal projection of $\mathbf{p}$ onto the column space of A.

II. MODEL

We are now ready to consider a real estimation problem. We can develop a model using the familiar computed tomography problem. The unknown signal is a set of cross-sectional attenuation coefficients. The data are the projection samples which are linear combinations of the attenuation coefficients. We shall ignore more complicated considerations such as beam hardening. Since the measurement process is not perfect, it introduces some noise. The goal of the reconstruction process is to produce an estimate of the unknown attenuation coefficients from the measured values.

We can use the methods of linear algebra to express this problem (see Chapter 8). The unknown signal is represented by the vector, $\mathbf{f}$; the measurement process is represented by a linear system, A; the measurement noise is represented by a random vector, $\mathbf{n}$; and the measurement is represented by the random vector $\mathbf{p}$. We can express the model of the measurement process mathematically as:

$$\mathbf{p} = A \cdot \mathbf{f} + \mathbf{n} \qquad\qquad (25.21)$$

Since the measurement noise and consequently the measured values vary from experiment to experiment, $\mathbf{n}$ and $\mathbf{p}$ are random vectors. The attenuation coefficients, $\mathbf{f}$, and the measurement process, A, are assumed to be fixed, deterministic entities. One should note the similarity between this equation and Equation 12.45. Instead of a single unknown, f, we now have an unknown signal, $\mathbf{f}$. Instead of representing the measurement process by a vector, $\mathbf{a}$, we now have a matrix, A.

In linear algebra texts this same problem is often presented as a set of inconsistent linear equations. Recall from Chapter 9 that inconsistent equations do not have a solution which satisfies all of the equations. In the computed tomography problem the set of equations are:

$$\mathbf{p} = A \cdot \mathbf{f} \qquad\qquad (25.22)$$

$\mathbf{f}$ are the unknowns and $\mathbf{p}$ are the measurements. Because of noise, this set of equations is almost always inconsistent. In this chapter, we shall use the random vector notation where the noise is included explicitly in the problem.

In this chapter, we shall consider linear estimates of the unknown signal. Any linear estimate can be written:

$$\hat{\mathbf{f}} = H \cdot \mathbf{p} \qquad\qquad (25.23)$$

From the estimate of the unknown, an estimate of the data is given by:

$$\hat{\mathbf{p}} = A \cdot \mathbf{f} \qquad\qquad (25.24)$$

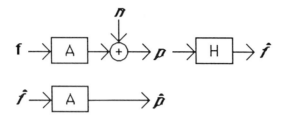

FIGURE 25.7.   Data collection, estimation model: this figure shows a diagrammatic representation of the data collection and estimation process. The unknown is represented by the vector, **f**. The data collection process, A, produces a linear combination of the unknown. The data, **p**, consists of A · **f** and additive noise, **n**. The data pass through the system, H, to produce the estimate of the unknown, $\hat{f}$. The estimate of the unknown, $\hat{f}$, passes through A to produce an estimate of the data, $\hat{p}$.

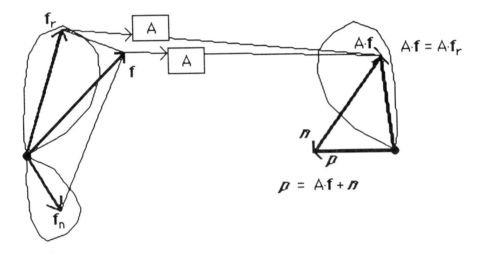

FIGURE 25.8.   Data collection model and associated vector spaces: the blobs represent the vector spaces associated with the data collection matrix, A. The upper left blob is the row space of A; the lower left blob is the null space of A; and the blob on the right is the column space of A. The data collection process, A, transforms the unknown, **f**, into A · **f** in the column space of A. The data, **p**, is the sum of A · **f** and the detector noise, **n**. The portion of **f** in the null space of A, $\mathbf{f_n}$, is mapped by A into the zero vector. The portion of **f** in the row space of A, $\mathbf{f_r}$ is mapped by A into the vector, A · **f**.

The reader should note the similarity between this model and the model given by Equations 12.28 and 12.29. As in Chapter 12, the estimate of the data is a set of values similar to the actual data, but consistent with the model.

Figure 25.7 shows these relationships diagrammatically. The unknown signal, **f**, passes through the system, A, and the noise, **n**, is added to it to produce the measurements, **p**. The measurements pass through the system, H, to produce the estimate of the unknown, $\hat{f}$, passes through the system, A, to produce the estimate of the data, $\hat{p}$.

It is not possible to draw a figure of a multi-dimensional vector space, but we shall again represent multi-dimensional vector spaces as blobs. Figure 25.8 shows the model of the system in terms of vector spaces associated with A, the system representing the data collection process. The unknown, **f**, is transformed by the system, A, into A · **f**. A · **f** must be in the column space of A. The noise, **n**, adds to A · **f** to produce, **p**, the data.

The unknown, **f**, can be divided into two parts, $\mathbf{f_r}$, the part in the row space of A, and $\mathbf{f_n}$, the part in the null space of A. The part of the signal in the row space of A will be passed by the system, A, to A · **f**. The part in the null space of A will be stopped by the system. These relations are also shown in Figure 25.8. Since no information about $\mathbf{f_n}$ passes

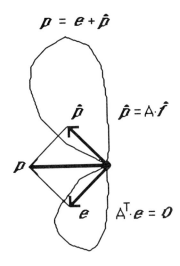

FIGURE 25.9. Orthogonality principle: the upper blob represents the column space of A; and the lower blob represents the null space of A^T. The data, p, consists of two components, the estimate of the data, $\hat{p}$, and the error, e. The model says that the estimation, $\hat{p}$, is in the column space of A. The orthogonality principle says that the error vector, e, is in the null space of A^T.

to the data, this part of **f** cannot be estimated. If the null space of A has a dimension greater than zero, then there is some aspect of the input which will not be represented in the data. In the terminology of simultaneous equations, the system is under determined. In the computed tomography problem, this situation could occur because of an inadequate set of projections.

III. ESTIMATION OF THE DATA

The goal of this chapter is to derive a linear, mean square estimate, $\hat{p}$, of the data which is consistent with the model given above. The error in this estimate is defined:

$$e = p - \hat{p} \tag{25.25}$$

The error is defined in terms of the data. Recall from Chapter 12, that when the error is defined in terms of the data, we refer to the estimate as an estimate of the data.

We could solve this problem algebraically by differentiating the mean square error with respect to each of the factors, h_{ij}. However, we shall take the simpler geometric approach of using the orthogonality principle. We know that the error must be orthogonal to the estimation space. The estimation space is the column space of A. All vectors in the column space of A can be written as $A \cdot \mathbf{f}'$, where $\mathbf{f}'$ is an arbitrary vector in the row space of A. Thus, orthogonality means that:

$$(A \cdot \mathbf{f}')^T \cdot e = \mathbf{f}'^T \cdot (A^T \cdot e) = \mathbf{0} \tag{25.26}$$

However, since the $\mathbf{f}'$ is an arbitrary vector, the second term must be zero and the orthogonality principle can be written:

$$A^T \cdot e = \mathbf{0} \tag{25.27}$$

Figure 25.9 shows the relations between p, $\hat{p}$, and e, diagrammatically. The model (Equation 25.24) states that the estimate, $\hat{p}$, must lie in the column space of A. The or-

$$n = e + (\hat{p} - A \cdot f)$$

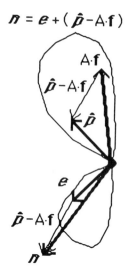

FIGURE 25.10.   Noise components: the upper blob represents the column space of A; and the lower blob represents the null space of A^T. The noise, n, consists of two components, e in the null space of A^T and $\hat{p} - A \cdot f$ in the column space of A.

thogonality principle (Equation 25.27) says that the error vector, e, must be in the null space of A^T. Thus, $\hat{p}$ is the projection of p onto the column space of A; and e is the projection of p onto the null space of A^T.

The noise can be divided into two parts, the part in the column space of A and the part in the null space of A. From Equations 25.21 and 25.25:

$$e + \hat{p} = p = A \cdot f + n \tag{25.28}$$

Solving for n:

$$n = e + (\hat{p} - A \cdot f) \tag{25.29}$$

The noise in the column space, $\hat{p} - A \cdot f$, is consistent with the model and it is not removed by the estimation process. The noise in the null space of A^T, e, is inconsistent with the model and it is removed by the estimation process. These relations are shown in Figure 25.10.

We can use the orthogonality principle to derive the normal equations. Substituting Equation 25.25 into 25.27 gives:

$$A^T \cdot (p - A \cdot \hat{f}) = A^T \cdot p - A^T \cdot A \cdot \hat{f} = 0 \tag{25.30}$$

Therefore,

$$A^T \cdot A \cdot \hat{f} = A^T \cdot p \tag{25.31}$$

The set of equations represented by this matrix equation are the **normal equations** of linear algebra. We have already derived exactly this same relationship (Equation 25.9) in the geometrical problem of finding the best estimate of a vector in terms of a set of vectors.

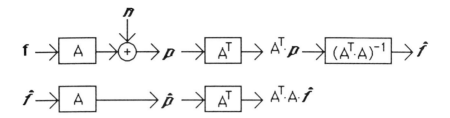

FIGURE 25.11. Data collection, reconstruction model: this figure is similar to Figure 25.7 except that the reconstruction matrix, H, has been replaced by $A^T \cdot (A^T \cdot A)^{-1}$. The data, $\boldsymbol{p}$, is equal to the unknown, $\mathbf{f}$, passed through the system, A, plus the detector noise, $\boldsymbol{n}$. The data, $\boldsymbol{p}$, is transformed by A^T into the vector, $A^T \cdot \boldsymbol{p}$. $A^T \cdot \boldsymbol{p}$ is then transformed by $(A^T \cdot A)^{-1}$ into the estimate of the unknown, $\hat{f}$. The estimate of the data, $\hat{p}$, is obtained by passing $\hat{f}$ through A. The estimate of the data, $\hat{p}$, is transformed by A^T into $A^T \cdot A \cdot \hat{f}$. The normal equations equate the data and the estimate of the data after transformation by A^T.

The normal equations are usually presented from the point of view of providing a least mean square solution to the set of inconsistent equations:

$$\mathbf{p} = A \cdot \hat{\mathbf{f}} \qquad (25.32)$$

These equations may be inconsistent since the vector $A \cdot \hat{\mathbf{f}}$ must be in the column space of A, while the vector $\mathbf{p}$ can be any vector. Thus it may not be possible to choose an $\hat{\mathbf{f}}$ which satisfies this equation. The normal equations provide a solution to this problem:

$$A^T \cdot \mathbf{p} = A^T \cdot A \cdot \hat{\mathbf{f}} \qquad (25.33)$$

The row space of A^T is the column space of A; therefore, A^T passes only the portion of $\mathbf{p}$ which is in the column space of A. All vectors of the form $A^T \cdot \mathbf{p}$ can be written in the forms $A^T \cdot A \cdot \hat{\mathbf{f}}$. Therefore, the normal equations are a consistent set of equations. If $A^T \cdot A$ does not have an inverse, there will not be a unique solution to this equation, but the equation is always true.

Since the orthogonality principle is the same for this problem and for the projection problem (Equations 25.31 and 25.9) the solution is the same.

$$H = (A^T \cdot A)^{-1} \cdot A^T \qquad (25.34)$$

The estimate of the unknown is:

$$\hat{f} = (A^T \cdot A)^{-1} \cdot A^T \cdot \boldsymbol{p} \qquad (25.35)$$

And the estimate of the data is:

$$\hat{p} = A \cdot (A^T \cdot A)^{-1} \cdot A^T \cdot \boldsymbol{p} \qquad (25.36)$$

The estimate of the data is the projection of the actual data onto the estimation space using the projection matrix:

$$A \cdot (A^T \cdot A)^{-1} \cdot A^T \qquad (25.37)$$

Using the definition of the matrix, H, from Equation 25.34, the diagrammatic model of the system can be expanded as shown in Figure 25.11. p is mapped by A^T into vector

$$A^T \cdot A \cdot \hat{f} = A^T \cdot p$$

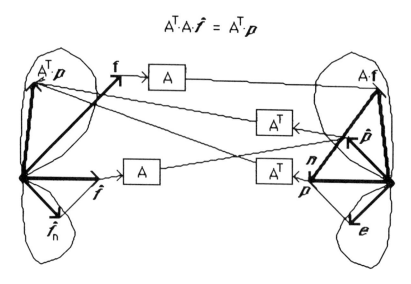

FIGURE 25.12.   The vector spaces associated with estimation of the data: the upper left blob represents the row space of A; the lower left blob represents the null space of A; the upper right blob represents the column space of A; and the lower right blob represents the null space of A^T. The data collection process, A, maps the unknown, **f**, to A · **f** in the column space of A. The data, **p**, is the sum of A · **f** and the detector noise, **n**. A maps the estimate of the unknown, $\hat{f}$, to the estimate of the data, $\hat{p}$, in the column space of A. The normal equations say that A^T maps the data, **p**, and the estimate of the date, $\hat{p}$, to the same vector, $A^T \cdot p$, in the row space of A. The portion of the estimate of the unknown in the null space of A, $\hat{f}_n$, does not contribute to the estimate of the data. The portion of the noise in the data which is inconsistent with the model, **e**, is in the null space of A^T. The normal equations discard this portion of the noise.

$A^T \cdot p$ in the row space of A. This vector is then mapped by $(A^T \cdot A)^{-1}$ to $\hat{f}$. Similarly, the estimate $\hat{p}$ is mapped by A^T to $A^T \cdot A \cdot \hat{f}$. In this diagram we can see that the normal equations relate the data and the estimate of the data after being mapped to the row space of A by A^T.

Figure 25.12 shows these relationships in terms of the vector spaces associated with the matrix, A. The model says that the unknown, **f**, is mapped into the vector, A · **f**, by the data collection process A. A · **f** is in the column space of A. The noise, **n**, is added to A · **f** to produce the data, **p**. Similarly, the estimate of the unknown, $\hat{f}$, is mapped to an estimate of the data, $\hat{p}$, by A. The orthogonality principle states that $\hat{p}$ is the projection of **p** on the column space of A.

As shown in Figure 25.9, **p** consists of two parts, $\hat{p}$, the projection of **p** on the column space of A and **e**, the projection of **p** on the null space of A^T. The normal equations compare **p** and the estimate $\hat{p}$ in the row space of A. In Figure 25.12, **p** is mapped into a vector, $A^T \cdot p$, in the row space of A by A^T. The portion of **p** in the null space of A^T, the error, **e**, is stopped by A^T; the portion of **p** in the row space of A^T, $\hat{p}$, is passed by A^T. Thus, both **p** and $\hat{p}$ are mapped by A^T into the same vector, $A^T \cdot p$.

The relationship given by the normal equations can be traced through the mappings shown in Figure 25.12. The mapping of the estimate of the unknown, $\hat{f}$, into the estimate of the data, $\hat{p}$, in the column space of A by the system A, followed by mapping back to the row space of A by the system A^T, results in the vector $A^T \cdot A \cdot \hat{f}$. The normal equations say that this vector is equal to the mapping of the data **p** into the row space of A by the system, A^T. The mapping of $\hat{f}$ into $\hat{p}$, zeroes $\hat{f}_n$; therefore, the normal equations are not concerned with estimation of the null space component of the unknown. The mapping of p and $\hat{p}$ back to the row space of A, zeroes e, the portion of the noise which is inconsistent with the model. The estimation removes the noise which is inconsistent with the model.

The difference between $\mathbf{f}$ and the estimate $\hat{f}$ can be divided into two parts, the difference in the null space of A and the difference in the row space of A. The normal equations give no indication of the relation between $\mathbf{f}$ and $\hat{f}$ in the null space. The normal equations are a linear, least mean square estimate of the data; since the null space does not affect the data, the family of solutions includes vectors with any null space components. In the row space the difference between $\mathbf{f}$ and $\hat{f}$ is due to the component of the noise which is consistent with the model, the portion of the noise in the column space of A.

Let us summarize the results of this section:

$$\text{Measurement:} \qquad p = A \cdot \mathbf{f} + n \qquad\qquad (25.38)$$

$$\text{Estimate:} \qquad \hat{p} = A \cdot \hat{f}, \quad \hat{f} = H \cdot p \qquad\qquad (25.39)$$

$$\text{Error:} \qquad e = p - \hat{p} \qquad\qquad (25.40)$$

$$\text{Orthogonality:} \qquad A^T \cdot e = 0 \qquad\qquad (25.41)$$

$$\text{Solution:} \qquad H = (A^T \cdot A)^{-1} \cdot A^T \qquad\qquad (25.42)$$

The model used in this problem is that a signal, $\mathbf{f}$, is transformed by a system, A. The transformed signal, $A \cdot \mathbf{f}$, is measured with a measurement noise, n, to produce data, p. Linear, least mean square estimation of the data, p, leads to the orthogonality principle — the error must be orthogonal to the estimation space, the column space of A. The orthogonality principle can be used to derive the normal equations of linear algebra:

$$A^T \cdot A \cdot \hat{f} = A^T \cdot p \qquad\qquad (25.43)$$

The estimated data, $\hat{p}$, is the orthogonal projection of p onto the column space of A. The estimate removes the portion of the noise which is inconsistent with the model. If the data collection process is under determined, then a portion of the unknown, the portion in the null space of A, has no affect on the data. Since this model estimates the data, it does not specify the portion of the unknown in the null space of A.

IV. ITERATIVE SOLUTION

Equation 25.35 is a practical solution to the estimation problem for very small matrix sizes. However, for radiological imaging applications the solution has two major problems. First, the matrices are often on the order of 64k × 64k. The matrix inversion is a very time-consuming problem. Second, the inverse matrix rarely exists. Thus, although this solution provides an interesting theoretical frame work, it is not of practical use for imaging problems.

A common practical method of solving large matrix problems is to use an iterative solution. Iterative solution is particularly useful when the matrix is sparse — when the matrix contains a high proportion of zeros. An iterative solution assumes that we have a good model of the data collection process, A, and an approximate solution of the reconstruction, H. The reconstruction, H, does not have to be very accurate so long as it produces a reasonable estimate.

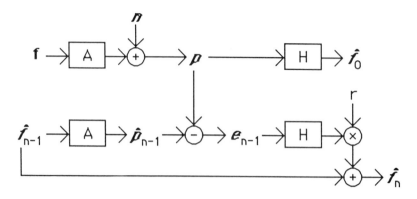

FIGURE 25.13. Iterative reconstruction model: the data, p, is equal to the sum of the unknown, $\mathbf{f}$, passed through the data collection system, A, plus noise, $\mathbf{n}$. The initial estimate of the unknown, $\hat{f}_0$, is produced from the data, p, by the approximate reconstructor, H. The $n - 1^{st}$ estimate of the data, $\hat{p}_{n-1}$, is obtained by passing the $n - 1^{st}$ estimate of the unknown, $\hat{f}_{n-1}$, through the data collection process, A. The $n - 1^{st}$ estimate of the data, $\hat{p}_{n-1}$, is compared to the actual data, p. The error, e_{n-1}, which is the difference between the data, p, and the estimate of the data, $\hat{p}_{n-1}$, is reconstructed with the approximate reconstructor, H. The reconstructed error correction is scaled with the relaxation factor, r. The correction is added to the $n - 1^{st}$ estimate of the unknown, $\hat{f}_{n-1}$, to produce the nth estimate of the unknown, $\hat{f}_n$.

Figure 25.13 shows the basic iterative algorithm. The top line shows the model of the data collection process. The vector, $\mathbf{f}$, goes through the data collection process, A. Then detector noise, $\mathbf{n}$, is added to the signal to produce the data, p. The approximate solution, H, produces a first approximation, $\hat{f}_0$, of the unknown.

The iterative step is shown by the loop at the bottom. The approximate solution, $\hat{f}_{n-1}$, is put through the data collection process to produce a set of estimated data, $\hat{p}_{n-1}$. The estimated data is compared with the actual data, p, to produce an error, e_{n-1}. The error is passed through the approximate reconstruction, H, to produce a set of correction factors. These correction factors are multiplied times a **relaxation factor**, r, and added to the estimate, $\hat{f}_{n-1}$, to produce the new estimate, $\hat{f}_n$. The iteration is repeated a number of times.

On each iteration the previous estimate is corrected using only the error, e_{n-1}. If the approximate reconstruction, H, is a reasonable estimate of the reconstruction process, then the error term will be small. Only the error is reconstructed on each iteration; therefore, the correction factors are relatively small. The key feature in arriving at an accurate result is that the model of the data collection process, A, is accurate. So long as A is accurate, then the accuracy of H is less important. The corrections become smaller as the estimates, $\hat{f}_n$, more closely approximate the unknown, $\mathbf{f}$.

There are several important aspects of iterative solution which we shall ignore. For example, mathematicians are very concerned about whether the iterative solution converges on the correct solution. In practice, it usually does. Ill-conditioned problems often result in mark noise sensitivity. In practice, simple solutions such as stopping the iteration after a few steps can limit noise sensitivity. It is possible for the successive estimates to oscillate around the proper solution. In practice, the relaxation factor, r, can be used to damp these oscillations. These interesting and important issues are beyond the scope of this book.

Although the formalism describe by Figure 25.13 aids understanding, the implementation of an iterative solution may not actually use matrix multiplication. In the case of radiological problems,the matrices are massive, often 64k $\times$ 64k. But, they are usually quite sparse. Special purpose operations which are equivalent to matrix multiplication can often be performed much more efficiently.

V. SUMMARY

This chapter is concerned with the data collection problem shown in Figure 25.7. An unknown object, $\mathbf{f}$, is sampled with a data collection system, A, with additive detector noise, $\mathbf{n}$, to produce data, $\mathbf{p}$. The goal is to derive an estimate, $\hat{f}$, of the unknown, $\mathbf{f}$, which combines the *a priori* information about the model with the data, $\mathbf{p}$.

An estimate of the data, $\hat{p}$, can be derived from the estimate of the unknown, $\hat{f}$, using the model. The error, $\mathbf{e}$ is defined as the difference between the data, $\mathbf{p}$ and the estimate of the data, $\hat{p}$. This algorithm produces estimates of both the unknown and the data; however, since the error is defined in terms of the data, we refer to this type of estimation problem as estimation of the data. In Chapter 12, we found that estimation of the data problems do not use *a priori* information about the unknown. Therefore, we have used a deterministic model, $\mathbf{f}$, of the unknown.

As we discovered several times in Chapter 12, least mean square estimation results in the orthogonality principle, the error, $\mathbf{e}$, is orthogonal to the estimation space. In this case the estimation space is the column space of A. The error, the difference between the data and the estimate of the data, must lie in the null space of A^T. (The null space of A^T is orthogonal to the column space of A.)

The orthogonality principle leads directly to the normal equations of linear algebra. The normal equations equate the data, $\mathbf{p}$, and the estimation of the data, $\hat{p}$, after they have been mapped by A^T to the row space of A. The solution to the normal equations is that the estimate, $\hat{p}$, is the orthogonal projection of $\mathbf{p}$ onto the column space of A.

The portion of the unknown which is in the null space of A, $\mathbf{f}_n$, does not pass into the data. Similarly, the portion of the estimate of the unknown which is in the null space of A, $\hat{f}_n$, does not affect the estimate. If the null space of A has a dimension greater than zero, then there is a family of solutions with different $\hat{f}_n$ components.

The portion of the noise in the null space of A^T is inconsistent with the model. This portion of the noise is equal to the error, $\mathbf{e}$; it is removed by the estimation process. The portion of the noise in the column space of A is consistent with the model. It cannot be removed by the estimation process.

This chapter has been concerned with linear, least mean square estimation of the data. The next chapter will be concerned with linear, time invariant, least mean square estimation of the unknown. Time invariance greatly simplifies the estimation process, but estimation of the unknown instead of the data makes the problem more difficult.

VI. FURTHER READING

Most descriptions of the normal equations of linear algebra are somewhat different from this chapter in that they do not explicitly include noise. A good description of the normal equations from this point of view can be found in Chapter 3 of the book by Strang.[1] Chapter 2 of that book also has an excellent discussion of the four vector spaces associated with a matrix. The more advance book by the same author[2] provides further understanding of this problem. A more complete description of iterative solution methods in the radiological context can be found in the books by Herman[3] and by Barrett and Swindell.[4]

REFERENCES

1. **Strang, G.,** *Linear Algebra and its Applications,* Academic Press, New York, 1980.
2. **Strang, G.,** *Introduction to Applied Mathematics,* Wellesley-Cambridge Press, Wellesley, MA, 1986.
3. **Herman, G. T.,** *Image Reconstruction from Projection,* Academic Press, New York, 1980.
4. **Barrett, H. H. and Swindell, W.,** *Radiological Imaging: The Theory of Image Formation, Detection, and Processing,* Vol. 2, Academic Press, New York, 1981.

Chapter 26

WIENER FILTERING

Wiener filtering is a linear, time invariant method of least mean square estimation of a stochastic process from a noisy sample of the stochastic process. Wiener filtering is important for several radiological applications. It will be particularly important in understanding the different filters used for image reconstruction in Chapter 32. The Wiener filter combines the concept of filtering a stochastic process introduced in Chapter 24 with the concept of linear, least mean square estimation introduced in Chapter 12.

This chapter is somewhat difficult. It may be easier to understand this chapter after reviewing Chapter 12 (Linear, Least Mean Square Estimation) and Chapter 24 (Filtering Stochastic Processes). It might be best to skim this chapter the first time through. However, this chapter is an important chapter to come back to later. The concepts derived in this chapter are essential to understanding the reconstruction of images in the presence of noise, the major goal of this book.

In Chapter 12, we found that one difficulty in understanding estimation was keeping track of the various different models which are used for different problems. A major distinction between the models was whether the data or the unknown was being estimated. Estimation of the data was less complicated than estimation of the unknown; however, it did not allow *a priori* information about the unknown to be used in the estimation.

The normal equations of linear algebra, described in the last chapter, provide a linear method for estimation of the data. The Wiener filter provides a linear, time invariant method for estimation of the unknown. The Wiener filter is less complicated than the normal equations in that it is both linear and time invariant instead of just linear. The Wiener filter is more complicated than the normal equations in that it estimates the unknown instead of the data. Both methods are similar in that they are linear, least mean square estimates.

I. MODELS

Most of the problems which will be discussed in this book involve the estimation of a signal from a single measurement of the signal. For example, consider a nuclear medicine liver, spleen scan. From a single experimental image of the liver, spleen scan, the goal is to obtain the best estimate of the distribution of activity in the liver and spleen. We wish to estimate the "true" liver spleen scan from a single image. The single image is different from the "true" liver spleen scan since the single image has measurement noise.

This experiment can be modeled with the equation:

$$p(t) = f(t) + n(t) \tag{26.1}$$

where f(t) is the "true" image, $n(t)$ is the measurement noise, and $p(t)$ is the measured signal. We have used t as a generalized independent variable. In the case of liver spleen scanning, t stands for x,y. f(t) is a deterministic signal; $n(t)$ and $p(t)$ are stochastic processes.

The problem with this model is that it assumes that the signal f(t) is known. This model is not useful for most radiological problems since usually f(t) is an unknown. (The model given by Equation 26.1 is used frequently in communications theory. Given that f(t) is known, the task is to detect f(t) in $p(t)$. This model leads to a result known as the **matched filter**.)

A more realistic model for most radiological imaging problems is given by:

$$p(t) = f(t) + n(t) \tag{26.2}$$

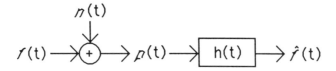

FIGURE 26.1. Wiener filter model: the model used in Wiener filtering is that data, $p(t)$, are equal to the unknown, $f(t)$, plus noise, $n(t)$. The Wiener filter, $h(t)$, is linear and time invariant. The estimate, $\hat{f}(t)$, is obtained by passing the data, $p(t)$, through the filter, $h(t)$.

where $f(t)$, $n(t)$, and $p(t)$ are all stochastic processes. The statistics of $f(t)$ and $n(t)$ are used to define the *a priori* information about the signal and the noise. The statistics of $f(t)$ contain the information provided by knowing that it represents a liver spleen scan. The statistics of $n(t)$ provide information about the character of the detector noise. This model will be used in the discussion of Wiener filtering.

As described in Chapter 12, knowing that an image is a liver spleen scan provides considerable *a priori* information. The various points in a liver spleen scan are not independent. For example, if we know all but one point in a scan, then we can predict the value of that point with good accuracy. Some of this information can be modeled in terms of statistical properties. An important property is the power spectral density functions of the signal, $f(t)$, and the noise, $n(t)$. From Chapter 24, one might guess that an important parameter will be the signal to noise ratio as a function of spatial frequency.

Any linear, time invariant estimation can be modeled as a convolution of a set of factors, $h(t)$, with the data, $p(t)$:

$$\hat{f}(t) = h(t) * p(t) \tag{26.3}$$

where $\hat{f}(t)$ is an estimate of the unknown, $f(t)$, from the data $p(t)$. The set of factors, $h(t)$, define the linear, time invariant estimation. This model of the data collection and estimation process is shown in Figure 26.1.

A liver spleen scan is a relatively simple example of the measurement process. More generally, the measurements may be made up from a combination of the unknown signal values. For example, in computed tomography the measurements are line integrals through the unknown cross-sectional image values.

A linear, time (or space) invariant data collection process can be modeled as a convolution:

$$p(t) = a(t) * f(t) + n(t) \tag{26.4}$$

where $a(t)$ represents the measurement process; $f(t)$, $n(t)$, and $p(t)$ are stochastic processes; $a(t)$ is a deterministic system. The noise is modeled as an additive factor after the convolution. This noise model is reasonably representative of the detector noise in computed tomography.

As above, any linear, time invariant estimate can be modeled:

$$\hat{f}(t) = h(t) * p(t) \tag{26.5}$$

This model of the data collection and estimation process is shown in Figure 26.2. In addition to estimating the unknown, the data can be estimated as:

$$\hat{p}(t) = a(t) * \hat{f}(t) \tag{26.6}$$

The estimate of the data, $\hat{p}(t)$, is obtained by passing the estimate of the unknown through the measurement process, $a(t)$.

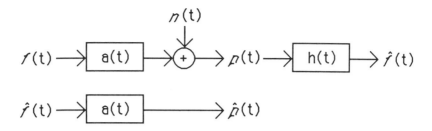

FIGURE 26.2. Wiener deconvolution model: the data collection process is modeled by a linear, time invariant system, a(t). The unknown, f(t), passes through the data collection process. The data, p(t), are equal to the unknown after passing through, a(t), plus the detector noise, n(t). The estimate, $\hat{f}$(t), is obtained by passing the data, p(t), through the filter, h(t). An estimate of the data, $\hat{p}$(t), is obtained by passing the estimate of the unknown through the data collection process.

The model in Figure 26.1 is very similar to the model in Figure 26.2. The major difference is that in the former the noise is added directly to the signal while in the latter the noise is added to the signal after it has passed through the system, a(t). The former can be used to model planar imaging while the latter is similar to models of tomographic imaging. The former will be used in describing Wiener filtering; the latter will be used in describing Wiener deconvolution. We shall find that there is a great similarity to the solution of these two problems.

Since the Wiener filter will be defined in terms of the power spectral density functions, we shall assume that the signal and the noise are jointly stationary. Furthermore, we shall assume that the power spectral density functions are known. The major value of this model is that it incorporates *a priori* information about the power spectral density functions into the estimate. The Wiener filter model is particularly useful when this type of information is known about the problem. As we shall see, this is frequently the case in radiological problems.

The assumption that the signal and the noise are jointly stationary is not strictly true. Imaging systems almost always have limited fields of view. Outside the field of view, the signal is zero. This problem is the same problem which arose when using shift-invariant models of imaging systems. As is the case with shift invariance, what is usually done is to use a stationary model, but then limit the region over which the model is valid to the field of view of the imaging system.

Furthermore, medical images are almost always in the center of the field of view. Consequently, the edges of the field of view rarely have much signal power. The expected value of the power at the edge is less than the power in the center; therefore, the stochastic process is not stationary. By using a stationary model, we discard the ability to include information about the position of the image in the field of view in the estimation. This limitation is frequently not too severe.

II. WIENER FILTERING

A. HEURISTICS

There was considerable similarity between estimation of the data for a single random variable described in Chapter 12 and derivation of the normal equations described in the last chapter. The estimation process was the same, but random vectors were used to replace random variables, and matrices replaced vectors. We shall see that there is also considerable similarity between estimation of the unknown for a single random variable (also described in Chapter 12) and Wiener filtering. The random variables are replaced by stochastic processes and linear, time invariant systems replace the vectors which defined the data collection and estimation.

Recall from Chapter 12 that the estimation of the unknown resulted in a factor which was the power in the unknown, divided by the sum of the powers in the unknown and the noise. If there is only a small amount of noise, then the data provides a good estimate of the unknown. If there is a great deal of noise, then the data provided misleading data, and it is better to assume the unknown is zero. We shall find a very similar result for Wiener filtering.

B. ORTHOGONALITY

Linear, mean square estimation problems lead to the orthogonality principle — the error in the estimate is orthogonal to the estimation space. The estimation space defines the estimates which are allowed by the model. Estimation projects the data onto the estimation space. The estimate is the point in the estimation space which is closest to the data. The model (Equation 26.3 or 26.5) defines the estimation space as a linear combination of the data. Therefore, the error is orthogonal to (uncorrelated with) the data. The estimate removes all of the information about the unknown from the data.

In Chapter 12, it was easy to draw a diagram of estimation of the data since the orthogonality principle was true for each measurement. It was more difficult to draw a diagram of estimation of the unknown since the orthogonality was in a statistical sense. Because of the complexity of the Wiener filtering model, we shall not try to draw a diagram of the orthogonality principle for Wiener filtering. A geometric sense of the orthogonality principle can be obtained by analogy to the results in Chapter 12.

C. MATHEMATICAL DERIVATION OF THE ORTHOGONALITY PRINCIPLE

The error for the Wiener filtering problem is defined as the difference between the unknown stochastic process, $f(t)$, and the estimate, $\hat{f}(t)$:

$$e(t) = f(t) - \hat{f}(t) \tag{26.7}$$

The error is also a stochastic process. The mean square error is given by:

$$|e|^2 = E\{|e(t)|^2\} \tag{26.8}$$

Since we have assumed that the process is stationary, the mean square error will not be a function of time.

The minimum of the mean square error can be found by setting the derivative of Equation 26.8 with respect to the estimation parameters equal to zero. Mathematically:

$$\partial|e|^2/\partial h(\alpha) = 0, \quad \text{for all } \alpha \tag{26.9}$$

where we have used α as a time variable. Equation 26.9 represents an infinite set of equations, one equation for each estimation parameter, $h(\alpha)$.

Equation 26.8 can be substituted into Equation 26.9 and the partial differentiation can be moved inside the expectation. From Equations 6.90 and 6.91, a sufficient condition for Equation 26.9 to be true is:

$$E\{2 \cdot e(t) \cdot [\partial e(t)/\partial h(\alpha)]^*\} = 0, \quad \text{for all } \alpha \tag{26.10}$$

Dividing by 2 gives:

$$E\{e(t) \cdot [\partial e(t)/\partial h(\alpha)]^*\} = 0, \qquad \text{for all } \alpha \qquad (26.11)$$

The partial derivative, $\partial e(t)/\partial h(\alpha)$ can be expanded using Equation 26.7:

$$\partial e(t)/\partial h(\alpha) = \partial f(t)/\partial h(\alpha) - \partial \hat{f}(t)/\partial h(\alpha) \qquad (26.12)$$

In the first term of Equation 26.12, $f(t)$, the unknown, is not a function of the estimation; therefore, its derivative is zero. The second term can be expanded using Equation 26.3:

$$\partial \hat{f}(t)/\partial h(\alpha) = \partial \left[\int_{-\infty}^{+\infty} p(t - \tau) \cdot h(\tau) \, d\tau \right] / \partial h(\alpha) \qquad (26.13)$$

The only value in the integral which is a function of $h(\alpha)$ is when τ is equal to α; therefore:

$$\partial \hat{f}(t)/\partial h(\alpha) = p(t - \alpha) \qquad (26.14)$$

Equations 26.12 and 26.14 can be used to rewrite Equation 26.11:

$$E\{e(t) \cdot p^*(t - \alpha)\} = 0, \qquad \text{for all } \alpha \qquad (26.15)$$

The error and the data are orthogonal in the statistical sense. Equation 26.15 is the orthogonality principle for Wiener filtering. It is very similar to Equation 12.87; the only difference is that random variables have been replaced by stochastic processes. There are an infinite number of orthogonality conditions parameterized by α.

When estimating the unknown, the orthogonality principle says that the error and the data are orthogonal. There is no mutual power between the error and the data. All of the information has been removed from the data by the estimation.

D. SOLUTION

As in previous problems, we can use the orthogonality principle to derive the solution to the estimation problem. The goal is to determine the value of the Wiener filter, $h(t)$. The Wiener filter is a set of estimation parameters.

Equation 26.7 can be substituted in Equation 26.15:

$$E\{[f(t) - \hat{f}(t)] \cdot p^*(t - \alpha)\} = 0, \qquad \text{for all } \alpha \qquad (26.16)$$

This equation can be expanded:

$$E\{f(t) \cdot p^*(t - \alpha)\} - E\{\hat{f}(t) \cdot p^*(t - \alpha)\} = 0, \qquad \text{for all } \alpha \quad (26.17)$$

The first term can be recognized as a cross correlation function of $f(t)$ and $p(t)$. Therefore:

$$R_{fp}(\alpha) - E\{\hat{f}(t) \cdot p^*(t - \alpha)\} = 0, \qquad \text{for all } \alpha \qquad (26.18)$$

where α is a dummy time variable.

The second term in Equation 26.18 can be further expanded using Equation 26.3:

$$E\{\hat{f}(t) \cdot p^*(t - \alpha)\} = E\left\{ \left[\int_{-\infty}^{+\infty} h(\tau) \cdot p(t - \tau) \, d\tau \right] \cdot p^*(t - \alpha) \right\} \qquad (26.19)$$

Since $p*(t - \alpha)$ is not a function of τ, it can be moved inside the integral. The order of integration and expectation can be switched, and the deterministic function $h(\tau)$ can be moved outside the expectation:

$$E\{\hat{f}(t) \cdot p*(t - \alpha)\} = \int_{-\infty}^{+\infty} h(\tau) \cdot E\{p(t - \tau) \cdot p*(t - \alpha)\} \, d\tau \quad (26.20)$$

The expectation can be recognized as the autocorrelation function of $p(t)$.

$$E\{\hat{f}(t) \cdot p*(t - \alpha)\} = \int_{-\infty}^{+\infty} h(\tau) \cdot R_p(\tau - \alpha) \, d\tau \quad (26.21)$$

The right side of this equality is recognized as the convolution of the autocorrelation function, $R_p(\alpha)$, with the Wiener filter, $h(\alpha)$, where again we use α as a time variable. Therefore:

$$E\{\hat{f}(t) \cdot p*(t - \alpha)\} = h(\alpha) * R_p(\alpha) \quad (26.22)$$

Substituting Equation 26.22 into Equation 26.18 gives an equation in terms of the Wiener filter and the second order statistics of the model:

$$R_{fp}(\alpha) - h(\alpha) * R_p(\alpha) = 0, \quad \text{for all } \alpha \quad (26.23)$$

In Chapter 24, the power spectral density function was defined as the Fourier transform of the autocorrelation function (Equation 24.7). The Fourier transform of Equation 26.23 gives:

$$S_{fp}(\omega) - H(\omega) \cdot S_p(\omega) = 0 \quad (26.24)$$

Solving for the Wiener filter:

$$H(\omega) = S_{fp}(\omega)/S_p(\omega) \quad (26.25)$$

The Wiener filter is equal to the ratio of the mutual power between the signal and the data divided by the power in the data. This result is very similar to the result given in equation 12.88. The estimate is related to how the power in the unknown, $f(t)$, is correlated with the power in the data, $p(t)$, normalized by the power in the data.

Much of the simplicity of the result in Equation 26.25 is due to the stationarity of the stochastic processes, $f(t)$, and $n(t)$, and to the linearity and time invariance of the estimation parameters, $h(t)$. Stationarity of the stochastic processes means that the statistics of the problem can be expressed in the frequency domain using the power spectral densities. Using a linear, time invariant estimation model means that the estimation can be expressed as a convolution in the time domain and consequently as a multiplication in the frequency domain.

We can further simplify the equation for the Wiener filter if the signal, $f(t)$, and the noise, $n(t)$, are uncorrelated. The cross correlation function can be expanded:

$$
\begin{aligned}
R_{fp}(\tau) &= E\{f(t - \tau) \cdot p*(t)\} \\
&= E\{f(t - \tau) \cdot [f*(t) + n*(t)]\} \\
&= E\{f(t - \tau) \cdot f*(t)\} + E\{f(t - \tau) \cdot n*(t)\} \\
&= R_f(\tau) + R_{fn}(\tau) \quad (12.26)
\end{aligned}
$$

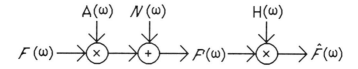

FIGURE 26.3. Frequency domain representation of Wiener deconvolution: the Wiener deconvolution model shown in the time domain in Figure 26.2 is shown in the frequency domain in this diagram. In the frequency domain, the operation of the linear, time invariant systems can be represented by multiplication. The data, $P(\omega)$, is equal to the unknown, $F(\omega)$, times the data collection process, $A(\omega)$, plus the noise, $N(\omega)$. The estimate of the unknown, $\hat{F}(\omega)$, is equal to the data modified by the parameters, $H(\omega)$.

(see Equation 11.11) If the signal and the noise are uncorrelated then $R_{fn}(\tau)$ is equal to zero; therefore:

$$R_{fp}(\tau) = R_f(\tau) \qquad (26.27)$$

The Fourier transform of this equation is:

$$S_{fp}(\omega) = S_f(\omega) \qquad (26.28)$$

Similarly, the autocorrelation function can be expanded:

$$R_p(\tau) = R_f(\tau) + 2 \cdot R_{fn}(\tau) + R_n(\tau) \qquad (26.29)$$

If the signal and the noise are uncorrelated,

$$R_p(\tau) = R_f(\tau) + R_n(\tau) \qquad (26.30)$$

The Fourier transform of this equation is:

$$S_p(\omega) = S_f(\omega) + S_n(\omega) \qquad (26.31)$$

Equation 26.28 and Equation 26.31 can be substituted into Equation 26.25:

$$H(\omega) = S_f(\omega)/[S_f(\omega) + S_n(\omega)] \qquad (26.32)$$

If the signal and the noise are uncorrelated, then the Wiener filter is equal to the ratio of the power spectral densities of the signal to the signal plus the noise. If the power spectral density in the signal is much larger than that in the noise, then the filter is approximately equal to one. If the power spectral density in the signal is much less than that in the noise, then the filter is approximately equal to zero.

When the signal to noise ratio is high, then $p(t)$ is nearly equal to $f(t)$. The data are a good estimate of the unknown. When the signal to noise ratio is low, then $p(t)$ is largely composed of noise. Zero is a better estimate of $f(t)$ than is $p(t)$. The Wiener filter estimates the unknown in terms of all of the angular frequencies, ω. It keeps those frequencies which provide a great deal of information about the unknown; it discards those frequencies which provide little information about the unknown.

Figure 26.2 shows the data collection, image reconstruction model in the time domain. Figure 26.3 shows the same model in the frequency domain. Because the model is linear and time invariant, the systems can be represented in the frequency domain by multiplication.

Using Figure 26.3 the analogy to the problem solved in Chapter 12 can be shown. The model shown in Figure 26.3 is analogous to the model shown in Figure 12.3. In Chapter 12 the solution given by Equation 12.89 was a ratio of the power in the signal to the power in the signal plus noise. The solution given by Equation 26.32 is the same ratio in the frequency domain. The Wiener filter is exactly the same problem as estimation of the data, but it is defined in the frequency domain.

It may be helpful to consider which elements are related directly to the stochastic processes and which are related to the square of the processes. The power spectral density function is a second-order statistic; it is related to the square of the stochastic process. The Wiener filter operates on a stochastic process; it is related directly to the process. However, the Wiener filter is defined in terms of the power spectral density functions. Although it operates directly on the process, it is defined in terms of the squared properties of the process.

E. SUMMARY OF WIENER FILTERING

Wiener filtering can be summarized as follows:

$$\text{Measurement:} \quad p(t) = f(t) + n(t)$$

$$f(t) \text{ and } n(t) \text{ jointly stationary} \tag{26.33}$$

$$\text{Estimate:} \quad \hat{f}(t) = h(t) * p(t) \tag{26.34}$$

$$\text{Error:} \quad e(t) = E\{f(t) - \hat{f}(t)\} \tag{26.35}$$

$$\text{Orthogonality:} \quad E\{e(t) \cdot p^*(t)\} = 0 \tag{26.36}$$

$$\text{Solution:} \quad H(\omega) = S_{fp}(\omega)/S_p(\omega) \tag{26.37}$$

$$\text{For } R_{fn}(\tau) = 0,$$

$$H(\omega) = S_f(\omega)/[S_f(\omega) + S_n(\omega)] \tag{26.38}$$

The Wiener filter model assumes additive noise where the signal and the noise are jointly stationary. Although the assumption of additive noise and of stationarity are not strictly accurate, this model is reasonable for many planar radiologic imaging applications. Since the error is defined in terms of the unknown, $f(t)$, it is the unknown which is estimated. The orthogonality principle says that the error is orthogonal to the data — the estimation removes all of the information about the solution from the data.

The Wiener filter is equal to the ratio of the mutual power spectral density of the signal and the data to the power spectral density of the data. If the signal and the noise are uncorrelated, then the Wiener filter is the ratio of the signal to the signal plus the noise power spectral density functions. For large signal to noise ratios, the filter is approximately equal to one. For small signal to noise ratios, the filter is approximately equal to zero.

The estimation depends upon having *a priori* knowledge of the signal and the noise power spectral densities. In many radiological applications we have this type of information. When there is no information about the power spectral densities of the signal and the noise, then the Wiener filter should not be used for estimation.

Figure 26.4 shows a typical example of an application of Wiener filtering. Suppose that the *a priori* information about the unknown is that the power spectral density falls off after a certain frequency. The top panel shows an example of such a power spectral density function. Suppose further that the noise is assumed to be white, as shown in the middle

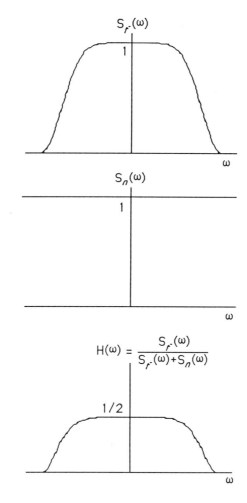

FIGURE 23.4. Example of a Wiener filter: the power-spectral density function shown in the top panel is typical of many unknowns. It is near unity at low frequencies and falls smoothly to zero around some cut-off frequency. For example, in imaging systems the response falls rapidly to zero above the resolution of the detector. Detector noise is often white, as shown in the second panel. In this case, the Wiener filter has the general shape of the power spectral density of the unknown with a magnitude determined by the signal to noise ratio.

panel. If the signal and the noise are uncorrelated, then the filter shown in the bottom panel is easily calculated from Equation 26.38.

Although the example in Figure 26.4 is described in terms of frequency, it should be easy to extend the description conceptually to spatial frequencies. The resolution of the "true" liver spleen scan image is often limited by the resolution of the gamma camera so that there is a rapid decline in power above some spatial frequency. The Poisson counting noise is independent from pixel to pixel; it is approximately white. Thus, a filter like that shown in Figure 26.4 will produce the best estimate of the "true" liver spleen scan from an experimental image.

III. WIENER DECONVOLUTION, SIMPLIFIED MODEL

In the Wiener filter model, the data are equal to the signal plus the noise (Equation 26.2, Figure 26.1). This model occurs frequently in planar imaging, when the noise in the image is primarily due to the detector. However, Part IV will be concerned with the model

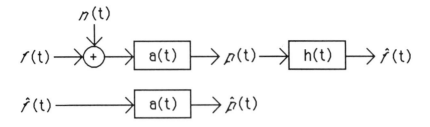

FIGURE 23.5. Simplified model of Wiener deconvolution: this diagram shows the simplified model of Wiener deconvolution. The difference between this model and the model shown in Figure 23.2 is that the noise enters the system before the data collection process, a(t), rather than after it. Notice the similarities of this model to the Wiener filter model shown in Figure 23.1.

given by Equation 26.4, shown in Figure 26.2. The data collection process involves sampling some combination of image values.

In the model shown in Figure 26.2, the noise is added after the signal passes through the system. This type of noise is a good model for the detector noise frequently encountered in radiology. It will be easier first to derive the solution to the simplified system shown in Figure 26.5 where the noise is added directly to the signal. This solution will then be used to solve the more typical model.

Mathematically the model in Figure 26.5 can be written:

$$p'(t) = f(t) + n(t) \tag{26.39}$$

$$p(t) = a(t) * p'(t) \tag{26.40}$$

The noise, $n(t)$, is added to the signal, $f(t)$, prior to convolution with the system, $a(t)$. We shall consider linear, time invariant estimation of the unknown from the data:

$$\hat{f}(t) = h(t) * p(t) \tag{26.41}$$

where the Wiener filter, $h(t)$, is used to derive an estimate, $\hat{f}(t)$, of the unknown from the data, $p(t)$.

The solution of this problem is easily derived from the Wiener filtering result above. The Fourier transform of Equation 26.40 is:

$$P(\omega) = A(\omega) \cdot P'(\omega) \tag{26.42}$$

For $A(\omega)$ not equal to zero:

$$P'(\omega) = P(\omega)/A(\omega) \tag{26.43}$$

The definition of $p'(t)$ in Equation 26.39 is exactly the same as the definition of the data for the Wiener filtering model. After dividing by $A(\omega)$, we are left with the problem which was already solved. Therefore, for $A(\omega)$ not equal to zero, the Wiener filter is given by:

$$H(\omega) = (1/A(\omega)) \cdot S_{fp}(\omega)/S_p(\omega) \tag{26.44}$$

When $A(\omega)$ is equal to zero, $P(\omega)$ is equal to zero, so the value of $H(\omega)$ will not matter, Formally, we could set $H(\omega)$ equal to zero for $A(\omega)$ equal zero. However, since the value for $A(\omega)$ equal to zero has no effect, we shall merely ignore this case.

The solution consists of two parts. The first part, $1/A(\omega)$, removes the effect of the system, $a(t)$. This part of the solution is a simple deconvolution. The second part is just the same Wiener filter as in the last problem.

Let us summarize these results:

$$\text{Measurement:} \quad p'(t) = f(t) + n(t)$$

$$p(t) = a(t) * p'(t)$$

$$f(t) \text{ and } n(t) \text{ jointly stationary} \tag{26.45}$$

$$\text{Estimate:} \quad \hat{f}(t) = h(t) * p(t) \tag{26.46}$$

$$\text{Error:} \quad e(t) = E\{f(t) - \hat{f}(t)\} \tag{26.47}$$

$$\text{Orthogonality:} \quad E\{p(t) \cdot e(t)\} = 0 \tag{26.48}$$

$$\text{Solution:} \quad H(\omega) = (1/A(\omega) \cdot S_{fp}(\omega)/S_p(\omega)) \tag{26.49}$$

$$\text{For } R_{fn}(\tau) = 0,$$

$$H(\omega) = \frac{1}{A(\omega)} \cdot \frac{S_f(\omega)}{S_f(\omega) + S_n(\omega)} \tag{26.50}$$

This model is exactly like the previous model except that the data are modified by $a(t)$. Thus, the solution involves deconvolution for $a(t)$ followed by the same filter as in the previous problem. In fact this problem is a trivial extension of the Wiener filtering problem. However, it helps to explain the Wiener deconvolution below.

IV. WIENER DECONVOLUTION

The next problem which we shall consider is shown in Figure 26.2. It is similar to the problem in Figure 26.5 except that the noise is added after system, $a(t)$, instead of before system. This model has similarities to the data collection process in several radiological applications. For example, in computed tomography the cross-sectional image is first projected, then noise is added to the projections by the detection process.

Mathematically, this model can be written:

$$p(t) = a(t) * f(t) + n(t) \tag{26.51}$$

As above, we shall be interested in linear, time invariant estimates:

$$\hat{f}(t) = h(t) * p(t) \tag{26.52}$$

This is a somewhat more complicated model in that the signal and the noise enter the image collection process at different points.

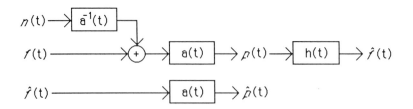

FIGURE 23.6.   Equivalent Wiener deconvolution model: the model shown in this diagram is equivalent to the model shown in Figure 23.2 for frequencies where $A(\omega)$ is not equal to zero. The noise enters the system at the same point as in the simplified model shown in Figure 23.5. However, since the noise is first filtered by the inverse of the data collection process, $a^{-1}(t)$, this model is equivalent to the Wiener deconvolution model. For frequencies where $A(\omega)$ is not zero, the inverse system, $a^{-1}(t)$, cancels the affect of the data collection system, $a(t)$.

We can transform this model into the form of the simplified model in the last section by deriving an expression for an equivalent noise. The Fourier transform of Equation 26.51 is:

$$P(\omega) = A(\omega) \cdot F(\omega) + N(\omega) \tag{26.53}$$

For $A(\omega)$ not equal to zero, this equation can be written:

$$P(\omega) = A(\omega) \cdot [F(\omega) + N(\omega)/A(\omega)] \tag{26.54}$$

This model is shown in Figure 26.6. We have used the potentially misleading symbol, $a^{-1}(t)$ to mean $FT\{1/A(\omega)\}$, the inverse Fourier transform of $a(t)$.

Equation 26.54 is in the form of Equation 26.42 with the noise replaced by a filtered version of the noise $N(\omega)/A(\omega)$. Similarly, the model in Figure 26.6 is in the form of the model in Figure 26.5 with the noise filtered by the system $a^{-1}(t)$. From Equation 24.28, the power spectral density function of the filtered noise is equal to $S_n(\omega)/|A(\omega)|^2$. Therefore, the Wiener filter for this model must

$$H(\omega) = (1/A(\omega)) \cdot S_f(\omega)/[S_f(\omega) + S_n(\omega)/|A(\omega)|^2] \tag{26.55}$$

The Wiener filter consists of two parts. The first part, $1/A(\omega)$, deconvolves the data for the effect of $a(t)$. The second part is a Wiener filter using noise which is filtered by the inverse system, $a^{-1}(t)$. This solution gives the flavor of many of the image reconstruction problems in Part IV. First, the effects of the data collection process must be undone. Second, the unknown image must be estimated based on the noisy data.

The trick to estimation is to compare the signal and the noise on equivalent footing. The noise needs to be modeled as if it were added to the signal. Depending upon where the predominant noise enters the system, it may be filtered by the inverse of the data collection process. Once an equivalent system is derived with the signal and the noise added directly, then the Wiener filter solution can be applied.

We have chosen to solve the Wiener deconvolution problem by analogy to the Wiener filter problem. A more mathematical approach would note that the derivation of Equation 26.25 is not dependent on the differences between the Wiener filtering and the Wiener deconvolution models. Thus, Equation 26.25 is also valid for Wiener deconvolution. The Wiener deconvolution filter is equal to the ratio of the power between the unknown and the data divided by the power in the data. Equation 26.55 can then be derived from Equation 26.25 using Equation 24.28.

The results of this section can be summarized:

$$\text{Measurement:} \qquad p(t) = a(t) * f(t) + n(t)$$

$$f(t) \text{ and } n(t) \text{ jointly stationary} \tag{26.56}$$

$$\text{Estimate:} \qquad \hat{f}(t) = h(t) * p(t) \tag{26.57}$$

$$\text{Error:} \qquad e(t) = E\{f(t) - \hat{f}(t)\} \tag{26.58}$$

$$\text{Orthogonality:} \qquad E\{p(t) \cdot e(t)\} = 0 \tag{26.59}$$

$$\text{Solution:} \qquad \text{For } R_{fn}(\tau) = 0,$$

$$H(\omega) = \frac{1}{A(\omega)} \cdot \frac{S_f(\omega)}{S_f(\omega) + S_n(\omega)/|A(\omega)|^2}$$

$$\tag{26.60}$$

Although this solution is quite complicated in the time domain, it is reasonably simple to understand in the frequency domain. It is a simple deconvolution, $1/A(\omega)$, and an estimation. The estimation is the ratio of the signal to the signal plus noise power spectral densities, where the noise is modeled as if it were added to the signal. In Chapter 32, we shall find that in computed tomography, the ramp filter is a simple deconvolution for the projection, back projection process, and that the roll-off of the ramp filter at high frequencies can be viewed as a Wiener filter. But more of this later.

V. SUMMARY

Wiener filtering is linear, time invariant, mean square estimation of the unknown. The normal equations of linear algebra are linear, mean square estimation of the data. The choice between the different models depends upon efficiency and how well each fits the problem. Many forms of estimation are used for the many different problems in radiology.

The key concept in this chapter is that when the signal and the noise are uncorrelated, then the linear, time invariant, least mean square estimate of an unknown is given by a filter which is the ratio of the signal to the signal plus the noise power spectral density functions. When the signal plus the noise power spectral density functions. When the signal power is large with respect to the noise power, then the signal to signal plus noise is about one. In this case the data are a good estimate of the unknown. When the signal power is small with respect to the noise power, then the signal to signal plus noise is about zero. In this case the data are largely noise, and zero is the best estimate of the unknown.

In Table 1.1, this chapter is seen to depend upon several previous chapters. This chapter has brought together many of the different concepts in the book. Linear systems theory has been key for modeling data collection and image estimation. Fourier transformation has been essential for understanding both data collection and image estimation. The stochastic process model has allowed us to consider the effects of noise. The concepts of estimation from the simple random variable model are remarkably similar in this much more complicated problem. With these many concepts, we are able to formulate the solution so that it is much more easily understood.

The results from this chapter will be very important for several of the chapters in Part IV. In particular Chapter 29 (Deconvolution: First Pass Radionuclide Angiocardiography) will use the results from Wiener filtering, and Chapter 32 (Reconstruction from Noisy Projection: Computed Tomography) will use the results from Wiener deconvolution.

VI. FURTHER READING

A concise development of the Wiener filter similar to that in this chapter can be found in Chapter 10 of the book by Papoulis.[1] Chapter 11 of a second book by the same author also describes the Wiener filter.[2] Another description of Wiener filtering can be found in Chapter 3 of the book by Mohanty.[3]

A major consideration in most engineering texts is implementation of Wiener filtering with a causal filter. (Recall that the output of a causal filter is due only to the previous inputs; future inputs have no affect on the output.) Since causality is of very little importance in image processing, we have not included a discussion of this topic.

Wiener filtering is placed in the context of image processing in Chapter 15 of the book by Pratt[4] and in Chapter 14 of the book by Castleman.[5] Also of interest are the references at the end of the chapters in Part IV.

REFERENCES

1. **Papoulis, A.,** *Signal Analysis,* McGraw-Hill, New York, 1977.
2. **Papoulis, A.,** *Probability, Random Variables, and Stochastic Processes,* McGraw-Hill, New York, 1965.
3. **Mohanty, N.,** *Random Signals Estimation and Identification: Analysis and Applications,* Van Nostrand Reinhold, New York, 1986.
4. **Pratt, W. K.,** *Digital Image Processing,* John Wiley & Sons, New York, 1978.
5. **Castleman, K. R.,** *Digital Image Processing,* Prentice-Hall, Englewood Cliffs, NJ, 1979.

Chapter 27

IMAGE ENHANCEMENT

This Chapter will discuss filtering images in order to enhance certain aspects of the images. The filtering described in this chapter is the same as any other filtering operation. The distinctive feature about image enhancement is conceptual. Image enhancement is processing which improves the quality of an image in some subjective sense. Enhanced images look "better" to the observer.

Image enhancement is an example of the application of signal processing techniques to a real problem. The major goal of this book, use of signal processing methods in image reconstruction, is covered in Part IV. This chapter gives a very brief indication of another area where these methods can be applied.

There are several types of image enhancement; this chapter presents a few very selected examples of image enhancement using filtering. The major examples which will be discussed are smoothing and edge enhancement. The introduction to filtering in Chapter 22 has already introduced several of these methods, and this chapter will make frequent references to Chapter 22.

I. IMAGE ENHANCEMENT AND IMAGE RESTORATION

Image processing techniques can be categorized in terms of the goal of the image processing task. Image enhancement refers to any operation which improves the quality of an image to the human observer. Image restoration refers to operations which attempt to correct for distortions caused by an imaging system. These terms are used somewhat loosely, but the basic idea is that enhancement is judged by some human observer, whereas restoration is judged by comparison to a "true" image. Often a restored image will have improved quality, but at other times theses two goals produce different results.

Many image enhancement operations have to do with gray scale operations such as windowing. The only image enhancement operations which are described in this chapter are filtering operations. We shall find that sometimes these operations are most easily understood as filtering in the frequency domain; other times they are most easily understood as convolutions in the space domain.

Image restoration is a related operation, but restoration assumes that there is an initial image which has been corrupted by some imaging system. The goal of restoration is to return the image to its original form. The estimation methods described in the last two chapters are techniques which can be used for image restoration. Deconvolution, which is described in Chapter 29, can also be classified as an image restoration operation.

The terms image enhancement and image restoration have to do with the goals of the image processing. Generally in this book we have separated topics based on the techniques which are used rather than the goals. However, categorizing image processing operations in terms of goals is also a useful way of understanding the difference between methods.

II. EXAMPLES OF IMAGE ENHANCEMENT

A. SMOOTHING

One of the most common image processing technique is smoothing. In Chapter 22 we introduced the idea of low pass filtering as a smoothing operation. In that chapter it was shown that low pass filtering can be implemented in the space domain by averaging surrounding pixels. To reduce dose or imaging time or both, radiological imaging is often photon limited. If the noise in adjacent pixels is uncorrelated, smoothing decreases the noise in the image. Noise reduction is accomplished at the expense of resolution.

B. EDGE ENHANCEMENT

A very common image processing operation is edge enhancement. The goal of edge enhancement is to make the edges in an image more conspicuous. Edge enhancement makes the detail in the image stand out; the image appears sharper to the observer.

A good heuristic about images is that the edges are formed by the high frequencies, and that the regions of more constant intensity are formed by the low frequencies. Thus, the edges in an image can be enhanced by increasing the amplitude of the high frequency components in an image.

Figure 22.8 shows the k_x axis of a high pass filter. This filter increase the amplitudes of the high frequencies making edges in the image more apparent. Figure 22.7 shows two nuclear magnetic resonance images. The image on the right is an edge enhanced version of the image on the left. The image on the right appears sharper; the edges in the image stand out. However, notice that the noise is also amplified.

C. UNSHARP MASKING

A somewhat similar type of effect is produced by an operation used in photography which is called unsharp masking. However, unsharp masking also has the effect of compensating for variations in the average intensity in different parts of the image. An unsharp masking operation is performed by making two transparencies. One of the transparencies is a negative; the other transparency is an out-of-focus positive. The image is made by printing using both the negative and the out of focus positive.

In regions of constant intensity, the negative and the positive tend to cancel, producing a mid-level gray in the print. On the dark side of an edge, the negative is relatively opaque. If the positive were in focus, then it would be relatively transparent; however, since it is out of focus, the region around the edge is at a mid level. Therefore, the out of focus positive will not cancel the negative, and the print will be very dark. On the bright side of an edge, the opposite effect makes the print very bright. Thus, the edge becomes more apparent.

Figure 27.1 shows the effect of the unsharp masking process on a delta function in one dimension. If the imaging system were perfect, then the negative would be a delta function. Any real negative will have some blurring. The top panel of Figure 27.1 shows the negative for a delta function input. Although the negative is of opposite intensity to the object, printing reverses the intensity, so the effect of the negative on the final image will be of the same intensity. Thus, the negative is shown with positive values in this figure.

The middle panel of figure 27.1 shows the out of focus positive. It is wider and the polarity is reversed. Again due to the reversal during printing, the effect of the positive on the intensities in the print is negative. Roughly speaking, the effect of printing an image using both the negative and the positive is to multiply the negative and the positive. The third panel shows the product of the negative and the positive. The print is positive in the center and negative in a surrounding region.

The effect of the unsharp masking process is similar to the high pass filtering process in that they both tend to emphasized edges. However, the unsharp masking process in not linear. The production of both the negative and the positive can be modeled using linear systems. However, the multiplication of the negative and the positive during printing is not a linear process. Below we shall see how this multiplication can be modeled using homomorphic signal processing methods.

D. LOW-FREQUENCY ATTENUATION

In photography, unsharp masking is used not only for edge enhancement, but also for compression of the dynamic range in an image. The dynamic range refers to the ratio of the largest intensity in a signal to the smallest. The dynamic range compression is accomplished by attenuation of the amplitudes of the lowest spatial frequency components.

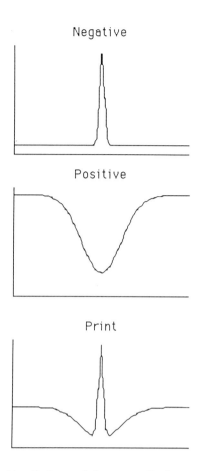

FIGURE 27.1.   Unsharp masking: the top panel shows a negative image of an object which is a delta function. Since the imaging system is not perfect, the negative has some width. The middle panel shows an out-of-focus positive of the same delta function. The positive has the opposite polarity. The bottom panel shows the product of the negative and the positive. It represents the unsharp masked print using both the negative and the positive.

In natural outdoor scenes, there can be a tremendous range in lighting conditions. The difference between bright sun light and a dark shadow can be a factor of ten thousand or more. However, the dynamic range which can be represented in a photographic print is often on the order of one hundred. Therefore, in order to represent an image which has both bright sun shine and dark shadows, the dynamic range of the image needs to be reduced.

The photographic solution is photograph the scene using a film with a very wide latitude, and then print the scene using unsharp masking. Wide latitude film has a large dynamic range and consequently low contrast. The unsharp masking process increases the contrast of the detail in the image. It enhances the edges. The unsharp masking process counteracts the effect of the low contrast film for the high spatial frequency data. However, the low spatial frequency data are further decreased in amplitude. The low spatial frequency data are very poorly represented in the output image.

Roughly speaking, we can identify the low spatial frequency data with the lighting conditions of different portions of the image. There are of course other contributions to the low spatial frequency components, but illumination is a major contributor. Even though the low spatial frequency data are very poorly represented in the image, unsharp masked images appear to the human to be very good representations of the natural scene. They can actually appear ''better'' to the human than the natural scene. In order to understand why images with such poor representation of the low spatial frequency components look so good, we must briefly describe some visual physiology.

III. SOME COMMENTS ABOUT VISUAL PHYSIOLOGY

The ganglion cells in the retina have a "center, surround" organization where the stimulation of a small central field is compared to the stimulation of a surrounding field. This early visual processing transforms the data from absolute intensities into the relative intensity of light in a small region compared to its surrounding. This processing is similar to unsharp masking. Information about detail is retained, and low frequency information is discarded.

Further, the visual system performs a considerable amount of higher level processing in order to compensate for the effects of variable lighting. One of the clearest examples of this processing is a feature known as color constancy. There is a strong tendency for colors to appear constant independent of the lighting conditions. Going from natural light, to incandescent light, to fluorescent light, there are only relatively minor fluctuations in the apparent color of objects to the human. By contrast there are marked changes in the colors recorded by film. Relatively strong filters need to be applied to correct photographs for these changes in lighting conditions. But the human visual system performs this task naturally.

Although the human is aware of the brightness of illumination of an object, there is a tendency to discount changes in the brightness. Generally speaking, the changes in illumination are of relatively low spatial frequency. Thus, attenuation of the effects of illumination has similarity to attenuation of the low spatial frequencies in an image. Teleologically, color constancy and the ability to discount brightness allows us to visualize the objects separate from the illumination. This ability greatly assists us in the important task of identifying objects.

In a certain sense our perception is very distorted. We do not see a natural scene as it is, rather we see it processed to eliminate the effects of the illumination. The processing which is performed by the unsharp masking operation is very similar to visual processing. This may explain why the images appear very natural to us, even though the low frequencies have been markedly altered.

IV. HOMOMORPHIC SIGNAL PROCESSING

The effects of variable illumination on a scene can be written mathematically as:

$$f'(x,y) = a(x,y) \cdot f(x,y) \qquad (27.1)$$

where $a(x,y)$ is the variations in illumination of the scene, $f(x,y)$ represents a uniformly illuminated scene, and $f'(x,y)$ represents the scene with variable illumination. In general, the illumination is a slowly varying function; it has predominately low spatial frequencies. The component of the image which is often of most interest is the detail, the high spatial frequencies.

Above, we have argued that by emphasizing the high spatial frequencies, we can emphasize the components of the image of most interest. However, we can look at this problem more analytically. In the frequency domain (Equation 16.9):

$$F'(k_x,k_y) = (1/2\pi) \cdot A(k_x,k_y) * F(k_x,k_y) \qquad (27.2)$$

In the spatial frequency domain, the scene, $F(k_x,k_y)$, is convolved with the illumination, $A(k_x,k_y)$. Thus, a simple filtering operation cannot completely remove the effects of the illumination.

The logarithm of Equation 27.1 is:

$$\log(f'(x,y)) = \log(a(x,y) \cdot f(x,y)) \tag{27.3}$$

The logarithm of the product can be written as the sum of the logarithms (Table 2.4):

$$\log(f'(x,y)) = \log(a(x,y)) + \log(f(x,y)) \tag{27.4}$$

The logarithms of the illumination and the scene are simply added; therefore, their Fourier transforms add. If the two signals have different spatial frequencies, then they can be exactly separated with a simple filtering operation.

The use of the logarithmic transformation is an example of homomorphic signal processing. When two signals are combined an operation of one type, then certain procedures may be viewed as transforming the operation to a new operation. For example, the logarithm of a product is equal to the sum of the respective logarithms. Thus there is a homology between the product of two signals and the sum of their logarithms. Conceptually, the product is transformed into a sum.

Nuclear magnetic resonance images at times show shading due to radio frequency inhomogeneities. This shading is a particular problem with surface coil images. This problem is analogous to the problem of variable illumination of a natural scene. The shading is generally of low spatial frequency while the data of most interest are high in spatial frequency. As with illumination of a natural scene, homomorphic signal processing using a logarithmic transformation can be used to separate the shading due to the radio frequency inhomogeneity from the tissue signal.

The unsharp masking process can also be simplified by homomorphic signal processing. The logarithm of the print is equal to the sum of the logarithms of the negative and the positive. If the original image contains mostly high spatial frequency, then the negative has high spatial frequencies. Because of the marked smoothing, the positive has predominantly low spatial frequency content. In a sense the positive is the reverse of the illumination. Under these conditions, unsharp masking can be used to compensate for the effects of the illumination in the image.

Figure 27.2 shows the effect of unsharp masking on a nuclear magnetic resonance image of a cervical spine obtained with a surface coil. Figure 27.2B has been processed with unsharp masking. The fall of in intensity is compensated by the unsharp masking. In addition, the edges in the image are sharpened.

V. IMAGE INFORMATION

The term image enhancement implies that the images are better after processing than they were before processing. However, it is important to understand in what way they are better. When the high frequencies are enhanced by a filter, the low frequencies are attenuated. In fact, except for an overall amplification, enhancement means increase in some frequencies relative to a decrease in some other frequencies. In other words, image enhancement is not adding anything new to the image, rather it is changing the ratio of components already in the image.

The information in an image can be defined mathematically. With the proper definition, all filtering operations can be shown to decrease the information in an image. From a common sense understanding of the information in an image, we can come to the same conclusion. Filtering is removing or decreasing some component of the image. Thus, the overall information in an image is decreased by all image processing operations. The unprocessed image has all of the information that the processed image has since the processed image can be

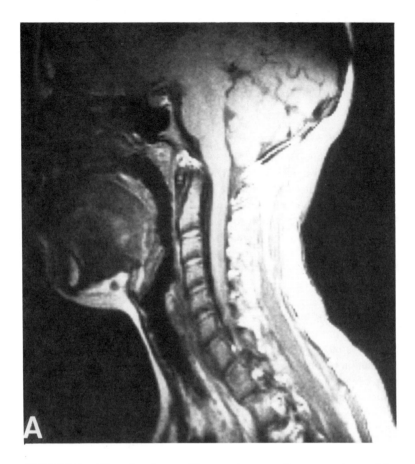

FIGURE 27.2.   Effect of unsharp masking: a nuclear magnetic resonance image of the cervical spine using a surface coil. There is marked fall-off in intensity in the anterior neck due to the inhomogeneity of the surface coil. Figure 27.2B was produced from (A) by unsharp masking. The effect of the coil inhomogeneity has been reduced. Also notice that there is some edge enhancement.

obtained from the unprocessed image. The reverse is not necessarily true; it may not be possible to retrieve the unprocessed image from the processed image.

If the processed image has less information, in what sense is it enhanced? It is enhanced to the extent that the uninteresting information, the "noise", is removed. The information of interest is made more conspicuous by removing the unwanted information. The image is enhanced in the sense that the information in the image is more conspicuous.

Whether a processed image is better than an unprocessed image has to do with what the processed image is used for. If the processed image is presented to a radiologist, then making the lesion more conspicuous may improve the accuracy of detection. In fact this is often the case. The goal of image enhancement in Radiology is to more accurately and efficiently present information to the radiologist.

Another example where processing is useful is when the image is being transferred to a medium with less information capacity than the original medium. Instead of discarding certain aspects of the image, they can be mapped to the range which is recorded on the output medium. In the case of photography, the negative has a much higher dynamic range than the final print. Unsharp masking transfers the information about the detail in the image to the dynamic range which can be accurately represented in the print. The final print produced by unsharp masking will retain more of the information about the detail at the expense of information about illumination. In most instances, this is a favorable trade off.

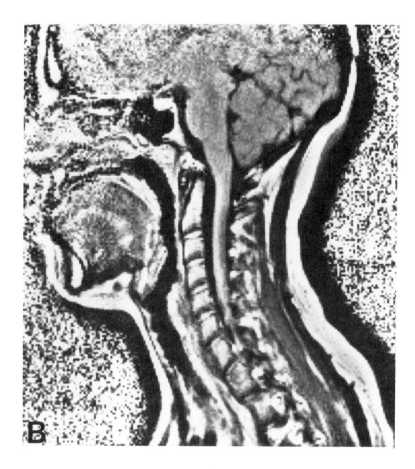

FIGURE 27.2B

VI. SUMMARY

Smoothing and edge enhancement are common examples of image enhancement operations. We have given a brief introduction to these operations. This chapter is not meant as a complete description of image enhancement or even of edge enhancement, but rather it shows how the filtering methods described in this part of the book can be put to use.

Image processing operations reduce the information in an image. If an image contains a great deal of irrelevant information, then the irrelevant detail may mask the observer's ability to identify the important information. Image enhancement is likely to improve the quality of the image in this case. When the original image contains little information, then image processing is unlikely to have an effect.

VII. FURTHER READING

Image enhancement is the topic of several books, for example see the books by Pratt,[1] Gonzalez and Wintz,[2] Andrews and Hunt,[3] Huang,[4] and Castleman.[5] Compilations of many good papers on signal processing methods[6] and image processing[7] are published by the Institute of Electrical and Electronics Engineers.

The goal of image enhancement is to make the images "better". What better means depends upon the use of the images. In radiology, better means that they transmit information more accurately and efficiently to the radiologist. Thus, in order to understand image enhancement in radiology, it is important to understand visual physiology. The reader is referred to the excellent books by Cornsweet[8] and Marr.[9]

Image enhancement has been used for many applications in radiology. For example, unsharp masking has been applied to chest radiographs.[10] Several methods have been applied to improved radionuclide imaging.[11,12] Image enhancement is often combined with image restoration. The image restoration takes into account the modulation transfer function of the imaging system.[13-16]

REFERENCES

1. **Pratt, W. K.**, *Digital Image Processing*, Johns Wiley & Sons, New York, 1978.
2. **Gonzalez, R. C. and Wintz, P.**, *Digital Image Processing*, Addison-Wesley, London, 1977.
3. **Andrews, H. C. and Hunt, B. R.**, *Digital Image Restoration*, Prentice-Hall, Englewood Cliffs, NJ, 1977.
4. **Huang, T. S., Ed.**, *Picture Processing and Digital Filtering*, Springer-Verlag, Berlin, 1979.
5. **Castleman, K. R.**, *Digital Image Processing*, Prentice-Hall, Englewood Cliffs, NJ, 1979.
6. Selected papers in digital signal processing, II. IEEE Press, New York, 1976.
7. **Chellappa, R. and Sawchuk, A. A.**, *Digital Image Processing and Analysis. Vol. 1. Digital Image Processing*, IEEE Computer Society Press, New York, 1985.
8. **Cornsweet, T. N.**, *Visual Perception*, Academic Press, New York, 1970.
9. **Marr, D.**, *Vision*, W. H. Freeman, San Francisco, 1982.
10. **Rogowska, J., Preston, K., and Sashin, D.**, Evaluation of digital unsharp masking and local contrast stretching as applied to chest radiographs, *IEEE Trans. Biomed. Eng. BME*, 35, 817, 1988.
11. **Miller, T. R. and Rollins, E. S.**, A practical method of image enhancement by interactive digital filtering, *J. Nucl. Med.*, 26, 1075, 1985.
12. **Ross, P. G. B., Sharp, P. F., and Undrill, P. E.**, A simple filtering routine for radionuclide bone images, *J. Nucl. Med.*, 26, 1081, 1985.
13. **Miller, T. R., Goldman, K. J., Epstein, D. M., Biellp, D. R., Sampathkumaran, K. S., Kumar, B., and Siegel, B. A.**, Improved interpretation of gated cardiac images by use of digital filters, *Radiology*, 152, 795, 1984.
14. **King, M. A., Doherty, P. W., Schwinger, R. B., Jacobs, D. A., Kidder, T. E., and Miller, T. R.**, Fast count-dependent digital filtering of nuclear medicine images, *J. Nucl. Med.*, 24, 1039, 1983.
15. **King, M. A., Schwinger, R. B., Doherty, P. W., and Penney, B. C.**, Two-dimensional filtering of SPECT images using the Metz and Wiener filters, *J. Nucl. Med.*, 25, 1234, 1984.
16. **King, M. A., Penney, B. C., and Glick, S. J.**, An image-dependent Metz filter for nuclear medicine images, *J. Nucl. Med.*, 29, 1980, 1988.

Chapter 28

SUMMARY OF FILTERING

One method of comparing the first three parts of the book is by their relation to the time (or space) and frequency (or spatial frequency) domains. Part I of this book describes several models of systems in terms of the time (or space) domain. Part II of the book presents methods of transforming back and forth between the time (or space) domain and the frequency or (spatial frequency) domain. Part III deals with a description of systems in terms of the frequency (or spatial frequency) domain.

This part of the book deals with two somewhat different issues. First, understanding filtering requires some familiarity with frequency domain operations, and the effects of these operations in the time domain. Chapters 22 and 27 deal with this issue. Second, filtering can be used as a method of including *a priori* statistical information into estimation of a signal. Chapters 24 to 26 deal with this issue. Chapter 23 (Sampling) conceptually belongs with the last part of the book, but filtering is needed to understand the inverse operation, interpolation.

A description of filtering is the goal of many image processing books. Various image modifications are useful for many image processing tasks. However, in this book, filtering is of most interest as a technique used during image reconstruction. Thus, the discussion of Wiener filtering in Chapter 26 is relatively detailed, and the discussion of image enhancement techniques in Chapter 27 is very superficial.

This part of the book has emphasized a few points. Filtering is the same operation as convolution, but it is viewed from the perspective of the frequency domain. Understanding aliasing is important for recognizing artifacts in under-sampled images. The normal equations of linear algebra combine the statistical model of signals with the linear algebra model of systems. The Wiener filter combine the statistical model of signals with the linear, time invariant model of systems using convolution. Use of both the time and frequency domain description of a problem often allows a better understanding of the overall problem.

I. FILTERING AND CONVOLUTION

Filtering is the modification of the amplitude of the frequency components of a signal. A filter can be written using Equation 22.1:

$$G(\omega) = H(\omega) \cdot F(\omega) \qquad (28.1)$$

where $F(\omega)$ is the original signal, $H(\omega)$ is the filter function, and $G(\omega)$ is the filtered signal. In the time domain this operation is equal to convolution, Equation 16.8:

$$g(t) = f(t) * h(t) \qquad (28.2)$$

Convolution and filtering are the same operation. Convolution is the time domain description and filtering is the frequency domain description. Any linear, time invariant system can be defined using convolution. Thus all linear, time invariant systems can be described as filters. However, it is typical to reserve the term filter for cases when it is most natural to conceptualize the operation as a modification of frequency domain components.

Filtering is not a new operation described in this part of the book. Rather it is a new perspective on an operation, convolution, which was presented in Chapter 3. It is the frequency domain description of a linear, time invariant system.

The dual operation is windowing. Windowing is defined by Equation 22.3:

$$g(t) = f(t) \cdot h(t) \qquad (28.3)$$

The frequency domain equivalent of this equation, given by Equation 16.9, is a convolution:

$$G(\omega) = (1/2\pi) \cdot F(\omega) * H(\omega) \qquad (28.4)$$

The windowing operation is very familiar, but its frequency domain consequences are not. The windowing operation can be used to help us understand the filtering operation, and the effects of filtering in the time domain can be used to help us understand the effects of windowing in the frequency domain.

II. SAMPLING

Sampling was described in Chapter 23. Sampling is very important in radiology since all of the computerized imaging modalities use sampling to transform continuous data to discrete signals. Sampling logically belongs with the discussion of the relation between the different types of transforms in Chapter 20; however, understanding sampling depends upon the ideas of filtering described in Chapter 22.

Although the purpose of sampling is to transform a continuous signal into a discrete signal, our description of sampling has been entirely in terms of continuous signals. We have represented discrete signals using a comb functions multiplied by the continuous signal. This approach provides a description of the effects of sampling in the frequency domain.

We have shown that the Fourier transform of a comb signal is also a comb signal, Equations 23.12 and 23.13:

$$\sum_{n=-\infty}^{\infty} \delta(t - n \cdot T) \leftrightarrow (2\pi/T) \cdot \sum_{k=-\infty}^{\infty} \delta(\omega - k \cdot 2\pi/T) \qquad (28.5)$$

The comb signal, Fourier transform pair has the familiar relationship between the time and frequency domain — as the delta functions in the time domain become more closely spaced, the delta functions in the frequency domain become more spread apart. This behavior is similar to the scaling property in Chapter 16 and especially similar to the properties of the transforms in Chapter 20.

Sampling is modeled in the time domain as a multiplication of the comb signal with the original signal. In the frequency domain, this is equivalent to a convolution of the signal with the frequency domain comb signal. Convolution with a comb signal results in replicates of the original frequency domain signal at the interval, $2\pi/T$ radians. Sampling in one domain replicates the signal in the other domain. These relations are analogous to the relations between the continuous Fourier transform, and the dual of the Fourier series.

A continuous signal can be though of as multiplication by a comb function where the interval between samples, T, is equal to zero. In that case the interval between the replicates in the frequency domain, $2\pi/T$, is infinity. A continuous signal has a transform which repeats at an interval of infinity, i.e., it is aperiodic. Similarly, in Chapter 20, it was noted that if a signal is continuous in one domain, its transform is aperiodic.

The Fourier transform of the original signal cannot be recovered from the transformed signal if the replicates overlap. The condition where the samples do not overlap is given by the sampling theorem. The sampling rate must be greater than twice the highest frequency in the original signal. This sampling rate is called the Nyquist rate. If the replicates do not overlap, then the original signal can be recovered from the sampled signal by ideal low pass filtering. In this case the ideal low pass filter is the inverse operation of sampling.

III. POWER SPECTRAL DENSITY FUNCTION

Chapter 24 introduced the power spectral density function, $S_f(\omega)$. The power spectral density function is defined for wide sense stationary stochastic processes. The power spectral density function is the Fourier transform of the autocorrelation function, $R_f(\tau)$. The Fourier transform is with respect to the variable, τ, the offset between two copies of the signal which is correlated with itself. It was shown in Chapter 24 that the power spectral density function gives the power in the stochastic process, $f(t)$, as a function of frequency.

The autocorrelation function, $R_f(\tau)$, is a second-order statistic of the stochastic process, $f(t)$, in the time domain. The power spectral density function is a second-order statistic of the stochastic process, $f(t)$, in the frequency domain. The major reason for introducing the frequency domain representation of signals in this book is that it greatly simplifies the understanding of linear, time invariant systems. Likewise, the effect of a linear, time invariant system on the statistics of a stochastic process is similarly simplified. In the time domain, the effect of a linear, time invariant system on the autocorrelation function is a double convolution (Equation 24.26). In the frequency domain, the effect of a linear, time invariant system on the power spectral density function is a simple multiplication (Equation 24.28):

$$S_g(\omega) = |H(\omega)|^2 \cdot S_f(\omega) \qquad (28.6)$$

Equation 28.6 is very important. If a system is modeled with stationary stochastic processes and linear, time invariant systems, then the second-order statistics are particularly simple in the frequency domain. The effect of a system is just a multiplicative factor. The values at one value of ω do not affect the values at any other ω. The similarity between the Wiener filter estimation of a signal, and the estimation of a single unknown in Chapter 12 is due to the simplicity of the model in the frequency domain.

IV. ESTIMATION OF A SIGNAL

Chapter 25 and 26 deal with similar models of data collection and estimation. The unknown, f or $f(t)$, passes through a data collection process, A or a(t), and then detector noise, n or $n(t)$, is added to produce the data, p or p(t). The estimate is produced by passing the data through the system, H or h(t). These models are shown in Figures 25.7 and 26.2.

Chapter 25 describes linear, least mean square estimation of the data, p, using the normal equation of linear algebra while Chapter 26 describes linear, time invariant, least mean square estimation of the unknown, $f(t)$ using the Wiener deconvolution filter. There are two major differences between these estimates. The normal equations are a linear estimation method whereas Wiener deconvolution filter is a linear and time-invariant estimation method. The normal equations estimate the data, whereas the Wiener deconvolution filter estimates the unknown.

A. ORTHOGONALITY PRINCIPLE

The estimation criteria used throughout this book is least mean square error. In both Chapter 12 and in this part of the book, the orthogonality principle has been emphasized. Least mean square estimation results in the orthogonality principle — the error is orthogonal to the estimation space.

In the case of estimation of the data, the orthogonality principle means that the estimate is the projection of the data on the estimation space defined by the model of the data collection process. The *a priori* information provided by the model is that data must lie in the estimation space. The orthogonality principle states that the estimate is a value in the estimation space which is closest to the data.

In the case of estimation of the unknown, the orthogonality principle means that the error is orthogonal to the data in a statistical sense. The estimation process removes all of the information about unknown from the data. The *a priori* information provided by the model is the relative power of the signal and the noise. These powers determine the statistical orthogonality.

B. NORMAL EQUATIONS OF LINEAR ALGEBRA

The normal equations of linear algebra provide a linear, least mean square estimation of the data. The normal equations bring together the random vector model of signals with the matrix model of systems. The normal equations are defined in the time domain; they are not a filtering operation. However, the normal equations are included in this part of the book in order to emphasize the analogies between the normal equations and the Wiener filter.

The error is defined as the difference between the data p and the estimate of the data $\hat{p}$, Equation 25.25:

$$e = p - \hat{p} \tag{28.7}$$

Definition of the error in terms of the data is very important. The error which is being minimized is the error between the data and the estimate of the data. Thus, we have referred to this problem as estimation of the data. The error for a single datum is defined analogously in Equation 12.47.

The normal equations of linear algebra are given by Equation 25.31:

$$A^T \cdot A \cdot \hat{f} = A^T \cdot p \tag{28.8}$$

The vector spaces associated with this solution are shown in Figure 25.12. $A \cdot \hat{f}$ is the estimate, $\hat{p}$, of the data from the unknown. The effect of this multiplication is that the portion of $\hat{f}$ which is in the null space of A does not affect the estimate of the data. Thus, the solution family includes contributions from any vector in the null space of A. $\hat{p}$ is compared to p after multiplication by A^T. The portion of the data in the null space of A^T is inconsistent with the model. Multiplication by A^T means that this portion of the data does not affect the result.

When $A^T \cdot A$ has an inverse, the solution to the normal equation is given by Equation 25.42:

$$H = (A^T \cdot A)^{-1} \cdot A \tag{28.9}$$

Notice the similarity of this result to the Equation 12.49. Equation 28.9 is the matrix analog of Equation 12.49.

Equation 28.9 is not useful for the image reconstruction problems in Part IV. The matrix sizes are immense, so that matrix inversion is not tractable. Furthermore, the solutions may be ill conditioned; a small amount of noise may result in a large error. The interative solution methods described at the end of Chapter 25 provide a solution to both of these problems. Iterative solution methods can be made almost as fast as linear, shift invariant solution methods. And, methods exist for avoiding ill conditioned solutions. Although the normal equations are not useful for imaging applications, they provide a good conceptual framework for understanding how the *a priori* information from the model of the data collection process can be used in the image reconstruction process.

C. WIENER FILTER

The Wiener filter provides a linear, time invariant, least mean square estimation of an unknown, stationary, stochastic process, $f(t)$, from data, $p(t)$. The data, $p(t)$, are the sum of the unknown and noise, $n(t)$. The solution of this problem is greatly simplified by the time invariance. In the frequency domain, the problem is exactly analogous to the solution given in Chapter 12. Notice the similarity of the models as shown in Figure 26.3 and 12.3.

The error is defined as the difference between the unknown, $f(t)$, and the estimate of the unknown, $\hat{f}(t)$, Equation 26.7:

$$e(t) = f(t) - \hat{f}(t) \qquad (28.10)$$

Since the error is defined in terms of the unknown, we have referred to this problem as an estimation of the unknown. Notice the similarity between this definition and the definition of the error in Equation 12.86.

The solution to the Wiener filter problem is given by Equation 26.37:

$$H(\omega) = S_{fp}(\omega)/S_p(\omega) \qquad (28.11)$$

In the frequency domain, the filter is the ratio of the mutual power in the signal and the data normalized by the power in the data. In the case where the signal and the noise are uncorrelated, this simplified result is given by Equation 26.38:

$$H(\omega) = S_f(\omega)/(S_f(\omega) + S_n(\omega)) \qquad (28.12)$$

The filter is the ratio of the power in the signal to the powers in the signal plus the noise. This is the same result that was obtained in Equation 12.89.

D. WIENER DECONVOLUTION

Wiener deconvolution is linear, time invariant, mean square estimation of the unknown, $f(t)$, from data, $p(t)$, which is the sum the unknown passed through a system, $a(t)$, and noise, $n(t)$. Except for time invariance, this model is analogous to the normal equation model.

For the case where the signal and the noise are uncorrelated, the solution to this problem is given by Equation 28.60:

$$H(\omega) = (1/A(\omega)) \cdot S_f(\omega)/[S_f(\omega) + S_n(\omega)/|A(\omega)|^2] \qquad (28.13)$$

The filter consists of two parts, deconvolution by $A(\omega)$ followed by a Wiener filter with the noise modified as if it were combined directly with the unknown.

Equation 28.13 provides a practical method for image reconstruction in radiology. We often have a good model of the data collection process as well as some *a priori* information about the power spectra of the signal and the noise. This equation will be used in Chapter 32 (Reconstruction from Noisy Projections: Computed Tomography).

V. IMAGE ENHANCEMENT

Chapter 27 is a brief introduction to image enhancement. Image enhancement is a major application of digital signal processing methods. However, it is not the focus of this book. Therefore, the chapter on image enhancement is very brief.

Many image enhancement methods fall into two categories, smoothing and edge enhancement. The former emphasizes the low frequencies while the later emphasizes the higher frequencies. Images with noisy, uncorrelated pixel values are often improved by smoothing.

High statistical quality images which have been smoothed during data collection often are improved with edge enhancement.

VI. SUMMARY

This section of the book has finished the development of basic mathematical techniques. It should provide the reader with some familiarity with the frequency domain and with operations in the frequency domain. Many of the filtering operations which are used in radiology can be understood as either smoothing or edge enhancement operations. More sophisticated image enhancement operations can also be useful, but they are not the focus of this book.

Chapter 23 (Sampling) is logically related to Chapter 20, which describes the relation between the various transform operations. However, filtering is important for understanding the inverse operation, interpolation. Understanding aliasing is important in recognizing the artifacts which can be produced from sampling below the Nyquist rate.

From Table 1.1, it can be seen that the various models remain largely separate until this part of the book. The linear systems and linear algebra models of systems are brought together with the statistical description of signals in this part of the book. The normal equations of linear algebra allow *a priori* information about the model of the data collection process to be used in estimation. The Wiener filter allows *a priori* statistical information about the power spectra of the signal and the noise to be used in estimation.

This section provides the tools which will be needed in understanding the reconstruction methods which are described in Part IV. Filtering will be important in noiseless reconstruction in computed tomography in Chapter 31. Statistical filtering will be important in understanding reconstruction from noisy data in Chapter 32. The normal equations of linear algebra will be important in understanding iterative reconstruction in Chapter 33.

IV. Reconstruction

Chapter 29

DECONVOLUTION: FIRST PASS RADIONUCLIDE ANGIOCARDIOGRAPHY

This part of the book describes several image reconstruction methods. Understanding image reconstruction is the major goal of the book. The first three parts have provided the mathematical tools and conceptual framework which will allow us to understand the image reconstruction described in this part.

This chapter describes the use of deconvolution in radionuclide angiocardiography. Although this application is not image reconstruction, the methods used are the same as those used for image reconstruction.

Chapter 30 shows that the data collected in nuclear magnetic resonance imaging are the spatial frequencies. Thus, image reconstruction is performed with the inverse Fourier transform. Chapter 31 and 32 describe the slightly more complicated reconstruction process in computed tomography. Chapter 33 describes nonshift invariant reconstruction which can be used for single photon emission computed tomography. Chapter 34 describes the combination of several different samples of a single cross-section obtained from a multi-detector scanner. Each of these application brings out different aspect of the reconstruction process.

We shall use both linear systems and linear algebra methods. Chapters 29 through 32 will emphasize linear system methods; linear algebra methods will be more important in Chapters 33 and 34. However, both methods provide insights about different aspects of the reconstruction problem. Statistical considerations will be the focus of Chapters 32 and 34, but the conclusions from these chapters are applicable to the topics discussed in the other chapters.

I. FIRST PASS RADIONUCLIDE ANGIOCARDIOGRAPHY

This chapter deals with the use of deconvolution to improve the calculation of shunts from first pass radionuclide angiocardiography. Deconvolution was briefly introduced in Chapter 16, and was considered more fully in Chapter 26 (Wiener Filtering). The Wiener deconvolution filter uses *a priori* statistical information about the signal and the noise to improve the deconvolution. In addition to the Wiener filter, this chapter will briefly describe other methods of including *a priori* information into the deconvolution process. These methods can greatly improve the accuracy of the deconvolution; however, a full discussion of these methods is beyond the scope of this book.

The first use of radionuclides in medicine was for radionuclide angiocardiography. Blumgart and Yens,[1] and Blumgart and Weiss[2] used Radium-C to measure the transit time from the antecubital fossa to the heart in 1927. The next use of radionuclides was by Prinzmetal[3] in 1949. He described the radiocardiogram — the time activity curve measured from the region of the heart. The first peak, the R wave, is due to the passage of activity through the right side of the heart. The second peak, the L wave, is due to the passage of activity through the left side of the heart.

If there is a left to right shunt, then the radiocardiogram will have a third peak due to the activity which is recirculated through the lung. However, this third peak may be difficult to identify on the radiocardiogram, and the magnitude of shunting cannot be easily calculated. Folse and Braunwald[4] simplified the first pass curve by moving the probe to a position over the lung. The curve over the lung in a patient with a left to right shunt shows a normal first peak and then an early recirculation peak due to the shunting.

The relative sizes of the first pass and early recirculation peaks can be used to quantify the size of the shunt. However, the two peaks have a considerable amount of overlap. Maltz and Treves[5] found that the curves could be successfully separated by fitting with a gamma variate function, $k \cdot (t - t_0)^\alpha \cdot e^{-\beta(t - t_0)}$. t_0 determines the position of the curve; k determines the overall amplitude of the curve. The more interesting parameters are α and β. α is largely responsible for fitting the up slope of the curve; and β is largely responsible for fitting the down slope of the curve. The shape of the top of the curve is related to both α and β.

With the advent of gamma cameras and computers, rapid sequence images of the first transit of activity through the central circulation can be collected and analyzed. Time activity curves are obtained from regions of interest drawn over the superior vena cava and the lung. The region from the lung is used to calculate the left to right shunting with the gamma variate technique. The region over the superior vena cava is used to evaluate the bolus.

Calculation of the left to right shunt ratio from a radionuclide angiocardiogram depends upon a good bolus injection. The top panel of Figure 29.1 shows the curve obtained in a patient with a moderate shunt after a poor bolus. The bolus was fragmented on its transit to the central circulation. The two portions of the bolus produced a curve which appears to have a large early recirculation peak. The bottom panel of Figure 29.1 show curves from the same patient on a repeat study with a good injection. On this study there is a much smaller early recirculation peak.

With careful attention to technique, a good bolus can be obtained in 90 to 95% of patients. However, there are still some occasions when a poor bolus is obtained. This chapter will present a method, deconvolution, which can be used to ameliorate the effects of a bad bolus. This method can reduce the number of repeat examinations. However, we shall see that when the bolus is too fragmented, the curves cannot be recovered.

II. MODEL

Left to right intracardiac shunts can be measured using the time activity curve over the lungs after injection of a bolus of activity into the superior vena cava.[6] A problem arises when the activity is injected into the antecubital fossa. By the time the activity reaches the superior vena cava, it may no longer represent a bolus of activity. In this case the lung time activity curve can be modeled using convolution. This model was described in Chapter 3. A system is used to model the transit of activity from the superior vena cava to the lungs. Time activity curves are obtained from both the superior vena cava and the lung. Deconvolution is used to determine the system function from these two curves.

The time activity curve at the level of the superior vena cava can be represented by a signal, f(t). The time activity curve from the lung can be represented by a second signal, p(t). The system representing the transit of activity to the lung can be represented by a signal, a(t). The output curve from the lung region will include some detector noise, n(t). These relations can be summarized with the equation:

$$p(t) = a(t) * f(t) + n(t) \qquad (29.1)$$

The noise is modeled as an additive term. In nuclear medicine the noise is best modeled as a Poisson process, but the additive noise model performs reasonably well.

All linear, time invariant deconvolution procedures can be modeled by convolution by a system, h(t). The estimate of the system, â(t), is given by:

$$\hat{a}(t) = h(t) * p(t) \qquad (29.2)$$

Deconvolution requires determination of the signal, h(t). In this problem, the system, a(t), is being estimated. In the subsequent chapters in this part, the input signal will be measured. However, it was shown in Chapter 3 that for systems modeled by convolution, the input

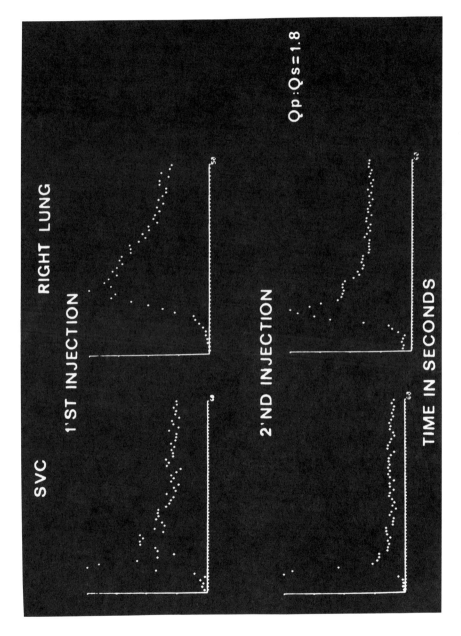

FIGURE 29.1. Effect of fragmented bolus: the top left graph shows the input signal from a region of interest over the superior vena cava. The input is fragmented due to poor injection technique. The output signal shown on the top right is compatible with a very large shunt. The bottom left graph shows a repeat study with a better bolus input. The bottom right shows the output signal obtained from this bolus. This output is a better representation of the system function. A moderate sized shunt, with $Q_p:Q_s$ equal to 1.8, was calculated using the gamma variate technique. (From Parker, J. A. and Treves, S., *Prog. Cardiovasc. Dis.*, 20, 121, 1977. With permission of W. B. Saunders Company.)

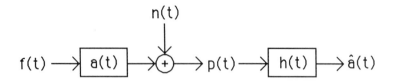

FIGURE 29.2.   Model: the input, f(t), is equal to the time activity curve over the superior vena cava. The transit of activity from the superior vena cava to the lungs is represented by the system, a(t). The time activity curve from the region of interest over the lungs, p(t), is the sum of the f(t)*a(t) and the detector noise, n(t). The estimate of the system, â(t), is obtained from the lung time activity curve with the estimation parameters given by the system, h(t).

and the system are equivalent (see Equations 3.4 to 3.10). Thus, these two problems are equivalent.

The data collection, system-estimation process is shown diagrammatically in Figure 29.2. Notice that the noise enters the process after the convolution. This figure is analogous to Figure 26.2, which describes the model for Wiener deconvolution, except that the roles of the input and the system are reversed.

In the frequency domain Equation 29.1 can be written:

$$P(\omega) = A(\omega) \cdot F(\omega) + N(\omega) \tag{29.3}$$

where the capital letter signals are the Fourier transforms of the signals written with small letters. Similarly, Equation 29.2 can be written in the transform domain as:

$$\hat{A}(\omega) = H(\omega) \cdot P(\omega) \tag{29.4}$$

III. NOISELESS DECONVOLUTION

Equation 29.3 can be substituted into Equation 29.4:

$$\hat{A}(\omega) = H(\omega) \cdot F(\omega) \cdot A(\omega) + H(\omega) \cdot N(\omega) \tag{29.5}$$

An obvious solution to this equation is given by:

$$H(\omega) = 1/F(\omega) \tag{29.6}$$

For $F(\omega)$ not equal to zero:

$$\hat{A}(\omega) = A(\omega) + N(\omega)/F(\omega) \tag{29.7}$$

In the absence of noise, the estimate $\hat{A}(\omega)$ is exactly equal to $A(\omega)$ when $F(\omega)$ is not equal to zero.

There is a problem when $F(\omega)$ is equal to zero — $H(\omega)$ is equal to infinity, and $\hat{A}(\omega)$ is not defined. When $F(\omega)$ is equal to zero, $P(\omega)$ contains no information about $A(\omega)$. Therefore, it makes sense that the estimate is not defined.

Because of the equivalence of the input and the system, we can conceptually reverse their roles. The system, a(t), can be considered to be filtered by the input, f(t). The input, f(t), does not pass any information about the system, a(t), to the output, p(t), for those frequencies for which $F(\omega)$ is zero. In the extreme case where the input is a constant, then the only nonzero $F(\omega)$ is at ω equal to zero. The shape of the bolus will determine what information can be obtained about the system from $p(t)$.

Since there is no information when $F(\omega)$ is equal to zero, some other rule must be used to establish these values. In the absence of some *a priori* information about the input, it is reasonable to set these frequencies to zero:

$$H(\omega) = \begin{cases} 1/F(\omega), & F(\omega) \neq 0 \\ \\ 0, & F(\omega) = 0 \end{cases} \tag{29.8}$$

In the absence of noise this filter will produce a good estimate of $a(t)$ so long as $F(\omega)$ is nonzero for the frequencies of interest.

IV. DECONVOLUTION WITH HIGH PASS FILTERING

In the presence of noise, deconvolution with Equation 29.8 results in a considerable amount of noise amplification. The problem with the deconvolution defined by Equation 29.8 comes from the second term in Equation 29.7. When $F(\omega)$ is small, $1/F(\omega)$ is large, and the noise term $N(\omega)/F(\omega)$ will dominate. When $F(\omega)$ is very small, this noise amplification can be very severe.

We have some *a priori* medical knowledge about the usual shapes of the system funciton and the input function. The system function, $a(t)$, is generally a relatively slowly varying function of time. Since $a(t)$ is slowly varying, the most important components of $A(\omega)$ are the low frequencies. We are interested in retaining the low frequency components of $A(\omega)$, but the higher frequencies are less important.

The shape of the input, $f(t)$, will determine the frequency components in $F(\omega)$. If $f(t)$ is a delta function, then $F(\omega)$ will have equal contributions from all frequencies. When $f(t)$ has the shape of a narrow bolus, $F(\omega)$ will be large for low frequencies and small for high frequencies. As $f(t)$ becomes wider, $F(\omega)$ will become narrower. For a reasonably narrow bolus, $F(\omega)$ will include the low frequency components contained in the system function.

Thus, an improved deconvolution could be obtained by using:

$$H(\omega) = \begin{cases} H_1(\omega)/F(\omega), & F(\omega) \neq 0 \\ \\ 0, & F(\omega) = 0 \end{cases} \tag{29.9}$$

where $H_1(\omega)$ is a low pass filter. An ideal low pass filter has been used,[7] but the sharp cut-off of an ideal low pass filter in the frequency domain will result in ringing in the time domain (see Chapter 16). An ideal low pass filter with a more gentle transition between the pass and stop zone has better results. Deconvolution with $H_1(\omega)$ defined in Equation 29.9 overcomes many of the problems with noise amplification.

V. WIENER FILTERING

The deconvolution problem was solved in Chapter 26 using the Wiener filter. The only difference between the models shown in Figure 29.2 and the model shown in Figure 26.2 is that the roles of the input and the system have been reversed. But, as we have already noted several times, the system and the input are equivalent for linear, time invariant systems.

Therefore, radionuclide angiocardiographic deconvolution could be performed with Wiener deconvolution.

In order to use the Wiener filter, the system and the noise must be modeled as stochastic processes, $a(t)$ and $n(t)$:

$$p(t) = a(t) \cdot f(t) + n(t) \tag{29.10}$$

Wiener deconvolution requires knowledge about the power spectral densities of the system, $S_a(\omega)$, and the noise, $S_n(\omega)$. (Recall that the power spectral density functions give the average power of the stochastic process as a function of frequency.)

The Wiener filter model is not a completely accurate representation of radionuclide angiocardiography. In Equation 29.10, the signal, $f(t)$, is deterministic. In first pass radionuclide angiocardiography, $f(t)$ represents the time activity curve from the region of the superior vena cava. Since it is measured, it will have some measurement noise. This model does not include this measurement noise. Since the activity comes through the superior vena cava as a compact bolus, $f(t)$, will be measured more accurately than $p(t)$. Thus, ignoring the statistical properties of $f(t)$, it may not be too severe a defect in this model.

If the system and the noise are uncorrelated, the Wiener deconvolution filter is given by Equation 26.60:

$$H(\omega) = [1/F(\omega)] \cdot S_a(\omega)/[S_a(\omega) + S_n(\omega)/|F(\omega)|^2] \tag{29.11}$$

The first factor $1/F(\omega)$ deconvolves the output for the effects of the bolus, $F(\omega)$. The second term filters the estimate statistically. For a very high signal to noise ratio, the second term is one; it has no effect. For a very low signal to noise ratio, the second term is zero. At intermediate signal to noise ratios, the second term depends upon how much information about the system is passed by the input, $F(\omega)$.

The number of counts in the study provide information about the overall signal to noise ratio. However, the signal to noise ratio is generally not precisely known as a function of frequency. It is usually assumed that the noise is uniform in frequency, and that $A(\omega)$ decreases at high frequency. Therefore, $S_a(\omega)/S_n(\omega)$ is flat at low frequency then falls off at higher frequencies.

VI. *A PRIORI* INFORMATION

There are two sources of information which we have about a radionuclide angiocardiography. One source is the information which is provided by the measured curves, $f(t)$ and $p(t)$. The other source of information is our medical knowledge about the cardiovascular system. This second type of information is independent of the results of a particular study. It is referred to as *a priori* information.

In Chapter 12, we emphasized that the purpose of the statistical model was to combine *a priori* information about the statistics of a signal with an outcome to produce a better estimate of the process. Above it was noted that we do not have particularly good information about the signal to noise ratio as a function of frequency. The major piece of medical information we have is about the shape of $a(t)$. This *a priori* information is not well captured by the statistics of $a(t)$.

The shape of the first pass radionuclide angiocardiogram is the sum of a small number of well-defined curves. The first transit of activity through the lungs and the early recirculation peaks are well modeled as gamma variate functions. Subsequent recirculation peaks are lower amplitude and wider gamma variate functions. The later recirculation peaks and systemic recirculation will merge to give a constant activity later in the study.

Thus, the first pass radionuclide angiocardiogram could be modeled as the sum of a small number of curves. Such a **low parameter model**, heavily constrains the solution. This type of model provides a great deal of *a priori* information about the problem. A much better deconvolution can be obtained by constraining the solution to be in the form of a low parameter model. There are good mathematical methods which determine a low parameter model using the least mean square error criterion. For example, modeling a(t) as a small number of lagged normal curves has been successfully applied to the first pass radionuclide angiocardiography.[8]

Although, low parameter models are useful in some image processing applications, the *a priori* information about images is usually not well captured by low parameter models. Therefore, we shall not cover this topic. The idea of using different models to capture different types of *a priori* information is, however, important. Many of the more advanced methods of reconstruction use image models which incorporate different varieties of *a priori* information. The key to understanding these methods is to understand how well the model matches the problem.

VII. LINEAR ALGEBRA MODEL

The cardiovascular system is pulsitile. Therefore, it is not time invariant. However, at the time scale used for left to right shunt calculation, it is well modeled as a linear, time invariant system. Thus, the convolution model provides a good description of the system. However, in order to discuss the constraints provided by *a priori* information, it is useful to use the terminology from linear algebra. Therefore, we shall describe a linear, nontime-invariant model for first pass radionuclide angiocardiography.

Although the model will be nontime invariant, it will take advantage of a time invariant feature — the equivalence of the input and the system. We shall model the system with a vector, a, and the input with a matrix, F. The roles of the system and the matrix have been interchanged. The model is given by:

$$p = F \cdot a + n \tag{29.12}$$

where p is the time activity curve over the lungs, and n is the measurement noise. The system, represented by the vector, a, goes through the input, represented by the matrix, F, to produce an output vector, p. The data, p, is transformed by the matrix, H, into a linear estimate, $\hat{a}$, of a:

$$\hat{a} = H \cdot p \tag{29.13}$$

The matrix equation 29.12 represents a series of simultaneous linear equations (see Chapter 8). The unknowns are represented by the vector, a, and the equations are represented by the matrix, F. If the number of independent equations is less than the number of unknowns, a, then the problem is said to be under determined. The problem is also under determined if the number of equations equals the number of unknowns, but the equations are not all independent. If Equation 29.12 is under determined, there is a family of solutions. A subspace of the unknown space satisfies Equation 29.12.

In the linear systems model, an under determined system is represented by cases where F(ω) is equal to zero. Any A(ω) is a valid solution when F(ω) is equal to zero. Thus, there is a family of valid solutions. In Equation 29.8, we have arbitrarily chosen the solution A(ω) equal to zero for the under determined case. Setting A(ω) equal to zero when F(ω) is equal to zero, introduces an additional constraint into the problem. The *a priori* information is that when there is no data, the best guess is that the value is zero.

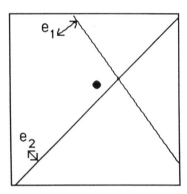

FIGURE 29.3.   Well-conditioned problem: a plane in the solution space is shown in this diagram. The two lines represent the intersection of two hyperplanes with the plane of solutions. The true solution is shown as a dot. Because of measurement errors, the intersection of the hyperplanes is not at the true solution. Because the hyperplanes are nearly orthogonal, the intersection is near to the true solution.

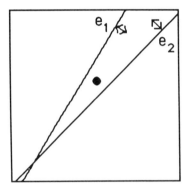

FIGURE 29.4.   Ill-conditioned problem: a plane in the solution space is shown in this diagram. The two lines represent the intersection of two hyperplanes with the plane of solutions. Since the hyperplanes are nearly parallel, the intersection point is far from the true solution.

Another problem which can occur is that the solution may be ill conditioned. Recall that each of the equations represented by the matrix equation given by Equation 29.12 can be viewed as defining a hyperplane of solutions. Any point in the hyperplane will satisfy the equation. The solution of the system of equations is the intersection of the hyperplanes.

Figure 29.3 shows a plane of possible solutions. The intersection of two hyperplanes with this plane of solutions are represented as lines. The intersection of the lines represents the solution of the equations in this plane. The true solution is shown as a point. Each of the hyperplanes is associated with some noise so that the planes do not intersect at the true solution. However, since the planes are approximately orthogonal, the intersection of the planes is near the true solution.

Figure 29.4 shows an ill-conditioned problem. Again, the two lines represent the two hyperplanes in a plane of solutions. The intersection of the lines represents the solution. The true solution is again indicated by a point. Since the lines are nearly parallel, the intersection of the lines is far from the true solution. Small errors in the data lead to very large errors in the solution. The ill-conditioned problem corresponds to the case where $F(\omega)$ is small.

As with the under-determined problem, additional constraints from *a priori* information need to be added to the problem. The Wiener filter makes the portions of the solution which are dominated by noise more ''zero like''. It would have the effect of moving the ill-

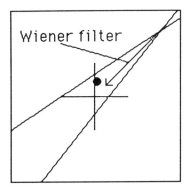

FIGURE 29.5.   Effect of a Wiener filter: the effect of the Wiener filter is to move the estimate from the intersection of the hyperplanes toward the origin. In this case, the estimate obtained with the Wiener filter is much closer to the true solution than the point of intersection of the hyperplanes.

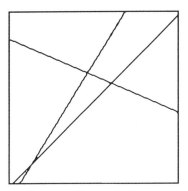

FIGURE 29.6.   Over-determined solution: this diagram shows a two-dimensional solution space. The three lines represent the solution of three independent equations. The three lines do not cross at a single point. The set of three equations represented by the three lines has no solution.

conditioned portions of the results toward the origin. In the case shown in Figure 29.5, this would improve the accuracy of the solution.

The way that additional constraints are added to the linear algebra model is that additional equations are added to Equation 29.12. The matrix, F, has additional rows. The additional constraints mean that there are more equations than unknowns. If the equations are independent, then the set of equations is inconsistent. Figure 29.6 show three solution hyperplanes. With the additional constraint, there is no longer a single point where all of the hyperplanes intersect.

For inconsistent equations, a rule is needed to determine the solution. The rule emphasized in this book is least mean square error. The least mean square error solution is provided by the normal equations of linear algebra. The normal equations find the position where the sum of the square of the distances to each of the hyperplanes is the least.

Inclusion of additional equations to the set of equations represented by Equation 29.12 is only one of many possible methods of including *a priori* information into the model. There are a number other methods, but a detailed discussion of these other models is beyond the scope of this book.

A. ITERATIVE SOLUTION

In Chapter 25, the iterative solution of equation 29.12 was described in general terms. The method by which the iterative steps are performed is very important, but beyond the

Well Conditioned

Ill Conditioned

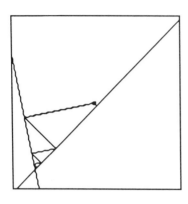 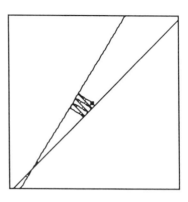

FIGURE 29.7. Limited number of iteration steps: this figure shows a diagrammatic representation of one iterative solution method. The starting point is represented by a small dot. From the starting point the solution moves orthogonally to one of the solution hyperplanes. From the point, the solution then moves orthogonally to the other hyperplane. And so on for a limited number of iteration steps. In the well-conditioned case, the solution moves rapidly toward the intersection point. In the ill conditioned case, the solution moves slowly toward the intersection point. After a small number of iterations, the solution will be strongly affected by the data for the well-conditioned case, and it will be strongly affected by the starting point for the ill-conditioned case.

scope of this book. One method of iteration is to successively determine the point in each of the hyperplanes which is the closest to the previous solution.

Figure 29.7 shows a well-conditioned and an ill-conditioned portion of a problem. Starting at zero, the constraints from each of the hyperplanes is successively applied four times. In the well-conditioned case, the solution rapidly approaches the intersection. In the ill-conditioned case, the solution approaches the intersection slowly. If a small number of iterations is performed, the well-conditioned case will be very close to the exact solution, while the ill-conditioned case will be close to the starting point.

If the initial position is determined by the *a priori* information about the solution, then the effect of using a small number of iterations is that the solution will reflect the *a priori* information in regions where there is little information provided by the data, and will reflect the data where there is a lot of information provided by the data.

Although this has not been a very mathematically rigorous description of iterative solutions, it may provide some understanding of why the initial guess at the solution is important, and why it is sometimes useful to stop the solution process after only a few iterations. Special iterative techniques can often be developed to provide efficient and accurate solutions to specific problems. A more complete discussion of these methods is beyond the scope of this book.

VIII. SUMMARY

Gamma variate analysis of first pass radionuclide angiography is probably the most accurate method of calculating the $Q_p:Q_s$ ratio in patients with left to right shunts. A poor bolus injection can make it impossible to analyze first pass radionuclide angiocardiography. If the distortion of the bolus is not too great, deconvolution will allow these curves to be analyzed.

Radionuclide angiocardiography is very different from the other applications in this part of the book; however, it is included in this part since the mathematical methods which are used are very similar. We shall see that several of the methods of radiological data collection can be modeled using convolution. Estimating the original signal from the data is then modeled as a deconvolution.

The Wiener filter is an optimal linear, time invariant, least mean square solution to the problem in Equation 29.10. Since it is an optimal solution, it would seem that this chapter should have stopped with the Wiener filter. However, the model is only optimal for (1) linear, (2) time invariant, (3) least mean square solutions to (4) the problem in Equation 29.10. The first three parts of the estimation model are reasonable assumptions about first pass radionuclide angiocardiography. Assumption number four is less accurate. Equation 29.10 is only a fair model of first pass radionuclide angiocardiography.

Equation 29.10 does not include the statistical nature of the time activity curve from the region of interest over the superior vena cava. More importantly, is does not capture the *a priori* medical knowledge about first pass radionuclide angiocardiography. We have a reasonable understanding of the shape of a(t), but mush less information about the power spectral densities of $a(t)$ and $n(t)$. It is always important to understand the model which is used and how the model relates to the real problem. A good solution for a particular model is important; however, throughout this book we emphasize that it is even more important to have a good the model of the problem.

IX. FURTHER READING

A review of shunt calculation methods written by Dr. Treves and myself[6] in 1977 contains a review of radionuclide angiocardiography. An up-to-date description of a low parameter model algorithm can be found in a paper by Kuruc et al.[9] Iterative techniques in image reconstruction are described in the book by Herman.[10]

A technique which has been used frequently in radiologic image processing is the maximum entropy method. Maximum entropy is a term from physics and information theory which refers to the values of the elements of the solution. If the sum of the pixel values is constant, the maximum entropy occurs when all values are equal. Very disparate values give a low entropy. Using a maximum constraint often results in an effect similar to smoothing. The maximum entropy method will not be covered in this book. An advanced description of the maximum entropy method can be found in a paper by Ulrych and Bishop.[11]

REFERENCES

1. **Blumgart, K. L. and Yens, O. C.,** Studies on the velocity of blood flow. I. The method utilized, *J. Clin. Invest.,* 4, 1, 1927.
2. **Blumgart, K. L. and Weiss, S.,** Studies on the velocity of blood flow. VII. The pulmonary circulation time in normal resting individuals, *J. Clin. Invest.,* 4, 399, 1927.
3. **Prinzmetal, M., Corday, E., Bergman, H. C., et al.,** Radiocardiography: A new method for studying the blood flow through the chambers of the heart in human beings, *Science,* 108, 340, 1948.
4. **Folse, R. and Braunwald, E.,** Pulmonary vascular dilution curves recorded by external detection in the diagnosis of left-to-right shunts, *Br. Heart J.,* 24, 166, 1962.
5. **Maltz, D. L. and Treves, S.,** Quantitative radionuclide angiocardiography: determination of $Q_p:Q_s$ in children, *Circulation,* 47, 1049, 1973.
6. **Parker, J. A. and Treves, S.,** Radionuclide detection, localization, and quantitation of intracardiac shunts and shunts between the great arteries, *Prog. Cardiovasc. Dis.,* 20, 121, 1977.
7. **Alderson, P. O., Douglass, K. H., Mendenhall, K. G., et at.,** Deconvolution analysis in radionuclide quantitation of left-to-right cardiac shunts, *J. Nucl. Med.,* 20, 502, 1979.
8. **Kuruc, A., Treves, S., Parker, J. A., et al.,** Radionuclide angiocardiography: an improved deconvolution technique for improvement after suboptimal bolus injection: experimental results in dogs with and without atrial septal defects, *Radiology,* 148, 233, 1983.
9. **Kuruc, A., Treves, S., Smith, W., and Fujii, A.,** An automated algorithm for radionuclide angiocardiographic quantitation of circulatory shunting, *Comp. Biomed. Res.,* 17, 481, 1984.
10. **Herman, G. T.,** *Image Reconstruction from Projections,* Academic Press, New York, 1980.
11. **Ulrych, T. J. and Bishop, T. N.,** Maximum entropy spectral analysis and autoregressive decomposition, *Rev. Geophys. Space Phys.,* 13, 183, 1975.

Chapter 30

RECONSTRUCTION FROM FOURIER SAMPLES: NUCLEAR MAGNETIC RESONANCE IMAGING

This chapter will describe image reconstruction in nuclear magnetic resonance imaging. We shall find that the data collected are samples of the Fourier transform of the image. Image reconstruction in nuclear magnetic resonance imaging is particularly simple; it is performed by the inverse Fourier transform operation.

The first paragraph has defined the entire image reconstruction algorithm — namely, it is an inverse Fourier transform operation. Almost all of this chapter will be devoted to describing how nuclear magnetic resonance imaging data are obtained. In part the emphasis on data collection in this chapter has to do with the simplicity of the reconstruction. However, in a more general sense it points out the importance of developing a good model of the data collection process. Often the most important part of understanding image reconstruction is developing a good model of the data collection process. The first task in each of the chapters in this part of the book will be to develop an accurate model of the image collection process.

I. PHYSICS AND INSTRUMENTATION

To understand image formation in nuclear magnetic resonance, we shall need to describe one relation from physics and one relation from instrumentation. There are many other important aspects of physics and instrumentation needed in order to understand the signal intensities in the resultant images, but this information will not be needed for understanding image formation. Thus, our description of nuclear magnetic resonance physics and instrumentation will be very brief.

Certain nuclei have intrinsic magnetic moments; they are "like" little bar magnets (well, not really). The magnetic moments of the nuclei precess (rotate) in a magnetic field the same way the angular momentum of a gyroscope precesses in the gravitational field of the earth. The only fact which is of importance to us is that the angular frequency of the precession is given by the Larmor equation:

$$\omega = \gamma \cdot B \tag{30.1}$$

where ω is the angular frequency of precession, γ is the gyromagnetic ratio for the nucleus, and B is the magnetic field. For a single nuclear species in a particular magnetic field, the rate of precession is called the Larmor frequency or the resonant frequency (see Chapter 7 for a description of resonance).

The gyromagnetic ratio, γ, is a fixed quantity for each nuclear species; it does not change. Therefore, from Equation 30.1 it can be seen that **the angular frequency is directly related to the magnetic field.** This fact is the only piece of physics which we shall need to know.

The feature which distinguishes nuclear magnetic resonance imaging instruments from nonimaging instruments is the gradient coils. A magnetic field gradient is the change in the magnetic field strength with respect to position. The gradient coils are set up so that they make the strength of the magnetic field vary with position. The key instrumental feature is that **the gradient coils make the magnetic field vary as a function of position.**

For conceptual purposes, the magnetic field strength is usually separated into three components — the static field, the gradient field, and the radio frequency field. The main magnet produces a large, fixed, homogeneous field called the static magnetic field, B_0. The static field induces a magnetic moment, M, in the sample. The gradient coils produce a magnetic field which varies with position. The gradient fields allow spatial localization of

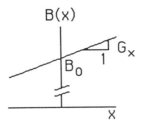

FIGURE 30.1.   Magnetic field gradient: the magnetic field gradient, G_x, gives the slope of the magnetic field strength, $B(x)$, as a function of position, x. B_0 is the main magnetic field.

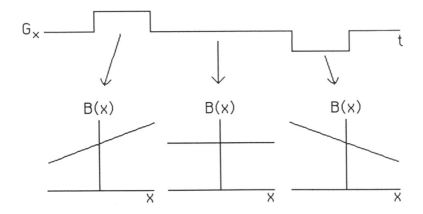

FIGURE 30.2.   Change in magnetic field gradient with time: the top panel shows the magnetic field gradient, G_x, plotted as a function of time. The bottom panel show the magnetic field strength, $B(x)$, as a function of position, x, at three points in time. As the gradient changes, the slope of the field strength vs. position changes.

the signal and are of most concern to us in this chapter. The radio frequency coils produce a field, B_1, which oscillates at the Larmor frequency. The radio frequency field manipulates the induced magnetization so that it can be measured. We shall not discuss the radio frequency field.

By definition, the direction of the main magnetic field is along the z axis. Although the direction of the magnetic field is always in the z direction, the strength of the field may vary in any direction. An imager has three sets of coils which can produce gradients in x, y, or z directions, or by combining the gradients, in any direction.

The strength of the magnetic field with a linear x gradient field can be written:

$$B(x) = B_0 + G_x \cdot x \qquad (30.2)$$

where $B(x)$ is the strength of the magnetic field, B_0 is the value of the static magnetic field, and G_x is the strength of the gradient. The magnetic field strength, $B(x)$, is given in units of Tesla or Gauss, and gradient strength, G_x, is given in Tesla/m or Gauss/cm.

Figure 30.1 shows the strength of the magnetic field as a function of x for a field with an x gradient. The gradient, G_x, is the slope of the line. For larger G_x, the slope would be larger; for negative G_x, the slope would in the other direction. Below we shall plot G_x as a function of time, in order to show a particular experiment is performed. This type of a timing diagram is a typical method of outlining a nuclear magnetic resonance imaging experiment, but it is not always clear to the novice what is meant by changes in the gradient strength. From Figure 30.2 it can easily be seen that the gradient strength, G_x, changes the slope of the field strength.

The physics relation given by Equation 30.1 states that the frequency is directly dependent on the magnetic field. The gradient field, produced by the instrument, makes the magnetic field a function of position. Combining these to relation gives:

$$\omega(x) = \gamma \cdot B_0 + \gamma \cdot G_x \cdot x \qquad (30.3)$$

Therefore, the angular frequency of precession is a function of position. This relation summarizes the key aspects of the physics and instrumentation which are needed to understand spatial localization in nuclear magnetic resonance imaging.

II. VECTOR ADDITION OF MAGNETIC MOMENTS

One important difference between nuclear magnetic resonance imaging and computed tomography is the way in which the signals from different portions of the cross section are combined. In computed tomography, the linear attenuation coefficients along a ray are summed. The data samples represent the sum of different combinations of pixel values. All of the values in the sum are positive; the linear attenuation coefficients never provide a negative contribution to the data values.

Since the data values represent sums of the cross-sectional data, we can predict that the data collection process tends to smooth the data. In the next chapter, we shall find that computed tomographic data tend to sample the low frequencies more accurately than the high frequencies. The basic reason that computed tomographic data are a sum of positive values is that the detector measures the energy in the ray (also called square law detector).

Nuclear magnetic resonance imaging is different. What is measured is the magnetic field produced by the precessing magnetic moment in the sample. The magnetic moments from different portions of the sample have both a magnitude and a direction. They are vector quantities. The total magnetic moment in the sample is the vector sum of the magnetic moments in the various portions of the sample. If the magnetic moments from two portions of the sample are pointing in different directions, then they will be subtracted from each other.

Another interesting aspect of the vector nature of the magnetic moment is that the signal has both a magnitude and a direction. If two coils are used, then the magnitude and the direction of the magnetization can both be measured. The basic signal in other fields of radiology is scalar. The vector nature of the nuclear magnetic resonance signal is unique in radiology.

Vector addition of the magnetic moments of the different portions of the samples is a major advantage of nuclear magnetic resonance imaging. Unlike computed tomography, it is not necessary to over sample the low frequencies. Below we shall see that by fooling around with the gradient fields, the vector orientations of the magnetic moments in the cross section can be used to sample any spatial frequency component of the object. We shall show how the Fourier transform of a cross section can be directly sampled.

III. FREE INDUCTION DECAY AND SPECTRUM

Nuclear magnetic resonance imaging is performed by inducing a magnetic moment, M, in the sample, manipulating the magnetic moment in a sometimes complicated manner, and then detecting the resulting signal. The signal produced is due to the precession of the magnetic moment induced in the sample. The rotating magnetic moment will produce a signal in a coil of wire surrounding the sample in the same way that power is generated in an electric generator. This signal is called the **free induction decay** (see Figure 14.4) — induction since the signal measures the induced magnetic moment, free since the radio frequency field is not manipulating the magnetic moment during read out, and decay since the most important part of the signal is how it decays over time.

The signal produced by the rotating magnetization will have a sinusoidal fluctuation at the Larmor frequency. If two coils are placed at right angles to each other, then the signal in the coils will be out of phase by $\pi/2$. In Chapter 6, we used an imaginary exponential to describe this type of signal:

$$f(t) = M \cdot e^{i\omega t} \tag{30.4}$$

where M is the magnetization induced in the sample and ω is the Larmor frequency. The signal in one coil is given by $Re[M \cdot e^{i\omega t}]$, and the signal in the other coil is given by $Im[M \cdot e^{i\omega t}]$.

Equation 30.4 gives the signal for a sample in a uniform magnetic field. In the presence of field variations, such as those caused by the gradient field, different portions of the sample will have different resonant frequencies. Above it was pointed out that the various magnetic moments add as vectors. The vector addition can be represented using complex notation. The signal can be written:

$$f(t) = \sum_i m_i \cdot e^{i\omega_i t} \tag{30.5}$$

where m_i is the induced magnetic moment in the tissue exposed to a field B_i, and ω_i is the Larmor angular frequency, $\gamma \cdot B_i$.

The free induction decay, f(t), is a time domain description of the nuclear magnetic resonance signal. The Fourier transform of the free induction decay is called the spectrum. From Equation 30.5 it is easy to identify the Fourier components, $F(\omega)$. The value of $F(\omega)$ is equal to the sum of the magnetic moments which are oscillating at angular frequency ω. This angular frequency is due to nuclei which are in a field given by ω/γ. Thus, each spectral component corresponds to nuclei which are in a specific magnetic field.

In chemical applications, the magnetic field that a nucleus experiences is due to the chemical environment of the nucleus. The nuclear magnetic resonance spectrum is used to show the number of nuclei in each chemical environment. In nuclear magnetic resonance imaging, the magnetic field is used to code the position. The spectrum is used to show the number of nuclei at various positions. For imaging, the conditions are usually adjusted so the chemical effects are relatively small. However, since both chemical and spatial effects are reflected through the magnetic field at the nucleus, differences in chemistry cause a shift in position, called **chemical shift artifact**.

IV. IMAGE, SPECTRUM DOMAIN

Figure 30.3 shows a simplified timing diagram for a one-dimensional nuclear magnetic imaging experiment. Since we are only concerned with image formation, the diagram does not include the radio frequency pulses. These pulses are essential to the nuclear magnetic imaging experiment, but they are not the focus of this discussion.

The top line of Figure 30.3 shows the x gradient strength as a function of time. There is an initial negative gradient followed by a positive gradient. We shall be interested in the signal at the center of the positive gradient. Later we shall explain the purpose of the initial negative gradient. The second line shows the free induction decay during the positive gradient.

Figure 30.4 shows the object which is being imaged. The values, f(x,y), represent the magnitude of the induced magnetization as a function of position. We have switched from the symbol, m_i, which emphasizes the fact that the parameter of interest is an induced

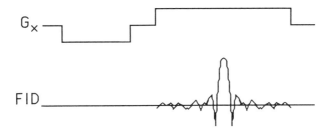

FIGURE 30.3. One-dimensional imaging experiment: the top panel shows the gradient strength, G_x, in the x direction as a function of time. The bottom panel shows the free induction decay (FID).

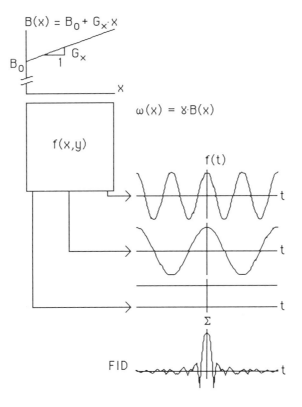

FIGURE 30.4. Image, frequency domain representation of position encoding: the spatial distribution of magnetic moments is represented by the signal, $f(x,y)$. The magnetic field gradient, G_x, changes the magnetic field, $B(x)$, as a function of x. Consequently, different frequency sinusoids are obtained from different columns of $f(x,y)$. The free induction decay, FID, is the sum of the sinusoids from each column of $f(x,y)$.

magnetization, to $f(x,y)$ in order to emphasize similarity to other imaging processing problems.

Because of the gradient in the x direction, all of the nuclei at a particular x position will oscillate at a frequency given by:

$$\omega(x) = \gamma \cdot B_0 + \gamma \cdot G_x \cdot x \qquad (30.6)$$

Figure 30.4 is a diagrammatic representation indicating that the signal from each column of the object will oscillate at a frequency proportional to its x position.

The free induction decay can be modeled as an audio frequency signal modulated by a radio frequency carrier. The radio frequency carrier is caused by the main magnetic field, B_0. The audio frequency variations are caused by the gradient field, G_x; the audio frequency variations contain the positional information. The first step in processing is to demodulate the audio frequency signal from the radio frequency carrier (see Equation 16.35). The demodulated signal is given by:

$$\omega(x) = \gamma \cdot G_x \cdot x \tag{30.7}$$

In all of our diagrams we shall show the demodulated audio frequency signal.

The gyromagnetic ratio, $\gamma/2\pi$, for protons is 42 MHz/T. The Larmor frequency, $\gamma \cdot B_0/2\pi$, for protons in a main magnetic field of 1.5 T magnet is in the radio frequency range, 65 MHz. The variations in frequency due to a gradient field are given by $\gamma \cdot G_x \cdot x/2\pi$. For a gradient field of .001 T/m over 25 cm, the frequency range is 11 kHz. These variations are in the audio frequency range.

Equation 30.7 and Figure 30.4 show that the frequency of oscillation of the induced magnetization is directly proportional to the position. The gradient field changes the field as a function of x, and hence the frequency changes as a function of x. Encoding the position in this fashion is called **frequency encoding,** the position is encoded by frequency.

The Fourier transform of the free induction decay is the spectrum, $F(\omega)$. From Figure 30.4 we can see that the magnitude of the various spectral frequencies will be equal to the sum of the magnetic moments in the corresponding columns of $f(x,y)$. The indented section shows this same relation mathematically.

The signal from each column in Figure 30.4 will be a single sinusoid. Mathematically:

$$f(x,y) \cdot e^{i\omega(x)t} \tag{30.8}$$

where $f(x,y)$ is the amplitude of the induced magnetization as a function of position and $\omega(x)$ is the angular frequency, $\gamma \cdot G_x \cdot x$. The free induction decay will be the sum of the sinusoids:

$$f(t) = \int_{-\infty}^{+\infty} \int_{-\infty}^{+\infty} f(x,y) \cdot e^{i\omega(x)t} \, dxdy \tag{30.9}$$

where $f(t)$ represents the time domain signal, and $f(x,y)$ represents the amplitudes of the induced magnetizations as a function of space.

Since $e^{i\omega(x)t}$ is not a function of y, Equation 30.9 can be rearranged:

$$f(t) = \int_{-\infty}^{+\infty} \left[(1/\gamma \cdot G_x) \cdot \int_{-\infty}^{+\infty} f(x,y) \, dy \right] \cdot e^{i\gamma G_x xt} \, d(\gamma \cdot G_x \cdot x) \tag{30.10}$$

Equation 30.10 is in the form of a Fourier transform. The x position is related to the frequency, ω, by Equation 30.7. The value of the Fourier transform $F(\omega)$ is proportional to the inner integral, the projection of $f(x,y)$ on the x axis.

$$F(\omega) = (1/\gamma \cdot G_x) \cdot \int_{-\infty}^{+\infty} f(x,y) \, dy \tag{30.11}$$

The application of a linear x gradient field makes the spectral values proportional to the projection of the cross section.

Figure 30.5 shows the relation between the Fourier transform of $f(x,y)$ and the free

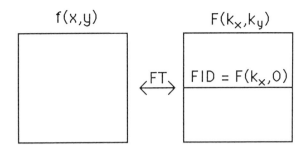

FIGURE 30.5. Data representation in the spatial frequency domain: the two-dimensional spatial frequency transformation of f(x,y) is given by $F(k_x,k_y)$. The free induction decay is proportional to the spatial frequency values along the k_x axis, $F(k_x,0)$.

induction decay. The free induction decay is equal to the values of $F(k_x, k_y)$ along the k_x axis.

In the next chapter we shall see that the primary data in computed tomography are the projections. By electronically rotating the gradient field, it is possible to collect nuclear magnetic resonance data similar to computed tomographic data. Therefore, the convolution, back projection algorithm described in the next chapter can be used in nuclear magnetic resonance imaging. However, unlike computed tomography, there are frequently spatial distortions in nuclear magnetic resonance images. Since the convolution, back projection algorithm tends to exaggerate errors due to inconsistencies in the projection values caused by spatial distortions, it is not commonly used for nuclear magnetic resonance imaging.

V. TIME, FREQUENCY, SPACE, AND SPATIAL FREQUENCY

In Chapter 15, we noted the very special relation between the time, frequency, space, and spatial frequency domains in nuclear magnetic resonance. It is worth reviewing this relation. Figure 15.1 shows the time, frequency, space, and spatial frequency domains. The space (image) domain is related to the frequency (spectrum) domain through Equation 30.7. The spatial frequency domain is the Fourier transform of the space domain, and the time (free induction decay) domain is the inverse Fourier transform of the frequency domain. Consequently, the spatial frequency domain is related to the time (free induction decay) domain.

For the radiologist, the image (or spectrum) domain is the primary domain. The spatial frequencies (or free induction decay) are in the transform domain. For the nuclear magnetic resonance scientist, the free induction decay (or spatial frequency) domain is the primary domain. The spectrum (image) is in the transform domain. In Chapter 15 it was pointed out that nuclear magnetic resonance imaging is one of the best examples of the duality between the domains. One domain is not primary; rather the domains are coequals.

Above we have described imaging from the image (spectrum) domain. It is best, however, to understand imaging from both domains. We shall find that the free induction decay (spatial frequency) domain is very useful for understanding encoding in more than one dimension.

VI. FREE INDUCTION DECAY, SPATIAL FREQUENCY DOMAIN

Instead of considering the encoding from the image, spectrum point of view, we can consider it from the free induction decay, spatial frequency point of view. Consider an object under the influence of a linear x gradient. Suppose that at time equal to zero the magnetic moments of all portions of the sample were pointing in the same direction. This is shown in the first snap shot in Figure 30.6

$$f(t) = \int\int f(x,y) \cdot e^{i \cdot k_x(t) \cdot x} \, dx \, dy$$

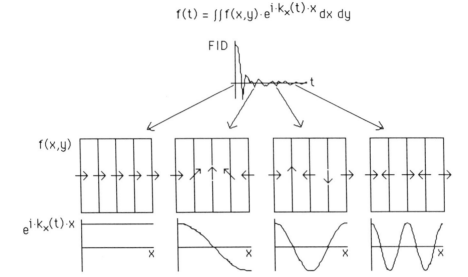

FIGURE 30.6. Time, spatial frequency domain representation of position encoding: the top panel shows the free induction decay (FID). The bottom panel shows snap shots of the sample at different points along the free induction decay. The phases of the magnetic moments vary sinusoidally as a function of the position, x. As time increases, the spatial frequency of the variation in the phases increases. The value of the free induction decay is the integral of the product of f(x,y) and the sinusoidally varying phases — namely, it is the spatial Fourier transform of the sample.

The phase angle of the magnetic moments after a period of time, t, will be:

$$\phi(x,t) = \int_0^t \omega(x,\tau) \, d\tau \qquad (30.12)$$

For the case where $\omega(x,t)$ does not vary with time:

$$\phi(x,t) = \omega(x) \cdot t \qquad (30.13)$$

Using Equation 30.6:

$$\phi(x,t) = \omega_0 \cdot t + \gamma \cdot G_x \cdot x \cdot t \qquad (30.14)$$

Demodulation cancels the first term so that in the audio signal, the phase is proportional to x and t.

Figure 30.6 shows snap shots of the phase angles of the object at several points in time. There is no change in angle for the column with x equal to zero. As x increases the phase angles increase. The phase angles change sinusoidally over the cross section. After a longer period of time, there is continued rotation of the induced magnetic moments. Again the phase angles change sinusoidally in the x direction, but at a higher spatial frequency. After still more time, there is more change in the phase angles. The spatial angular frequency of the oscillation in the phases at any point in time is:

$$k_x(t) = \gamma \cdot G_x \cdot t \qquad (30.15)$$

At any point in time, the total signal will be the sum of the individual amplitudes multiplied by $e^{i\gamma G_x x t}$. Above we have considered this imaginary exponential to be a function

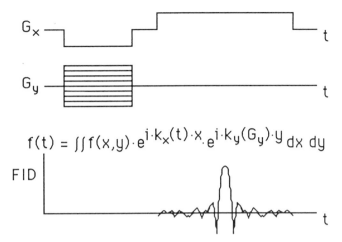

FIGURE 30.7. Two-dimensional imaging experiment: the gradient in the x direction, G_x, and the free induction decay (FID) are the same as in the one-dimensional experiment shown in Figure 30.6. The gradient in the y direction, G_y, varies over the range shown. A separate free induction decay is collected for each step of the y gradient. The value of the free induction decay is the two-dimensional Fourier transform of the sample, $f(x,y)$. The spatial frequency in the x direction is a function of time, $k_x(t)$. The spatial frequency in the y direction is a function of the y gradient strength, $k_y(G_y)$.

of t. However, for a given time, it can be considered a function of x. The spatial frequency, $\gamma \cdot G_x \cdot t$, is a function of t. For successive points in time the spatial frequency is higher and higher.

At each point in time, the signal, $f(t)$, is the sum of the magnitudes, $f(x,y)$, multiplied by the spatial sinusoid, $e^{i\gamma G_x x t}$. The sum of the product of two signals is the correlation of the signals. The correlation of $f(x,y)$ with a spatial sinusoid is the value of the spatial Fourier transform (see Chapter 14). The value of the free induction decay at each point in time is equal to the corresponding spatial frequency of the image.

Application of a gradient field for an appropriate period of time manipulates the phases into a spatial sinusoid. The value of the free induction decay at that point in time is just the spatial frequency represented by the phases. This result is not new, it is just a slightly different way of describing Equation 30.9.

VII. TWO-DIMENSIONAL ENCODING

The image, spectrum domain provides a very natural method of understanding one-dimensional spatial encoding. It is awkward for understanding two-dimensional encoding. (It is possible to introduce pseudo time variables t_1 and t_2, but these are not particularly simple concepts.) The free induction decay, spatial frequency domain description of one-dimensional encoding is a little awkward, although Chapter 14 may have made the association between a correlation and a Fourier transform more seem more natural. However, the free induction decay, spatial frequency domain greatly simplifies the understanding of two-dimensional encoding.

Figure 30.7 shows the timing diagram for a typical two-dimensional imaging sequence. The x gradient and the free induction decay are the same as in the one-dimensional experiment, but now there is also a y gradient. The diagram for the y gradient is a symbolic representation to indicate that the whole sequence is repeated a number of times; each time a different strength y gradient is used.

$$f(t) = \iint f(x,y) \cdot e^{i \cdot k_y(G_y) \cdot y} \, dx \, dy$$

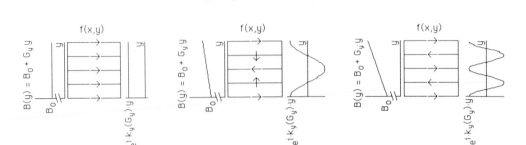

FIGURE 30.8. Position encoding prior to the free induction decay: this figure shows the phases of the sample, f(x,y), after application of different strength gradients in the y direction. The phase varies sinusoidally in the y direction. The value of the signal is proportional to the y spatial frequency component of the Fourier transform of f(x,y).

Figure 30.8 shows the phases of the induced magnetic moments after the application of different strength y gradients. When no magnetic moment is applied, then all of the moments point in the same direction. When a small gradient is used then the phases vary sinusoidally in the y direction. With larger gradients the variation in the y direction is more rapid. The spatial angular frequency of the variation is:

$$k_y(G_y) = \gamma \cdot G_y \cdot T_y \tag{30.16}$$

where T_y is the length of time the gradient is applied. The spatial frequency varies with the gradient strength, G_y.

After application of the gradient, the signal is:

$$f(t) = \int_{-\infty}^{+\infty} \int_{-\infty}^{+\infty} f(x,y) \cdot e^{i\gamma G_y T_y y} \, dx dy \tag{30.17}$$

Like Equation 30.9, this equation is in the form of a Fourier transform. But in this case, the Fourier transform is with respect to the y spatial direction. It is the correlation of the signal, f(x,y), with a sinusoid in the y direction. The spatial frequency is a function of G_y. Encoding using a gradient before the signal read out is often called **phase encoding.** The phases of the magnetic moments encode the position.

The two terms, frequency encoding and phase encoding, are often used to describe gradients used during read out and prior to read out, respectively. However, as we have seen the difference between frequency encoding of position and phase encoding of position has to do with whether the problem is viewed from the image, spectrum domain or from the spatial frequency, free induction decay domain, not with whether the gradient occurs before or during the free induction decay. Unfortunately, these misleading terms seem embedded in the vernacular.

Now let us return to the two-dimensional experimental design diagrammed in Figure 30.7. After application of the y and x gradients, there will be both a y and an x component to the phases of the induced magnetic moments. These two components will result in a sinusoid at some angle. The signal will be given by:

$$f(t) = \int_{-\infty}^{+\infty} \int_{-\infty}^{+\infty} f(x,y) \cdot e^{ik_x(t)x} \cdot e^{ik_y(G_y)y} \, dx dy \tag{30.18}$$

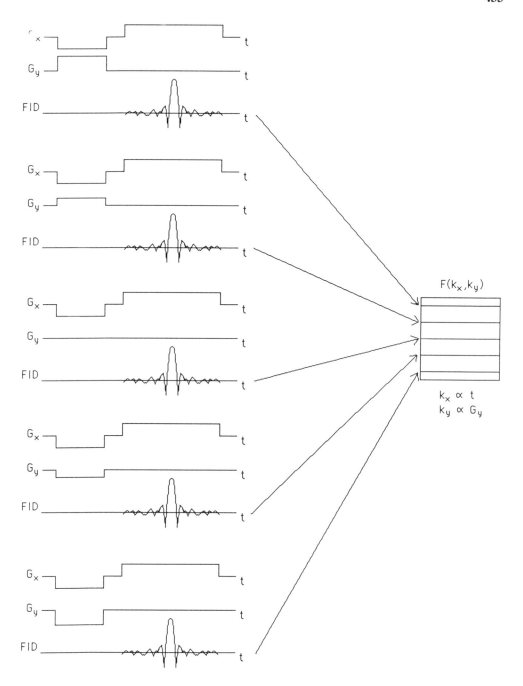

FIGURE 30.9. Spatial frequency representation of two-dimensional data: the free induction decays from the experiment shown diagrammatically in Figure 30.7 are lines in the Fourier transform of the sample. The position of the lines is related to the G_y gradient.

The time domain signal, $f(t)$, is the correlation of the image, $f(x,y)$, with a two-dimensional sinusoid; the time domain signal is the two-dimensional spatial Fourier transform of the image. The x spatial frequency, given by Equation 30.15, is a function of the time from the center of the echo. The y spatial frequency, given by Equation 30.16, is a function of the gradient strength, G_y. The sequence of experiments diagrammed in Figure 30.7 sample all of the values of the spatial frequencies of the image. The sampling is shown in the spatial frequency domain in Figure 30.9.

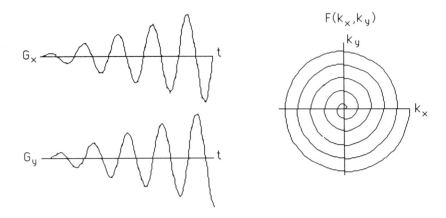

FIGURE 30.10.   Spiral data sampling: the x and y gradients, G_x and G_y, shown on the left causes data samples in the spatial frequency domain as shown on the right. The path of the samples is a spiral in the spatial frequency domain. All of the spatial frequencies can be sampled in a single free induction decay.

VIII. ALTERNATE DATA COLLECTION PROTOCOLS

The timing diagram shown in Figure 30.7 is a common method of collecting data during nuclear magnetic resonance imaging. However, there are many other methods of sampling the cross sectional data. The free induction decay, spatial frequency domain point of view is useful for understanding these alternate methods. At any point in time, the value of the free induction decay represents the correlation of the magnitude of the induced magnetic moments with the phases of the magnetic moments.

The spatial frequency of the variation in the phases will depend upon the strength of the gradient fields and the lengths of time over which they are applied. The spatial angular frequencies are equal to:

$$k_x(t) = \int_{-\infty}^{+\infty} \gamma \cdot G_x(t)\, dt \qquad (30.19)$$

$$k_y(t) = \int_{-\infty}^{+\infty} \gamma \cdot G_y(t)\, dt \qquad (30.20)$$

Equation 30.15 is the solution of Equation 30.19 and Equation 30.16 is the solution of Equation 30.20 given the experiment diagrammed in Figure 30.7. However, Equations 30.19 and 30.20 are much more general. They describe a method for moving around the spatial frequency domain in any pattern. Applying a positive x gradient moves the sample in the positive k_x direction at a rate determined by G_x; applying a positive y gradient moves the sample in the positive k_y direction at a rate determined by G_y.

In Figure 30.7, the movement along the k_y direction occurred prior to data collection and the movement along the k_x direction occurred during data collection. However, there is no reason why one gradient or the other is applied at any particular time.

Figure 30.10 shows an alternate timing diagram. The path traversed by the sampling point in the spatial frequency domain is a spiral. Using these gradients, samples throughout the spatial frequency domain can be obtained in a single read out. Similar types of gradient manipulations have been used to produce an entire nuclear magnetic resonance image in tens of a millisecond.

The initial negative gradient in the timing diagram shown in Figure 30.7 was not

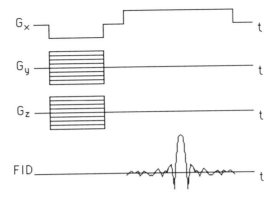

FIGURE 30.11. Three-dimensional imaging experiment: the timing diagram for a three-dimensional imaging experiment is shown in this figure. k_x is encoded at different points in time during the free induction decay. k_y and k_z are encoded by the gradient strengths during different free induction decays.

explained above. Its effect is to move in the negative k_x direction. The positive gradient moves back along the k_x axis. Since it is not possible to turn the gradients on and off instantaneously, it is best to sample data during the period that the gradient field is constant (or changing smoothly). The negative gradient moves to very negative k_x values. The positive gradient comes on and becomes stable before the data sampling takes place. During the time sampling takes place, the movement along the k_x direction is at a constant rate.

Slice selection was touched on very briefly in Chapter 16. That chapter described the effect of time, band width considerations on slice selection. For the purposes of this chapter we have assumed that the magnetization in a single slice has been selected by judicious application of radio frequency pulses without describing this process. Assuming that a slice has been selected, the methods described above can be used to reconstruct an image in that slice.

Alternately, the radio frequency pulses can be used to select a whole slab of tissue. Then a three-dimensional imaging sequence can be used to image a volume of tissue. Figure 30.11 shows the timing diagram for a three-dimensional imaging sequence. The only difference compared to Figure 30.7 is the inclusion of a variable gradient field in the z direction.

A separate free induction decay is collected for each combination of y and z gradient fields. The three-dimensional data collection time will be equal to the z resolution times the two-dimensional data collection time. The magnitude of the z gradient will determine which z spatial frequency, $k_z (G_z)$, is sampled during a particular free induction decay. The sequence of free induction decays will fill the three-dimensional spatial frequency domain.

IX. RECONSTRUCTION

Image reconstruction for the data collection scheme shown in Figures 30.7 and 30.11 is very simple; it is an inverse Fourier transform. For the more complicated data sampling methods such as that shown in Figure 30.10 it may be necessary first to interpolate the data to rectilinear coordinates. But the reconstruction is still just an inverse Fourier transform. Three-dimensional images are reconstructed with a three-dimensional inverse Fourier transform.

X. CHEMICAL SHIFT IMAGING

The resonant frequency for a nuclear magnetic moment is directly proportional to the magnetic field to which the nucleus is exposed (Equation 30.1). The magnetic field is due

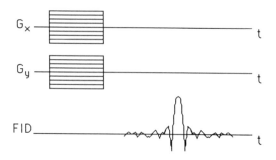

FIGURE 30.12. Imaging and chemical shift experiment: this timing diagram allows two spatial dimensions and chemical shift information to be collected. The chemical shift information is collected during the free induction decays. The k_x and k_y dimensions are sampled during different free induction decays.

to a number of sources. We have been most concerned with the main magnetic field and the gradient fields. However, there are also local effects. The magnetic moments of the surrounding electrons and the nearby nuclei affect the magnetic field experienced by a nucleus.

In nuclear magnetic spectroscopy, these local magnetic moments are used to understand the chemical environment of the nucleus. In Chapter 14, we briefly described nuclear magnetic resonance spectroscopy. The difference between spectroscopy and imaging is the gradient fields. A free induction decay collected with no imaging gradients will only show the effects of the chemical milieu. The spectrum will show the relative abundances of nuclei experiencing each magnetic field environment.

The spectroscopic experiment can be combined with the imaging experiment. Figure 30.12 shows a timing diagram for a three-dimensional experiment. The two space dimensions are encoded using the gradients, G_x and G_y, prior to the free induction decay. The chemical information is encoded by the local magnetic fields during the free induction decay. A two-dimensional cross section of spectra can be obtained using a three-dimensional inverse Fourier transform operation. A spectrum is obtained at each point in space.

At times we are interested in a relatively simple description of the spectrum. For example, in proton imaging we are typically interested in separating the "fat" from the "water" protons, where the terms, "fat" and "water" are used loosely. In this cases it is possible to devise more efficient methods for imaging this "low resolution" spectral information. One of the strengths of nuclear magnetic resonance imaging is the richness of the imaging protocols which can be developed.

XI. VELOCITY IMAGING

Equations 30.19 and 30.20 assume that the object of interest does not move. When portions of the sample move during imaging, these simple equations are no longer valid. Movement of portions of the object is commonly associated with image artifacts. However, with a well-designed experiment, the effects caused by movement can be used to measure velocity.

Consider the gradient shown in Figure 30.13. For an object which is stationary at position, $-x_0$, there is no net effect from this gradient. The negative portion of the gradient results in a phase change of $\gamma \cdot G_x \cdot x_0 \cdot T$; the positive portion of the gradient results in a phase change of $-\gamma \cdot G_x \cdot x_0 \cdot T$. The net phase angle is 0. Consider instead an object which jumps from $-x_0$ to x_0 as the gradient changes from negative to positive. For such an object the phase will add, and the net phase angle will be $2 \cdot \gamma \cdot G_x \cdot x_0 \cdot T$.

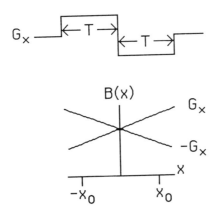

FIGURE 30.13. Velocity encoding gradient: the gradient on the top can be used to encode velocity. On the bottom the magnetic field strength for these gradients are shown.

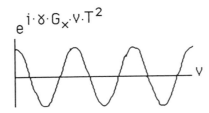

FIGURE 30.14. Velocity encoding: the gradient shown in Figure 30.13 will result in a sinusoidal phase shift which is a function of velocity. This diagram is analogous to Figure 30.4.

Instead of an object which jumps from $-x_0$ to x_0, let us consider an object which moves at a constant velocity from the left to the right passing through zero as the gradient switches from negative to positive. It will start at position $-v \cdot T$ and go to $v \cdot T$, where v is the velocity. The net phase angle will be $\gamma \cdot G_x \cdot v \cdot T^2$.

Figure 30.14 shows the phase angle as a function of the velocity. The signal which is received is the correlation of a sinusoid with the number of nuclei at each velocity. This situation is exactly analogous to the situation described above for position. For the gradient shown in Figure 30.13, the signal which is receive is the Fourier transform of the object with respect to the velocity components in the object. Thus, this type of gradient can be used to encode velocity.

Figure 30.15 shows a timing diagram for measuring the proton density as a function of x, y, z, v_x, v_y, v_z, and chemical shift — a seven-dimensional experiment. A separate free induction decay is collected for each combination of position and velocity for each gradient. For 256 resolution, 256^6 free induction decays are needed. If each free induction decay is collected in 1 sec, then this experiment would take 9,151,158 years!

The experiment diagrammed in Figure 30.15 is totally impractical. Rather than using this brute force experiment, more sophistication is needed. For example, the velocity within a pixel is often nearly a constant. In this case it is not necessary to obtain the intensity as a function of velocity, $f(x,y,z,v_x,v_y,v_z)$, but rather in is sufficient to obtain four values as a function of position, $f(x,y,z)$, $v_x(x,y,z)$, $v_y(x,y,z)$, and $v_z(x,y,z)$. There is a big difference between these two experiments. The first is a six-dimensional experiment, while the second is four three-dimensional experiments. The first provides the quantity of nuclei in each pixel which is traveling with a particular speed. The second provides a single velocity value for each pixel.

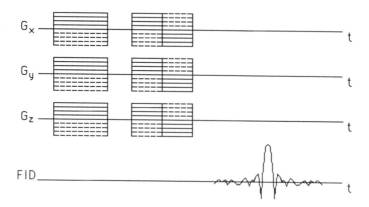

FIGURE 30.15. Seven-dimensional experiment: this figure shows the timing diagram for collection of data in the x, y, z, v_x, v_y, v_z, and chemical shift directions. Chemical shift data are collected during the free induction decay. The k_x, k_y, and k_z data are encoded by combinations of the unipolar gradients. The k_{vx}, k_{vy}, and k_{vz}, data are encoded by combinations of the bipolar gradients.

For a particular problem, only the axial velocity in a cross section may be of interest. Then, the problem amounts to measuring $v_z(x,y)$. This problem is a simple two-dimensional measurement. Rather than the intractable seven-dimensional experiment in Figure 30.15, the data of interest can be collected with a very practical two-dimensional experiment.

There is a wealth of information available from a nuclear magnetic resonance imaging experiment. Much of the trick to nuclear magnetic resonance imaging is understanding what information is most important for a particular problem. The data collection can then be limited to a practical experiment. Understanding how the data are collected allows the radiologist to design an experiment which will answer the clinical problem in an efficient manner.

XII. SUMMARY

The key to understanding nuclear magnetic resonance imaging is understanding the relation between the time (free induction decay), frequency (spectrum), space (image), and spatial frequency domains. Frequency is related to the magnetic field by the Larmor equation (Equation 30.1), and the magnetic field is related to the position by the gradient field (Equation 30.2). Therefore, the image positions are related to the spectral frequencies. These important relations are shown diagrammatically in Figure 15.1.

Spatial encoding during data sampling is most easily understood in the image, spectrum domain. However, it can also be understood from the spatial frequency, free induction decay domain. Figure 30.6 shows that at each point in time, the free induction decay is equal to the correlation of the image with a spatial sinusoid. Equations 30.19 and 30.20 show that the effect of the gradient fields is to move about in the spatial frequency domain. The advantage of this free induction decay, spatial frequency domain description is that it is best for understanding encoding prior to data sampling, and for understanding the more complicated encoding techniques.

This chapter deals almost exclusively with modeling the data collection process. The section on reconstruction is a single paragraph long. Since the data are samples in the spatial frequency domain, reconstruction can be done with an inverse Fourier transform. Although nuclear magnetic resonance imaging is a special case, it does point out the importance of having a good model of the data collection process. Development of an accurate model of data collection is the most important step in understanding image reconstruction.

XIII. FURTHER READING

This chapter has presented a very selective view of nuclear magnetic resonance imaging. It has only described image formation. It has not described how the radio frequency field, B_1, manipulates the magnetization. It has not discussed the mechanisms which lead to contrast between tissues such as relaxation times and flow. Most references include all of these topics.

The first eight chapters of the book by Stark and Bradley,[1] the first six chapters of the book by Kean and Smith,[2] and the book by Young[3] are among the radiologically oriented sources which present an introduction to nuclear magnetic resonance and to image formation. The physics on nuclear magnetic resonance is presented in the book by Farrar and Becker.[4]

REFERENCES

1. **Stark, D. D. and Bradley, W. G.,** *Magnetic Resonance Imaging,* C. V. Mosby, St. Louis, MO, 1988.
2. **Kean, D. M. and Smith, M. A.,** *Magnetic Resonance Imaging: Principles and Applications,* William & Wilkins, Baltimore, MD, 1986.
3. **Young, S. W.,** *Nuclear Magnetic Resonance Imaging: Basic Principles,* Raven Press, New York, 1984.
4. **Farrar, T. C. and Becker, E. D.,** *Pulse and Fourier Transform NMR,* Academic Press, New York, 1971.

Chapter 31

RECONSTRUCTION FROM NOISELESS PROJECTIONS

This chapter will describe reconstruction from noiseless projection data. The next chapter will consider the same problem with noise added during data collection. This type of reconstruction is used in X-ray computed tomography.

As in the last chapter, a very important step in understanding computed tomographic reconstruction will be development of a good model of the data collection process. The relationship between the cross-sectional object and the projection data is difficult to understand because the object and the data are defined in terms of different coordinate systems. We shall find that back projection of the data to the cross-sectional coordinate system simplifies the model of the data.

A second step in understanding reconstruction will be development of the projection, slice theorem. The projection, slice theorem explains how the projection data are related to the spatial frequency representation of the cross-sectional data. The projection, back projection model of the data and the projection slice theorem will make understanding image reconstruction relatively simple.

I. DATA COLLECTION MODEL

In X-ray computed tomography, the intensity of an X-ray beam is measured after it passes through a cross section. The beam is attenuated by the tissue in each pixel along the way. Mathematically:

$$I_{out} = I_{in} \cdot e^{-\mu_1 \Delta x} \cdot e^{-\mu_2 \Delta x} \cdot e^{-\mu_3 \Delta x} \ldots \tag{31.1}$$

where I_{in} is the intensity of the X-ray beam as it passes into the cross section, I_{out} is the intensity of the X-ray beam as it passes out of the tissue, the μ_i are the linear attenuation constants of the successive pixels, and Δx is size of the pixels.

The logarithm of the ratio of the output signal to the input signal has a particularly simple form:

$$\log(I_{out}/I_{in}) = -(\mu_1 + \mu_2 + \mu_3 + \ldots) \cdot \Delta x \tag{31.2}$$

The logarithm is a simple sum of the linear attenuation coefficients in the path of the beam. The first part of the data collection process is to take the logarithm of the ratio of the input and output intensity. This operation was used in Chapter 4 (see Equation 4.14 and 4.15) as a example of transforming a nonlinear problem into a linear problem.

We shall use the symbol, f(x,y), to represent the two-dimensional cross-section of linear attenuation coefficients, μ_i. The symbol, μ_i, emphasizes the physics, that the values are linear attenuation coefficients. In the following, we shall use f(x,y) to emphasize the similarity with other image reconstruction problems.

Figure 31.1 shows the data collected at a single angle, θ. After taking the logarithm and normalizing, the data values are the sum of the linear attenuation of the pixels along each X-ray beam. The data are given by p(x′,θ), where x′ is the distance from the origin, and θ is the angle. The data, like the object, are given by a two-dimensional function; however, the independent variables for the data are very much different than the object. The data are ray sums at a particular angle, θ, and distance, x′, from the origin. Below, the direction perpendicular to x′ will be called the y′ direction.

Because the data are a linear combination of the object values, the data collection process can be considered to be transform, the **Radon transform.** Image reconstruction in the absence

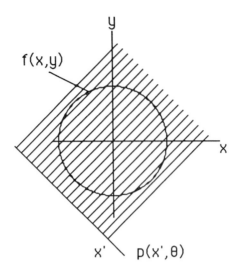

FIGURE 31.1. Projection: the projection of an object, f(x,y), at an angle, θ, results in data, p(x',θ). The lines represent the rays along which the data is summed.

of noise is then an inverse Radon transform. The Radon transform transforms a signal from the object domain into the ray sum domain. The inverse Radon transform transforms a signal from the ray sum domain back to the object domain. Radon[1] described the mathematics of transforming between these two domains in 1917. We shall not use this point of view; rather, we shall use an initial operation (back projection) so that we can consider the data collection process as a space domain operation.

Each pixel, f(x,y) contributes to the datum, p(x'θ), where x' is the projection of the position, x,y, onto the x' axis. The ray sum is the sum of pixel values for which the pixel location, x,y, projects to x'. The operation of projecting the point at x,y to the subspace defined by the x' axis was described in Chapter 8. In the mathematical sense, it is the pixel locations which are projected to determine the appropriate x', not the pixel values. However, in radiology, the term projection has come to be used to describe the ray summing operation. This usage is not mathematically correct, but it is prevalent.

There are several different geometries for collection of X-ray computed tomographic data. For example, it is more common to collect the data using a fan beam than the pencil beam used in Figure 31.1. Several interesting algorithms have been developed to deal directly with data in this format. However, the data can always be rearranged into the format shown in Figure 31.1, and this format is the easiest for understanding the basic principles of reconstruction.

We shall use the system, A{·}, to describe the data collection process:

$$p(x',\theta) = A\{f(x,y)\} \tag{31.3}$$

where f(x,y) is the cross-sectional object, p(x',θ) is the projection data, and A{·} is the projection operation. In vector, matrix notation we shall write:

$$\mathbf{p} = A \cdot \mathbf{f} \tag{31.4}$$

where $\mathbf{f}$ is the object, A is the projection operation (the Radon transform), and $\mathbf{p}$ is the projection data. The vector, matrix notation assumes that the system, A, is a linear system; the output values are a weighted sum of the input values.

II. BACK PROJECTION

One method of reconstructing the data is to back project the ray sums to the object space. Back projection is similar to projection in that the same pixels are related to the ray sum. From the single ray sum value, there is no information about which pixels along the ray contributed how much to the sum. Therefore, during back projection, the value of the ray sum is distributed equally to each pixel along the ray. At a single projection angle, the back projected data will vary along the x' direction, but not along the y' direction.

The projection, back projection operation is analogous to the original form of tomography used in radiology which we shall call **blurring tomography.** In blurring tomography, data are obtained at several different angles. The X-ray beam and film are manipulated so that only one plane is in focus and other planes are out of focus. Data in overlying planes are blurred. In a projection,, back projection image, the data from the different angles reinforce at the position of the original data, and are blurred at other positions.

We shall use the system, $B\{\cdot\}$, to describe the back projection operation:

$$g(x,y) = B\{p(x',\theta)\} \tag{31.5}$$

where $g(x,y)$ is the projected, back projected image. In vector matrix notation:

$$g = B \cdot p \tag{31.6}$$

where B is a matrix which performs the back projection operation and g is a vector representing the projected, back projected image. The back projection operation is not be used in the vector, matrix model during reconstruction, but it is included here to emphasize the analogies between these the two models.

The projection, back projection operation can be written:

$$g(x,y) = B\{A\{f(x,y)\}\} \tag{31.7}$$

We shall use the system $D\{\cdot\}$ to represent the projection, back projection operation:

$$g(x,y) = D\{f(x,y)\} \tag{31.8}$$

In linear algebra notation:

$$g = B \cdot A \cdot f = D \cdot f \tag{31.9}$$

where D represents the projection, back projection operation. Figure 31.2 shows a diagram of the projection, back projection operation in the linear system notation, and Figure 31.3 shows a diagram of this operation in the linear algebra notation.

In the next chapter when the effects of noise are considered, image reconstruction will be considered as an estimation problem. The original object is estimated from the projected data samples. In Chapter 34, we shall consider how to combine several different data values to a single estimate. In that chapter we shall see that the back projection operation can be viewed as an optimal method of combining the projection data. But more of that later.

Let us consider the point spread function of the projection, back projection operation. For each angle we can define a projection, back projection operation, $d_\theta(x,y)$, and an output, $g_\theta(x,y)$. For each angle the projection, back projection operation is equivalent to convolution with a one-dimensional delta function, $\delta(x')$:

$$g_\theta(x,y) = f(x,y) * \delta(x')/N \tag{31.10}$$

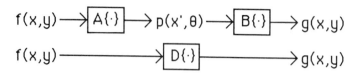

FIGURE 31.2.   Projection, back projection: the object, f(x,y), is projected with the system, A{·}, to produce the data, p(x',θ). The data, p(x',θ), is back projected with the system, B{·}, to produce the projected, back projected image, g(x,y). The system, D{·}, is equivalent to the projection, back projection operation, B{A{·}}.

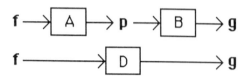

FIGURE 31.3.   Vector, matrix model of projection, back projection: the object represented by the vector, **f**, is projected by the system represented by the matrix, A, to produce the data represented by the vector, **p**. Back projection to the vector, **g**, is represented by the matrix, B. The matrix, D, represents the projection, back projection operation, B · A.

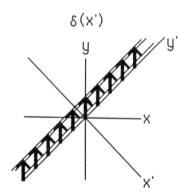

FIGURE 31.4.   One-dimensional delta function: the one-dimensional delta function, δ(x'), is equal to infinity along the y' axis and is equal to zero elsewhere. The integral of δ(x') in the x' direction is one.

where N is a normalization factor (for the discrete case N is equal to the number of pixels along the beam path).

Figure 31.4 shows a representation of δ(x') on the x,y coordinate system. δ(x') is infinite for x' equal to zero, zero elsewhere, and the one-dimensional integral along the x' axis is equal to one. The notation captures the key element — that δ(x') is a delta function in the x' direction.

Figure 31.5 shows a diagram of the projection operation for f(x,y) equal to δ(x,y). For each projection angle, there will be a single nonzero value in the signal, p(x',θ). The back projections of these projections, shown in Figure 31.6, results in a star pattern. All of the rays reinforce at the origin. The rays spread out as they move away from the origin. The distance between the rays increases with the distance, r, from the origin (where r is equal to $\sqrt{(x^2 + y^2)}$, see Chapter 6).

The density of the rays at distance, r, from the origin is given by 1/r. In the limit as the the number of angles becomes infinite, the point spread function can be given by:

$$d(x,y) = 1/r \tag{31.11}$$

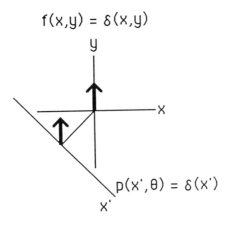

FIGURE 31.5. Projection of δ(x,y): the projection of δ(x,y) at angle, θ, has a single nonzero point at x' equal to zero.

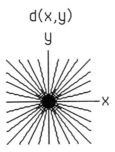

FIGURE 31.6. Projection, back projection point spread function: the point spread function of the projection, back projection operation is shown diagrammatically. The back projected rays reinforce at the origin. The intensity of point spread function decreases proportionally to the distance from the origin, r. The projection, back projection operation blurs the delta function.

There are a number of mathematical problems with this point spread function. It requires an infinite number of angles. It is infinite at the origin. And, it has an infinite extent.

In any real imaging system, X-ray beams are not infinitely thin. Therefore, a finite number of angles suffice, and the point spread function will not be infinite. However, the problem with the infinite extent of the point spread function is more complicated. The extent of the point spread function means that for any finite imaging system, the point spread function is not shift invariant. As the object is shifted in the field of view of the imaging system, the point spread function will vary significantly. Figure 31.7 shows the point spread function at the edge of the imaging system. It is obviously much different from Figure 31.6.

For now, we shall consider only infinite extent imaging systems. For an infinite extent imaging system, the point spread function, d(x,y), is shift invariant, so the projection back projection operation can be written as a convolution:

$$g(x,y) = f(x,y) * d(x,y) \qquad (31.12)$$

This relationship is shown in Figure 31.8. Below we shall see how the reconstruction process allows us to use this formulation with finite extent image systems. However, shift invariance is a property of the whole projection, back projection, reconstruction process, not the projection, back projection process itself. Making the process shift invariant is one of the key aspects of the reconstruction process.

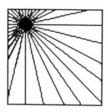

FIGURE 31.7.   Point spread function with a limited field of view: this figure shows the point spread function at the edge of the field of view. It is much different from the point spread function shown in Figure 31.6. The point spread function of the projection, back projection operation is not shift invariant when the field of view is noninfinite.

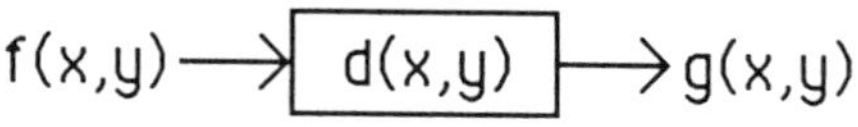

$$f(x,y) \longrightarrow \boxed{d(x,y)} \longrightarrow g(x,y)$$

FIGURE 31.8.   Linear, shift invariant projection, back projection model: d(x,y) is the system function for a linear, shift invariant model of the projection, back projection operation. The object, f(x,y), is convolved with d(x,y) to produce the projected, back projected image, g(x,y).

III. PROJECTION, SLICE THEOREM

The projection, $p(x',\theta)$, provides information about the variations of f(x,y) in the x' direction. It provides no information in the y' direction. For a single angle, the projection, back projection data, $g_\theta(x,y)$, has a constant value in the y' direction. Thus, we might expect that a projection will provide information about the spatial frequency variations along the $k_{x'}$ direction, but that it will only provide information for $k_{y'}$ equal to zero.

This heuristic conclusion can be derived mathematically. For angle θ equal to zero, the x' axis is colinear with the x axis. The projection is given by:

$$p_{\theta=0}(x) = \int_{-\infty}^{+\infty} f(x,y) \, dy \tag{31.13}$$

where $p_{\theta=0}(x)$ has been used instead of p(x,0) to emphasize that θ is being held constant. The projection is just the integral along the y axis.

The values of the Fourier transform of f(x,y) along the k_x axis are given by $F(k_x,0)$. Setting k_y equal to zero in Equation 14.33 gives:

$$F(k_x,0) = \int_{-\infty}^{+\infty} \int_{-\infty}^{+\infty} f(x,y) \cdot e^{ik_x x} \, dxdy \tag{31.14}$$

Since k_y is equal zero, the sinusoid in Equation 31.14 is not a function of y. Therefore, Equation 31.14 can be rearranged:

$$F(k_x,0) = \int_{-\infty}^{+\infty} \left[\int_{-\infty}^{+\infty} f(x,y) \, dy \right] \cdot e^{ik_x x} \, dx \tag{31.15}$$

Using Equation 31.13, the inner integral in Equation 31.15 can be identified as the projection $p_{\theta=0}(x)$. Therefore:

$$F(k_x,0) = \int_{-\infty}^{+\infty} p_{\theta=0}(x) \cdot e^{ik_x x} \, dx \tag{31.16}$$

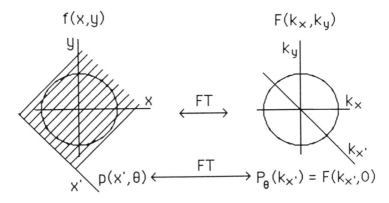

FIGURE 31.9.   Projection, slice theorem: on the left is the projection, p(x',θ), of the object, f(x,y). The Fourier transform of the projection with respect to x', $P_\theta(k_{x'})$, is equal to a slice of the Fourier transform of $F(k_x,k_y)$ in the θ direction.

The right side of Equation 31.16 is the Fourier transform of $p_{\theta=0}$ (x) with respect to x. Therefore:

$$F(k_x,0) = P_{\theta=0}(k_x) \tag{31.17}$$

The values of the Fourier transform of f(x,y) along the k_x axis are equal to the the Fourier transform of the projection of f(x,y) onto the x axis.

In Chapter 20, it was shown that rotation in the space domain results in the same rotation in the transform domain (Equation 20.16). Thus:

$$F(k_{x'},0) = P_\theta(k_{x'}) \tag{31.18}$$

where $k_{x'}$ is the spatial frequency variable in the x' direction. Let us define the one-dimensional set of points along the $k_{x'}$ axis as a slice of the Fourier transform. The projection, slice theorem says that **the Fourier transform of the projection of an object at angle, θ, is equal to a slice of the Fourier transform of the object along angle, θ.** The projection, slice theorem is shown diagrammatically in Figure 31.9.

The projection, back projection for a single angle, θ, is given by $g_\theta(x,y)$. The Fourier transform of $g_\theta(x,y)$ along the $k_{x'}$ axis is equal to the Fourier transform of the projection. By Equation 31.18, it is also equal to the Fourier transform of f(x,y) along the $k_{x'}$ axis. The projection, back projection operation does not alter the data along the x' direction. Since $g_\theta(x,y)$ is constant in the y' direction, the Fourier transform is nonzero only for $k_{y'}$ equal to zero. Therefore,

$$G_\theta(k_{x'},k_{y'}) = F(k_{x'},k_{y'}) \cdot \delta(k_{y'}) \tag{31.19}$$

The projection, back projection operation removes all of the frequencies in the object along the $k_{y'}$ direction except for those at $k_{y'}$ equal to zero.

The one-dimensional delta function, $\delta(k_{y'})$, is the Fourier transform of the one-dimensional delta function, $\delta(x')$. Convolution with the delta function, $\delta(x')$, in the space domain results in a constant in the y' direction. The constant in the y' direction results in a delta function, $\delta(k_{y'})$, in the spatial frequency domain. Convolution by $\delta(x')$ in the space domain is equivalent to multiplication by $\delta(k_{y'})$ in the spatial frequency domain.

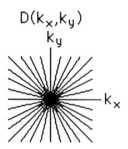

$$D(k_x, k_y)$$

FIGURE 31.10. Spatial frequency representation of the projection, back projection point spread function: the spatial frequency domain representation of the point spread function of the projection, back projection operation is $D(k_x, k_y)$. For an infinite number of angles, $D(k_x, k_y)$ is equal to $1/k$.

IV. PROJECTION, BACK PROJECTION AS SPATIAL FREQUENCY SAMPLES

In the space domain, the projection, back projection data are relatively complex. It is the convolution of the cross-sectional data with the one-dimensional delta functions, $\delta(x')$. The projected, back projected image is a complicated linear combination of the cross-sectional object. In the spatial frequency domain, the projection, back projection data for each angle are equal to the cross section along the $k_{x'}$ direction. The computed tomographic data can be view as samples of the spatial frequency of the object.

Figure 31.10 shows the data from a series of projections in terms of the spatial frequencies. The data samples form a star pattern in the spatial frequency domain. The samples are closest together near the origin and they spread out with increasing distance. The distance between the samples in the radial direction increases as k where k is the distance from the origin, $\sqrt{(k_x^2 + k_y^2)}$. (k Is the radial, polar, spatial frequency variable analogous to r in the space domain.)

The sum of the projection, back projection data from each angle is equal to data from the original cross section at the points shown in Figure 31.10. The density of samples decreases with the distance, k, from the origin. The low spatial frequencies are sampled more finely than the high spatial frequencies. Because there is a greater contribution from the low spatial frequencies, the projection back projection data are a smoothed version of the cross section.

This conclusion is not new. In the last chapter we argued that since computed tomographic data are a sum of positive values, the data collection process tends to smooth the data. However, Figure 31.10 shows exactly how the data are sampled. We can see that the projection, back projection operation is equivalent to multiplying the spatial frequency representation of the cross section by $1/k$. For an infinite number of angles the projected, back projected image can be given mathematically:

$$G(k_x, k_y) = F(k_x, k_y) \cdot (1/k) \tag{31.20}$$

Comparing Equations 31.12 and 31.20 we can see that:

$$D(k_x, k_y) = 1/k \tag{31.21}$$

Above, it was shown that in the space domain the projection, back projection system function is given by:

$$d(x, y) = 1/r \tag{31.22}$$

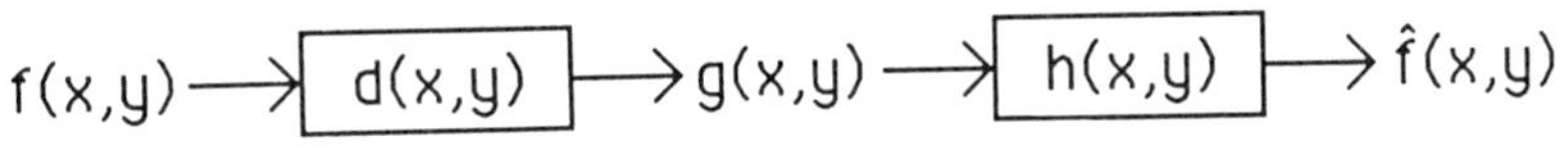

FIGURE 31.11. Data collection, reconstruction model: this figure shows a linear, shift invariant model of the data collection reconstruction process. The projection, back projection operation is represented by $d(x,y)$. The reconstruction is represented by the filter, $h(x,y)$. The object, $f(x,y)$, passes though the system, $d(x,y)$, to produce the projected, back projected image, $g(x,y)$. $g(x,y)$ is filtered by $h(x,y)$ to produce the estimate, $\hat{f}(x,y)$, of the original object.

In Chapter 14, it was stated that in two dimensions the Fourier transform of $1/r$ is equal to $1/k$ (Equation 14.35). Similarly, this Chapter has shown that the system function of the projection, back projection operation is $1/r$ in the space domain, and it is $1/k$ in the spatial frequency domain.

V. RECONSTRUCTION FILTER

We have shown that the data collection process smooths the data. The projected, back projected image is smoothed by a filter given by $1/r$ in the space domain and $1/k$ in the spatial frequency domain. In the absence of noise, the original image can be reconstructed by sharpening the projected, back projected image. Reconstruction amounts to deconvolving the effects of $d(x,y)$ on $g(x,y)$.

Figure 31.11 shows the image collection, reconstruction process diagrammatically. The projected, back projected image, $g(x,y)$ is filtered with the system, $h(x,y)$, to produce the output, $\hat{f}(x,y)$. The reconstructed image, $\hat{f}(x,y)$, is an estimate of the original cross section, $f(x,y)$.

The system function, $H(k_x,k_y)$, can be determined from Equation 31.20 by inspection:

$$H(k_x,k_y) = k \tag{31.23}$$

The system function increases linearly with distance from the origin. The estimate, $\hat{F}(k_x,k_y)$, is equal to:

$$\hat{F}(k_x,k_y) = k \cdot (1/k) \cdot F(k_x,k_y) \tag{31.24}$$

Thus,

$$\hat{F}(k_x,k_y) = F(k_x,k_y) \tag{31.25}$$

Except for the point at the origin, the estimate is equal to the object.

The system function, $H(k_x,k_y)$, given by Equation 31.23 is called a **ramp filter**. There are some problems with this function. As k increases in any direction, the function goes to infinity. In any practical implementation, the X-ray beams will not be infinitely thin. Therefore, the resolution of the data collection will be limited. Above the limit of resolution, $H(k_x,k_y)$, can be set equal to zero.

Figure 31.12 shows this type of $H(k_x,k_y)$ and its Fourier transform, $h(x,y)$. $h(x,y)$ has the shape of a sharpening filter. It is positive in the center with negative side lobes.

Equation 31.20 is a model of data collection. From this model, we were able to determine how the image is reconstructed by inspection. Almost all of the work is developing a good model of the data collection process. Given a good model, reconstruction is very easy to understand.

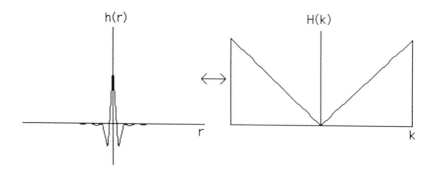

FIGURE 31.12.   Ramp filter: the ramp filter is shown on the right. It increases in direct proportion to the spatial frequency, k, up to a cut-off frequency. On the left is the inverse Fourier transform of the ramp filter.

VI. FOURIER TRANSFORM RECONSTRUCTION

Image reconstruction can be implemented using a number of methods. Above we have described filtering of projected, back projected data. However, for noninfinite image systems, projection, back projection is not shift invariant. Although it is easy to understand reconstruction in terms of a projection, back projection, filter model, filtering a back projection image is not a practical algorithm.

A more practical algorithm is called Fourier transform reconstruction. Since Fourier transforms are used in a variety of reconstruction methods, this name is not very descriptive, but there is no other commonly used name for this algorithm. Fourier transform reconstruction takes advantage of the relation between the Fourier transform of the projection data and the object. From Equation 31.18, the Fourier transform of a projection, $P_\theta(k_{x'})$, is equal to the Fourier transform of the object, $F(k_{x'}, \theta)$, in terms of a polar coordinate system.

The samples, $F(k_{x'}, 0)$ of the Fourier transform are on a polar grid. The fast Fourier transform algorithm is defined for a rectangular coordinate system. Therefore, in order to determine the Fourier transform, the points must be interpolated to a rectangular coordinate system. After interpolation, a Fourier transform can be performed. Figure 31.13 shows the steps in this algorithm diagrammatically.

The Fourier transform method does not include an explicit ramp filtering operation. However, the interpolation accomplishes an equivalent effect. The samples are farther apart as the distance, k, from the origin increases. Therefore, a single sample is used in estimating a number of rectilinear samples proportional to the distance, k. The reproduction of a single sample in proportion to k is analogous to ramp filtering. The interpolation makes the density of data points uniform.

VII. CONVOLUTION, BACK PROJECTION RECONSTRUCTION

Image reconstruction can also be performed in the space domain using a convolution, back projection algorithm. The reconstruction filter can be expanded to emphasize the contributions from the different angles:

$$\hat{F}(k_x, k_y) = H(k_x, k_y) \cdot \sum_\theta G_\theta(k_x, k_y) \qquad (31.26)$$

where $G_\theta(k_x, k_y)$ is the projected, back projected image for a single angle, θ. The only nonzero data in, $G_\theta(k_x, k_y)$, is along the k_x' axis.

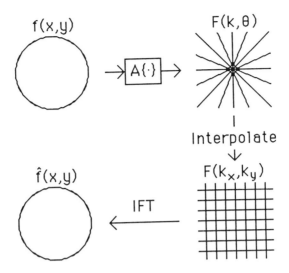

FIGURE 31.13. Fourier transform reconstruction: the spatial frequency domain representation of the projection data are polar samples of the Fourier transform of the object. The polar samples are interpolated to a rectilinear grid. The estimate, $\hat{f}(x,y)$, of the object, $f(x,y)$, is produced by an inverse Fourier transform operation.

$H(k_x,k_y)$ can be moved inside the summation:

$$\hat{F}(k_x,k_y) = \sum_{\theta} H(k_x,k_y) \cdot G_{\theta}(k_x,k_y) \qquad (31.27)$$

Filtering $G(k_x,k_y)$ is equivalent to filtering each of the slices, $G_{\theta}(k_x,k_y)$ separately. Filtering the slice of the transform is the same as filtering the Fourier transform of the projection, $P_{\theta}(k_x)$ with a ramp. Therefore, reconstruction can be performed by filtering each of the projections prior to back projection.

In general it is more efficient to perform a filtering operation by transforming to the frequency domain, multiplying, and inverse transforming. However, when the extent of the space domain representation is small and when special convolution hardware is available, it may be more efficient to filter by convolving in the space domain. In Figure 31.12, the extent of $h(x)$ can be seen to be relatively small. For this reason, most computed tomographic systems implement reconstruction using convolution of each of the slices followed by back projection.

VIII. SUMMARY

Image reconstruction in computed tomography is somewhat more complicated than in nuclear magnetic resonance. It involves a filtering operation instead of just an inverse Fourier transformation. In both cases the description of reconstruction was very simple once a good model of the data collection process is developed.

The description of reconstruction in this chapter relies heavily on the projection, slice theorem. The Fourier transform of a projection is equal to a slice in the spatial frequency domain. This theorem can be used to show that computed tomographic data collection over-samples the low spatial frequencies. The number of samples in the spatial frequency domain decreases with spatial frequency, k. Image reconstruction is performed by filtering by 1/k, the ramp filter.

Linear algebra methods are not used for understanding reconstruction in this chapter.

They will be used in Chapter 33 to explain iterative reconstruction methods. The linear algebra model has been included in parallel with the linear systems model so that the information in this chapter can be correlated with the information in Chapter 33.

The next chapter will consider the effects of noise on reconstruction. Chapter 33 will use a linear model of data collection instead of the linear, shift invariant model used in this chapter. Chapter 34 will use a linear, shift invariant model, but will include several different samples of the data. Each of these models helps to explain different aspects of the reconstruction problem.

IX. FURTHER READING

There are several mathematical difficulties with reconstruction as described in this chapter. For example, the projection, back projection point spread function is infinite at the origin, and it has an infinite extent. A rigorous mathematical demonstration that a cross section could be reconstructed from line integrals was given in 1917 by Radon.[1] The Radon transform and the inverse Radon transform were described briefly in Chapter 20.

The approach in the chapter has been to use the back projection operation to transform the projection data from the x',θ coordinate system to the x,y coordinate system. The projected, back projected data are the starting point for most of the discussion in this chapter. This approach allows the reader to visualize the data in the object coordinate space. The book by Barrett, and Swindell[2] gives more equal weighting to the projection space. It attempts to give the reader a better understanding of the data in that space.

Filtering with the ramp filter was described by Shepp and Logan,[3] and the ramp filter is often referred to as a Shepp and Logan filter. A good description of the projection, slice theorem was given in a review paper by Mersereau and Oppenheim.[4] That paper also discusses ''Fourier transform reconstruction'', and the issues associated with interpolation of the spatial frequency samples. A more recent source for this material is Chapter 7 of the book by Dudgeon and Mersereau.[5]

The goal of this chapter has been to develop a basic understanding of the reconstruction process. There are several practical considerations which have been ignored. For example, in the convolution, back projection algorithm, the method of interpolating from the x',θ coordinate system to the x,y coordinate system has important effects on efficiency and on the accuracy of reconstruction. The discussion in this chapter has assumed that the data are collected as a parallel projection. In actuality, most computed tomography data are collected with fan beam geometry. The reader interested in these and other issues not covered in this chapter should is referred to the book by Kak and Slaney,[6] and the books by Herman.[7,8]

REFERENCES

1. **Radon, J.,** Uber die bestimmung von funktionen durch ihre integralwerte langs gewisser mannigfaltigkeiten, *Ber. Verh. Sachs. Akad. Wiss. Leipzig,* 69, 262, 1917.
2. **Barrett, H. H. and Swindel, W.,** *Radiological Imaging: The Theory of Image Formation, Detection, and Processing,* Academic Press, New York, 1981.
3. **Shepp, L. A. and Logan, B. F.,** The Fourier reconstruction of a head section, *IEEE Trans. Nucl. Sci.,* NS-21, 21, 1974.
4. **Mersereau, R. M. and Oppenheim, A. V.,** Digital reconstruction of multidimensional signals from their projections, *Proc. IEEE,* 62, 1319, 1974.
5. **Dudgeon, D. E. and Mersereau, R. M.,** *Multidimensional Digital Signal Processing,* Prentice-Hall, Englewood Cliffs, NJ, 1984.
6. **Kak, A. C. and Slaney, M.,** *Principles of Computerized Tomographic Imaging,* IEEE Press, New York, 1987.
7. **Herman, G. T.,** *Image Reconstruction from Projections: Implementation and Applications,* Springer-Verlag, Berlin, 1979.
8. **Herman, G. T.,** *Image Reconstruction from Projections: The Fundamentals of Computerized Tomography,* Academic Press, New York, 1980.

Chapter 32

RECONSTRUCTION FROM NOISY PROJECTIONS: COMPUTED TOMOGRAPHY

This chapter will describe image reconstruction from noisy projections similar to those found in computed tomography. The difference between this chapter and the last is that a statistical model of the imaging process will be used.

The model used in this chapter will be the same model used in Chapter 26 for the Wiener deconvolution filter. As in that chapter the deconvolution filter will consist of two parts — deconvolution for the effect of the system and a noise suppression filter. The deconvolution operation will be the same as in the last chapter, and the noise filter will be the Wiener filter from Chapter 26. The results of this chapter bring together the results of these two chapters. The new feature in this chapter will be development of a model for the noise in computed tomography.

I. MODEL

A. DATA COLLECTION

The model of the data collection process will be similar to the model in the last chapter, except that noise will be included. In computed tomography most of the noise occurs during measurement of the ray sums. The noise can be modeled:

$$p(x',\theta) = A\{f(x,y)\} + n'(x',\theta) \tag{32.1}$$

where $p(x',\theta)$ is the projection data, $A\{\cdot\}$ is the projection operation, $f(x,y)$ is the cross-sectional object, and $n'(x',\theta)$ is the noise. Equation 32.1 is analogous to Equation 31.3 except for the noise term, and the statistical nature of the model.

The model is Equation 32.1 uses stochastic processes for both the unknown signal, $f(x,y)$, and the noise, $n'(x,y)$. We shall assume that the stochastic processes are wide sense stationary; in other words, the statistics of the processes do not vary with position. The statistics of the unknown signal allow *a priori* medical information about the cross-sectional object to be used in the reconstruction. This model is most useful when the *a priori* knowledge is well captured by the power spectral density function.

In Chapter 29 we noted that the second-order statistics are not a particularly good method of capturing the *a priori* knowledge about first-pass radionuclide angiocardiography. In that case, constraints on the shape of the curve provide the most useful information. Constraining the shape of the curve can markedly improve the accuracy of the deconvolution.

Usually, there is less *a priori* information about the mathematical form of a cross-sectional object, so the model in Equation 32.1 performs well for computed tomographic reconstruction. However, it is important to remember that in cases where there is considerable *a priori* information about the cross section which is not captured by the second-order statistics, other reconstruction methods may give better results.

The *a priori* information about the instrumentation is provided by the statistics of the noise. Knowledge of the signal to noise ratio as a function of frequency, in the form of the power spectral density functions, will allow the effects of noise to be suppressed.

Equation 32.1 models the noise as an additive term. In computed tomography the noise is not strictly additive. It is related to the intensity of the ray, $p(x',\theta)$. However, it is much simpler to work with the additive noise model, and the results using the additive noise model produce accurate reconstructions.

We shall assume that the expected value of the power of the noise is the same for all

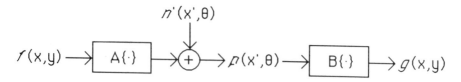

FIGURE 32.1. Data collection model: the projection data, $p(x',\theta)$, are the sum of the cross section, $f(x,y)$, projected by the operator, $A\{\cdot\}$, and the noise, $n'(x',\theta)$. The back projection operator, $B\{\cdot\}$, produces the back projected image, $g(x,y)$, from the data $p(x',\theta)$.

ray sums. The noise for each ray sum is largely independent of the other ray sums. Therefore, the autocorrelation function can be modeled as:

$$R_{n'}(x',\theta) = N^2 \cdot \delta(x',\theta) \tag{32.2}$$

where N is the noise intensity. This model states that the noise for each ray sum is independent of the noise for all other ray sums. However, below we shall find that in the back projected image the noise in one pixel is not independent of noise in other pixels.

In this chapter, the same variables, x' and θ, are used for positions in the stochastic processes and for offsets in the autocorrelation function. In previous chapters we have used t for the stochastic processes and τ for the autocorrelation functions. Hopefully the dual use of the independent variables will not be a source of confusion.

The power spectral density function was defined in Chapter 24 as the Fourier transform of the autocorrelation function (Equation 24.7). The noise power spectral density function is:

$$S_{n'}(k_{x'})|_\theta = N^2 \tag{32.3}$$

where $S_{n'}(k_{x'})|_\theta$ is the one-dimensional power spectral density with respect to the spatial frequency variable, $k_{x'}$, for fixed projection angle, θ. Equation 32.3 states that the noise has equal power at all frequencies. This type of noise process was defined in Chapter 24 as a white noise process.

B. BACK PROJECTION

As in the last chapter, back projection of the data to the original coordinate system will aid the understanding of the model. The back projected image, $g(x,y)$ is defined as:

$$g(x,y) = B\{A\{f(x,y)\}\} + B\{n'(x',\theta)\} \tag{32.4}$$

where $B\{\cdot\}$ is the back projection operator described in the last chapter. This equation is similar to Equation 31.7 except for the noise term. Figure 32.1 shows a diagram of this model.

In the last chapter the projection, back projection operator, $D\{\cdot\}$, was defined. $D\{\cdot\}$ has the advantage that both the input and the output are defined in terms of the object coordinate system. Using this operator, Equation 32.4 can be written:

$$g(x,y) = D\{f(x,y)\} + B\{n'(x',\theta)\} \tag{32.5}$$

This equation is similar to Equation 31.8 except for the noise term.

C. BACK PROJECTED NOISE

One of the conceptual difficulties with reconstructions from projections is that the projection space is defined in terms of coordinates, x',θ, while the object and image spaces

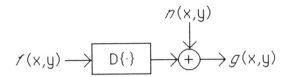

FIGURE 32.2. Modified data collection model: the noise, $n(x,y)$, enters the modified data collection model after the projection, back projection operator, $D\{\cdot\}$. The data, $f(x,y)$, and the back projected image, $g(x,y)$, are the same as in the model shown in Figure 32.1.

are defined in terms of coordinates, x,y. By using the back projection operator, it was possible to define the image data in terms of the x,y coordinates in Chapter 31 (see Equation 31.8). Unfortunately, the model given by Equation 32.5 mixes the x,y and x',θ coordinate systems.

Figure 32.2 shows a model of the data collection process with the noise added after the back projection. The noise, $n(x,y)$, is defined to be equal to the back projected noise, $B\{n'(x',\theta)\}$. This model can be written:

$$g(x,y) = D\{f(x,y)\} + n(x,y) \tag{32.6}$$

However, there is still a considerable amount of work to be done. The statistics of $n(x,y)$ need to be determined in terms of the statistics of $n'(x',\theta)$.

D. BACK PROJECTED NOISE POWER SPECTRAL DENSITY

The back projected noise is the sum of the back projected noises at each angle:

$$n(x,y) = \sum_{\theta} n_\theta(x,y) \tag{32.7}$$

where $n_\theta(x,y)$ is the back projected noise for the data from a single projection angle, θ. The autocorrelation function for $n_\theta(x,y)$ is equal to the autocorrelation function for $n'(x',\theta)$ in the x' direction. In the y' direction the noise is perfectly correlated. Therefore, the auto-correlation function is constant in the y' direction:

$$R_{n_\theta}(x',y') = R_{n_\theta}(x',0) = R_{n'}(x',\theta)|_\theta \tag{32.8}$$

where $R_{n'}(x',\theta)|_\theta$ is the autocorrelation function of $n'(x',\theta)$ for a fixed projection angle, θ.

The power spectral density function for $n_\theta(x,y)$ will be equal to $S_{n'}(k_{x'})|_\theta$ along the $k_{x'}$ axis:

$$S_{n_\theta}(k_{x'},0) = S_{n'}(k_{x'})|_\theta \tag{32.9}$$

Elsewhere it will be equal to zero. The back projected noise power spectral density function for a single projection angle is nonzero along a slice in the spatial frequency domain. In back projecting from the x',θ coordinates to the x,y coordinates, the notation has become a bit obscure, but the concepts should not be obscure. The power spectral density function for back projected noise from a single projection angle is a two-dimensional function, $S_{n_\theta}(k_x,k_y)$. Equation 32.9 states that along the $k_{x'}$ axis it is equal to the one dimensional power spectral density function of the noise defined in the projection space.

The autocorrelation function, $R_n(x,y)$, for the back projected noise from all projection angles is a sum of terms of the form $E\{n_{\theta i}(\cdot) \cdot n_{\theta j}(\cdot)\}$, where $n_{\theta i}(\cdot)$ is the back projected noise for projection θ_i. Since the noise is uncorrelated with respect to projection angle, θ, the only nonzero terms are for θ_i equal to θ_j. The terms, $E\{n_{\theta i}(\cdot) \cdot n_{\theta i}(\cdot)\}$ give the noise power for a single projection angle. Thus, the noise power in $n(x,y)$ is the sum of the noise powers for each back projection angle, $n_\theta(x,y)$. The key point in simplifying this description is the fact that the noise is not correlated with projection angle.

In the last paragraph we have argued that the noise autocorrelation function, $R_n(x,y)$, is the sum of the autocorrelation functions for the noise at each angle, $R_{n_\theta}(x,y)$. Since the Fourier transform is a linear operation, the power spectral density function, $S(k_x,k_y)$, is the sum of the power spectral density functions at each angle:

$$S_n(k_x,k_y) = \sum_\theta S_{n_\theta}(k_x,k_y) \qquad (32.10)$$

Above it has been shown that the power spectral density functions for the back projected noise at each angle, $S_{n_\theta}(k_x,k_y)$, is nonzero only along the $k_{x'}$ axis.

As described in the last chapter, the slices in the spatial frequency domain are closer together near the origin, and farther apart at high frequency. For an infinite number of angles, the density of slices along which the noise is defined falls of by $1/k$, where k is the radial spatial frequency variable. If the noise is not a function of the angle, the power spectral density function for the back projected noise is given by:

$$S_n(k_x,k_y) = S_{n'}(k)/k \qquad (32.11)$$

where $S_{n'}(k)$ is the one-dimensional noise power spectral density function defined in the projection space.

In Equation 32.3, the noise added to each projection is assumed to be white. Substituting Equation 32.3 into Equation 32.11 gives:

$$S_n(k_x,k_y) = N^2/k \qquad (32.12)$$

If the noise added to the image is white, the noise in the back projected image is not white. In the back projected image the noise is scaled by $1/k$.

E. BACK PROJECTED SIGNAL POWER SPECTRAL DENSITY

The last chapter showed that the projection, back projection operation, $D\{\cdot\}$, could be model as a linear, time invariant system. Therefore, Equation 32.6 can be written:

$$g(x,y) = f(x,y) * d(x,y) + n(x,y) \qquad (32.13)$$

In the last chapter it was shown that the system function, $d(x,y)$, is equal to $1/r$ where r is the radial, polar variable. The two-dimensional Fourier transform of $1/r$ is $1/k$ (see Equations 14.34 and 14.35). Thus, the system, $d(x,y)$, has the affect of filtering the data by $1/k$.

In Chapter 24, the affect of a filter on a stationary stochastic process was found by multiplying the power spectral density function by the squared magnitude of the filter. Thus, the power spectral density of the back projected image can be given by:

$$S_g(k_x,k_y) = S_f(k_x,k_y)/k^2 + S_n(k_x,k_y) \qquad (32.14)$$

The first term, $S_f(k_x,k_y)/k^2$, is the power spectral density of the signal. The second term, $S_n(k_x,k_y)$, is the power spectral density of the noise.

The projection, back projection operation scales the power spectral density function of the signal by $1/k^2$. Equation 32.12 shows that the back projection operation scales the noise by $1/k$. The difference between these two operations is that the contribution of the signal

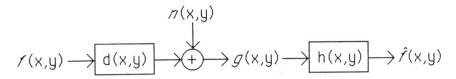

FIGURE 32.3. Linear, shift invariant reconstruction model: the projection, back projection operator is modeled as a linear, shift invariant system, d(x,y). The back projected image, g(x,y), is the sum of the projected, back projected cross-sectional object, f(x,y)*d(x,y), and the noise, n(x,y). The linear, shift invariant system, h(x,y), produces the estimate, $\hat{f}$(x,y) from the back projected image.

to the data is correlated between projections, whereas the noise is uncorrelated between projections.

F. RECONSTRUCTION MODEL

This chapter will consider linear, shift invariant reconstruction. Any linear, shift invariant reconstruction can be modeled as convolution with a function, h(x,y):

$$\hat{f}(x,y) = g(x,y) * h(x,y) \tag{32.15}$$

where $\hat{f}$(x,y) is the estimate of the object, f(x,y). h(x,y) are the estimation factors.

The model given by Equations 32.13 and 32.15 is shown diagrammatically in Figure 32.3. The projection, back projection operation, d(x,y), is equal to 1/r. The noise is added after the projection, back projection operation. h(x,y) is the image reconstruction filter. The model shown in Figure 32.3 is similar to the model show in Figure 26.2 which was used for Wiener deconvolution.

II. IMAGE RECONSTRUCTION

The image collection, reconstruction model given in Figure 32.3 is the same model given for Wiener deconvolution in Chapter 26. Therefore, the solution to that problem can be used directly. With appropriate substitution of variables, Equation 26.60 can be written:

$$H(k_x,k_y) = 1/D(k_x,k_y) \cdot S_f(k_x,k_y)/[S_f(k_x,k_y) + S_n(k_x,k_y)/|D(k_x,k_y)|^2] \tag{32.16}$$

The system function $D(k_x,k_y)$ is equal to 1/k, the radial, spatial frequency variable. Thus, Equation 32.16 can be rewritten:

$$H(k_x,k_y) = k \cdot S_f(k_x,k_y)/[S_f(k_x,k_y) + k^2 \cdot S_n(k_x,k_y)] \tag{32.17}$$

The first factor in Equation 32.17 is the ramp filter, k. It deconvolves the data for the effect of the projection, back projection operation. The second factor is a Wiener filter. It is in the form of a ratio of the signal over the signal plus the noise. Equation 32.17 can be written:

$$H(k_x,k_y) = H_1(k_x,k_y) \cdot H_2(k_x,k_y) \tag{32.18}$$

where $H_1 (k_x,k_y)$ is equal to the ramp filter k, and $H_2 (k_x,k_y)$ is equal to the Wiener filter $S_f(k_x,k_y)/[S_f(k_x,k_y) + k^2 \cdot S_n(k_x,k_y)]$. Image reconstruction consists of two factors — one undoes the smoothing due to the data collection process, the other filters the noise.

In Chapter 26, it was shown that multiplication of the noise by $1/|D((k_x,k_y)|^2$ was needed since the signal and the noise enter the model at different points. Division by $1/|D((k_x,k_y)|^2$ is equivalent to moving the noise to the other side of the projection, back projection operator where it can be compared directly to the signal.

As in the previous chapters, image reconstruction is simple to derive once we have developed a good model of the system. Some of the simplicity in this chapter relates to the fact that the solution to a problem of the form given by Equation 32.6 has already been derived in Chapter 26. However, one of the values of developing a good model is that it allows one to notice the analogies between problems. If the analogies between problems are noted, previously derived solutions can be applied to new problems without need to rederive the solution.

In order to solve Equation 32.17 we need a model of the power spectral density functions of the signal and the noise. Above we have assumed that the noise added to the projection data is white (Equation 32.3). The noise power is the same at all spatial frequencies. The power spectral density function for the back projected noise, $n(x,y)$, is given by Equation 32.12.

$$S_n(k_x,k_y) = N^2/k \qquad (32.19)$$

In the back projected image, the noise is not white.

It is very reasonable to assume that the signal power spectral density function is radially symmetric:

$$S_f(k_x,k_y) = S_f(k) \qquad (32.20)$$

In other words, the average signal intensity is the same at all distances from the origin in the spatial frequency domain. As a general rule, the power in a cross section decreases rapidly with increases in spatial frequency.

Substituting Equations 32.19 and 32.20 into Equation 32.17 gives:

$$H(k) = k \cdot S_f(k)/[S_f(k) + k \cdot N^2] \qquad (32.21)$$

The second factor in Equation 32.21 is the Wiener filter, $H_2(k)$. When k is small, $H_2(k)$ is equal to one. When k is large, $H_2(k)$ is equal to $S_f(k)/k \cdot N^2$. The transition between these two forms is determined by the signal to noise ratio, $S_f(k)/k \cdot N^2$. $H_2(k)$ is equal to 1/2 when k is equal to $S_f(k)/N^2$.

Figure 32.4 shows the signal and the noise power spectral density functions and the Wiener filter, $H_2(k)$. The signal power spectral density function falls off with increasing frequency. The noise power spectral density function is white; it is equal to N^2 at all frequencies. The Wiener filter, $H_2(k)$, is equal to one for low k. It then falls off around k equal to $S_f(k)/N^2$. For large k, where it is equal to $S_f(k)/k \cdot N^2$, it falls off more rapidly than $S_f(k)$.

Figure 32.5 shows the two components of H(k). The ramp filter, $H_1(k)$, is shown in the top panel, the Wiener filter, $H_2(k)$, is shown in the middle panel, and their product, H(k), is shown in the bottom panel. At low frequency, the filter, H(k), goes up like the ramp, k. At high frequency, the filter is equal to $S_f(k)/N^2$. At high frequency it falls off like the signal power spectral density function.

The data, $g(x,y)$, is the sum of the projected, back projected object, $f(x,y)*d(x,y)$, and the noise, $n(x,y)$. The low spatial frequencies in the cross section, $f(x,y)$, are sampled more densely than the high spatial frequencies. There is more information about the low spatial frequencies in the data. At the low spatial frequencies, the reconstruction filter is equal to the ramp filter — the reconstruction filter used in noiseless reconstruction. The reconstruction ignores the noise. At the higher frequencies, the data are sampled less densely; there is less information about the object. Thus, the noise suppression is more important.

It is sometimes said that the projection reconstruction algorithm tends to amplify the high frequencies in the noise. As we have modeled the system, it is more appropriate to

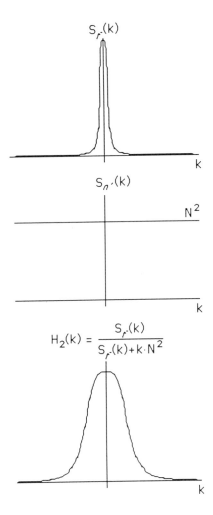

FIGURE 32.4. Wiener filter: the top panel shows the power spectral density function, $S_f(k)$, of the cross-sectional object. Most of the power in the object is at low frequencies. The middle panel shows the noise power spectral density, $S_{n'}(k)$. $S_{n'}(k)$ is a white noise process. The bottom panel shows the Wiener filter, $H_2(k)$, used for reconstruction.

say that the projection reconstruction samples the high frequencies in the object less accurately.

III. IMPLEMENTATION

Image reconstruction in the presence of noise can be implemented in the same way as reconstruction in the absence of noise. The filter given by Equation 32.21 can be used instead of the ramp filter in the filtered back projection algorithm. Applying the filter to each projection prior to back projection filters the final image. In the "Fourier method", the second factor, the Wiener filter, can be applied to the spatial frequencies in either the polar or the rectilinear format.

Figure 32.6 shows both the space and spatial frequency representations of the ramp filter and the Wiener filter modified, ramp filter. They have generally the same shape, except that the ramp filter has an oscillatory behavior not seen with the Wiener filter modified, ramp filter. The oscillations in the space domain are due to the sharp cut-off of the filter in the spatial frequency domain (see Chapter 16).

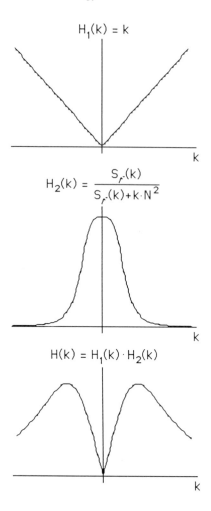

FIGURE 32.5.   Reconstruction filter: the reconstruction filter, H(k), is the product of the ramp filter, $H_1(k)$, and the Wiener filter, $H_2(k)$.

Figure 32.6 shows one of the difficulties with the ramp filter. With perfect data, the ramp filter results in exact reconstruction. With less than perfect data, the sharp transition at the cut-off frequency can produce ringing in the space domain. This ringing can be seen in computed tomographic images near the edge of high contrast edges such as those seen near bones. One of the advantaages of the Wiener filter is that it rolls off the sharp transition at the cut-off frequency.

The Wiener filter provides the best linear, shift invariant, least mean square estimate of the object. For a particular application, this may or may not provide the best image. For example, it may be desirable to perform some edge enhancement or smoothing of the image of the object, particularly, when the goal is to present the object to the radiologist. Although the higher spatial frequencies may have less power thant the lower frequencies, they may be of most use in a particular interest. If this is the case it may be desirable to modify the filter, H(k), to include an additional image enhancement filter, $H_3(k)$. Many image recon-struction algorithms may allow an adjustable filter. The adjustment is not to change the reconstruction, but to allow for other types of filtering.

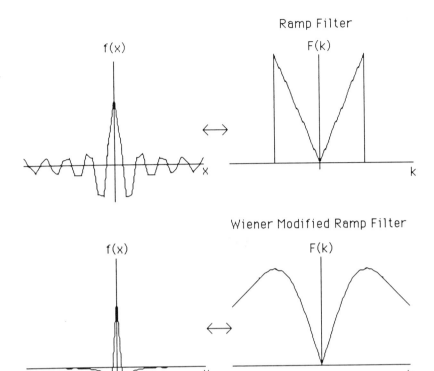

FIGURE 32.6. Comparison of reconstruction filters: the top panel shows the space and spatial frequency domain representations of the ramp filter. The bottom panel shows the space and spatial frequency domain representations of the reconstruction filter shown in Figure 32.5. The sharp cut off of the ramp filter results in oscillations in the space domain which are not seen with the Wiener modified ramp filter.

IV. SUMMARY

Data collection in computed tomography can be most easily understood by comparison of the models shown in Figure 32.1 and 32.2. The noise enters the system after the projection operation. The most difficult problem with using the projection, back projection model from the last chapter is understanding the power spectral density function of the noise in the back projected image.

Because the noise from different projections is uncorrelated, the back projected noise power spectral density is the sum of the power spectral densities of the noise for each angle. Since the density of the samples in the spatial frequency domain is equal to 1/k, the back projected noise power spectral density function is related to the noise power spectral density function in the projection space divided by k.

In Figure 32.3 reconstruction is modeled as linear, shift invariant filtering of the back projected data. The filtering consists of two or three factors. The first factor in the filter is the ramp filter, k, which performs the reconstruction; it corrects for the high sampling density at the low frequencies.

The second factor is a Wiener filter which reduces the noise. The Wiener filter attenuates the higher frequencies where the noise may predominate with respect to the signal. There may be a third factor which performs an image enhancement operation such as edge enhancement. Although image enhancement is not part of the reconstruction process, it is convenient to include it with the reconstruction filter.

Although the filter is generally implemented in a single filtering operation, it is easiest to understand these various functions as separate factors. The ramp portion of the filter will always predominate in the low frequency, densely sampled region. The noise reduction filter will predominate at high frequencies where the signal has less power and is less densely sampled. The image enhancement filter is less clearly defined, and selection of the ideal filter may involve some empirical determination of image quality. However, an understanding of the factors involved may aid in directing an empirical search.

V. FURTHER READING

The model of the computed tomographic noise in this chapter is quite simple. It is also somewhat inexact. For a more careful discussion of the noise in computed tomography, the reader is referred to the article by Riederer.[1]

This chapter has separated the problem of reconstruction from noisy projections into two parts — exact reconstruction with with $H_1(k)$, and noise suppression with $H_2(k)$. The references to exact reconstruction are found in the last chapter, and the references to noise suppressions are found in Chapter 26 (Wiener Filtering). The references in the last chapter also generally include some discussion on noise in computed tomography (see for example, the book by Kak and Slaney[2]).

A discussion which is beyond the scope of this book is the choice of an image enhancement filter, $H_3(k)$. The reconstruction and noise enhancement filters are choosen by minimizing the mean square error between the estimate of the object and   true object. Criteria for the image enhancement filter are much less straight forward. The simplest criteria are subjective — the image should look better after filtering. More objective criteria require use of performance measurements such as receiver operating characteristic, ROC, curves.

REFERENCES

1. **Riederer, S. J., Pelc, N. J., and Chesler, D. A.,** The noise power spectrum in computed x-ray tomography, *Phys. Med. Biol.,* 23, 446, 1978.
2. **Kak, A. C. and Slaney, M.,** *Principles of Computerized Tomographic Imaging,* IEEE Press, New York, 1987.

Chapter 33

ITERATIVE RECONSTRUCTION: SINGLE PHOTON EMISSION COMPUTED TOMOGRAPHY

The last three chapters have dealt with linear, shift invariant reconstruction. In this chapter we shall consider linear, nonshift invariant reconstruction applied to single photon emission computed tomography. Since shift invariance greatly simplifies the model of a system, it is always best to try to formulate a problem so that it is shift invariant. When the deviations from shift invariance are small, it may be possible to use a shift invariant model with a correction. However, the deviation from shift invariance are so great with single photon emission computed tomography, that a nonshift invariant model provides the most realistic description of the problem.

Linear, nonshift invariant systems were presented in the description of linear algebra in Chapters 8, 9, 19, and 25. It might be best to review these chapters prior to reading the current chapter. In Chapter 25 the normal equations of linear algebra were described. The normal equations provide a linear; mean square estimation of a signal based on data which are linear combinations of the unknown signal. The normal equations are a linear system analog of linear, shift invariant estimation using the Wiener filter.

In Chapter 25, we argued that algorithmic solution of the normal equations is not practical for the large vectors and matrices used in imaging. A more practical solution is the iterative solution, described at the end of that chapter. Iterative methods were applied to deconvolution in first pass radionuclide angiocardiography in Chapter 29. In this chapter we shall apply the iterative solution for image reconstruction.

I. SINGLE PHOTON EMISSION COMPUTED TOMOGRAPHY

In emission computed tomography, a radiopharmaceutical is injected into a patient, and the distribution of the radioactivity in a cross section is derived from measurements made from various positions around the patient. There are two broad categories of emission computed tomography — positron emission tomography and a single photon emission computed tomography. In positron tomography, two photons are given off at nearly a 180 degree angle; by contrast, in other modes of radioactive decay a single photon is emitted.

In X-ray computed tomography, the goal is to measure the attenuation of the pixels in the cross section. In emission computed tomography, the goal is to measure the activity of a radionuclide which is distributed in the cross section. The activity from each pixel undergoes attenuation as it traverses the cross section. There may be a considerable amount of attenuation of the signal before it reaches the detector. In computed tomography, the attenuation is the parameter of interest. In emission computed tomography, the attenuation is a confounding factor making measurement of the activities difficult.

In positron emission computed tomography, the sum of the paths of the two photons is equal to the thickness of the cross section, independent of the position of the source. Thus, a source can be placed outside the cross section and the attenuation can be measured in a separate data collection process. This attenuation measurement scheme is not possible in single photon emission computed tomography. In the next chapter we shall briefly touch on another interesting potential with positron emission tomography, time of flight measurement. But more of this later. In this chapter we shall be concerned with the effects of attenuation of image reconstruction in single photon emission computed tomography.

Typically, single photon emission computed tomographic data are collected using a rotating gamma camera. The gamma camera rotates around the patient over 180 or 360°. In X-ray tomography and in positron tomography, there is no difference between views from

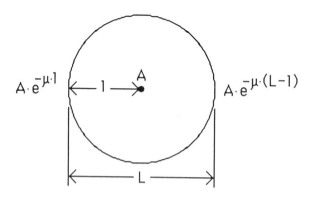

FIGURE 33.1. Point source attenuation: a point source of activity, A, is located at depth, 1, in a cross section of thickness, L. The measured activity at the front is $A \cdot e^{-\mu l}$, and the measured activity at the back is $A \cdot e^{-\mu(L-1)}$.

opposite sides of the cross section. Because of attenuation, the opposing view in single photon emission computed tomography may be very different.

A single row of pixels in the field of view of the gamma camera sees the same cross section at each angle. A cross section is reconstructed from the samples within this row at the various angles. The data for reconstructing other cross sections is obtained simultaneously at other rows in the field of view of the gamma camera. The data from a single rotation of the gamma camera can be used to reconstruct multiple cross sections. However, the data from one cross section does not interact with the data from another cross section. Therefore, our description of reconstruction will describe a single cross section.

To a first approximation, the data obtained from a gamma camera are the sum of the pixels along a line similar to that X-ray computed tomography. Attenuation causes the major deviation from this simple model. However, there are other important effects. The resolution of a gamma camera decreases rapidly with depth. Gamma camera nonuniformity and errors in the center of rotation can affect data collection. Although a gamma camera tries to reject scattered radiation, there is still an important contribution from scattered radiation in the data. All of these effects have important consequences for reconstruction; but, this chapter will use a simplified model which only includes the effects of attenuation.

Rotating gamma camera data are the most common form of single photon emission computed tomography, but there are several other interesting methods of collecting the raw data. The next chapter describes one method, the multidetector scanner. Other methods include the rotating slant hole collimator, the seven pin hole collimator, and coded apertures. The interested reader may wish to investigate the special problems introduced by these other forms of data collection in the references at the end of this chapter.

II. POINT SOURCE ATTENUATION CORRECTION

In order to understand the effects of attenuation, it is useful to start with a very simple model. Assume that the goal is to measure the activity of a point source of activity located at an unknown depth in a patient. There is a very simple algorithm for exactly correcting for the attenuation using opposing views.[1] Figure 33.1 shows a body cross-section with a source of activity, A, located at an unknown depth, 1, in the tissue. The activity is measured using opposing view from the front and from the back of the patient.

The activity measured from the front will be equal to $A \cdot e^{-\mu l}$, where μ is the linear attenuation coefficient, and 1 is the distance from the point source to the front of the cross section. The distance from the source to the back of the cross section will be L − 1, where

L is the thickness of the cross section. The activity measured from the back will be equal to $A \cdot e^{-\mu(L-1)}$. The geometric mean of the two measurements is defined as the square root of the product of the measurements:

$$\sqrt{(A \cdot e^{-\mu l} \cdot A \cdot e^{-\mu(L-1)})} = A \cdot e^{-\mu L/2} \qquad (33.1)$$

The geometric mean is dependent only on the total thickness of the cross section, L. Since it is simple to measure L, the effect of the attenuation can be calculated.

The geometric mean has a very special property — it is independent of l, the depth of the source. In the product, $A \cdot e^{-\mu l} \cdot A \cdot e^{-\mu(L-1)}$, the exponents add, and the distance, l, cancels. As the depth increases, the increased attenuation for the measurement from the front is exactly balanced by the decreased attenuation from the back. The geometric mean is used in studies such as gastric emptying where the activity can be reasonably modeled as a point source. The geometric mean has been used to correct for attenuation in emission computed tomography; however, it performs poorly for a distributed source.

There are two problems with this algorithm. The first problem is that it only works for a single source of activity. If there are two sources of activity, A_1 and A_2, located at depths, l_1 and l_2, then the geometric mean is:

$$\sqrt{[(A_1 \cdot e^{-\mu l_1} + A_2 \cdot e^{-\mu l_2}) \cdot (A_1 \cdot e^{-\mu(L-l_1)} + A_2 \cdot e^{-\mu(L-l_2)}]} = \qquad (33.2)$$
$$(A_1 + A_2) \cdot e^{-\mu L/2} + \sqrt{[(A_1 \cdot A_2) \cdot (e^{-\mu(L-l_1+l_2)} + e^{-\mu(L+l_1-l_2)}]}$$

The first term on the right hand side of Equation 33.2 is the sum of the two activities times $e^{-\mu L/2}$. This term is independent of the depths, l_1 and l_2, as in the case where there is a single source (Equation 33.1). But the second term is a complicated cross term. For two sources of activity the attenuation is not independent of depth, but related to depth by a complicated cross term.

The second problem with this simple algorithm has to do with noise. If a source of activity is located at the front surface, then the activity measurement from the back may be a small fraction of the activity measured from the front. Due to statistical noise, the measurement from the front will be more accurate than the measurement from the back. In the geometric mean, both measurements contribute equally. The statistical accuracy of the geometric mean will be dominated by the least accurate measurement. The accuracy of the final estimate of the activity is dominated by the least accurate measurement.

These two problems with the geometric mean are typical of the problems which occur with attenuation during reconstruction. While the attenuation for a single source of activity is easily compensated, attenuation correction for a distributed source is very complicated. Noise amplification can be a severe problem. Several of the simpler attenuation correction algorithms give the most weight to measurements which are the least accurate.

III. IMAGE COLLECTION MODEL

In this chapter image reconstruction will be implemented with an iterative algorithm using a vector, matrix model. However, we shall use the linear system model to understand the data collection process and to develop a heuristic understanding of image reconstruction. Therefore, we shall describe the data collection operation using both models.

This chapter will borrow ideas from the previous chapters which depend upon the notion of least mean square estimation. However, we shall not formally use least mean square estimation to derive the reconstruction algorithm. Therefore, the stochastic process, random vector notation will not be used. An extension of this chapter would be to more fully consider the statistics of reconstruction in the face of attenuation.

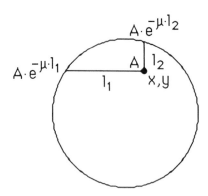

FIGURE 33.2. Attenuation in different projections: if the distance from a pixel, x,y, with activity, A, to the surface of the cross section is l_1 for one projection and l_2 for another projection, then the measured activities will be $A \cdot e^{-\mu l_1}$ and $A \cdot e^{-\mu l_2}$, respectively.

A. LINEAR SYSTEM MODEL

The attenuation for a single pixel can be calculated from the linear attenuation coefficient, μ, and the thickness of overlying tissue. The thickness of overlying tissue is different for each projection angle, θ. Figure 33.2 shows a pixel at position, x,y, and the attenuation at two different angles. If the activity at position, x,y, is A, then the measured activities will be $A \cdot e^{-\mu l_1}$ and $A \cdot e^{-\mu l_2}$, where l_1 and l_2 are the distances from x,y to the boundary for the two projections. The measured values are no longer a simple projection of the cross section, but rather they are modified by a multiplicative attenuation factor.

The attenuation for each pixel for each view can be given by a three-dimensional signal, $\mu(x,y,\theta)$. If the attenuation is uniform, and if the body contour is known, then the attenuations, $\mu(x,y,\theta)$, can be calculated from μ and the distance from the pixel at position x,y to the edge of the cross section along the direction, θ.

We can define a three-dimensional signal, $f'(x,y,\theta)$, which is the product of the attenuations, $\mu(x,y,\theta)$, and the cross sectional values, $f(x,y)$:

$$f'(x,y,\theta) = \mu(x,y,\theta) \cdot f(x,y) \tag{33.3}$$

The simple projection of $f'(x,y,\theta)$ produces values, $p(x',\theta)$, which are equal to the attenuated projection of $f(x,y)$. The three-dimensional function, $f'(x,y,\theta)$, is more complicated than the original two-dimensional function, $f(x,y)$. But this more complicated function transforms the attenuated projection operation into a simple projection operation. The simple projection of $f'(x,y,\theta)$ is similar to the operations in the last two chapters.

Using linear system methods, the data collection operation can be modeled as:

$$p(x',\theta) = A\{f'(x,y,\theta)\} + n(x',\theta) \tag{33.4}$$

where $p(x',\theta)$ are the projection values, $A\{\cdot\}$ is the projection operation, and $n(x',\theta)$ is the detector noise. Using Equation 33.3 we can expand Equation 33.4:

$$p(x',\theta) = A\{\mu(x,y,\theta) \cdot f(x,y)\} + n(x',\theta) \tag{33.5}$$

This model is analogous to the model given by Equation 32.1, except that the system, $A\{\cdot\}$, is replaced by the system, $A\{\mu(x,y,\theta) \cdot \}$. This model is shown in Figure 33.3.

In Chapter 31, it was shown that the Fourier transform of a projection is equal to a slice of the Fourier transform of the cross section. This relation is called the projection, slice

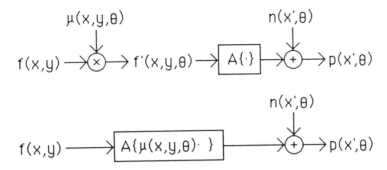

FIGURE 33.3.   Data collection model: the attenuated projection of a cross-sectional object, f(x,y), can be modeled as multiplication by attenuation factors, $\mu(x,y,\theta)$, followed by the usual projection operation, $A\{\cdot\}$. The attenuation factors, $\mu(x,y,\theta)$ and the attenuated cross section, $f'(x,y,\theta)$, are functions of the projection angle, θ. The projection data, $p(x',\theta)$, is the sum of the attenuated projection and the noise, $n(x',\theta)$. The attenuated projection operation can be modeled by an operator, $A\{\mu(x,y,\theta) \cdot \}$, which includes the attenuation factors.

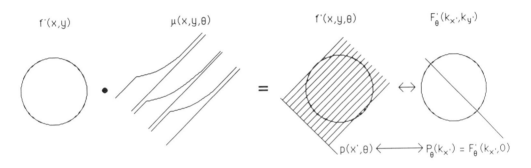

FIGURE 33.4.   Attenuated projection model: the cross sectional object, f(x,y), times the attenuation factors, $\mu(x,y,\theta)$, gives the attenuated cross section, $f'(x,y,\theta)$. The attenuated projection of f(x,y) or equivalently, the unattenuated projection of $f'(x,y,\theta)$, gives the projection data, $p(x',\theta)$. The one-dimensional Fourier transform of the projection data with respect to x' is given by $P_\theta(k_{x'})$. $P_\theta(k_{x'})$ is equal to a slice, $F'_\theta(k_{x'},0)$, of the Fourier transform of the attenuated cross section.

theorem, Equation 31.18. Therefore, the Fourier transform of $p(x',\theta)$ is equal to a slice from the transform of $f'(x,y,\theta)$. Mathematically,

$$P_\theta(k_{x'}) = F'_\theta(k_{x'},0) \tag{33.6}$$

where $P_\theta(k_{x'})$ is the one-dimensional Fourier transform of $p(x',\theta)$ with respect to x', and $F'_\theta(k_{x'},0)$ is the two-dimensional Fourier transform of $f'(x,y,\theta)$ with respect to the x' and y' axes. $k_{y'}$ is set equal to zero to indicate that the slice is along the $k_{x'}$ axis. We have used θ as a subscript for the Fourier transforms instead of including it as a variable to emphasize the fact that θ is held constant in the transform.

Figure 33.4 shows these relations diagrammatically. The cross-sectional object, f(x,y), is multiplied by the attenuation, $\mu(x,y,\theta)$, to produce, $f'(x,y,\theta)$. The projection of $f'(x,y,\theta)$ at angle, θ, or equivalently the attenuated projection of f(x,y) at angle, θ, is given by $p(x',\theta)$. The Fourier transform of the projection, $P_\theta(k_{x'})$, is equal to a slice of $F'_\theta(k_x,k_y)$ along the $k_{x'}$ axis. As the angle, θ, changes, $\mu(x,y,\theta)$, $f'(x,y,\theta)$, and $F'_\theta(k_x,k_y)$ change; of course, the cross section, f(x,y), remains constant.

The back projected image for the data obtained at angle, θ, is given by:

$$g_\theta(x,y) = B_\theta\{p(x',\theta)\} \tag{33.7}$$

where $B_\theta\{\cdot\}$ is the back projection operation at angle, θ. In this back projection operation, the angle, θ, is held constant. The one-dimensional set of projection values is back projected to the two-dimensional image. The back projected image, $g(x,y)$, is the sum of the back projections from all of the angles:

$$g(x,y) = B\{p(x',\theta)\} \tag{33.8}$$

where the system, $B\{\cdot\}$, is equal to the sum of the back projections at all angles:

$$B\{\cdot\} = \sum_\theta B_\theta\{\cdot\} \tag{33.9}$$

The projection, back projection operation for a single angle can be given by an operator defined as:

$$D_\theta\{\cdot\} = B_\theta\{A\{\cdot\}\} \tag{33.10}$$

For the case of attenuation, the projection, back projection operation can be defined by:

$$D_\theta\{\mu(x,y,\theta)\cdot\} = B_\theta\{A\{\mu(x,y,\theta\cdot\}\} \tag{33.11}$$

The operators, $A\{\cdot\}$, $B_\theta\{\cdot\}$, and $D_\theta\{\cdot\}$, are the same operators used for the case where there is no attenuation. The attenuation is included explicitly as multiplication with $\mu(x,y,\theta)$.

Using Equations 33.4, and 33.7, and 33.11, the back projected image at angle, θ, is given by:

$$g_\theta(x,y) = D_\theta\{\mu(x,y,\theta)\cdot f(x,y)\} + B_\theta\{n(x',\theta)\} \tag{33.12}$$

The noise in the back projected image is modified by the back projection operation.

The projection, back projection operation for all of the angles, $D\{\cdot\}$, is given by:

$$D\{\cdot\} = B\{A\{\mu(x,y,\theta\cdot\}\} \tag{33.13}$$

The back projected image can be obtained from the original cross section using $D\{\cdot\}$:

$$g(x,y) = D\{\mu(x,y,\theta)\cdot f(x,y)\} + B\{n(x',\theta)\} \tag{33.14}$$

Except for the attenuation factor, this equation is analogous to Equation 31.5.

For an infinite field of view with an infinite number of angles, it was shown in Chapter 31 that the system, $D\{\cdot\}$ (without attenuation), is linear and shift invariant. A system function, $d(x,y)$, was defined and Equation 31.8 was written as a convolution in Equation 31.12. With attenuation, the system, $D\{\mu(x,y,\theta)\cdot\}$, is no longer shift invariant. The intensity of the rays in the point spread function vary with the position of the point.

Figure 33.5 shows a diagrammatic representation of the point spread function for the projection back projection operation at two different points in the cross section. The point spread function varies markedly with position. The marked variation of the point spread function with position indicates that a shift invariant model will not adequately model single photon emission computed tomography.

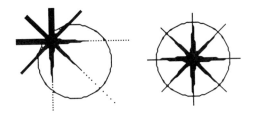

FIGURE 33.5. Nonshift invariance of the point spread function for the attenuated projection, back projection operation: on the left is a diagrammatic representation for the point spread function of the attenuated projection, back projection operation near an edge of the cross section. On the right is the point spread function for the same operation near the center of the cross section. The point spread function is much different in these two positions.

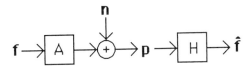

FIGURE 33.6. Data collection reconstruction model: the vector **f**, represents the cross-sectional object. The matrix, A, represents the attenuated data collection process. The projectional data represented by the vector, **p**, are the sum of the measurement noise represented by the vector, **n**, and A · **f**. The estimate, $\hat{\mathbf{f}}$, of the cross section is obtained by passing the data, **p**, through the system, H.

B. LINEAR ALGEBRA MODEL

Using linear algebra methods, a cross-sectional object is represented by a vector, **f**. The data collection operation is represented by matrix, A. The noise is represented by a vector, **n**. The projection data are represented by the vector, **p**. the linear algebra model can be described by:

$$\mathbf{p} = A \cdot \mathbf{f} + \mathbf{n} \tag{33.15}$$

where we have again assumed an additive noise model. This model is shown diagrammatically in Figure 33.6.

The capital letter, A, has been given three different meanings in this section. A has been used to represent the activity of a single source, e.g., A · $e^{-\mu l}$. This usage is common in nuclear medicine. A{·} has been used to represent the projection operation in the linear systems model. And A has been used to represent the data collection process in the linear algebra model. The latter two usages are similar, but there is an important difference. The matrix, A, is analogous to the system, A{μ(x,y,θ)·}. The matrix, A, includes both the attenuation factors, μ(x,y,θ), and the projection operation A{·}. The multiple usage can be a source of confusion; the reader should pay special attention to the difference between the projection operation, A{·}, without attenuation and the matrix, A, which includes attenuation.

In Chapter 31, the back projection operation was used in order to define a linear, shift invariant system. Since the linear algebra method is not shift invariant, the back projection operation is not usually a part of the description. Below, a type of back projection operation will be defined using A^T:

$$\mathbf{g} = A^T \cdot \mathbf{p} \tag{33.16}$$

where A^T is the transpose of the data collection operation, and **g** is a back projected vector. There are important differences between this operation and B{·}. Understanding the differ-

$$f(x,y) \cdot \mu(x,y,\theta) \longleftrightarrow F(k_x,k_y) * M_\theta(k_x,k_y)$$

FIGURE 33.7. Attenuated cross section: the attenuated cross section is equal to the cross section, $f(x,y)$, multiplied by the attenuation factors, $\mu(x,y,\theta)$. In the frequency domain, this multiplication is represented by the convolution of the cross section, $F(k_x,k_y)$, and the attenuation factors, $M_\theta(k_x,k_y)$.

ences between the models will help understanding the reconstruction process. The next chapter will shed additional light on these differences.

IV. HEURISTICS

We can develop some heuristics to understand the projection values, $p(x',\theta)$. The heuristics will help to explain how these data values relate to the cross section, $f(x,y)$. First it will be shown how the Fourier transforms of the attenuated and unattenuated cross sections are related. Then, the interesting effect of making the attenuation constant both inside and outside the cross section will be examined.

A. ATTENUATION VIEWED AS SMOOTHING OF THE SPATIAL FREQUENCIES

The Fourier transform of the projection, $P_\theta(x')$, is a slice of $F'_\theta(k_x,k_y)$ along the $k_{x'}$ axis (Equation 33.6). Since $f'(x,y,\theta)$ is equal to the product of $\mu(x,y,\theta)$ and $f(x,y)$, $F'_\theta(k_x,k_y)$ is equal to the convolution of $M_\theta(k_x,k_y)$ and $F(k_x,k_y)$:

$$F'_\theta(k_x,k_y) = M_\theta(k_x,k_y) * F(k_x,k_y) \tag{33.17}$$

where $M_\theta(k_x,k_y)$ is the two-dimensional Fourier transform of $\mu(x,y,\theta)$. This relation is another example of the important relationship between multiplication in one domain and convolution in the other domain (Equation 16.8). Figure 33.7 shows this relationship diagrammatically.

In the spatial frequency domain, the effect of the attenuation can be viewed as a smoothing of the cross section, $F(k_x,k_y)$, by convolution with $M_\theta(k_x,k_y)$. In order to understand the relation of $F'_\theta(k_x,k_y)$ to $F(k_x,k_y)$, let us examine the form of $M_\theta(k_x,k_y)$. For θ equal to zero, a typical set of attenuations, $\mu(x,y,0)$, and the Fourier transform, $M_\theta(k_x,k_y)$, are shown in Figure 33.8. The changes in $\mu(x,y,0)$ in both the x and the y direction are reasonably slow; therefore, $M_\theta(k_x,k_y)$, is relatively narrow in both the k_x and the k_y directions. ($M_\theta(k_x,k_y)$ is shown on a logarithmic scale since the values near the origin are so much larger than the other values.) $F'_\theta(k_{x'},0)$ is similar to $F(k_x,k_y)$ along the $k_{x'}$ axis; along that slice, it is a smoothed version of $F(k_x,k_y)$, smoothed in both the k_x and k_y directions.

The data, $P_\theta(k_{x'})$, are a slice of $F'_\theta(k_x,k_y)$ along the $k_{x'}$ axis. Since $F'_\theta(k_x,k_y)$ is a reasonable estimate of $F(k_x,k_y)$, we would expect that a reasonable estimate of the cross section can be obtained. The major effect will be a smoothing of the spatial frequencies. However, since the data are not exact, the estimates will not be exact. Using the X-ray computed tomographic reconstruction algorithm on the attenuated projection data produces a surprisingly good first estimate of a cross section. As described below, simple corrections can be used to produce useful image reconstructions.

B. CONSTANT ATTENUATION

An interesting modification can be made to the projection data in order to simulate the case where the attenuation is constant not only within the cross section, but also outside the cross section. The modification is the mathematical equivalent of placing a water bath between the patient and the detector. In order to perform the calculation, we shall assume that the cross section is convex; that the boundary of the cross section is known; and that the linear attenuation coefficient, μ, is constant throughout the cross section.

Each projection value, $p(x',\theta)$, is multiplied by a value equal to the attenuation from the boundary to the detector:

$$p'(x',\theta) = e^{-\mu l(x',\theta)} \cdot p(x',\theta) \qquad (33.18)$$

where $p'(x',\theta)$ are the modified projection data, $l(x',\theta)$ are the distances between the boundary and the detector, and $p(x',\theta)$ are the raw projection data. Figure 33.9 shows the distance factors $l(x',\theta)$ for a typical convex cross section.

Equation 33.18 can be expanded using Equation 33.5:

$$p'(x',\theta) = e^{-\mu l(x',\theta)} \cdot A\{\mu(x,y,\theta) \cdot f(x,y)\} + e^{-\mu l(x',\theta)} \cdot n(x',\theta) \qquad (33.19)$$

Multiplying the projection data by $e^{-\mu l(x',\theta)}$ is equivalent to using a modified model:

$$p'(x',\theta) = A\{\mu'(x,y,\theta) \cdot f(x,y)\} + e^{-\mu l(x',\theta)} \cdot n(x',\theta) \qquad (33.20)$$

where:

$$\mu'(x,y,\theta) = e^{-\mu l(x',\theta)} \cdot \mu(x,y,\theta) \qquad (33.21)$$

The modified attenuation factors decrease exponentially from the detector along the y' direction.

Figure 33.10 shows a comparison between the unmodified attenuation factors, $\mu(x',y',\theta)$, and the modified attenuation factors, $\mu'(x',y')$ in the x',y' coordinate system. The unmodified attenuation factors are different values of x' and for different values of θ. The modified attenuation factors are much simpler. They can be given by:

$$\mu(x',y') = e^{-\mu(y'-y_0)} \qquad (33.22)$$

where y_0 is the position of the detector. The factors depend upon y', the distance from the detector, but not on x'. They are the same for all positions, x', along the projection. Furthermore, except for rotation, the factors are the same for all values of θ. In the x,y coordinate system the modified attenuations, $\mu'(x,y,\theta)$ are a function of θ. In the x',y' coordinate system the modified attenuations, $\mu'(x',y')$, are not a function of θ.

$\mu'(x',y')$ and the magnitude of its Fourier transform $|M'(k_{x'},k_{y'})|$ are shown diagrammatically in Figure 33.11. Since $\mu'(x',y')$ does not change in the x' direction, the Fourier transform $M'(k_{x'},k_{y'})$ is a delta function in the $k_{x'}$ direction. Multiplying the projection values to simulate uniform attenuation throughout the cross section simplifies the attenuations in both the space, $\mu'(x',y')$, and the spatial frequency, $M'(k_{x'},k_{y'})$, domains.

As above, we can consider the effect of the attenuations in the spatial frequency domain. Multiplication by $\mu'(x',y')$ is equivalent to convolution by $M'(k_{x'},k_{y'})$. $M'(k_{x'},k_{y'})$ is simplified with respect to $M_\theta(k_{x'},k_{y'})$ since $M'(k_{x'},k_{y'})$ is a delta function in the $k_{x'}$ direction. Therefore, the effect of the attenuation is to smooth in the spatial frequency domain only along the $k_{y'}$ direction, not along the $k_{x'}$ direction. Figure 33.12 shows this smoothing operation diagrammatically. The smoothing is orthogonal to the direction of the slice. The direction of the smoothing changes with projection angle. For large k, the direction of the smoothing is in the θ direction.

The smoothing is somewhat unusual. Nevertheless, much of the effect of the attenuation can be described by a smoothing operation in the θ direction. Since the modified attenuations, $M'(k_{x'},k_{y'})$, are the same for all values of θ, the smoothing is shift invariant in the θ direction. As k increases, the distance over which the smoothing takes place is constant, but the angular

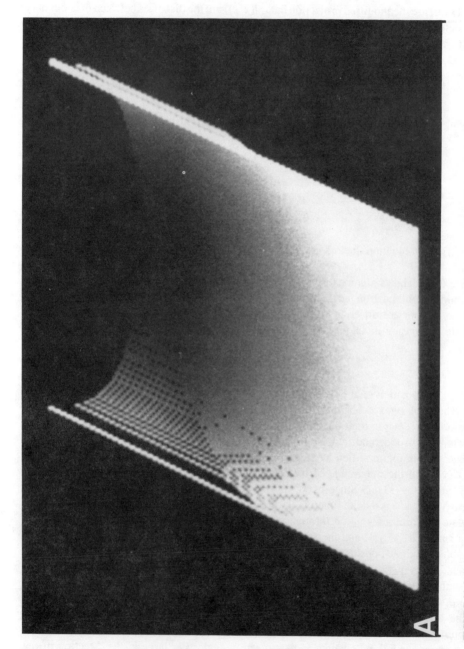

FIGURE 33.8.   Attenuation factors: (A) the attenuation factors, $\mu(x,y,\theta)$, for a circular cross section; (B) the magnitude of the Fourier transform, $|M_\theta(k_x,k_y)|$, of this object is shown on the right.

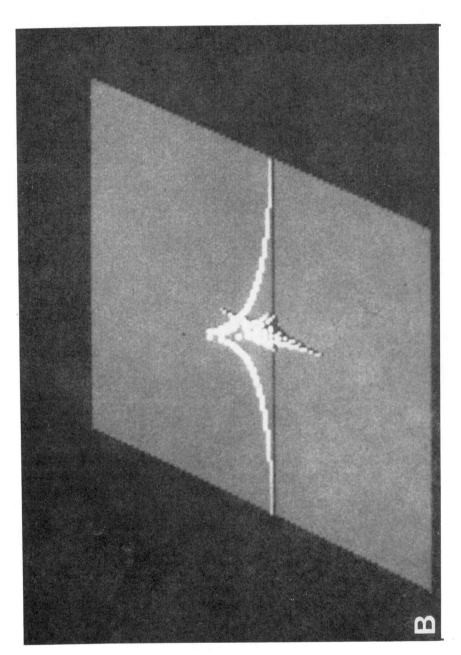

FIGURE 33.8 (continued).

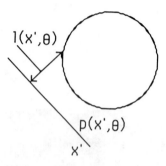

FIGURE 33.9.   Distance from the detector to the boundary of the cross section: the distance from the detector to the boundary of a convex cross section is given by $l(x',\theta)$.

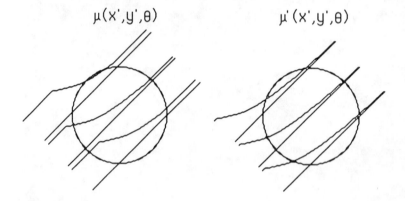

FIGURE 33.10.   Modified attenuation factors: on the left is a diagrammatic representation of the attenuation factors for one projection, $\mu(x',y',\theta)$. On the right is a diagrammatic representation of modified attenuation factors, $\mu'(x',y')$ which have been multiplied by $e^{-\mu l(x',\theta)}$. The modified attenuation factors simulate uniform attenuation throughout the imaging field of view.

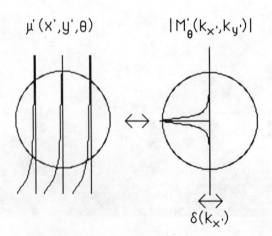

FIGURE 33.11.   Spatial frequency representation of the modified attenuation factors: on the left is a diagrammatic representation of the modified attenuation factors, $\mu'(x',y')$. On the right is a diagrammatic representation of the magnitude of the Fourier transform of the modified attenuation factors, $|M'(k_{x'},k_{y'})|$. In the spatial frequency domain the modified attenuation factors are a delta function in the $k_{x'}$ direction, and a narrow function in the $k_{y'}$ direction.

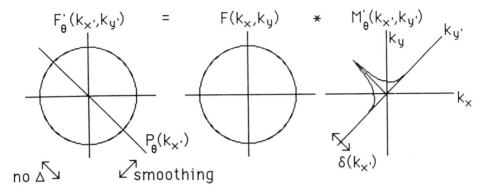

FIGURE 33.12. Spatial frequency representation of the attenuated cross-sectional object: in the spatial frequency domain, the attenuated cross sectional object, $F'_\theta(k_x,k_y)$, is the convolution of the cross sectional object,
$F(k_x,k_y)$, and the modified attenuation factors, $M'(k_{x'},k_{y'})$. The modified attenuation do not affect the cross-
sectional object along the direction of the projectional data (along the $k_{x'}$ axis). They tend to smooth the object
in a direction perpendicular to the slice defined by the projection.

spatial frequency decreases. Using the proper scaling, the smoothing is a one-dimensional,
shift invariant process.

In Equation 33.20, the modified model has a modified noise term, $e^{-\mu l(x',\theta)} \cdot n(x',\theta)$.
If the detector noise is the same for all samples, then this modification of the noise will
lead to some noise amplification. The different samples of a pixel value will not enter into
the estimate equally, but rather will be weighted by an arbitrary factor related to the distance
between the detector and the cross-section boundary. In the next chapter we shall return to
a consideration of how different samples of a single value should be combined.

The attenuated projection model is not shift-invariant (see Figure 33.5). Modification
of the attenuation values has transformed the problem into a quasi shift-invariant problem.
It is shift invariant in the θ direction for large k. The cost of transforming this to the quasi
shift-invariant model is a certain amount of noise amplification.

V. LINEAR, SHIFT INVARIANT RECONSTRUCTION METHODS

Most linear, shift invariant reconstruction methods are not truly shift invariant. Instead
these algorithms use a linear, shift invariant method in spite of the fact that the reconstruction
is not shift invariant. Some type of correction is performed during the process which ame-
liorates the most egregious effects of assuming that the process is shift invariant. In limited
domains, these methods often perform satisfactorily.

A. MODIFICATION OF THE PROJECTION VALUES

The most interesting modification to the projection values is that described above —
mathematically making the attenuation constant both inside and outside the cross section.
We have seen that the effect of this modification is to smooth the data in the θ direction.

In order to estimate the unattenuated data, the attenuated data must be unsmoothed in
the θ direction. A more complicated sharpening operation must be performed on values near
the origin. This process transforms the attenuated reconstruction problem into the nonattenuated reconstruction problem.

This outline of a reconstruction algorithm is interesting theoretically, but it has not been
implemented practically to determine its performance on real images. Some algorithms
modify the filtering operation prior to back projection. To some extent, these modifications
approximate the required sharpening. In some situations, this simple modification works
well.

Several other techniques have been developed which correct the projection data prior to back projection. The simplest is to use the geometric mean of orthogonal views. However, we have already shown that this method does not perform well for a distributed source. In some circumstances the arithmetic mean will out perform the geometric mean. But neither of these methods produce particularly good results.

B. POST-RECONSTRUCTION CORRECTION

If the cross section is reconstructed without consideration to attenuation, the center pixels experience considerable attenuation in all projections, while there are at least some projections where the peripheral pixels are seen without attenuation. As a result, the center will tend to have lower values that the periphery. A simple attenuation correction is to multiply the pixel values by a factor after reconstruction. Chang defined the attenuation correction factor for a pixel as the sum of the attenuation values for all of the projections.[2]

If a uniform flood source is reconstructed without attenuation, the center values will be less than the edges. Sources with high frequency detail will be better represented in the reconstruction, than low frequency objects. The major effect of a post-reconstruction correction is to make the values in a uniform flood source end up uniform.

Post-reconstruction correction can be used as part of any approximate algorithm. For example, with the algorithm above, a post-reconstruction correction can be used at the end to improve the uniformity of the reconstruction for flood sources.

C. EXPONENTIAL BACK PROJECTION

Tretiak and Delaney[3] proposed a modification to the back projection operation, which makes the projection, back projection operation truly shift invariant. The algorithm assumes that the cross section is convex, that the boundary of the cross section is known, and that the attenuation coefficient is uniform throughout the cross section. The first step in the process is the same as that described above. The projection data are multiplied by $e^{-\mu l(x',\theta)}$, where $l(x',\theta)$ is the distance to the boundary of the cross section. The effect of this operation is the same as if a tissue attenuator was placed between the boundary and the detector.

The more important step in this algorithm is the modification of the back projected data by the inverse of the attenuation, $1/\mu'(x,y,\theta)$. At each angle, the modified back projection data are equal to:

$$g_\theta(x,y)/\mu'(x,y,\theta) = B_\theta\{A\{\mu'(x,y,\theta) \cdot f(x,y)\}\}/\mu'(x,y,\theta)$$

$$+ B_\theta\{e^{-\mu l(x',\theta)} \cdot n(x',\theta)\}/\mu'(x,y,\theta) \tag{33.23}$$

where $g_\theta(x,y)$ is the back projected image at angle, θ, $\mu'(x,y,\theta)$ are the modified attenuation values described by Equation 33.21, and $n(x',\theta)$ is the measurement noise.

In the case where there is a single source of activity located at position, x_0,y_0, then the first term in Equation 33.23 is very simple. There is a single nonzero ray in the projection equal to $\mu(x_0,y_0,\theta) \cdot f(x_0,y_0)$. The back projected ray is equal to $\mu(x_0,y_0,\theta) \cdot f(x_0,y_0)/\mu(x,y,\theta)$. At the position where x,y is equal to x_0,y_0, the value is equal:

$$\mu(x_0,y_0,\theta) \cdot f(x_0,y_0)/\mu(x_0,y_0,\theta) = f(x_0,y_0) \tag{33.24}$$

Figure 33.13 shows the back projected ray.

The point spread function for this algorithm is very strange. It is the sum of increasing exponentials. At one angle, the sum of the exponentials increasing from the two sides is a hyperbolic cosine function.

$$e^{\mu(r+R)} + e^{-\mu(r-R)} = e^R \cdot (e^{\mu r} + e^{-\mu r}) = e^R \cdot \cosh(\mu \cdot r) \tag{33.25}$$

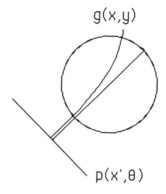

FIGURE 33.13. Exponential back projection: the exponential back projection operation amplifies the back projected value as the distance from the detector increases.

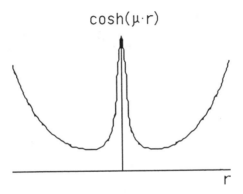

FIGURE 33.14. Point spread function for exponential back projection: the point spread function of the exponential back projection algorithm for an infinite number of angles is equal to $\cosh(\mu \cdot r)/r$.

where r is the distance from the origin, and R the distance to the detector. The overall point spread function is a sum of these hyperbolic cosines. For an infinite number of angles the point spread function is proportional to $\cosh(\mu \cdot r)/r$. A single slice of the point spread function is shown in Figure 33.14. The interesting feature is that the value at the position of the point source is independent of position. Therefore, the point spread function is shift invariant.

This algorithm has the very attractive feature that it makes the point spread function shift invariant. For a single source of activity, the projection, exponential back projection is the same at any point. Therefore, the projection, exponential back projection system can be modeled as a linear, shift invariant system. The projection data can be filtered as in the nonattenuated case to produce a simple projection, filter, exponential back projection algorithm. Some special considerations in the design of the filter are discussed by Gullberg.[4]

Equation 33.23 shows the problem with this algorithm. For pixels with a large amount of attenuation, $\mu'(x,y,\theta)$ is very small, and the noise term is very large. The contribution of these pixels to the projection data is very small; however, in Figure 33.14 we can see that the projection contributes most heavily to these pixels. The data values are used most heavily to estimate pixels about which they have the least information.

A heuristic described in the next chapter is that the data should be put back where it comes from. In other words, the data value should be distributed to the pixels in proportion to the relative contribution of the pixel to the data value. The reason that this algorithm performs so badly is that it puts most of the data where they did not come from.

The worst noise amplification occurs at the pixels at the edge of the image. This has led to modification of this algorithm to use a modified weighting of the two projections so that the projection closest to the detector is weighed most heavily.[5] This modification removes much of the noise amplification of this algorithm. There is still some noise amplification, and the algorithm is not truly shift invariant.

VI. ITERATIVE RECONSTRUCTION

The exponential back projection algorithm makes the reconstruction process truly shift invariant; however, the noise amplification makes this algorithm unusable. The modifications of the exponential back projection algorithm improve the noise amplification, but result in some degree of nonshift-invariance. Shift invariant reconstruction with a nonshift-invariant model results in some errors. Similarly, the other shift invariant algorithms which we have described trade errors due to the correctness of the model for error due to noise amplification.

In practice, these algorithms may be adequate for some applications, but when more accuracy is required, it is necessary to use a nonshift-invariant model, such as the linear algebra model shown diagrammatically in Figure 33.6. A further advantage of the linear algebra model is that the requirements for a convex boundary and for uniform attenuation can be removed. We shall continue to assume that the attenuations are known.

The model of the data collection process was given above in Equation 33.15:

$$\mathbf{p} = A \cdot \mathbf{f} + \mathbf{n} \tag{33.26}$$

where the vector, $\mathbf{p}$, represents the projection data, the matrix, A, represents the data collection process, the vector, $\mathbf{f}$, is the cross section, and $\mathbf{n}$ is the detector noise. Linear, nonshift-invariant image reconstruction can be modeled by:

$$\hat{\mathbf{f}} = H \cdot \mathbf{p} \tag{33.27}$$

where $\hat{\mathbf{f}}$ is the estimate of the cross-sectional image and H is the reconstruction process.

In Chapter 25, using an analogous statistical model the linear mean square estimation of the data resulted in the normal equation of linear algebra (Equation 25.31):

$$A^T \cdot A \cdot \hat{\mathbf{f}} = A^T \cdot \boldsymbol{p} \tag{33.28}$$

When $A^T \cdot A$ has an inverse, the solution is given by Equation 25.42:

$$H = (A^T \cdot A)^{-1} \cdot A^T \tag{33.29}$$

The purpose of defining a back projected image, $g(x,y)$, in the cross-sectional coordinate system was to transform the problem to a shift invariant format. Since the linear algebra formulation is nonshift invariant, the back projection is not part of the formulation. Thus, H is not analogous to H{·}. H operates directly on $\mathbf{p}$, whereas H{·} operates on $g(x,y)$.

In order to bring out the analogy between the two models, a back projected image vector can be defined:

$$\mathbf{g} = A^T \cdot \mathbf{p} \tag{33.30}$$

Since the column space of A^T is equal to the row space of A, the back projected vector, $\mathbf{g}$, is in the same vector space as $\mathbf{f}$ (or more precisely in a subspace of the cross-sectional space).

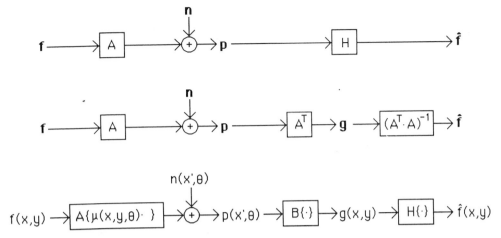

FIGURE 33.15. Comparison of linear algebra and linear systems models: the linear algebra model of the system is shown in the top two panels. The data, **p**, are equal to the cross-sectional object, **f**, projected with the system, A, plus noise, **n**. The estimate, $\hat{\mathbf{f}}$, of the cross section is obtained by passing the data through the system, H. The system, H, can be divided into two systems — A^T, which is similar to a back projection operation, produces image, **g**, and $(A^T \cdot A)^{-1}$ estimates the cross section from **g**. The linear systems model is shown on the bottom panel. Again, the data, $p(x',\theta)$, are equal to the cross sectional object, $f(x,y)$, projected by the system, $A\{\mu(x,y,\theta) \cdot \}$, plus noise, $n(x',\theta)$. The back projection operation, $B\{\cdot\}$, produces the back projected image, $g(x,y)$. The system, $H\{\cdot\}$, produces the estimate, $\hat{f}(x,y)$, of the cross section from the back projected image, $g(x,y)$. The back projection operation, $B\{\cdot\}$, is analogous to, but not identical with A^T. The linear algebra estimation matrix, H, is analogous to the combination of the linear systems back projection operation and the estimation operation, $H\{B\{\cdot\}\}$.

The matrix, A^T, is analogous to, but not identical to the back projection operator, $B\{\cdot\}$. The estimate, $\hat{\mathbf{f}}$, is given by:

$$\hat{\mathbf{f}} = (A^T \cdot A)^{-1} \cdot \mathbf{g} \tag{33.31}$$

From Equation 33.31, it can be seen that the matrix $(A^T \cdot A)^{-1}$, is analogous to the system, $H\{\cdot\}$. The matrix, H, is analogous to $H\{B\{\cdot\}\}$. The different uses of H and $H\{\cdot\}$ can be a source of confusion if the reader does not take special note of the differences between the two models. Figure 33.15 shows a comparison of the two models.

In Chapter 25 several reasons were given why direct solution of Equation 33.29 is not tractable. Instead an approximate solution is needed. In Chapter 29, we considered several approximate solutions to the first pass radionuclide angiocardiographic deconvolution problem. Several of the considerations which apply in that case also apply in the case of reconstruction. In addition, since images contain a large number of data points, efficiency is also an important consideration.

The most common method of solution is to use an iterative reconstruction. An example of an iterative reconstruction scheme is shown in Figure 33.16. Some type of approximate reconstruction is used to derive a zero-order estimate of the original cross section:

$$\hat{\mathbf{f}}_0 = H \cdot \mathbf{p} \tag{33.32}$$

Successive estimates are produced by reprojecting the previous estimate, comparing it to the data, and correcting the estimate with the difference between the reprojected estimate and the data:

$$\hat{\mathbf{p}}_{n-1} = A \cdot \hat{\mathbf{f}}_{n-1} \tag{33.33}$$

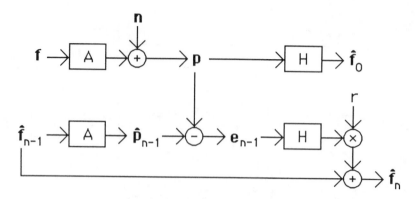

FIGURE 33.16. Iterative reconstruction: the data, **p**, are the sum of A · **f** plus **n**. The initial estimate, $\hat{\mathbf{f}}_0$, of **f** is obtained by passing **p** through H. The estimated data, $\hat{\mathbf{p}}_{n-1}$, on the n − 1st iteration is compared to the actual data, **p**. The difference between the data, **p**, and the estimate of the data, $\hat{\mathbf{p}}_{n-1}$ is reconstructed with H and scaled by r to obtain a correction to the estimate. The nth estimate, $\hat{\mathbf{f}}_n$, of the cross section is the sum of the n − 1st estimate, $\hat{\mathbf{f}}_{n-1}$, and the correction, r · H · (**p** − $\hat{\mathbf{p}}_{n-1}$).

$$\hat{\mathbf{f}}_n = \hat{\mathbf{f}}_{n-1} + r \cdot H \cdot (\mathbf{p} - \hat{\mathbf{p}}_{n-1}) \qquad (33.34)$$

This algorithm was described in Chapter 25.

The most important part of the iterative reconstruction is the model of the data collection operation. On each iteration, the current estimate is passed through the data collection model to produce an estimate, $\hat{\mathbf{p}}_{n-1}$, of the data (Equation 33.33). The model, A, of the data collection process is much more important than the reconstructor, H. Generally speaking, the reconstructor affects how rapidly the estimate approaches the correct answer, but the model of the data collection determines how accurate the reconstruction will be.

The description of iterative reconstruction methods in this book is very simplified. There are several important issues such as the convergence of the estimate to the true answer, oscillation of the estimate, etc. which have been ignored. The interested reader should pursue this topic in other sources.

One of the major problems with linear, nonshift-invariant reconstruction as compared to shift invariant reconstruction is efficiency. Linear, shift invariant reconstruction uses convolution which can be performed in N · log(N) time. Linear, nonshift-invariant reconstruction requires N^3 time for calculation of H. Even in the case where H can be precomputed for standard geometries, N^2 time is required for calculation of the estimate from the data.

There are two steps in the iterative algorithm shown in Figure 33.16 which require N^2 time — reprojection, A · $\hat{\mathbf{f}}_{n-1}$, and reconstruction H · $\hat{\mathbf{p}}_n$. One of the shift invariant, approximate reconstructors from the first part of this chapter can be used to transform the reconstruction step into an N · log(N) process. The reprojection step cannot be transformed into a shift invariant process. However, the projection matrix A, is sparse; most of the values are zero. The number of pixels which contribute to each data value is proportional to $\sqrt{N}$, the distance across the cross section. Thus, special purpose projection algorithms require only N · $\sqrt{N}$ time.

Iterative reconstruction requires more time, N · $\sqrt{N}$, than shift invariant reconstruction, N · log(N), but considerably less time than generalized, nonshift invariant reconstruction, N^3 if H must be calculated, N^2 otherwise. An N · $\sqrt{N}$ iterative reconstruction is practical for clinical application.

VII. SUMMARY

The bulk of this chapter has dealt with understanding the deviations from shift invariance caused by attenuation in single photon emission computed tomography. The attenuation is modeled using a three-dimensional multiplicative signal, $\mu(x,y,\theta)$. This model has been used to consider attenuation as a smoothing operation.

Premultiplication of the projection values removes the smoothing in the $k_{x'}$ direction at the expense of some noise amplification. For large k, the smoothing is in the θ direction. Reconstruction requires a θ sharpening operation.

The various shift invariant methods all have problems associated with them. Either they are not truly shift invariant, or they cause noise amplification. They can be made reasonably accurate especially with corrections either to the projection data or to the estimate. However, the best reconstruction is provided by nonshift invariant methods. This chapter has briefly outlined an iterative reconstruction algorithm.

One of the many important issues in single photon emission computed tomography which this chapter has not considered is determination of the attenuation factors, $\mu(x,y,\theta)$. For a convex cross section of uniform attenuation, these factors can be calculated from the contour of the cross section. However, the attenuation may not be uniform, the cross section may not be convex, and the boundary may not be accurately known. Other important issues which have not been covered are the change in the resolution of a gamma camera with depth, and the effect of scattered radiation. These other issues have important effects on the accuracy of reconstruction, but they are beyond the scope of this book.

VIII. FURTHER READING

A quite readable source on single photon emission computed tomography is the book by Croft.[6] A more mathematical discussion can be found in the chapter by Budinger, Gullberg, and Huesman in the book by Herman.[7] Single photon emission computed tomography with a discussion of various coded apertures can be found in the book by Barrett and Swindell.[8]

REFERENCES

1. **Sorenson, J. A.,** Quantitative measurement of radioactivity in vivo by whole-body counting, in *Instrumentation in Nuclear Medicine*, Hine, G. J. and Sorenson, J. A., Eds., Academic Press, San Diego, 1974, 311.
2. **Chang, L.-T.,** A method for attenuation correction in radionuclide computed tomography, *IEEE Trans. Nucl. Sci.,* NS-25, 638, 1978.
3. **Tretiak, O. J. and Delaney, P.,** The exponential convolution algorithm for emission computed axial tomography, in *Review of Information Processing in Medical Imaging*, Brill, A. B. and Price, R. R., Eds., Oak Ridge National Laboratory Report ORNL/BCTIC-2, 1978, 266.
4. **Gullberg, G. T. and Budinger, T. F.,** The use of filtering methods to compensate for constant attenuation in single-photon emission computed tomography, *IEEE Trans. Biomed. Eng.,* BME-28, 142, 1981.
5. **Tanaka, E.,** Quantitative image reconstruction with weighted back projection for single photon emission computed tomography, *J. Comput. Assist. Tomogr.* 7, 692, 1983.
6. **Croft, B. Y.,** *Single-Photon Emission Computed Tomography*, Year Book Medical, Chicago, Il, 1986.
7. **Budinger, T. F., Gullberg, G. T., and Huesman, R. H.,** Emission computed tomography, in *Image Reconstruction from Projections: Implementation and Applications*, Herman, G. T., Ed., Springer-Verlag, Berlin, 1979.
8. **Barrett, H. H. and Swindell, W.,** *Radiological Imaging: The Theory of Image Formation, Detection, and Processing*, Academic Press, New york, 1981.

Chapter 34

RECONSTRUCTION FROM MULTIPLE SAMPLES: MULTI-DETECTOR SCANNER

A linear, shift invariant model of the data collection process was described in Chapters 31 and 32. A linear, nonshift invariant model was described in Chapter 33. This chapter will describe a model which consists of multiple linear, shift invariant samples. The radiological example will be the multi-detector scanner. Although the multi-detector scanner is an uncommon single photon emission computed tomographic device, the principles derived from consideration of this model have a broader application in radiology.

The major issue addressed in this chapter will be how to combine a sequence of estimates of a single cross section. In the case of X-ray tomography, we shall find that the best method of combining the estimates is the back projection operation which we have already described in Chapters 31 and 32. The results this chapter will also be applied to reconstruction of time of flight information in positron emission tomography.

This chapter will begin with a brief description of the multi-detector scanner. Then, the multiple sample, linear, shift invariant model of data collection will be presented. This model is very simple in the spatial frequency domain — each spatial frequency domain component is estimated separately. In Chapter 12, the estimation of a random variable from multiple samples was performed by scaling the samples by their variance. Scaling by the variance in the frequency domain results in a convolution in the space domain. We shall find that the result of this convolution is to "put the data back from where it came."

I. MULTI-DETECTOR SCANNER

The multi-detector scanner described by Stoddart[1] uses multiple rectilinear scanner detectors to sample the radioactivity in a cross section. Each sodium iodide scintillation detector, equipped with a focused collimator, scans back and forth over the slice and moves in and out with respect to the slice. The scanning action for a single detector is shown in Figure 34.1. The focal point of one collimator traverses half of the cross section, and the focal point of the collimator from the opposite side of the cross section traverses the other half of the cross section.

A focused collimator has a series of holes at various angles which all point at a single location called the focal point of the collimator. A focused collimator is most sensitive to activity placed at the focal point; however, it will detect activity over a broad area surrounding the focal point. The sensitivity of a focused collimator is best described by the collimator response function, the response of the collimator to a point of activity as a function of the positions of the activity.

A typical collimator response function, $a(x,y)$, is shown in Figure 34.2. The lines are a contour map of the isosensitivity of the collimator. The collimator response function falls off more rapidly in the axial than the radial direction.

The collimator response function is represented by a signal, $a(x,y)$. The point spread function of the data obtained from scanning the detector is inverted with respect to the collimator response function. As the detector moves up, the source moves down on the collimator response function. As the detector moves to the right, the source moves to the left on the collimator response function. The point spread function of a scan is equal to $a(-x, -y)$. The point spread function is equal to the collimator response function mirrored about both the x and the y axes.

When a distributed source of activity is viewed with a focused collimator, the count rate of the detector is proportional to the integral of the product of the source activity and the collimator response function which has been shifted appropriately. This operation is

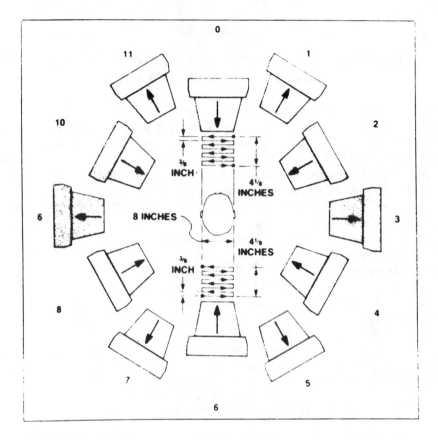

FIGURE 34.1. Multi-detector scanner: this figure is a diagrammatic representation of the multi-detector scanner. Each of the focused collimator detectors scans back and forth, and in and out. The motion of one opposing pair of detectors is shown. (Reprinted from Zimmerman, R. E., Kirsch, K.-M., Lovett, R., and Hill, T. C., in *Single Photon Emission Computed Tomography and Other Selected Computer Topics,* 147—157. Society of Nuclear Medicine, New York, 1980. With permission.)

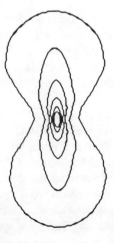

FIGURE 34.2. Collimator response function: the isosensitivity lines of the collimator response function for a focused collimator are shown. The collimator is most sensitive at the focal point. However, the response extends over a large region.

readily recognized as a convolution. Thus, the data obtained from the scanning motion shown in Figure 34.1 are the convolution of the collimator response function and the activity distribution.

The multi-detector scanner has 12 focused collimator detectors positioned around the cross section. In addition, the gantry rotates by one-half the detector spacing and then repeats the scanning process. Twenty-four scans of half the object are produced. If the opposing detectors are similar, then this is equivalent to 12 full scans of the cross section, where each scan is equal to the convolution of the detector and the activity distribution.

There are several important considerations which will not be discussed in this chapter. Because of the axial dimension of the detectors, the multi-detector scanner has high single slice sensitivity. However, this leads to interesting effects along the axial direction (perpendicular to the cross section). The multi-detector scanner is a single photon emission computed tomographic device. The last chapter described the importance of including attenuation in the data reconstruction process. In this chapter, attenuation will be ignored in order to simplify the model. Thus, the multi-detector scanner is more of a point of departure than the topic of this chapter.

II. MODEL

In this chapter, the data collection process will be modeled using a series of linear systems. Each of the systems will produce a set of measurements which can be written:

$$p_i(x',y') = A_i\{f(x,y)\} + n_i(x',y') \qquad (34.1)$$

where $p_i(x',y')$ are the data for one of the measurements, $A_i\{\cdot\}$ is the system representing the measurement process, and $n_i(x',y')$ is the measurement noise. The set of data obtained from the two opposing detectors in a multi-detector scanner could be modeled approximately using $p_i(x',y')$. There are several sets of measurements, each set represented by a value of the index, i. For the multi-detector scanner, the index, i, would relate to the different angles, θ, at which scans are obtained.

Separating the data into a series of signals, $p_i(x',y')$, is a bit artificial. Instead, the data could be defined by a three-dimensional function where i is an additional variable. Since the emphasis in this chapter is on combinations of different measurements into a single estimate, it is useful to maintain the concepts of a number of signals, $p_i(x',y')$. We shall refer to the signal, $p_i(x',y')$, as a projection since it is analogous to the projection data, $p(x',\theta)$, in Chapter 31. However, these projection data have very little relation to the mathematical concept of the projection.

The first step in the reconstruction process is defined to be a transformation of the signal back to the object coordinate system:

$$g_i(x,y) = B_i\{p_i(x',y')\} \qquad (34.2)$$

The back projected signals are then summed:

$$g(x,y) = \sum_i g_i(x,y) \qquad (34.3)$$

Since this operation is analogous to the back projection operation in X-ray computed tomography described in Chapter 31, we shall refer to $g(x,y)$ as the back projected image. However, this image may only be vaguely related to the ideas of back projection used in Chapter 31.

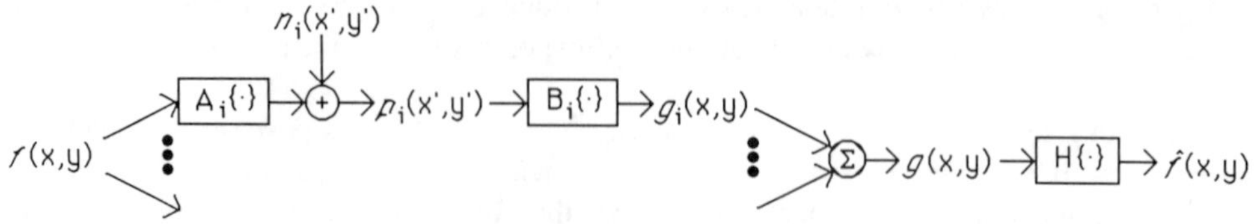

FIGURE 34.3.   Multiple sample model: this figure shows a diagrammatic representation of the multiple sample model. $f(x,y)$ is the unknown object. The system, $A_i\{\cdot\}$, is one of several data collection processes. Each of the samples, $p_i(x',y')$, consists of $A_i\{f(x,y)\}$ plus the measurement noise, $n_i(x',y')$. The system, $B_i\{\cdot\}$, "back projects each of the data samples, $p_i(x',y')$, to $g_i(x,y)$ in the object coordinate system. The "back projected" image $g(x,y)$ is the sum of the $g_i(x,y)$. The estimate, $\hat{f}(x,y)$, of the unknown is obtained by passing the back projected image through the reconstruction system, $H\{\cdot\}$.

We can define a projection, back projection system:

$$D_i\{\cdot\} = B_i\{A_i\{\cdot\}\} \tag{34.4}$$

An overall system is given by:

$$D\{\cdot\} = \sum_i D_i\{\cdot\} \tag{34.5}$$

Using this system the back projected image can be written:

$$g(x,y) = D\{f(x,y)\} + \sum_i B_i\{n_i(x',y')\} \tag{34.6}$$

This equation is similar to Equations 31.8 and 33.14. Image reconstruction is modeled as:

$$\hat{f}(x,y) = H\{g(x,y)\} \tag{34.7}$$

where $\hat{f}(x,y)$ is an estimate of a cross section from the process, $g(x,y)$.

The model of the image reconstruction process requires that the projection data first be combined in the coordinate space of the cross section, x,y, by a back projection operation (Equation 34.6). Then the back projected data are used in the estimation step (Equation 34.7).

This model of the data collection, back projection, estimation process is shown in Figure 34.3. The cross section is sampled with a number of systems, $A_i\{\cdot\}$, to produce projection data, $p_i(x',y')$. The detection process is associated with additive noise, $n_i(x',y')$, in the projection space. The data are combined after being modified by a back projection operation, $B_i\{\cdot\}$. Finally, the system, $H\{\cdot\}$, forms an estimate.

The focus of this chapter will be on selection of the back projection operation, $B_i\{\cdot\}$. What is the best method of combining a sequence of measurements, $p_i(x',y')$? In Chapters 31 and 32, the back projection operation was given by definition. The reconstruction, $H\{\cdot\}$, given $g(x,y,)$ was determined. This goal of this chapter will be to determine the best back projection operation.

III. LINEAR, SHIFT INVARIANT MODEL

The problem can be simplified by restricting the model to linear, shift invariant systems. Then, the data are given by:

$$p_i(x,y) = f(x,y) * a_i(x,y) + n_i(x,y) \tag{34.8}$$

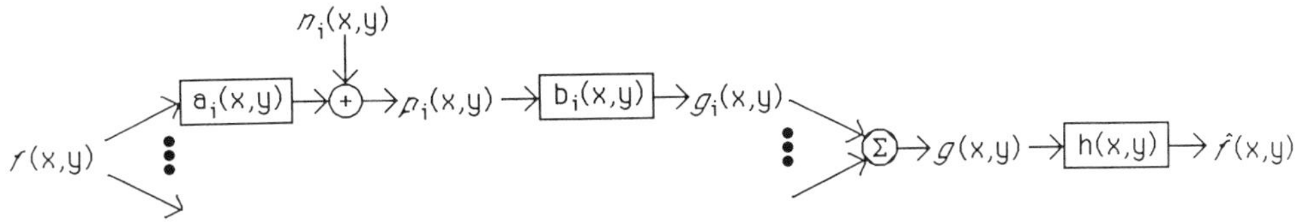

FIGURE 34.4. Linear, shift invariant, multiple sample model: the model shown in this figure is a shift invariant example of the more general model shown in Figure 34.3. The linear, shift invariant systems, $a_i(x,y)$, $b_i(x,y)$, and $h(x,y)$ are used instead of the systems, $A_i\{\cdot\}$, $B_i\{\cdot\}$, and $H\{\cdot\}$. Because the systems are represented by convolution, the data samples, $p_i(x,y)$, are expressed in the same coordinate system as the object.

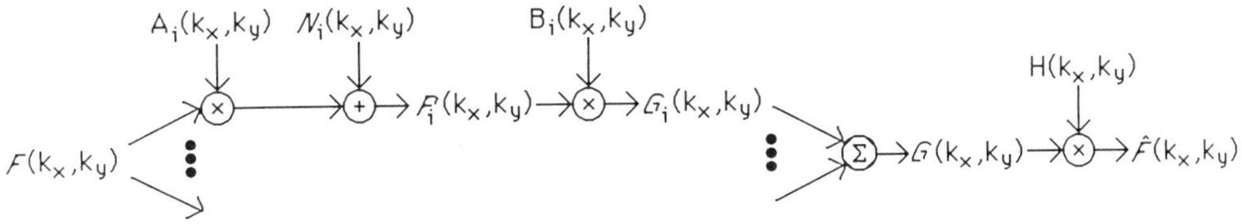

FIGURE 34.5. frequency domain representation of the linear, shift invariant, multiple sample model: the model shown in this figure is the spatial frequency domain representation of the model shown in the space domain in Figure 34.4. The linear, shift invariant systems are represented by multiplication in the spatial frequency domain. It can be seen from this model that each of the spatial frequency components is estimated independently from all other spatial frequencies.

The back projection is given by:

$$g_i(x,y) = p_i(x,y) * b_i(x,y) \tag{34.9}$$

And the estimate is given by:

$$\hat{f}(x,y) = g(x,y) * h(x,y) \tag{34.10}$$

The linear, shift invariant model is shown in Figure 34.4.

The model is even more simple in the spatial frequency domain. The convolution operations are replaced by multiplication:

$$P_i(k_x,k_y) = F(k_x,k_y) \cdot A_i(k_x,k_y) + N_i(k_x,k_y) \tag{34.11}$$

$$G_i(k_x,k_y) = P_i(k_x,k_y) \cdot B_i(k_x,k_y) \tag{34.12}$$

$$\hat{F}(k_x,k_y) = G(k_x,k_y) \cdot H(k_x,k_y) \tag{34.13}$$

The model is shown in the spatial frequency domain in Figure 34.5. In the spatial frequency domain the problem is very simple. Since the spatial frequencies do not interact, the estimate for a particular value of k_x,k_y can be considered separately from all the other values of k_x,k_y. The simplicity of this model comes from the representation of the signals in terms of the eigenfunctions of the linear, shift invariant systems used in the model (see Chapter 4).

For each spatial frequency, we have a number of samples from which we wish to estimate a single random variable:

$$G_i(k_x,k_y) = F(k_x,k_y) \cdot A_i(k_x,k_y) \cdot B_i(k_x,k_y) + N_i(k_x,k_y) \cdot B_i(k_x,k_y) \tag{34.14}$$

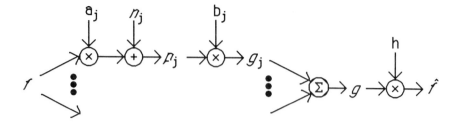

FIGURE 34.6.   Equivalent estimation problem: the estimation problem shown in this diagram is equivalent to the estimation problem shown in Figure 34.5. Since each of the spatial frequency components is estimated independently, the stochastic process can be replaced with random variables representing a single spatial frequency, k_x, k_y.

The samples, $G_i(k_x,k_y)$, for each spatial frequency, k_x,k_y, are independent of the other spatial frequencies. Therefore, in the spatial frequency domain, this problem is very simple — it is the estimation of a random variable, $F(k_x,k_y)$, from multiple scaled and noisy samples of $F(k_x,k_y)$. Each spatial frequency can be separately estimated. This problem is exactly analogous to the problem given by Equation 12.84.

Use of the linear, shift invariant model has greatly simplified the problem. Now the only issue is how to combine a series of estimates of the frequency domain variable. Use of the frequency domain has transformed this very complex problem into a much simpler problem.

IV. REVIEW OF ESTIMATION OF AN UNKNOWN FROM MULTIPLE SAMPLES

Equation 34.14 is analogous to estimation of an unknown from multiple samples described in Chapter 12. We shall repeat the derivation in Chapter 12 for the case that the signal and noises are uncorrelated, but we shall use slightly different notation. Unlike Chapter 12, complex notation will be maintained in this derivation.

Although the goal is to apply estimation to multiple samples in the spatial frequency domain, we shall derive the estimation using the same lower case, random variable notation used in Chapter 12. The model of the data samples is:

$$p_j = a_j \cdot f + n_j \qquad (34.15)$$

where p_j are the data samples, a_j is a scale factor, f is the unknown, and n_j is an additive noise term.

The linear estimate is given by:

$$\hat{f} = h \cdot \sum_j b_j \cdot p_j \qquad (34.16)$$

where the estimate has been divided into two factors, h and b_j; b_j, represent the portion of the estimate which is different for each data value and h represents an overall scaling term. We shall be most interested in the values, b_j, which change for each data value. They determine how the data values are combined. Equation 34.16 is different from Equation 12.85 in that the estimation has been separated into two factors.

We can define a "back projected" random variable, g:

$$g = \sum_j b_j \cdot p_j \qquad (34.17)$$

The factors, b_j, are used to combine the data samples into the back projected random variable. Figure 34.6 shows a model of this estimation process.

The error is defined as:

$$e = f - \hat{f} \tag{34.18}$$

The least mean square error criterion leads to the orthogonality principle (Equation 12.87):

$$E\{e \cdot p_i^*\} = 0, \quad \text{for all i} \tag{34.19}$$

The orthogonality principle uses orthogonal in the statistical sense. Over a series of experiments the error will be uncorrelated for each of the measured data values, p_i.

The orthogonality principle can be expanded using Equations 34.16 and 34.18:

$$E\{f \cdot p_i^*\} - E\left\{h \cdot \sum_j b_j \cdot p_j \cdot p_i\right\} = 0, \quad \text{for all i} \tag{34.20}$$

The order of the expectation and the summation can be changed, and the deterministic quantity $h \cdot b_j$ can be moved outside the expectation. Using the second moment notation defined in Equation 10.31:

$$h \cdot \sum_j b_j \cdot R_{p_j p_i} = R_{f p_i}, \quad \text{for all i} \tag{34.21}$$

Equation 34.21 is analogous to Equation 12.88. It represents a set of simultaneous equations for the factors, $h \cdot b_j$. The estimation factors, $h \cdot b_j$, are determined from the relationship of the cross powers of various combinations of the data values and the unknown. The key factor is the mutual power, $R_{f p_i}$, between the signal and the noise compared to the total power in the signal., $R_{p_j p_i}$, in the data including the noise. This equation was shown to be a relative of the Wiener filter in Chapter 26.

Equation 34.21 can be simplified if we assume that the unknown is uncorrelated with the noise:

$$R_{f n_i} = 0, \quad \text{for all i} \tag{34.22}$$

and that the noise from different measurements is uncorrelated:

$$R_{n_j n_i} = 0, \quad j \neq i \tag{34.23}$$

The cross power of the data can be expanded using Equation 34.15:

$$
\begin{aligned}
R_{p_j p_i} &= E\{(a_j \cdot f + n_j) \cdot (a_i \cdot f + n_i)^*\} \\
&= a_j \cdot a_i^* \cdot R_f + a_j \cdot R_{f n_i} + a_i^* \cdot R_{n_j f} + R_{n_j n_i}
\end{aligned} \tag{34.24}
$$

The second and third terms in Equation 34.24 are always zero; the fourth term is nonzero only when j is equal to i. Thus,

$$R_{p_j p_i} = \begin{cases} a_j \cdot a_i^* \cdot R_f, & j \neq i \\ |a_i|^2 \cdot R_f + R_n, & j = i \end{cases} \tag{34.25}$$

and:

$$R_{fg_i} = a_i^* \cdot R_f \tag{34.26}$$

Using Equations 34.25 and 34.26, Equation 34.21 can be expanded:

$$h \cdot \sum_j b_j \cdot a_j \cdot a_i^* \cdot R_f + h \cdot b_i \cdot R_{n_i} = a_i^* \cdot R_f, \qquad \text{for all i} \tag{34.27}$$

This equation can be solved for the estimation factors $h \cdot b_i$:

$$h \cdot b_i = (a_i^*/R_{n_i}) \cdot R_f \cdot \left(1 - h \cdot \sum_j b_j \cdot a_j\right), \qquad \text{for all i} \tag{34.28}$$

Already at this point we can tell a great deal about the estimation factors. The first factor in Equation 34.28 varies for each data value. The second factor is the same for all values. Thus, the first factor is equal to b_i:

$$b_i = a_i^*/R_{n_i} \tag{34.29}$$

The second factor is equal to h. b_i must be applied individually to each data value. It governs the relative scaling of the data values.

The most important point of this chapter is contained in Equation 34.29. The data values are scaled by the complex conjugate of a_i and divided by the variance of the noise. Scaling the values by the inverse of the variance of the noise means that the data values with the least noise are used most heavily in the estimate. Scaling by the factor, a_i^*, means that the data values which have the greatest effect from the unknown are used the most heavily in the estimate.

The second term in Equation 34.28, equal to h, is not in a very useful form. It includes the estimation factors, $h \cdot b_j$, which are being determined. With some tricky algebraic manipulations, it can be expressed in terms of known quantities. We shall start with Equation 34.27. In order to keep our notation straight we shall substitute the variable k for i. Multiplying by a_k/R_{n_k} and summing over k gives:

$$h \cdot \sum_j b_j \cdot a_j \cdot R_f \cdot \sum_k |a_k|^2/R_{n_k} + h \cdot \sum_k a_k \cdot b_k = R_f \cdot \sum_k |a_k|^2/R_{n_k} \tag{34.30}$$

The second factor in Equation 34.30 is the sum of the estimation factors scaled by a_j. Equation 34.30 is the sum of all of the simultaneous equations represented by Equation 34.28. Thus, we might expect that we are on the right track. The summations in the different terms in Equation 34.30 are independent; therefore, the variable in the second term can be changed from k to j. With this change, the second term is seen to also be a factor in the first term. Thus,

$$h \cdot \sum_j a_j \cdot b_j \cdot \left(R_f \cdot \sum_k |a_k|^2/R_{n_k} + 1\right) = R_f \cdot \sum_k |a_k|^2/R_{n_k} \tag{34.31}$$

Dividing by the factor in parenthesis gives:

$$h \cdot \sum_j a_j \cdot b_j = R_f \cdot \sum_k |a_k|^2/R_{n_k} / \left(R_f \cdot \sum_k |a_k|^2/R_{n_k} + 1\right) \tag{34.32}$$

One can be subtracted from both sides of Equation 34.32. The right side of the equation can be simplified if 1 is expressed as $(R_f \cdot \Sigma |a_k|^2/R_{n_k} + 1)/(R_f \cdot \Sigma |a_k|^2/R_{n_k} + 1)$:

$$1 - h \cdot \sum_j a_j \cdot b_j = 1/\left(R_f \cdot \sum_k |a_k|^2/R_{n_k} + 1\right) \tag{34.33}$$

The left side of Equation 34.33 is equal to the term in parenthesis in Equation 34.28.

Substitution of Equation 34.33 in Equation 34.28 gives:

$$h \cdot b_i = (a_i^*/R_{n_i}) \cdot \left[R_f/\left(R_f \cdot \sum_k |a_k|^2/R_{n_k} + 1\right)\right], \qquad \text{for all i} \tag{34.34}$$

The top and the bottom can be divided by $\Sigma |a_k|^2/R_{n_k}$. With some rearrangement:

$$h \cdot b_i = (a_i^*/R_{n_i}) \cdot \left(1/\sum_k |a_k|^2/R_{n_k}\right)$$
$$+ \left[R_f/\left(R_f + 1/\sum_k |a_k|^2/R_{n_k}\right)\right], \qquad \text{for all i} \tag{34.35}$$

Equation 34.35 gives the value of $h \cdot b_i$ in terms of three factors. The first factor is different for each data value. As noted above:

$$b_i = a_i^*/R_{n_i} \tag{34.36}$$

The last two factors are the same for all data values. Thus,

$$h = \left(1/\sum_k |a_k|^2/R_{n_k}\right) \cdot \left[R_f/\left(R_f + 1/\sum_k |a_k|^2/R_{n_k}\right)\right], \qquad \text{for all i} \tag{34.37}$$

The first factor in Equation 34.37 undoes the overall scaling caused by a_i and b_i. In the absence of noise, multiplication by the first factor will return the original value. The first term is analogous to an exact reconstruction algorithm.

In order to make sense of the second factor in Equation 34.37, it is useful to consider the noise power in the random variable after multiplication by the first factor. At that point, the noise is given by:

$$\sum_i n_i \cdot a_i^*/R_{n_i} \cdot \left(1/\sum_k |a_k|^2/R_{n_k}\right) \tag{34.38}$$

Recall that the power is multiplied by the square of the signal scaling factor. Thus, the power at this point is:

$$\sum_i R_{n_i} \cdot \left(|a_i|^2/R_{n_i}^2\right) \cdot \left(1/\sum_k |a_k|^2/R_{n_k}\right)^2 = 1/\sum_k |a_k|^2/R_{n_k} \tag{34.39}$$

Thus, the second factor in Equation 34.37 is the ratio of the power in the signal to the sum of the power in the signal and the power in the noise. It is analogous to a Wiener filter.

Figure 34.7 shows how Equations 34.36 and 34.37 could be implemented. The different rows show the different samples of the unknown, f. The data values are "back projected" with the factor, a_i^*/R_{n_i}. The "back projected" values are added together. The effect of the back projection operation is removed with the "noiseless reconstructor" given by the first factor in Equation 34.37, $1/\Sigma |a_k|^2/R_{n_k}$. Then the result is filtered with a Wiener like factor given by $R_f/(R_f + 1/\Sigma |a_k|^2/R_{n_k})$.

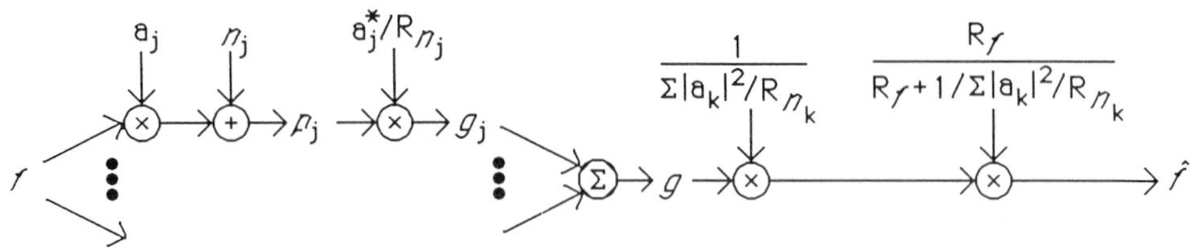

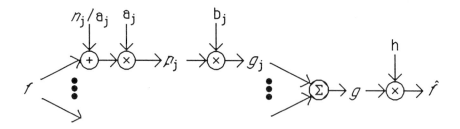

FIGURE 34.7. Solution to the estimation from multiple samples: this figure shows a diagrammatic representation of the solution to the estimation problem shown in Figure 34.6 and by analogy to the problem shown in Figures 34.4 and 34.5. Before combining the data samples, they are scaled ("back projected") by a_j*/R_{n_j}. The estimation factor, h, can be separated into two factors, an exact reconstructor which undoes the effect of the projection, back projection operation, and a Wiener-filter-like noise reduction factor.

FIGURE 34.8. Equivalent multiple sample model: if a_j is not equal to zero, the model shown in this diagram is equivalent to the model shown in Figure 34.6. In this diagram, the noise enters the system before scaling by a_j. In this form the noises for each of the sampling operations can be compared directly.

Adding noise, n_i, after scaling by a_i is equivalent to adding an amount of noise n_i/a_i prior to scaling. Figure 34.8 shows this model. Moving the noise to the other side of the scaling operation is analogous to transforming into the "unknown space". The power of n_i/a_i is given by $R_{n_i}/|a_i|^2$. The "projected", "back projected", data are added combined after being multiplied by $|a_i|^2/R_{n_i}$, the inverse of the power of n_i/a_i. Using the model with the noise added directly to the unknown, it can be seen that the samples are combined after being scaled by the inverse of the power in the noise. This is the same result obtained in Chapter 12.

One interesting feature of this derivation is the fact that b_i includes a factor which is a complex conjugate, a_i*. Usual estimation problems involve real quantities, so that the complex conjugate has no effect. Since our goal is to estimate spatial frequency components which are generally complex numbers, the complex conjugate will have an important effect.

V. RECONSTRUCTION OF MULTIPLE LINEAR, SHIFT INVARIANT SAMPLES

The model shown in Figure 34.5 is analogous to the model shown in Figure 34.6. Therefore we can apply the results of the last section to reconstruction from multiple linear, shift invariant samples of an image. The back projection operation is given by:

$$B_i(k_x,k_y) = A_i^*(k_x,k_y)/S_{n_i}(k_x,k_y) \qquad (34.40)$$

where the power spectral density function, $S_{n_i}(k_x,k_y)$, which gives the power as a function of the spatial frequency, k_x,k_y, has been used in place of the power, R_{n_i}.

Recall from Chapter 16, that the complex conjugate in one domain results in a time reversed complex conjugate in the other domain (Equation 16.71). Using the two headed arrow notation:

$$a_i^*(-x,-y) \leftrightarrow A_i^*(k_x,k_y) \tag{34.41}$$

The collimator response function is a real valued function, therefore $a_i^*(-x,-y)$ is equal to $a_i(-x,-y)$. Thus the back projection operation is a space inverted version of the data collection operation. The data collected with $a_i(x,y)$ are put back by $b_i(x,y)$ to where they came from after scaling by the power in the noise.

The back projected image, $g(x,y)$, is the sum of the back projected samples:

$$g(x,y) = \sum_i a_i^*(-x,-y) * p_i(x,y) \tag{34.42}$$

The estimate, $\hat{f}(x,y)$, is obtained from $g(x,y)$ by filtering with $h(x,y)$. In the spatial frequency domain, the filter, $H(k_x,k_y)$, is given by:

$$H(k_x,k_y) = \left[1/\sum_j |A_j(k_x,k_y)|^2/S_{n_j}(k_x,k_y) \right]$$
$$\cdot \left[S_f(k_x,k_y)/\left(S_f(k_x,k_y) + 1/\sum_j |A_j(k_x,k_y)|^2/S_{n_j}(k_x,k_y) \right) \right] \tag{34.43}$$

Equation 34.43 appears to be very complicated; however, two familiar factors can be readily recognized. The first factor simply undoes the effect of the projection, back projection operation. It is an exact reconstructor. The second term is the ratio on the signal power to the signal plus noise power of the signal after exact reconstruction. It is just a Wiener filter term. Thus, $H(k_x,k_y)$, inverts the projection, back projection system and filters the noise with a Wiener filter.

This algorithm is interesting theoretically; however, it is not particularly useful for implementation. The back projection operation involves convolution with a signal, $a_i^*(-x,-y)$, which may have considerable extent. The back projected image may be considerably larger than the original image. During the back projection process, the image may extend well outside the object space. Reconstruction may be inefficient. Recall from Chapter 31 that the finite extent of the reconstruction process was a special property of the entire projection, back projection, reconstruction process, not just the back projection.

One source of *a priori* information that is almost always true is that the object is within the field of view of the imaging equipment. Using this algorithm, the reconstructed image may extend outside of the field of view of the imager. Thus, the *a priori* information about the field of view is not well captured by this algorithm.

VI. COMPARISON TO THE NORMAL EQUATIONS OF LINEAR ALGEBRA

The normal equations of linear algebra were derived in Chapter 25. The normal equations were given by Equation 25.43:

$$\mathbf{A} \cdot \mathbf{A}^T \cdot \hat{\mathbf{f}} = \mathbf{A}^T \cdot \mathbf{p} \tag{34.44}$$

Image reconstruction is performed with the matrix, H, defined by Equation 25.42:

$$H = (A^T \cdot A)^{-1} \cdot A^T \qquad (34.45)$$

when the inverse $(A^T \cdot A)^{-1}$ exists.

The matrix, A^T, transforms the data, **p**, from the projection space back to the image space. The matrix, A^T, in the linear algebra formulation is analogous to the back projection operation, $b_i(x,y)$, in the linear systems formulation. In Chapter 33, we noted the difference between $h(x,y)$ and H. Although we have used the same letter for these two operations, they are not analogous. The matrix, $A^T \cdot A$, is analogous to the reconstruction operation, $h(x,y)$. The matrix, H, is analogous to $\Sigma b_i(x,y)*h(x,y)$.

With both the linear algebra and linear systems methods, the projection data must be transformed from the projection space back to the image space. In the former case, the transformation is done with A^T, in the later case, it is done with $b_i(x,y)$. The transformation operation is similar. After moving back to the image space, the resulting image is filtered to produce an estimate of the object. The filtering operations are different since the normal equations estimate the data and the Wiener filter estimates the unknown.

VII. X-RAY COMPUTED TOMOGRAPHY

In Chapters 31 and 32, the back projection operation was given as a part of the model. We did not consider whether it was the best back projection operation. If the model of the data collection process given in Figure 34.4 is applied to X-ray computed tomography, then the best back projection operation can be determined.

The data collection process for X-ray computed tomography can be modeled by a delta function:

$$a_\theta(x',y') = \delta(x') \qquad (34.46)$$

where $a_\theta(x',y')$ is convolved with $f(x,y)$ to produce the projection data $p_\theta(x',y')$. The two-dimensional function $p_\theta(x',y')$ is the data obtained at one angle, θ.

The two-dimensional function, $p_\theta(x',y')$, varies along the x' axis, but not along the y' axis. Since it is constant in the y' direction, it provides only one dimension worth of information, but we shall consider it a two-dimensional function to show the analogies to the previous section. This two-dimensional function is equivalent to the one-dimensional set of points given by $p(x',\theta)$ for θ equal to a constant.

If the noise is unity for all projection, then Equation 34.40 states that the back projection operation is given by:

$$b_\theta(x',y') = \delta(-x') \qquad (34.47)$$

But this is just another way of writing the standard back projection operation.

Thus, the results of this chapter show that the best back projection operation is in fact the back projection operation which was used in Chapters 31 and 32. The filtering operation is performed after the back projection in Figure 34.4; however, as has been pointed out a number of times, filtering prior to the back projection operation is mathematically equivalent to filtering after it. Thus, the usual convolution, back projection operation is the best method of combining the multiple samples obtained in X-ray computed tomography.

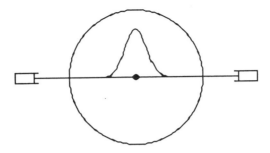

FIGURE 34.9. Time-of-flight positron emission tomography: this figure shows a diagrammatic representation of the point spread function for two detectors in a positron camera using time-of-flight information. The position of the positron decay is along a line between the two detectors. The difference in the time of arrival of the photons provides information about the depth of the decay within the cross section. The depth information is not as accurate as the position information.

VIII. TIME-OF-FLIGHT POSITRON EMISSION COMPUTED TOMOGRAPHY

The multi-detector scanner is a good example where $a_i(x,y)$ is extended in both the x and the y direction. That is why we have used the multi-detector scanner to motivate the multiple sample model. However, the model of the data collection process used in this chapter is not very accurate for single photon emission computed tomography. It leaves out attenuation. The last chapter pointed out the importance of attenuation in single photon emission computed tomography.

The multiple sample model shown in Figure 34.4 is a reasonably good model for time-of-flight, positron emission computed tomography. When a positron annihilates an electron, two photons are given off simultaneously at approximately 180°. Detectors on opposite sides of the patient record the two photons. With very fast detectors, it is possible to obtain information about the depth of positron decay from the difference in arrival time of the two photons. The depth positioning is, however, not very accurate.

Figure 34.9 shows a diagrammatic representation of the results obtained for a point source of activity from two opposing detectors. The position of the two detectors localizes the annihilation along a line through the cross section. The time of flight information provides depth information. However, since the depth information is not very accurate, there is considerable spread along the line between the detectors.

The various detector pairs which are in coincidence can be assembled into parallel projection data (not an entirely trivial task, but not the subject of this discussion). The data obtained at each angle can be modeled as the convolution of the activity distribution with a signal $a_i(x,y)$, which is equal to the reverse of the curve in Figure 34.9 in the y' direction and is a delta function in the x' direction.

If the noise is the same at all angles, then the back projection operation is proportional to $a_i^*(-x,-y)$. The projection, back projection operation at each angle has the affect of multiplying the image by $|A_i(k_x,k_y)|^2$ in the spatial frequency domain. Reconstruction from the back projected image is performed by some reconstructor, $H\{\cdot\}$.

The exact method of reconstruction used is not the point of this chapter. Rather, the combination of the data from the different angles is the focus. In the spatial frequency domain the data samples are combined with factors, $A_i^*(k_x,k_y)/S_{n_i}(k_x,k_y)$.

IX. SUMMARY

The goal of this chapter is to determine how multiple measurements of a cross section should be combined during the reconstruction process. The data collection model used in this chapter separates the data into a series of samples, $p_i(x,y)$. Separating the data into a series of samples is somewhat artificial, but it is conceptually useful. The reconstruction process can be separated into factors that are different for each of the data samples, $p_i(x,y)$, and factors that are the same for all samples. In this chapter, the factors that are different for each sample are referred to as the back projection operation.

The assumption that the data collection, image reconstruction process is linear and shift invariant is key to the simplification of the problem. The eigenfunctions of linear, shift invariant systems are the imaginary exponentials. The spatial frequency components are the eigenvalues for these eigenfunctions. Since the eigenfunctions pass through the system independently, each of the eigenvalues can be estimated separately. The eigenfunction description changes the complicated reconstruction problem into the much simple problem of estimation of a single random variable, $F(k_x,k_y)$, from several data samples.

For the linear, shift invariant case, the back projection operation in the spatial frequency domain is equal to a multiplication by $A_i^*(k_x,k_y)/S_{n_i}(k_x,k_y)$. The model in Figure 34.8 shows that the back projection operation scales the samples by the inverse of the variance of their noise. In the space domain, the numerator, $A_i^*(k_x,k_y)$, is equal to the complex conjugate of the space inverted collection operation. The effect of this factor is to put the data back to the position from which it came.

The results of this chapter are useful for many reconstruction problems. They indicate that the back projection operation which was used in Chapters 31 and 32 for X-ray computed tomography is in fact the best algorithm. The results of this chapter suggest how the time-of-flight information in positron emission computed tomography can be used during reconstruction. In general, the results of this chapter are useful for understanding the back projection step in any reconstruction operation.

X. FURTHER READING

The approach taken in this chapter is somewhat unique. Separating the data into a set of two-dimensional projections is somewhat artificial, but the goal was to show how the different data are combined. As such, there are no direct references to this material; however, the references at the end of the last chapter deal with some of the issues brought up in this chapter.

A more complete description of reconstruction from the multi-detector scanner with inclusion of axial reconstruction of a number of slices can be found in an article by Moore and Mueller.[2] A description of time-of-flight positron emission computed tomography can be found in the article by Ter-Pogossian et al.[3]

REFERENCES

1. **Stoddart, H. F. and Stoddart, H. A.,** A new development in single gamma transaxial tomography: union carbide focused collimator scanner, *IEEE Trans. Nucl. Sci.*, NS-26, 2710, 1079.
2. **Moore, S. C. and Mueller, S. P.,** Inversion of the 3D Radon transform for a multidetector, point-focused SPECT brain scanner, *Phys. Med. Biol.*, 31, 207, 1986.
3. **Ter-Pogossian, M. M., Mullani, N. A., Ficke, D. C., Markham, J., and Synder, D. L.,** Photon time-of-flight-assisted positron emission tomography, *J. Comput. Assist. Tomogr.*, 5, 227, 1981.

Chapter 35

SUMMARY OF RECONSTRUCTION

Part IV of this book has described image reconstruction in several fields of radiology. Description of image reconstruction is the major goal of this book. The first three parts of the book were a prologue; they developed the techniques which were needed to understand reconstruction.

Part I (System Models) presented three major methods for modeling systems — the convolution model from linear system theory, the vector, matrix model from linear algebra, and the random process model from stochastic analysis. Part II (Transforms) presented the Fourier transform, the major tool used for both understanding and implementing reconstruction. Part III (Filtering) described modification of signals in the frequency domain. A very important filter in this book is the Wiener filter. The Wiener filter and similar operations are used to reduce the noise in reconstructed images. This part of the book brings together the different methods described in the other sections in order to understand reconstruction.

There are several themes which have been developed in this part of the book. Development of a good model of the data collection process is a large part of the task of understanding reconstruction. Use of *a priori* information can markedly improve the accuracy of reconstruction. Comparison between the different models provides a better understanding of the reconstruction process. Use of eigenfunctions greatly simplifies the description of reconstruction. The ''back projection'' operation helps to explain the process of combining different data samples. The separation of the reconstruction process into back projection, exact reconstruction, and noise reduction aids understanding of reconstruction. This chapter will review these themes.

I. MODELS

A recurring theme in this part of the book is the importance of a good model of the data collection process. In Chapter 30, which described nuclear magnetic resonance imaging, almost all of the chapter was spent on describing the model of the data collection process. In nuclear magnetic resonance imaging, the data samples are equal to spatial frequency components of the object. Once this relation between the data and the spatial frequencies of the object is clearly understood, reconstruction is trivial — it is an inverse Fourier transform. The major issue in understanding reconstruction is the development of the model of the data collection process.

Chapter 31 described image reconstruction in computed tomography. Again the major task in understanding computed tomographic reconstruction is to understand the relation of the projection data to the cross-sectional object. The back projection operation was important in our description of this relation. The projection, back projection model explains the data in terms of the object coordinate system. The projection, back projection operation has the effect of smoothing the cross section by convolution with a function equal to 1/r. With this model of the data collection process, understanding image reconstruction is simplified — reconstruction is performed by deconvolution for the 1/r point spread function of the projection, back projection operation.

Chapter 32 dealt with image reconstruction from noisy projections. Careful development of the data collection model allowed us to note the similarity between this problem and the problem solved in Chapter 26 (Wiener Filtering). With this model, image reconstruction could be understood in terms of two factors — exact reconstruction as in Chapter 31, and noise reduction with a Wiener filter.

Chapter 33 described single photon emission computed tomography. Due to attenuation, single photon emission computed tomography can not be modeled using a shift invariant system. However, it is possible to develop a shift invariant model for the data in a single projection. This model was useful in understanding the data, and in understanding the effects of the attenuation on the data. Actual reconstruction is performed by applying an iterative algorithm to a nonshift invariant model. The nonshift invariant, iterative algorithm is more easily understood by carefully developing both models.

Chapter 34 described a model for combining multiple data samples. The goal of this model is to determine the best method for combining different samples of the same cross section. The result is logical. The combination could be performed by putting the data back from where it came. This model can be used in understanding not only the multidetector scanner and positron emission computed tomography, but also to understanding the back projection process used in computed tomography. The key to solving this problem is that the model allowed us to recognize the similarity of this model to the simpler random variable problem solved in Chapter 12.

II. *A PRIORI* INFORMATION

In several chapters in this part of the book, the importance of *a priori* information has been noted. A very important part of the reconstruction process is how well the model reflects the *a priori* information about the system. The difference between the performance of various reconstruction methods is often largely dependent upon how well this *a priori* information is captured by the model which is used.

The first chapter in this part of the book, Chapter 29, described deconvolution of radionuclide angiocardiography. One reason for including this problem was to show the similarlity of one-dimensional signal processing methods with two-dimensional image reconstruction methods. Another reason for including this relatively simple problem was to provide some indication of how *a priori* information could be incorporated in the deconvolution process. For real problems, the best results are obtained by including as much *a priori* information as possible.

Although this part has mentioned *a priori* information several times, it has included relatively few methods for inclusion of *a priori* information. The advantages of several of the methods which have not been described in this book have to do with how they model different forms of *a priori* information. Understanding how different reconstruction methods allow *a priori* information to be incorporated is a valuable direction for further study.

III. CORRELATION BETWEEN MODELS

The three approaches to modeling — linear systems, linear algebra, and stochastic processes — were treated separately in the first two parts of the book. In Part III, Wiener filtering brought together the linear systems and stochastic process models. Similarly, the normal equation brought together linear algebra and random vectors. Throughout the book we have tried to emphasize the similarities between the linear systems and linear algebra approaches. But, it is this part of the book which has really brought together these methods in the explanation of image reconstruction.

The linear systems approach was used in explaining nuclear magnetic resonance imaging, X-ray computed tomography, and the multi-detector scanner. Linear algebra was used to explain deconvolution in first pass radionuclide angiocardiography and reconstruction in single photon emission computed tomography. More generally, it can be used to solve nonshift invariant problems which arise in any of these applications. Stochastic processes were used most in Chapters 32 and 33, but again the result from these chapters provides a back drop for the other reconstruction techniques. In fact, each of these methods helps to explain the others.

Combination of so many techniques into one book is a bit unusual. The description of each method is of necessity somewhat abbreviated. And even so, the book is very long. However, the reason for including these various methods in a single book with a consistent notation is that each method best explains certain aspects of the reconstruction problem. The combination provides a better understanding of reconstruction than any one method would provide.

IV. EIGENFUNCTIONS

The value of eigenfunctions in understanding systems was first pointed out in Chapter 5. Part II of the book dealt with the transformation of signals into a description in terms of the imaginary exponentials, the imaginary exponentials are the eigenfunctions of linear, time or shift invariant systems. The major value of the Fourier transform is that signals and systems can be expressed using this eigenfunction description.

The linear, shift invariant models of reconstruction in this part of the book take advantage of this eigenfunction description. For example, a large part of the simplicity of the description of computed tomography has to do with the fact that the spatial frequency domain is an eigenfunction description for the projection, back projection operation.

Part IV has emphasized the linear system model over the linear algebra model. Even in Chapter 33, which used a nonshift invariant model, much of the discussion was in terms of the linear system theory. The major reason for this emphasis is that the eigenfunctions simplify the description. (There are eigenvector methods which can be used with the linear algebra methods, but they are beyond the scope of this book.)

The most complicated model of reconstruction was given in Chapter 34. This model is shown in the spatial frequency domain in Figure 34.5. In the spatial frequency domain, it can be seen that each of the eigenfunctions traverses the system independently. The problem reduces to estimation of each of the eigenvalues independently of all the other values. This problem is analogous to estimation of a single random variable described in Chapter 12. There is some algebraic complexity in keeping all the factors straight, but the basic problem is reasonably simple. By expressing this very complicated model of data collection and reconstruction using eigenfunctions, the model reduces to the much simpler problem of estimation of a single unknown at a time from several data samples.

The convolution model from Part I together with the transform method from Part II has allowed the complicated reconstruction problem to be separated into two parts. The spatial frequency description is used to understand the model in terms of its eigenfunctions. Then, the least mean square estimation method can be used to obtain an estimate of each of the eigenvalues.

V. BACK PROJECTION

This book provides an unusually heavy emphasis on the back projection operation. It is possible to describe reconstruction without back projection. Radon's original description transformed directly between a function with limited support and the set of line integrals through that function. It did not use a "back projection" of the line integrals. Most authors do use the back projection operation in describing computed tomographic reconstruction, but it is very unusual to consider a "back projection" type of operation in other models.

Separation of the back projection operation from the rest of the reconstruction process provides some insights. In the case of computed tomography, back projection transforms the data from the less concrete projection space, x',θ, to the more easily understood object space, x,y. Back projection allows direct comparison of the data with the object. From the back projected image, it is easy to understand that the data collection process samples the lower spatial frequencies more heavily than the higher spatial frequencies. The origin of the ramp filter becomes obvious.

In Chapter 33, the "back projection like" process is multiplication with A^T. Back projection transforms vectors to the row space of A, where the unknown, **f**, is defined (at least the part of **f** which can be measured by the data collection process). The normal equations of linear algebra say that the "back projected" estimate of the data $A^T \cdot (A \cdot \hat{f})$ is equal to the "back projected" data $A^T \cdot \mathbf{p}$. The portion of the data which is inconsistent with the model is due to measurement noise. The back projection operation discards the part of the noise which is inconsistent with the model.

The back projection operation was the topic of Chapter 34. The goal of that chapter was to determine how to select the back projection operation. For the linear, shift invariant model, the back projection operation was given by $A_i^*(k_x,k_y)/S_{n_i}(k_x,k_y)$. This result shows that the data are combined after normalizing for the noise variance. In the case that the measurement noise is the same for all of the samples, the effect of this multiplication in the spatial frequency domain is a convolution by $a_i^*(-x,-y)$ in the space domain. This convolution has the effect of putting the data back from where it came — a very logical result. The back projection operation is a way of combining data samples on an equal footing.

VI. EXACT RECONSTRUCTION, NOISE REDUCTION, AND IMAGE ENHANCEMENT

In Chapter 32, the reconstruction from noisy computed tomographic projections was divided into three factors. The first factor was the ramp filter; the same reconstruction used in Chapter 31. The ramp filter performs an exact reconstruction. The second factor was equal to a Wiener filter. The Wiener filter part of the reconstruction process suppresses noise. A third factor was included for image enhancement. The image enhancement filter is not really a part of the reconstruction process, but it can be used to improve the appearance of the image.

Image enhancement was described very briefly in Chapter 27. The goal of image enhancement is often to produce a more pleasing image. However, it has also been used to attempt to improve lesion detection by the radiologist. The criteria used in this book to select the reconstruction filter is least-mean-square error between the estimate and the object being estimated. Once the radiologist is made part of the image processing model, this criteria is no longer satisfactory. It needs to be replaced with a measure of performance such as that provided by receiver operating characteristic methods. A discussion of these methods is beyond the scope of this book, but these methods are a direction for further study.

The reconstruction process at first seems complicated. However, it can be separated into a sequence of steps — back projection, exact reconstruction, noise reduction, and image enhancement. Each of these steps is relatively straight forward. Dividing the process into a series of steps simplifies understanding of the reconstruction process.

VII. SUMMARY OF DATA COLLECTION AND IMAGE RECONSTRUCTION

The most complete form of the linear systems model was that given in the last chapter. It will be restated here in a compact form. The cross sectional object, $f(x,y)$, is sampled by convolution with several systems, $a_i(x,y)$. The measurement noise enters the system after convolution with $a_i(x,y)$. Equation 34.8 gives this model:

$$p_i(x,y) = f(x,y) * a_i(x,y) + n_i(x,y) \tag{35.1}$$

The first step in the process is to back project the data:

$$g(x,y) = \sum_i p_i(x,y) * b_i(x,y) \tag{35.2}$$

In Chapter 34, it was shown that if the noise power spectrum is the same for all of the projections, then the back projection operation should "put the data back from where it came":

$$b_i(x,y) = a_i^*(-x,-y) \tag{35.3}$$

The back projection system function is the complex conjugate of a space-inverted version of the data collection system function.

The reconstruction is performed by filtering (Equation 34.10):

$$f(x,y) = g(x,y) * h(x,y) \tag{35.4}$$

The filter can be divided into two factors (Equation 34.43). The first factor undoes the effect of the projection, back projection operation:

$$1/\sum_j |A_j(k_x,k_y)|^2/S_{n_j}(k_x,k_y) \tag{35.5}$$

The second factor is in the form of a Wiener filter:

$$S_f(k_x,k_y)/\left[S_f(k_x,k_y) + 1/\sum_j |A_j(k_x,k_y)|^2/S_{n_j}(k_x,k_y) \right] \tag{35.6}$$

The first factor is an exact reconstructor, the second factor is a noise reduction filter.

The data collection, image reconstruction model is shown in Figure 34.4. The overall projection, back projection operation is modeled as a linear, shift invariant system. Those spatial frequencies which are passed by the system can be exactly reconstructed by use of an inverse system. A Wiener filter is used to improve the signal to noise in the reconstructed image. The *a priori* information included by this model is the statistics of the power in the signal and the noise.

The most complete form of the linear algebra method is the iterative reconstruction scheme given in Chapter 33. The cross section, f, is sampled using a data collection process represented by the system, A. The measurement is associated with detector noise, n:

$$p = A \cdot f + n \tag{35.7}$$

Exact reconstruction with the normal equations is not practical. Thus, reconstruction is performed with an approximate iterative reconstruction process. We assume that there is a reasonable reconstruction operator, H. H does not have to be very good, it only needs to have some relation to a reconstruction process. For example, it could be a simple back projector. What is required is very accurate knowledge of the data collection opperation, A.

The process starts with a zero order approximation of the unknown:

$$\hat{f}_0 = H \cdot p \tag{35.8}$$

The successive estimations of the projection data are produced by passing the approximation of the unknown through the model of the data collection process, A:

$$\hat{p}_{n-1} = A \cdot \hat{f}_{n-1} \tag{35.9}$$

The estimates are corrected at each stage by the difference between the estimated data and the actual data:

$$\hat{f}_n = \hat{f}_{n-1} + r \cdot H \cdot (p - \hat{p}_{n-1}) \tag{35.10}$$

r, the relaxation factor, is typically somewhat less than one e.g., 0.7. Values of r closer to one cause faster reconstruction, but may lead to oscillations in the successive estimations.

This reconstruction algorithm is shown in Figure 33.16. Notice that the operation of the algorithm reflects the data collection process. Unlike the Wiener filter which estimates the unknown, this algorithm estimates the data (as do the normal equations). The *a priori* information included in this algorithm is that the data must be consistent with the data collection process, A. If the reconstruction process is ill conditioned, it may converge to a result which has considerable effect from noise. One frequent solution is to stop the iteration after only a few steps. Then, an initial estimate can be used to include additional *a priori* information.

The description of linear algebra methods of reconstruction has been more superficial than the discussion of linear systems methods. There are a large number of methods available, each with unique properties. The interesting issues presented by these methods are beyond the scope of this book, but they suggest an important area of further study.

Linear, shift invariant reconstruction can be performed in an amount of time proportional to $N \cdot \log(N)$, where N is the number of pixels in the image. Reconstruction with the normal equations requires an amount of time proportional to N^2 if the matrix, H, is precalculated and an amount of time N^3, if H must be calculated during reconstruction. The iterative algorithm requires an amount of time N^2 at each step; however, since the matrices, A and H, are often sparse (mostly zeroes), there are often application-specific methods which are much faster than N^2. Iterative algorithms developed for particular applications are often nearly as fast as shift invariant algorithms.

VIII. SUMMARY

The goal of this book has been to provide the reader with ... understanding of the image reconstruction process. General principles have been emphasized at the expense of detailed description of the particular applications. The applications in this part have served as a point of departure. Whenever the application and the model differed, we chose to consider the model. The goal of this book is to provide a framework for understanding reconstruction. With this framework, the reader interested in a particular application should be able to understand the more detailed descriptions available in other sources.

Hopefully this book has raised more questions than it has answered, and has stimulated the reader to further study of the image reconstruction problem.

APPENDIX: SYMBOLS

The following is a list of symbols used in this book along with their usual meaning. A few of the symbols are used for more than one purpose; however, the context in which they are used should make their meaning apparent.

O	Zero vector
A	Matrix representing measurement process
A_0	Activity present at time zero
$A(\cdot)$	Fourier transform of the measurement process
$A\{\cdot\}$	General measurement process
$a(\cdot)$	Linear measurement process
$B(\cdot)$	Fourier transform of data sample combining process
$B\{\cdot\}$	General data sample combining process
$b(\cdot)$	Data sample combining process
B	Magnetic field
B_0	Main magnetic field
B_1	Radio frequency magnetic field
c	Speed
$c(\cdot)$	Cost function
$\cos(\cdot)$	Cosine
γ	Gyromagnetic ratio
D	Diagonal matrix
D	Matrix representing projection, back projection
$D(\cdot)$	Fourier transform of projection, back projection
$D\{\cdot\}$	General projection, back projection process
$d(\cdot)$	Projection, back projection system function
$d(\cdot)/dt$	Derivative with respect to time
$\partial(\cdot)/\partial t$	Partial derivative with respect to time
d	Cononical basis vector
$\delta(\cdot)$	Delta function
Δt	Small time increment
$E\{\cdot\}$	Expectation operator
e	Base for exponentials, equal to approximately 2.7183
e	Error value
e	Error random value
e	Error vector
$FT\{\cdot\}$	Fourier transform operation
$FT^{-1}\{\cdot\}$	Inverse Fourier transform operation
$F(\cdot)$	Fourier transform of an input signal
$F[\cdot]$	Discrete Fourier transform of an input signal
$F_\theta'(k_x,k_y)$	Fourier transform of attenuated cross section
$F_e(\cdot)$	Fourier transform of $f_e(\cdot)$
$F_0(\cdot)$	Fourier transform of $f_0(\cdot)$
$f(\cdot)$	Continuous input signal
$f[\cdot]$	Discrete input signal
$f_e(\cdot)$	Even part of $f(\cdot)$
$f_0(\cdot)$	Odd part of $f(\cdot)$
$f'(x,y,\theta)$	Attenuated cross section, equal to $f(x,y)\cdot\mu(x,y,\theta)$

f	Length of **f**
f	Input vector
f	Random variable
f	Random vector
$\hat{f}$	Estimate of a random variable
$\hat{\boldsymbol{f}}$	Estimate of a random vector
$f(\cdot)$	Input random process
$\hat{f}(\cdot)$	Estimate of the input random process
$G(\cdot)$	Fourier transform of the output signal
$G[\cdot]$	Discrete Fourier transform of the output signal
$g(\cdot)$	Continuous output signal
$g(\cdot)$	Back projected image
$g[\cdot]$	Discrete output signal
g	Length of **g**
g	Output vector
g	Random variable
$g(\cdot)$	Random process
H	Matrix representation of a system
$H(\cdot)$	Fourier transform of the system function
$H[\cdot]$	Discrete Fourier transform of the system function
$H\{\cdot\}$	System operator
$h(\cdot)$	Continuous system function
$h[\cdot]$	Discrete system function
i	$\sqrt{(-1)}$
I	Identity matrix
$Im\{\cdot\}$	Imaginary part of a complex number
k	Spring constant
k	Wave number
k,θ	Polar spatial frequency variables
k_x,k_y	Spatial frequency variables
$\ln(\cdot)$	Natural logarithm
Λ	Diagonal matrix of eigenvalues
λ	Eigenvalue
λ	Decay constant
λ	Wave length
M	Bulk magnetic moment
$M_\theta(k_x,k_y)$	Fourier transform of attenuation values
m	Mass
m	Mean of a random variable
m_i	Bulk magnetic moment of region i
$m(t)$	Mean of a stochastic process
μ	Sample mean
μ	Linear attenuation constant
$\mu(x,y,\theta)$	Attenuation values
$n(\cdot)$	Noise signal
n	Noise vector
ν	Frequency variable
$P_\theta(k_{x'})$	Fourier transform of projection
$p(x',\theta)$	Projection
$p(\cdot)$	Random process representing projection data
$p'(\cdot)$	Random process representing modified projection data

$\hat{p}(\cdot)$	Estimate of the data
$\mathbf{p}$	Data vector
p	Random variable
$\hat{p}$	Estimate of p
π	Pi, equal to approximately 3.1416
r	Rank of a matrix
r	Relaxation factor
r,θ	Polar spatial variables
R	Second moment of a random variable
$R(\cdot)$	Correlation of a random process
$Re\{\cdot\}$	Real part of a complex number
S	Matrix with orthonormal rows
$S(\cdot)$	Power spectral density function
s	Complex exponential variable
s^2	Sample variance
$\sin(\cdot)$	Sine
σ	Standard deviation
σ^2	Variance
Σ	Summation operator
T	Period
$(\cdot)^T$	Transpose operator
$T_{1/2}$	Half life
T_1	Spin lattice relaxation time
T_2	Spin-spin relaxation time
T_2^*	Instrumetnal T_2 time
t	Time variable
$\tan^{-1}(\cdot)$	Arctangent
τ	Alternate time variable
τ_c	Correlation time
θ	Phase variable
$u(\cdot)$	Step function
$u[\cdot]$	Discrete step function
W	Matrix which performs a discrete Fourier transform
x,y	Spatial variables
x',y'	Spatial variables, rotated with respect to x,y
x',y'	Spatial variables for the projection space
ω	Angular frequency variable
z	Complex number
z*	Complex conjugate of z
$|z|$	Magnitude of z
*	Convolution operation
$\int_{-\infty}^{+\infty}$	Integration operation

Index

INDEX

A

Absorptive signals, 239
Adding in convolution, 30
Addition of matrices, 101
Additivity in linearity, 44—46
Algebraic derivation
  in least mean square estimation of the data, 170—171
  in least mean square estimation of the unknown, 179—180
Aliasing, 335—339, 346, 348
AM modulation, 231, 233
Analytic functions, 77
Angiogiocardiography, first pass radionuclide, 411—420
Angular frequency, 72, 423
Applications of complex numbers, 62—63
A priori information, 416—417, 498
Associative property defined, 102
Attenuation
  constant, 470—475
  low frequency, 396—398
  point source, 464—465
Attenuation factors, 472—474
Audio amplifier signals, 49—50
  eigenfunctions, 53—54
  filtering in, 319
  Fourier transform in, 225—226
Autocorrelation of stochastic processes, 155, 355—356

B

Back projection, 443—446, 448—449, 499—500
  in computed tomography, 454
  exponential, 476—478
  in X-ray computed tomography, 494
Band pass filters, 329, 357—358
Bar phantom aliasing, 336, 338—339
Base of the exponential, 22
Basic concepts, 9—27
Basis functions, 33—35
  in discrete Fourier transform, 261—262
  eigenfunctions as, 56—58
  of Fourier transform, 309
  representation of signals, 185—186
  sum of in Fourier transform, 264—265
Basis vectors, 119—124
Blood activity curves, 29—30
Blurring tomography, 443
Bolus imaging, 29, 32, 413
Boundary conditions, 90
Butterworth filter, 331—332

C

Cardiovascular system, nontime invariance of, 417

Carrier modulation, 231—233
Cauchy-Rieman equations, 77
Causal signals, 238—239
Change in scale, 233—234, 307
Chemical shift, 125, 426, 435
Closed spaces, 111
Coefficient domain, 249
Coefficients in linear differential equations, 82, 90—94
Comb signal, 337—345
Commutative property, 102—103
Complex conjugates, 66
Complex exponentials, 66—70
  mathematical operations, 70—71
  plane waves, 74—75
  sinusoidal functions, 71—73
  tissue impedance to ultrasound, 75—76
  trigonometric relationships, 70
Complexity of system models, 50—51, 186—187
Complex numbers, 4, 61—62
  applications of, 62—63
  in eigenfunctions of linear time invariant systems, 78
  functions of complex variable, 76—78
  operations on, 65—70
  representations of, 63—64
  uses of complex exponential, 70—76
Complex plane integration transforms, 299—301
Complex valued functions, 76
Complex variables
  derivatives of, 77—78
  functions of, 76—78
Computed tomography
  image reconstruction, 457—459
  implementation, 459—460
  linear, shift invariant model in, 119
  linearization in, 46
  model, 453—457
  as model of estimation process, 371—373
  positron emission time-of-flight, 495
  single photon emission, 463—481, see also Single photon emission computed tomography
  standard deviation in, 147
  uncertainty principle in, 244
  X-ray, 348—349, 441—451
Conservation of energy, 242
Constant coefficients in linear differential equations, 82, 90—94
Continuous functions, 11
Continuous signals, 312
Continuous systems, 183
Continuous vs. pulsed inputs, 55—56
Continuous vs. pulsed NMR, 195—196
Convolution, 3
  description of, 29—31
  discrete, 118
  examples of, 38—42
  filtering and, 403—404

in linear, time invariant systems, 47—50
mathematical description of, 31—38
one-dimensional, 37
two-dimensional, 36—38
in X-ray computed tomography, 450—451
Convolution integrals, 35
Correlation, 35, 188—189
between models, 498—499
Fourier transform as, 200—202
Crosscorrelation of stochastic processes, 156
Cross power (mutal power), 143—144
CT scanning, see Computed tomography

D

Data estimation, 373—379
least mean square estimation of, 170—174
linear mean square estimation of, 373—379
Data collection, see also Sampling
alternative protocols in NMR imaging, 434—435
in computed tomography, 453—457
summary of, 500—502
Decibel values, 363
Deconvolution, 5
in first pass radionuclide angiocardiography, 411—420
high pass filtering and, 415
models for, 412, 414, 417—420
noiseless, 414—415
Wiener, 389—393, 407
Delta functions, 25—26, 33, 47, 225
unsharp masking and, 396
Demodulation, 327—329
Dependent variables, 9
Derivatives of complex variables, 17—18, 77—78
Deterministic systems, 185
Deterministic values, 139—140
Deviations, see also Standard deviation
correlation of, 143—144
Diagonal of matrices, 100
Difference operation, 17
Differential equations
additional constraints, 89—90
defined, 81—82
eigenfunctions, 92—94
linear, with constant coefficients, 82, 90—94
mapping to polynomial equations, 234—235
systems described by, 82—89
Digital functions, 12
Dimension
of matrices, 100
of vector space, 124
Discrete convolution, 118
Discrete Fourier transform, 257, 292
basis functions in, 261—262
inverse, 261—262
N point intervals, 263—264
of pairs, 260—261
periodicity of, 262—263
periodic signals in, 258—260
proof of, 265—266

relation to continuous, 291—297
as rotation, 277—279
sum of basis functions in, 264—265
Discrete functions, 11
Discrete signals, 312
Discrete systems, 183
Dispersive signals, 239
Domain multiplexing, 327
Domain of the mapping, 129
Doppler principle, 244
Duality, in Fourier transform, 212—213, 306
Dual of the Fourier series, 291, 294—296
Dummy variable of the integration, 20
Duration band width, 243

E

Edge enhancement, 396
Eigenfunctions, 4, 187—188, 499
as basis functions, 56—58
defined, 53
differential equation, 92—94
examples, 53—56
in Fourier transform, 311
of linear, time invariant systems, 58—59
of linear, time variant systems, 78—79
Eigenvalues, 53, 92—93
Eigenvectors, 56, see also Eigenfunctions
linear systems, 131—134
rotation to, 281—284
Energy, 188—189
conservation of, 242
defined, 142—143
Energy relationship of Fourier transform, 306
Equations
differential, see Differential equations
Euler, 67—70
linear, see Linear equations
normal, see Normal equations
simultaneous linear, 97—98, see also Simultaneous linear equations
Equilibrium solutions, see Forced solutions
Equivalence of input signal and system function, 35—36
Ergodicity in stochastic processes, 157—158
Error vectors, 367
Estimation, 189, 405—407, see also Data estimation
least mean square, see Least mean square estimation
model of, 369, 371—373
of unknown from multiple samples, 488—492
Estimation subspace, 175
Euler's equation, 67—70
Evaluation, 250—251
Even and odd signals, 235, 238, 307
Expectation operators, 138—140
Experiment vs. measurement distinction, 161—162
Exponential back projection, 476—478
Exponentials, 22, see also Imaginary exponentials
complex, 66—76
logarithms and, 22—25

F

Factorial notation, 27
Fast Fourier transform, 267—268
Film exposure, linearization in, 46
Filtering, 5, see also Windowing, specific types of
        filtering
    convolution and, 403—404
    defined, 317—318
    image enhancement, see Image enhancement
    implementation of, 318—319
    normal equations, see Normal equations
    ramp, 449—450
    sampling, see Sampling
    spatial, 320—323
    stochastic processes, 5, 351—364
    summary of, 411—408
    Wiener, see Wiener filtering
Filters, types of, 326—332
First moment of random variable, see Mean
First order statistics, 138
FM modulation, 231
Forced solutions, 91—92
Fourier analysis, see Fourier transform
Fourier sample reconstruction in NMR imaging,
        423—438
Fourier series, 291—297
Fourier synthesis, see Inverse Fourier transform
Fourier transform, 4, 133, see also Inverse Fourier
        transform
    analogy with sight and hearing, 193—194
    autoregulation in, 159
    basis functions of, 309
    calculation of, 200
    of comb function in time domain, 342
    completeness of, 220—221
    as correlation, 200—202
    of correlation function, see Power spectral density
        function
    correspondence between continuous and discrete,
        291—297
    discrete, 4
    duality of, 212—213
    eigenfunctions in, 311
    fast, 227—228
    image reconstruction by, 450—451
    linearity of, 211
    magnitude and phase of, 205—207
    of odd and even signals, 235—239
    orthogonality of imaginary exponentials, 213—217
    proof of relationships, 219—220
    properties of
        change in scale, 233—234
        conservation of energy, 242
        heuristics, 245
        mapping of convolution to multiplication, 223—
            228
        mapping of deconvolution to division, 228—229
        mapping of differential equations to polynomial
            equations, 234—235
        shift/modulation, 229—233

    summary of, 306—308
    uncertainty principle, 243—245
    value at origin and integral in other domain,
        241—242
    real and imaginary parts of, 203—205
    in response to imaginary exponential, 202—203
    selected pairs, 308—309
    sinc function in, 240—241
    slice theorem and, 447
    two-dimensional, 4, 208, 288
    two domains of, 199—200
Free induction decay, 55, 196, 425—426
Frequency, 71—73
Frequency domain
    aliasing in, 346
    multiplexing, 327
    signal representation, 196—199
    transforms in, 305—306
Frequency encoding, 432
Functionals, see Systems
Functions, 9—11
    analytic, 77
    basis, see Basis functions
    complex valued, 76
    continuous, 11
    delta, 25—26
    digital, 12
    discrete, 11
    linear, time invariant, 49—50
    line spread, 203
    modulation transfer, 203
    multidimensional, 13—14
    special, 25—26
    step, 25
    support of, 258
    two-dimensional, 12—13

G

Gamma variant analysis in radionuclide angiocardi-
        ography, 420—421
Gaussian functions, 201
    as filter, 332
    Fourier transform of, 244—245
Gaussian processes, 157
Generalized systems, 44
Geometric derivation in least mean square estimation,
        171—172, 176—178
Geometric representation of vectors, 99

H

Hamming window, 331—332
Hankel's transform, 302
Hanning window, 330—331
Hearing and sight analogy with Fourier transform,
        193—194
Heisenberg's uncertainty principle, 243
Hertz, 71
Heuristics
    about images, 396

Fourier transform and, 245
in single photon emission computed tomography, 470—475
in Wiener filtering, 383—384
High pass filtering, 326, 415
Hilbert transform, 239
Homogeneous solutions, see Natural solutions
Homomorphic signal processing, 398—399
Hook's law of the spring, 85—86

I

Ill-conditioned problems, 418—420
Image arithmetic, 103
Image collection in single photon emission computed tomography, 465—470
Image enhancement, 408, 500
    examples of, 395—398
    homomorphic signal processing, 398—399
    visual physiology and, 398
Image information, 399—401
Image reconstruction
    in computed tomography, 457—461
    importance of exact, 500
    from multiple samples, 483—496
    noise reduction in, 500
    from noisy projections, 453—462
    in NMR imaging, 435
    summary of, 497—502
    in X-ray computed tomography, 449—450
Image restoration, 395
Image vs. matrix, 100
Imaginary exponentials, 68—69, 197
    Fourier transform in, 202—203
    integral of, 217—219
    orthogonality of, 213—217
Inconsistent linear equations, 98
Independent variables, 9, 15—16
Infinity and powers of t, 249
Initial conditions, 89—90, 94
Input signals, 29—31
Input signal/system function equivalence, 35—36
Integrals, 19—22
    convolution, 35
    of imaginary exponentials, 217—219
Integration in the complex plane, 299—301
Interpolation, 251—252, 345—347
Intervals, N point and discrete Fourier transform, 263—264
Intracardiac shunting measurements, 411—420
Inverse Fourier transform, 199—200
    discrete, 261—262
    polynomial representation similar to, 247
Inversions, 103—105
    pseudo, 128
Iterative reconstruction, 5, 478—480
Iterative solutions, 377—378
    in radionuclide angiocardiography, 419—420

K

Kidney excretion of radiopharmaceutical, 29—31

L

Laplace transform, 4, 78, 297—299
Larmor frequency, 426
Least mean square error, 164—165
Least mean square estimation
    of the data, 170—174
    model of, 161—162
    from multiple measurements, 168—170
    of the unknown, 174—181
Limited extent signal, 258
Linear, shift invariant samples, multiple, 492—493
Linear algebra
    description of systems, 117—134
    matrix operations, 101—109, see also Matrices
    model of a system, 117—118
    in multidetector scanning, 493—494
    normal equations of, see Normal equations
    in single photon emission computed tomography, 469—470
    solution of simultaneous linear equations, 97—98
    in two-dimensional signals, 119
    vector and matrix notation, 99—101
    vector space, 109—114
Linear equations, 98
    differential, 82, 90—94
    simultaneous, see Simultaneous linear equations
    time invariant, 118—119
Linear estimation, 162—164
    least mean square, see Least mean square estimation
Linear independence, 124
Linearity, 44—46
    in Fourier transform, 211, 306
Linearizable systems, 46
Linear mean square estimation of data, 373—379
Linear phase shift, 230
Linear shift invariant reconstruction, 475—478
Linear system function, 48
Linear systems, 184, see also Linear, time invariant systems
    compared with linear, time invariant, 118—119
    eigenvectors, 131—134
    matrix rotations analogous to, 284—285
    response calculation in, 49
    theory, 3
    in single photon emission computed tomography, 466—467
Linear, time invariant functions, 49—50
Linear, time invariant systems
    differential equations with constant coeffients in, 90—91
    eigenfunctions of, 58—59
Line spread function, 203
Liver spleen scan
    as model of Wiener filtering, 381—383
    stochastic processes in, 152—153
Logarithms, 22—25
Low frequency attenuation, 396—398
Low parameter models, 417
Low pass filters, 327—332, 395
Lung time activity curve, 38—39

M

Magnetic field gradient in NMR imaging, 423—425

Magnitude and phase, of Fourier transform, 205—207

Mapping, 129
  convolution to multiplication, 223—228, 253—255, 306, 311—312
  deconvolution to division, 228—229
  differential equations to polynomial equations, 234—235, 307

Mass on a spring example, 85—89

Matched filter, 381

Mathematical descriptions
  of convolution, 31—38
  of systems, 43

Matrices
  associated with vector spaces, 125—131
  diagonal of, 100
  dimension of, 100
  inversion of, 103—105
  notation in simultaneous linear equations, 103
  operations with, 101—103
  rotation of, 279—281, 284—285
  singular, 126
  square, 100

Matrix addition, 101

Matrix algebra, 97—114

Matrix multiplication, 101—103

Mean, 137—139
  of stochastic process, 151—152, 354—355

Measurement subspace, 175

Measurement vs. experiment distinction, 161—162

Memoryless systems, 183—184

Modeling, 417, 497

Modulation, 203, 327—329

Moire patterns, 336, 338

Multidetector scanning, 483—488

Multidimensional Fourier transform, 287—291

Multidimensional functions, 13—14

Multiple sample reconstruction, 5, 483—496

Multiplexing, 327—329

Multiplication
  matrix, 101—102
  polynomial, 252
  scalar, 101

Mutal power (cross power), 143—144

Mutual energy, 168

Mutual power and Wiener filter, 386

N

Natural solutions, 91—92

Newton's second law, 86

NMR imaging, see Nuclear magnetic resonance imaging

Noise, 359—362, 374, see also Signal:noise ratio
  back projected, in computed tomography, 454—456
  measurement of, 173—174

Noiseless projection reconstruction, 441—451

Noisy measurements, 4

Noisy projections, 5, 453—462

Nonhomogeneous solutions, see Forced solutions

Nonlinear systems, 45—46, 184

Nontime invariant systems, 184

Normal equations, 365—379, 406—407
  compared with Wiener filtering, 365
  in multidetector scanning, 493—494

Normally distributed random variables, 149

N point intervals and discrete Fourier transform, 263—264

Nuclear magnetic resonance imaging
  continuous, 55, 93, 195—196
  duality in, 213
  edge enhancement in, 324—326
  eigenfunctions, 54—56
  filtering in, 320—322
  as four-dimensional, 109
  Fourier transform in, 213
  free induction decay in spatial frequency domain, 429—431
  frequency domain, 428—429
  image reconstruction, 435
  linear least mean square estimation in, 161
  liver spleen scan as model of Wiener filtering, 381—383
  optical, 195
  physics and instrumentation, 423—425
  position aliasing, 340
  pulsed, 55, 195—196
  quadrature detection, 231—232
  7-dimensional imaging, 438
  similarity to mass on a spring, 85—89
  time, frequency, space, and spatial frequency domains, 429
  spectrum domain, 426—428
  two-dimensional encoding in, 431—434
  unsharp masking in, 400
  vector addition of magnetic moments, 425

Nuclear magnetic resonance spectrum, 54—55

Null space, 126

Number systems, 61—63

Nyqvist rate, 347

O

One-dimensional convolution, 37

Operations
  complex number, 65—70
  derivative, 17—18
  difference, 17
  exponentials and logarithms, 22—25
  on independent variable, 15—16
  integral, 19—22
  partial derivative, 18
  powers and roots, 22
  sum, 18—19

Optical spectroscopy, 195

Orthogonality, 126—127, 188—189, 373, 405—406
  of imaginary exponentials, 213—217
  in least mean square estimation, 167
  mathematical derivation of principle, 384—386
  vectors, 113—114

in Wiener filtering, 384
Orthogonal random variables, 145
Output functions, 29—31
Over-determined linear equations, 98
Over-determined solutions in radionuclide angiocardiography, 419

P

Parent/daughter decay, see Radioactive decay
Parseval's relation, 242, 306
Partial derivatives, 18
Periodicity of discrete Fourier transform, 262—263
Periodic signals, 258—260
Phantom bars, 336, 338—339
Phase encoding, 432
Physiology of vision, 398
Plane waves, 74—75
Point source attenuation, 464—465
Poisson distribution, 158—159
Polar notation, 64
Polynomial equations, mapping to differential equations, 234—235
Polynomial multiplication, 252
Polynomial transform, 247—256
Position aliasing in NMR imaging, 340
Positron emission computed tomography, time-of-flight, 495
Postreconstruction correction, 476
Power, defined, 142
Powers and roots, 22
Power series expansions, 26—27
Powers of t, 248—249
Power spectral density, 352—353, 405
  of back-projected noise, 454—456
  of stochastic output process, 356—357
Power spectral localization, 357—359
Probability density function, 135—136
  in radiological measurement, 139
  second moment of, 141
  in stochastic processes, 151—152
  for sum of two random variables, 138
Problems, well- and ill-conditioned, 418—420
Product of two vectors, 108
Projection, 442
  back, 443—446, 448—449
  slice theorem, 446—448
  vector, 111—112
    onto second vector, 165—168
    onto subspace, 365—371
Projection values modification, 475—476
Pseudoinverses, 128
Pulsed inputs, 55—56
Pythagorean theorem, 107

Q

Quadrature detection, in NMR imaging, 231—232
Quadrature signals, 238—240

R

Radioactive decay, 82—85
Radio frequency pulses, 244
Radiological measurement, probability density function in, 139
Radionuclide angiocardiography, 411—420
Radon filtering, 449—450, 460—461
Radon transform, 302, 441—442
Random variables, see also Deviations
  first moment of, see Mean
  multiple, 147—148
  normally distributed, 149
  orthogonal, 145
  single, 136—143
  statistically independent, 145
  sum of two, 136—137
  two, 143—147
  uncorrelated, 145, 146
Random vectors, 147—148
Range, of a mapping, 129
Real number systems, 61
Reconstruction, 5, see also specific methods
  deconvolution: first pass radionuclide angiocardiography, 411—420
  emission computed tomography, 463—480
  iterative reconstruction, single photon emission computed tomography, 463—480
  multiple samples, multiple detector scanner, 483—495
  noiseless projections, 441—451
  noisy projections, computed tomography, 453—459
  reconstruction from Fourier samples, NMR imaging, 423—437
Relaxation factor, 378
Renal excretion of radiopharmaceutical, 29—31
Representations of complex numbers, 63—64
Resonance, 81, 92—93
Rotation
  discrete Fourier transform as, 277—279
  to eigenvector's basis, 281—284
  examples of, 271—274
  matrix, 279—281
  signal and its Fourier transform, 288—291
  of vector space, 271, 275—277
Row space, 126
Row (transposed) vectors, 105

S

Sample representation of a signal, 249—250
Sampling, 404
  aliasing, 335—337, 348
  alternative protocols in NMR imaging, 434—435
  average value, 349
  comb signal, 337—345
  in computed tomography, 453—457
  implementation of, 348—349
  interpolation, 345—347
  multiple linear, shift invariant, 492—493
  in X-ray computed tomography, 441—442

Sampling theorem, 347—348
Scalar multiplication, 101
Scaling
  in convolution, 30
  Fourier transform, 233—234
  of independent variable, 16
  in linearity, 44—46
Second moment of probability density function, 141
Second order statistic, 140, 144
Sequence of systems, 226—228, 312
Seven-dimensional imaging in NMR imaging, 437—438
Shifting, 16, 30, 259—260
Shift invariance, 46—47, 118, see also Time invariance
Shift/modulation, 229—233, 307
Shunting, intracardiac, 411—420
Sight and hearing analogy with Fourier transform, 193—194
Signal:noise ratio, 173—174, 181, 362
  Wiener filter and, 387
Signal power spectral density, back projected, 456—457
Signal processing, 3, 398—399
Signals
  absorptive, 239
  basis function representations, 185—186
  comb, 337—345
  complexity vs. vector space, 109—110
  discrete, 257, 266—267
  dispersive, 239
  estimation of, see Estimation
  frequency domain representation, 196—199
  limited complexity, 247
  limited extent, 258
  passing through linear system, 125—130
  periodic, 258—260
  polynomial, representation of, 247—249
  quadrature, 231—232, 238—240
  rotation of signal and its transform, 288—291
  sample representation of, 249—250
  undersampled, 348
  value at origin and integral in other domain, 241—242
Simultaneous linear equations, 4, 97—98, 103
Sinc function, 240—241
Sine and cosine transformations, 237
Single photon emission computed tomography
  heuristics in, 470—475
  image collection model, 465—470
  iterative reconstruction, 478—480
  linear, shift invariant reconstruction methods, 475—478
  point source attenuation correction, 464—465
Single-valued functions, 9
Singular matrices, 126
Sinusoidal functions, complex exponentials in, 71—73
Slice selection, 435
Slice theorem projection, 446—448
Smoothing, 323, 395, 470

Spatial filtering, 320—323
Spatial frequency projection, 448—449, 474—475
Spectroscopy, nuclear magnetic resonance, see Nuclear magnetic resonance imaging
Spiral data sampling, 434
Square matrix, 100
Standard deviation, 141—142
State of a system, 81, 93—94, 188
Stationarity of stochastic processes, 156—157
Statisically independent random variables, see Independent variables
Statistical signals, 4, see also Stochastic processes
Statistical systems, 185
Statistics
  first order, 138
  second order, 140, 144
Step functions, 25
Stochastic processes, 351—352
  autocorrelation, 155—156, 355—356
  crosscorrelation, 156
  definition of filtering, 351—364
  ergodicity, 157—158
  examples of, 152—155
  mean, 155
  mean of output process, 354—355
  Poisson, 159
  power spectral density function of output process, 356—357
  probability density function, 151—152
  stationarity, 156—157
Stochastic signal filtering, 5
Strict sense stationarity, 157
Subspace projection of vectors, 365—371
Summing in linearity, 45
Sums, 18—19, 136—137
Support of function, 258
Symbols chart, 503—505
System function/input signal equivalence, 35—36
System functions, 29, 93
System models, 3, 9—189
  complex numbers, 61—78
  convolution, 29—42
  differential equations, 81—93
  eigenfunctions, 53—58
  introduction, 1—7
  linear algebra, 97—113
  linear algebra description of systems, 117—131
  linear, least mean square estimation, 161—180
  random variables, 135—149
  review of basic concepts, 9—26
  stochastic processes, 151—160
  systems, see Systems
Systems
  complexity of, 50—51, 186—187
  examples of, 43—44
  generalized, 44
  linear, see Linear systems
  linear, time-invariant, 47—50
  linearizable, 46
  mathematical description of, 43
  number, 61—63

properties of, 44—47
sequence of, 312
summary of, 183—193

T

Taylor series expansions, 26—27
Three-dimensional imaging in NMR imaging, 435
Time domain of signal, 212, 429
Time invariance, 46—47, see also Shift invariance
Time invariant linear systems, 47—50
Time invariant systems, 184
Time-of-flight positron emission computed
    tomography, 495
Time reversal, 16
Tissue impedance to ultrasound, 75—76
Tomography
  blurring, 443
  computed, see Computed tomography; X-ray
    computed tomography
  limited angle, 130
Transformations, 4, 310—311, see also specific
    transforms
Transforms, see also specific transforms by name
  complexity of signals represented, 301—302
  in complex plane integration, 299—301
  Hankel, 302
  Hilbert, 239
  Laplace, 297—299
  multidimensional Fourier, 287—291
  polynomial, 247—256
  Radon, 302
  summary of, 305—313
Transient solutions, see Natural solutions
Transpose of vector (row vector), 105
Transposition of matrices, 105—106
Treble and bass accentuation, 319
Trigonometric relationships of complex exponentials,
    70
Two-dimensional convolutions, 36—38
Two-dimensional Fourier transform, 208
Two-dimensional functions, 12—13
Two-dimensional imaging in nuclear magnetic
    resonance imaging, 431—434
Two-dimensional signals and linear algebra, 119

U

Ultrasonography, 244
Ultrasound, tissue impedance to, 75—76
Uncertainty principle, 243—245
Uncorrelated random variables, 145—146
Under-determined linear equations, 98
Unknowns
  estimation of from multiple samples, 488—492
  least mean square estimation of, 174—181
Unknown subspace, 175
Unsharp masking, 396

V

Variance, 140—141
Vector notation, 99—101

Vectors, 14—15
  addition of in nuclear magnetic resonance imaging,
    425
  analogy with discrete signals, 266—267
  basis, see Basis vectors
  error, 367
  geometrical representation of, 99
  length of, 107
  multiplication of, 103, 106—109
  orthogonality, 113—114
  product of two, 108
  projection of, 111—113
    onto subspace, 365—371
    onto second vector, 165—168
  random, 147—148
  transposed (row), 105
Vector spaces, 109—113
  associated with matrix, 125—131
  complexity versus a signal, 109—110
  defined by basis vectors, 122—124
  dimension of, 124
  in linear mean square data estimation, 376
  rotation of, 4, 271, 275—277
Vector subspace, 110—111
Velocity imaging in NMR imaging, 436—438
Visual physiology, 398

W

Wagon wheel aliasing, 337
Wave number, 74
Well-conditioned problems, 418—420
White noise, 360—361
Wide sense stationarity, 157
Wiener deconvolution, 389—393, 407
Wiener filtering, 407, 461
  compared with normal equations, 365
  heuristics in, 383—389
  models of, 381—383
  in radionuclide angiocardiography, 415—416, 419
Windowing, 323—327, see also Filtering

X

X-ray cassette imaging, 39
X-ray computed tomography
  back projection in, 443—446, 494
  convolution and back projection reconstruction,
    450—451
  data collection model, 441—442
  Fourier transform reconstruction, 450
  projection and back projection as spatial frequency
    samples, 448—449
  reconstruction filtering, 449
  slice theorem, 446
x,y plane, 110

Z

Z transform, 4, 291, see also Fourier series